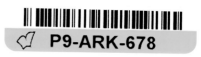

Wolf-Heidegger's

Atlas of
Human Anatomy

Volume 2

Petra Köpf-Maier, Berlin

Wolf-Heidegger's

Atlas of Human Anatomy

Volume 2
**Head and Neck, Thorax, Abdomen,
Pelvis, CNS, Eye, Ear**

5th, completely revised
and supplemented edition, 2000

866 figures of which 677 are in color

KARGER

Editor
Univ.-Prof. Dr. med. Petra Köpf-Maier
Professor of Anatomy
Freie Universität Berlin
Königin-Luise-Strasse 15
D–14195 Berlin (Germany)

This Atlas is published in two volumes:
Volume 1: Systemic Anatomy, Body Wall, Upper and Lower Limbs
Volume 2: Head and Neck, Thorax, Abdomen, Pelvis, CNS, Eye, Ear

Until 1989 the Atlas was published as
'Atlas of Systematic Human Anatomy', vol. I–III
1st edition 1954
2nd edition 1960
3rd edition 1972
Spanish translation: Salvat Editores S.A., Barcelona
Portuguese translation: Editors Guanabara Koogan S.A., Rio de Janeiro

4th edition 1990
Published as 'Wolf-Heidegger's Atlas of Human Anatomy'
Japanese translation: Nishimura Co., Ltd., Tokyo
Indonesian translation: Penerbit Widya Indonesia, Jakarta

Library of Congress Cataloging-in-Publication Data

Wolf-Heidegger's atlas of human anatomy. — 5th, completely rev. and
supplemented [English] ed. / [editor] Petra Köpf-Maier.
p.   cm.
"The original Latin nomenclature version with German and English captions
is available under the titles: 'Wolf-Heideggers Atlas der Anatomie des Menschen'/
'Wolf-Heidegger's Atlas of Human Anatomy'" — T.p. verso.
Includes bibliographical references and index.
Contents: v. 1. Systemic anatomy, body wall, upper and lower limbs —
        v. 2. Head and neck, thorax, abdomen, pelvis, CNS, eye, ear.
ISBN 3–8055–6852–5 (v. 1: hardcover). – ISBN 3–8055–6853–3 (v. 2: hardcover) –
ISBN 3–8055–6854–1 (complete set: hardcover)
1. Human anatomy Atlases.   I. Wolf-Heidegger, G. (Gerhard)
II. Köpf-Maier, P. (Petra)   III. Title: Atlas of human anatomy.
[DNLM: 1. Anatomy atlases.   QS 17 W859 1999]
QM25.W633   1999b
611'.022'2—dc21
DNLM/DLC
for Library of Congress
                                                    99-33383
                                                    CIP

The original Latin nomenclature version with German and English captions is also
available under the titles: "Wolf-Heideggers Atlas der Anatomie des Menschen"/
"Wolf-Heidegger's Atlas of Human Anatomy"
Bd./Vol. 1: Allgemeine Anatomie, Rumpfwand, obere und untere Extremität/Systemic
Anatomy, Body Wall, Upper and Lower Limbs: ISBN 3–8055–6754–5
Bd./Vol. 2: Kopf und Hals, Brust, Bauch, Becken, ZNS, Auge, Ohr/Head and Neck,
Thorax, Abdomen, Pelvis, CNS, Eye, Ear: ISBN 3–8055–6755–3
Complete set: ISBN 3–8055–5442–7

KARGER

Basel · Freiburg · Paris · London · New York · New Delhi · Bangkok · Singapore ·
Tokyo · Sydney

© Copyright 2001 by S. Karger AG,
P.O. Box, CH–4009 Basel (Switzerland)
Printed in Switzerland on acid-free paper by Reinhardt Druck, Basel
ISBN 3–8055–6853–3

The editor dedicates
this book to her grandson

Leander Leonin

Homage to Those Who Bequeathed Their Bodies to Science

'Hic locus est ubi mors gaudet succurrere vitae'

'This is the place where death delights in helping life'
(Inscription above the Anatomical Theatre of Bologna)

The present atlas of human anatomy shall not begin without paying due homage and returning thanks to those who freely bequeath their bodies to anatomy. Such donations testify to an admirable, unselfish, and idealistic sense of sacrifice and nothing can compensate for the invaluable service rendered to science and society. Anatomy and medicine owe these individuals a tremendous debt of gratitude. By bequeathing their bodies, they enable medical students to learn through real observation and direct 'grasping', and even now, at the end of the twentieth century, there is no alternative to this. Thus, even beyond death, these altruistic people help the living – medical students, physicians, and their patients alike. This is how the above inscription should be interpreted. Students should make every endeavour to be worthy of these voluntary and generous body donations by respecting and honoring the dead as well as by working hard and learning eagerly.

Contents

Contents of Volume 1:
Systemic Anatomy, Body Wall, Upper and Lower Limbs

Preface to the 5th Edition

Macroscopic anatomy is a fundamental branch of medicine without which clinical facts cannot be understood.

Throughout history, the importance of anatomy for medicine – and thus for medical studies – has fluctuated considerably. Five hundred years ago, at the end of the Renaissance, Leonardo da Vinci and Andreas Vesal laid the foundation stones of modern anatomy and modern medicine. In those days, anatomy – then exclusively macroscopic – was the only fundamental speciality medical students were confronted with during their studies, along with the clinical subjects internal medicine, surgery and botany (in the meaning of use of herbal drugs).

The first half of the twentieth century saw the development of microscopic anatomy besides macroscopic anatomy; physiology became an independent speciality and physiological chemistry and biochemistry made huge progress. Research in these fields provided new knowledge on functional and molecular interactions in the mammalian organism which fundamentally altered our understanding of diseases and opened new perspectives in clinical diagnosis and therapy. As a consequence of these developments, macroscopic anatomy was somehow relegated to the background during the 1960s and 1970s, and seemed to have retained its essential importance only for surgical specialities.

Apart from these developments, new diagnostic imaging technologies have become clinically established in the second half of the twentieth century: computed tomography, magnetic resonance imaging, and ultrasonography. These imaging techniques opened up new visions of the morphology of the living organism, enabled a very detailed identification of structures and thus laid the foundation stone of rapid and unexpected progress in clinical diagnosis. However, the interpretation of normal and pathologically altered structures in two-dimensional images of the human body with all these techniques demands extremely precise anatomical knowledge. In recent years, this has led to the revival and to a considerable increase in the significance of macroscopic anatomy both for clinical medicine and the education of medical students.

Successful clinical work without well-founded knowledge in topographical and sectional anatomy is thus no longer possible. This is the reason why the editor urges present and future medical students to study macroscopic anatomy intensively.

As a matter of fact, it is the establishment of the new imaging techniques in clinical medicine that prompted this new revised version of Professor Wolf-Heidegger's Atlas of Human Anatomy, which had been continued by H. Frick, B. Kummer, and R. Putz in its 4th edition, and the supplementation of its 5th edition with numerous anatomical sections, computed and magnetic resonance imaging tomograms and ultrasonograms. Such a new design of an atlas of the anatomy of the whole human body is only possible with the collaboration of many enthusiastic forces. Thus I am deeply indebted to Dr.

R. Andresen and Priv.-Doz. Dr. D. Banzer (Berlin) for most of the new radiographs as well as the computed and magnetic resonance tomograms included in this atlas. Prof. Dr. G. Bogusch (Berlin), Prof. Dr. E. Fleck (Berlin), Dr. M. Jäckel (Göttingen), Dr. H. Kellner (Munich), Priv.-Doz. Dr. T. Riebel (Berlin), Priv.-Doz. Dr. C. Sohn (Heidelberg), Dr. D. Zeidler (Berlin) and Prof. Dr. W.G. Zoller (Munich) contributed some further radiographs, tomograms and ultrasonograms for which I would like to thank them.

I am moreover deeply indebted to Prof. Dr. M. Herrmann (Ulm) who provided the anatomical sections for most of the computed and magnetic resonance tomograms of the present atlas and thus considerably enriched it. The sections on which these illustrations are based were prepared and photographed by Mr. E. Voigt (Ulm), whom I would like to thank as well.

Valuable help in translating the Latin terms of the original Latin nomenclature version into English equivalents was contributed by Prof. A.W. English, Ph.D. (Atlanta, Georgia, USA). I thank him very much for his engagement.

I also express my thanks to Mrs. G. Heymann-Monhof, Mr. H. Jonas, Mrs. H. Heinen, Mrs. I. Tripke, Mrs. C. Naujok and Mr. F. Geisler who prepared about 230 new anatomical drawings for the present edition.

My special thanks go to Dr. h.c. Th. Karger for his constructive collaboration during the past years. Dr. Karger always lent an understanding ear to my concepts, which were often difficult and expensive to realize, and was a partner whose expert advice and understanding always helped me in my work with the atlas. Many thanks in particular to Mr. B. Pfäffli as well as to all the personnel of S. Karger Publishers and Neue Schwitter AG who helped in the production of Wolf-Heidegger's atlas.

Mrs. M. Risch, my secretary, has been a great and dependable help over the past years, which has eased my work in many respects. I would like to thank her as well.

This new edition of Wolf-Heidegger's *Atlas of Systematic Human Anatomy* has been supplemented by numerous new anatomical drawings, radiographs, tomograms, ultrasonograms and anatomical sections. As the editor, I am confident that this new edition will indeed 'help one to see' – one of the most difficult things, according to the quote from Goethe, which Wolf-Heidegger chose as the motto for the first edition of his atlas – and that it will give medical students better access to anatomy and clinical medicine:

'What is the hardest of aught? What seemeth the simplest to you: With your eyes to see that which is in front of your eyes.'

Johann Wolfgang von Goethe,
Distichon 155 of the *'Xenien'* (translated by M. Pfister, Berlin)

Berlin, Spring 1999   Petra Köpf-Maier

Preface to the 1st Edition

«Was ist das Schwerste von allem? Was dir das Leichteste dünket:
Mit den Augen zu sehn, was vor den Augen dir liegt.»*

Accustomed during his school years to place greater trust in the written word than in his own senses, the young medical student in his first pre-clinical term is faced with a problem which Goethe aptly describes as 'hardest of all': He has to learn how to see. To teach him to do so, by the aid of anatomical preparations and plates as the most effective means at his disposal, is the foremost task of the pre-clinical instructor. The aim of the present Atlas is to give to the medical student and to the physician wishing to revise his anatomical knowledge a picture, as true and exact as possible, of the organs of our human body. The drawings were made partly from specimens preserved in the large collection of the Basle Anatomical Institute, partly from special preparations. Nearly all the plates in the section on muscles were drawn from fresh preparations in order to exclude the deformities caused by preservation. Our aim was always to avoid individual peculiarities and, by using a larger number of similar preparations, to produce as general and universal a picture as possible. With a few exceptions, noted in the legends, the right side of the body was always chosen in all bilaterally symmetrical organs or parts.

We were for a long while undecided whether or not the illustrative material should be accompanied by a short written text. As stated above, we are of the opinion that the Atlas is the primary aid in anatomical instruction, but it neither can nor should be a substitute for the detailed textbook and the spoken word; these are indispensable in preparing the student for what he is to see and in fixing what he has seen firmly in his mind. Students tend to regard a short Atlas text as a source of information sufficient for their needs, but it can never deal exhaustively with all noteworthy and necessary aspects of the subject; we therefore decided finally to publish the present volume without text, but to pay great attention to the labelling of the separate illustrations. The Atlas can thus be used in combination with any textbook of anatomy. On the other hand, for the sake of clarity, care was taken not to overload the separate plates with too many pointers; thus, parts and details which have already been shown are not re-labelled in plates in which they are not important for purposes of instruction. Sketches of the body surface, copied partly from well-known sculptures, have been inserted beside the plates showing the superficial muscular layers; it is hoped that these will help the student and qualified doctor to fit the muscle relief into the body of the patient. X-ray photographs of all important skeletal parts and junctures have been included with the intention of preparing the student for a form of examination which is of vital importance in clinical medicine and only possible on the basis of a sound knowledge of the normal anatomical picture. We had also planned, and partly completed, some treatment of general morphology, constitutional types, evolution, and the mechanics of joints, also a summarising survey in tabular form of the musculature; but all this had to be omitted in order to keep the volume of handy size and accessible price for the student.

Pending the establishment — we hope at a not too distant date — of a standard anatomical nomenclature, internationally recognised and scientifically and linguistically acceptable, we have made use in the present work of the Jena nomina anatomica; this is the terminology most widely used in the German-speaking countries. The Basle nomenclature has, however, been substituted for a few linguistically incorrect or in our opinion inappropriate terms.

I wish to take this oppportunity of expressing once again may sincere thanks to the publisher, Dr Heinz Karger, who by his energy and expert knowledge, his optimism and kindly, confident encouragement has made possible the wearisome and costly realisation of this work. I wish to thank further my faithful artistic collaborators: Mr Adolph Dressler (junctures), Mr Rolf Muspach (osteology), and above all Mr Robert Schlumpf (myology), who as sculptor with many years' dissecting room experience has in the course of our prolonged collaboration far surpassed his original function as artist and become a knowledgeable and indispensable scientific colleague, invaluable at every stage of the work from the preparation of muscle specimens to the typographical composition of the plates and the correction of proofs. For untiring and invaluable help I owe sincere thanks to my former Viennese assistant, Dr Arthur von Hochstetter (now Fribourg, Switzerland). Nearly all the X-ray photographs I owe to the kindness of Dr Emil A. Zimmer (Basle/Berne). For important suggestions and active help I wish to thank in particular my kind and highly esteemed anatomy instructor, Professor Eugen Ludwig, M.D. (Basle), and also Dr Walter Bejdl (Vienna/Basle), Dr Leopold Drexler (Vienna), Mr Willy Jäggi of S. Karger Ltd., Dr Walter Krause (Vienna), Dr Kurt S. Ludwig (Basle), Dr Carl Rudolf Pfaltz (Basle), Professsor Joseph Tomasch, M.D. (Kingston, Canada; formerly Vienna/Basle), Mr Armin Wolf, dissector (Basle), and Dr Wolfgang Zürcher (Basle).

In deep gratitude I wish finally to pay tribute to the memory of my mother who by her devoted and untiring energy made it possible for me, after the early death of my father, to follow the profession of my choice and thus to bring this Atlas into being.

Basle, Autumn 1953   Gerhard Wolf-Heidegger

---

* J.W. Goethe: 'Xenien.' From the posthumous papers.
  Weimar Edition, Vol. 5, part 1, p. 275, No. 45, 1893.

Concept of the New Version of the Atlas and Illustration Credits

The present 5th edition of the *Atlas of Human Anatomy,* published in 1954, 1960, and 1972 by Professor Dr. Gerhard Wolf-Heidegger and edited in 1990 by Prof. Dr. H. Frick, Prof. Dr. B. Kummer, and Prof. Dr. R. Putz, has been thoroughly revised in several aspects and supplemented in comparison to the previous four editions.

1. Retained Anatomical Drawings

The classical drawings of the three previous editions prepared by Wolf-Heidegger and his illustrators have been retained, recolored and – in the case of black-and-white drawings – colored didactically in order to make them clear also for beginners. Moreover, most of the figures prepared by Frick, Kummer, and Putz for the 4th edition, were revised and incorporated into the current 5th edition.

2. New Anatomical Pictures

The original illustrations of the previous four editions have been supplemented with about 230 new, mostly topographical drawings. These drawings were realized by six illustrators from Berlin, whom I would like to thank here for their enthusiasm. First of all, Mrs. Gertrud Heymann-Monhof, who possesses the talent to represent anatomical situations both true to detail and in an aesthetically convincing fashion. Mr. Hendrik Jonas drew most of the new illustrations of the locomotor apparatus and the head and succeeded very well in maintaining them in the style of the earlier editions. Mrs. Hildegard Heinen prepared numerous schematized drawings in a didactically clear manner. Other, mostly smaller drawings were done by Mrs. Ilona Tripke; three illustrations whose originals had been lost where painted in water colors by Mrs. Corinna Naujok. Mr. Frank Geisler prepared some new pictures and revised several others of the last edition.

Mrs. Gertrud Heymann-Monhof
Volume 1: Cover picture; Figs. 18, 19, 20, 21, 48b,c, 54b, 59, 60c, 75, 77a,b, 79a, 82, 83, 87a, 134a, 170, 171, 244a, 246a–c, 253, 254
Volume 2: Cover picture; Figs. 79, 95a, 107a, 113, 115b, 118a, 160c, 166, 172, 209a–c, 211b, 227, 243a, 250a,b, 251a,b, 256a–c, 285a, 336a, 342, 352, 382a, 395c

Mr. Hendrik Jonas
Volume 1: Figs. 90a,b, 99a, 103a, 123b, 125a–c, 127a–c, 131a–d, 137b,c, 138a,b, 155a, 163a, 167c–e, 175b, 176c, 177b, 181e, 189a–c, 191a,b, 193c, 196a,b, 200b–e, 201b–e, 209b, 213b, 220b, 221a,b, 225a,b, 226b, 249b,c, 250a,b, 257a–c, 280b
Volume 2: Figs. 264a,b, 265a, 276b, 277b, 281a,b, 290a,b, 292a, 321a,b, 324b, 325b, 329a,b, 332a,b, 368a, 369a,b, 394a,b, 395a, 399a

Mrs. Hildegard Heinen
Volume 1: Figs. 40b,c, 41b,c, 67a,b, 69b,c, 71c, 73a
Volume 2: Figs. 95b,c, 106b, 114c, 122b, 123b, 137a–c, 144a–c, 145a–c, 146a,c, 147a,c, 178b, 212a, 235b,c, 237b, 246b,c, 247a,b, 272a–e, 273a,b, 392a,b,d

Mrs. Ilona Tripke
Volume 1: Figs. 5c, 23b, 24, 63b, 79, 134b, 244b, 248b, 249a
Volume 2: Figs. 45b, 49b, 60a,b, 80a, 81a, 84a,b, 86b, 87b, 88b, 89b, 90b,c, 183c, 184a,b, 199b, 214b–e, 231b, 249, 293a–c, 371d, 379a, 382b, 383b

Mrs. Corinna Naujok
Volume 1: Fig. 252
Volume 2: Figs. 320a,b

Mr. Frank Geisler
Volume 1: Figs. 6a–c, 18, 19, 20, 21
Volume 2: Figs. 27b, 53a,b, 405a

Other anatomical illustrations, that is 3D reconstructions of the coronary arteries (Vol. 2, Figs. 148a–d), were contributed by Prof. Dr. Eckart Fleck and Dr. Helmut Oswald, Deutsches Herzzentrum Berlin. I acknowledge Dr. Martin Jäckel, Universitätsklinik Göttingen, for the laryngoscopic pictures in Volume 2 (Figs. 69a–d) of the present atlas, and Prof. Dr. Dieter Sasse, Universität Basel, for giving us access to the Anatomical Collection of the University of Basel and allowing Hansjörg Stöcklin to photograph the corrosion casts of the pulmonary, hepatic and renal vessels for the present atlas (Vol. 2, Figs. 115a, 119a, 183a, 213c, 214a).

3. Presentation of Imaging Techniques

The present atlas also aimed at giving imaging techniques due attention. Most radiographs, CT[1] and MRI[2] images published in the previous edition were technically superseded and, thus, replaced by new pictures. Besides conventional radiographs, the editor was anxious to incorporate computed and MRI tomograms of the whole human body and to represent ultrasonography by some selected images. For an anatomist, this could only be achieved by the close collaboration with enthusiastic radiologists: two radiologists from Berlin, Dr. Reimer Andresen and Priv.-Doz. Dr. Dietrich Banzer, Krankenhaus Zehlendorf, Behring-Krankenhaus Berlin. They have both untiringly searched for 'normal' anatomical images, which proved much more difficult and time-consuming than expected. Most MRI tomograms were done by use of a Philips Gyroscan ACS-NT MRI tomograph which had fortunately been installed a few years ago in the Zehlendorf Hospital.

---

[1] CT = Computed tomography, computed tomogram
[2] MRI = Magnetic resonance imaging, magnetic resonance image

Nearly 200 radiographs, CT and MRI tomograms as well as ultrasonograms were taken from Dr. Reimer Andresen's and Priv.-Doz. Dr. Dietrich Banzer's 'treasury':

Volume 1: Figs. 3a,b, 7b, 8d, 33b, 36a,b, 37b, 38a,b, 39b, 43, 45d, 51a,b, 55c, 71a,b, 73b, 85b, 87b, 91a,b, 93a,b, 97a,b, 100a,b, 101a,c, 103c, 106b, 120, 121, 123a, 129b, 137a, 139, 144b, 145b, 146b, 147b, 149a–c, 151b, 155b, 156b, 157b, 158b, 159b, 163b, 164b, 166a, 167a, 173a,b, 181f, 185, 188c, 194a,b, 195a–c, 197a,b, 202a–c, 203a–c, 204a,c,e, 205, 208b, 209a, 210a,b, 247a,b, 251, 258c,d, 259b, 260b, 261b, 262b, 263b, 264b, 265b, 269, 272b, 273b, 274b, 275b, 276a–c, 281a,b

Volume 2: Figs. 5, 7, 12b, 26c,d, 41b, 43c, 53c,d, 59a, 61a,b, 71a–c, 72a, 75a, 78, 110a, 118b, 119b, 126, 127, 128a, 129a, 130a, 131a, 156a, 157a, 159a,b, 175a–c, 182a,b, 186b,d, 188b, 189c,d, 194b, 197a,b, 198b, 201a,b, 203b, 208c, 215a–e, 217a,b, 218c, 219, 221, 223b, 224b, 229, 244b, 253a,b, 255a,b, 257a–c, 259a–c, 261a,b, 271b, 278a,b, 287a–c, 305, 336b, 339, 341, 343, 347, 349, 367b, 378b, 385a,b, 387a,b

Moreover, I gratefully acknowledge the following colleagues for other radiographs and ultrasonograms:

Prof. Dr. Eckart Fleck and Dr. Helmut Oswald, Deutsches Herzzentrum Berlin:
Volume 2: Figs. 136a–c, 138a–h, 146b,d, 147b,d

Dr. Martin Jäckel, HNO-Klinik, Universität Göttingen:
Volume 2: Figs. 9, 11, 395b, 406a–c, 407a–c

Dr. Herbert Kellner, Medizinische Poliklinik, Klinikum Innenstadt, Universität München:
Volume 1: Fig. 173c

Priv.-Doz. Dr. Thomas Riebel, Strahlenklinik, Virchow-Klinikum, Humboldt-Universität Berlin:
Volume 1: Fig. 177a

Priv.-Doz. Dr. Christof Sohn, Frauenklinik, Universität Heidelberg:
Volume 2: Figs. 74a, 238b, 242a–d, 245b,c

Dr. Diethmar Zeidler, dentist, Berlin:
Volume 2: Figs. 40e,f

Prof. Dr. Wolfram Zoller, Medizinische Poliklinik, Klinikum Innenstadt, Universität München:
Volume 2: Figs. 185a, 186c, 199c, 210e, 218b, 236b,c

I thank Prof. Dr. Gottfried Bogusch, formerly Institut für Anatomie der Freien Universität Berlin, now Humboldt-Universität Berlin, for giving me the permission to inspect the collection of radiographs and tomograms set up by him and to use the following pictures for the atlas:
Volume 1: Figs. 194a, 199a,b, 214b, 222b
Volume 2: Figs. 23c, 59b, 73a, 74a, 107a, 158a,b, 160a,b 161a,b, 176b, 213a, 222b, 225b, 278c,d, 301b, 302a,b

4. Anatomical Sections

In order to facilitate the understanding of the radiological sections (CTs and MRIs), the present atlas was designed to enable direct comparison with anatomical sections. While many institutes of anatomy pay attention to sectional anatomy, only few institutes possess complete series of sections of the whole human body. I would like to thank very much Prof. Dr. Martin Herrmann and Mr. Ernst Voigt, Abteilung Anatomie der Universität Ulm, for these illustrations; Mr. Voigt prepared and photographed all the sections.

A total of 90 anatomical sections contributed by Prof. Dr. M. Herrmann, Universität Ulm, have been included in the present new edition of Wolf-Heidegger's atlas:

Volume 1: Figs. 37a, 39a, 60b, 101b,d, 103b, 129a, 144a, 145a, 146a, 147a, 148a,b, 156a, 157a, 158a, 159a, 166b, 167b, 204b,d,f, 208a, 211, 258a,b, 259a, 260a, 261a, 262a, 263a, 264a, 265a, 272a, 273a, 274a, 275a, 277a–c

Volume 2: Figs. 62a,b, 63a,b, 68c, 72b, 73b, 74b, 75b, 128b, 129b, 130b, 131b, 156b, 157b, 158c, 159c, 164, 165, 213b, 220, 222a, 223a, 224a, 225a, 252a,b, 254a,b, 258a–c, 260a,b, 355a,b, 356a,b, 357a,b, 358a,b, 359a,b, 360a,b, 361a,b, 362a,b, 386a,b, 400b,c, 408a,b

5. Organization

The first three editions of Wolf-Heidegger's *Atlas of Systematic Human Anatomy* were published in three volumes organized in a somewhat modified manner according to the classical division into three parts:
Volume 1: Bones, joints, muscles
Volume 2: Viscera, skin, sensory organs
Volume 3: Nervous system, vascular system

In the 4th edition, prepared by H. Frick, B. Kummer, and R. Putz, the main contents of the previous three volumes were concentrated into one volume and reorganized according to topographical aspects.

The present 5th edition is divided into two volumes; the topographical arrangement of the illustrations has been taken over from the 4th edition, but the chapters have been arranged as follows:
Volume 1: Systemic anatomy, body wall, upper and lower limbs
Volume 2: Head and neck, thorax, abdomen, pelvis, central nervous system, eye, and ear.

This arrangement is based on the organization of the dissection courses into two main parts in many institutes of anatomy:
Part 1 – dissection of the locomotor apparatus: Ventral and dorsal body wall, upper and lower limbs
Part 2 – dissection of the viscera: Thorax, abdomen, pelvis, neck, head, brain

This division of the atlas into two volumes should make it easier for students to carry the atlas around during the dissection course and should moreover facilitate future supplementations.

Information for Users

1. Anatomical Nomenclature

In the present atlas, the designation of anatomical structures follows the most current international anatomical nomenclature, the *Terminologia Anatomica* (TA), in its latest edition of 1998. In this edition of the TA, a list of English terms in common usage was taken up for the first time. The American English variants of these terms (e.g., cecum instead of caecum, esophagus instead of oesophagus, fiber instead of fibre, gray instead of grey, tenia instead of taenia) were used throughout in the present atlas. Many of the synonyms that appear in the TA are listed in the subject index, an arrow referring to the main term given by the TA.

2. Abbreviations

In some cases, the following abbreviations were used:

Singular			Plural		
a.	=	artery	aa.	=	arteries
br.	=	branch	brr.	=	branches
cut.	=	cutaneous			
eth.	=	ethmoidal			
fem.	=	femoral			
inf.	=	inferior			
lig.	=	ligament	ligg.	=	ligaments
m.	=	muscle	mm.	=	muscles
n.	=	nerve	nn.	=	nerves
post.	=	posterior			
r.	=	ramus	rr.	=	rami
rad.	=	radiation			
rt.	=	right			
sup.	=	superior			
v.	=	vene	vv.	=	venes

3. Brackets

Parentheses ( ) are used to note terms also shown in parentheses in the TA, and for designating varieties, additional information, and explanations. Moreover, in the legends, the relative size of images referred to the originals is given as percentage in parentheses.

Commonly used, but not official TA terms are noted in pointed parentheses ⟨ ⟩.

Numbers of vertebrae and cranial nerves are placed in square brackets [ ], as in the TA.

4. Dashes

A dash *following* (left column) or *preceding* (right column) an entry indicates that one or several specific entries for the same body part will follow. The generic term is shown above it – usually without a pointer:

Examples	*Body of fibula*	or	*Infraclavicular part*
	Lateral surface –		*of brachial plexus*
	Anterior border –		*– Lateral cord*
	Medial surface –		*– Medial cord*
	Interosseous border –		*– Posterior cord*

5. Pointers and Dots

If dots on a pointer identify two or more anatomical structures or if several dots appear on a pointer, the various designations are separated by a comma; their order follows that of the arrangement of the anatomical structures in the figure. In both columns, the labelings are arranged according to the following principle: left first, then right; in the case of branched pointers, above first, then below.

6. Notation of Sizes

Unless otherwise indicated in the legends, the anatomical drawings in the present atlas always represent the situation in adults; the percentages given in parentheses in the legends denote the relative size of the image referred to the original. With a view to the considerable biological variations in body size, the percentages have been rounded off and should only be considered as indicative.

7. MRI Tomograms

Enhancement of the tissue-specific relaxation parameters T_1 and T_2 in MRI tomograms is noted in the legends as T_1 or T_2 weighting. T_1- and T_2-weighted tomograms represent the various structures of the human body in different brightnesses and different contrasts. Thus, in T_1-weighted tomograms, liquid-filled spaces are shown black, muscles dark, and the bone marrow white. In T_2-weighted tomograms, liquid-filled spaces appear white, bones dark, and muscles light gray.

8. Tomograms and Anatomical Sections

In current clinical practice, transverse computed and magnetic resonance imaging tomograms of the human body are always viewed from caudal, that is from below and looking up. This is the reason why, in the present atlas, the anatomical sections – with the few exceptions noted in the legends – are also viewed from caudal, that is from the feet of the patient. While this view of the tomograms and sections is doubtless difficult for beginners, it does correspond to the physician's perspective when he approaches the supine patient from the foot end of the patient's bed. The accompanying figure illustrates this view from caudal (bottom) to cranial (top) and makes clear that in this perspective the organs located on the patient's right (R) side appear on the left in the figure and the organs located on the left (L) side appear on the right side of the figure.

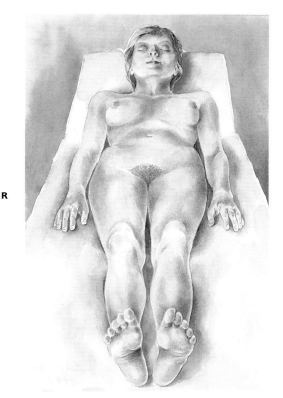

R   L

(Painted by G. Heymann-Monhof, Berlin)

Head and Neck

a

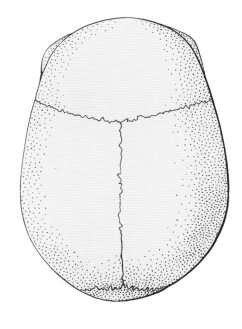

b

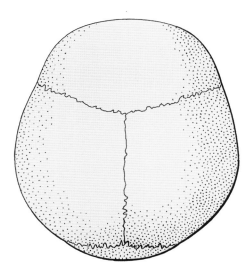

c

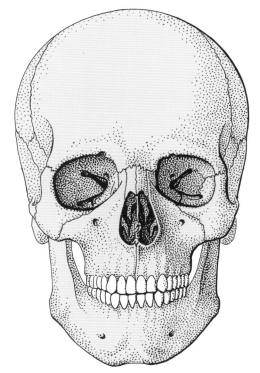

d

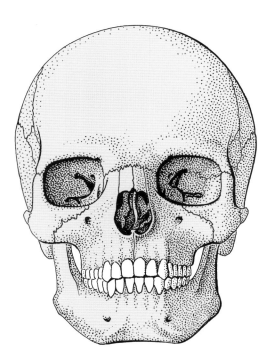

2 Shape differences of skull (= cranium)

a, b   Skull cap = calvaria, superior aspect (vertical aspect)
c, d   Skull = cranium, facial aspect (frontal aspect)
   a   Long (dolichocephalic) skull
   b   Broad (brachycephalic) skull
   c   Long (dolichocephalic) skull with a narrow face (leptoprosopia)
   d   Broad (brachycephalic) skull with a broad face (euryprosopia)

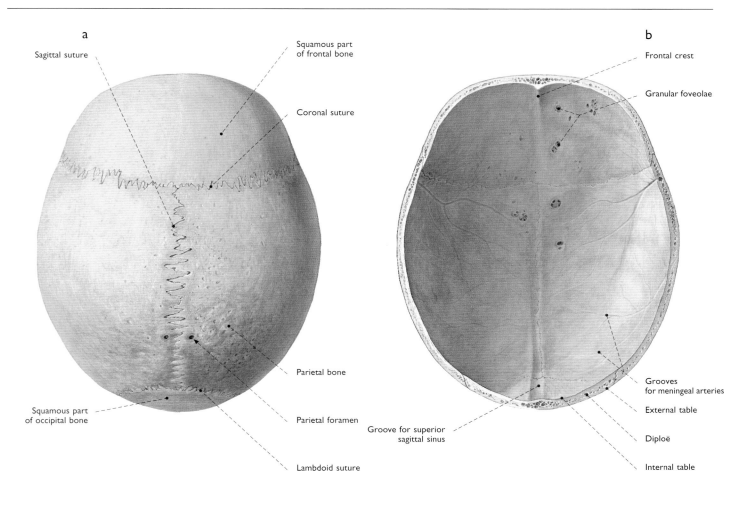

a
Sagittal suture
Squamous part of frontal bone
Coronal suture
Squamous part of occipital bone
Parietal bone
Parietal foramen
Lambdoid suture

b
Frontal crest
Granular foveolae
Grooves for meningeal arteries
External table
Diploë
Internal table
Groove for superior sagittal sinus

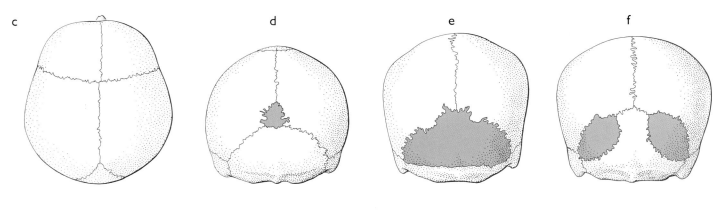

c   d   e   f

3 Skull cap (= calvaria) and sutural bones

a Superior aspect (vertical aspect) (50%)
b Inferior aspect (internal aspect) (50%)
c Persisting frontal suture
d Sutural bone (gray) in the sagittal suture
e Inca bone (interparietal bone) (gray)
f Sutural bones (gray) in the lambdoid suture

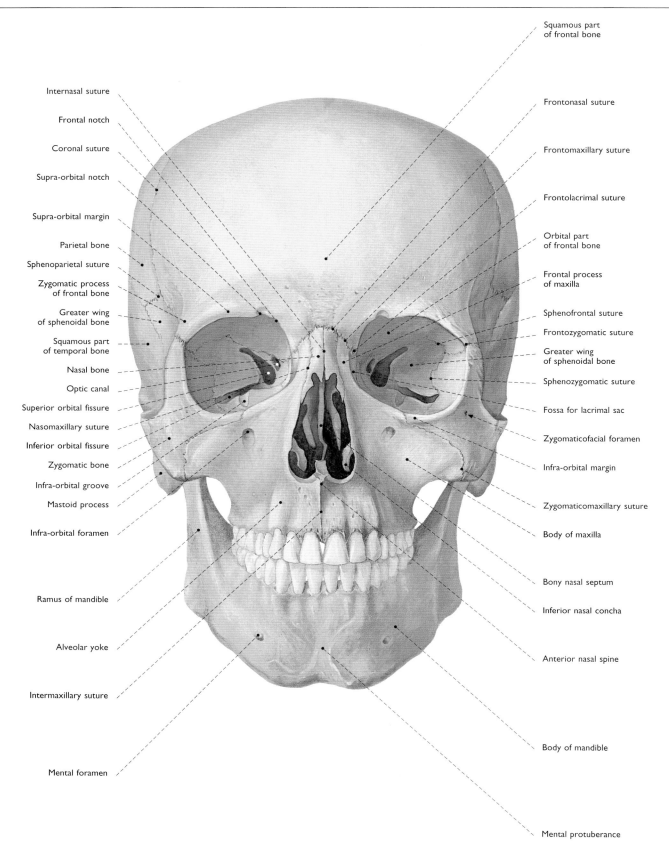

Squamous part
of frontal bone

Internasal suture

Frontal notch

Coronal suture

Supra-orbital notch

Supra-orbital margin

Parietal bone

Sphenoparietal suture

Zygomatic process
of frontal bone

Greater wing
of sphenoidal bone

Squamous part
of temporal bone

Nasal bone

Optic canal

Superior orbital fissure

Nasomaxillary suture

Inferior orbital fissure

Zygomatic bone

Infra-orbital groove

Mastoid process

Infra-orbital foramen

Ramus of mandible

Alveolar yoke

Intermaxillary suture

Mental foramen

Frontonasal suture

Frontomaxillary suture

Frontolacrimal suture

Orbital part
of frontal bone

Frontal process
of maxilla

Sphenofrontal suture

Frontozygomatic suture

Greater wing
of sphenoidal bone

Sphenozygomatic suture

Fossa for lacrimal sac

Zygomaticofacial foramen

Infra-orbital margin

Zygomaticomaxillary suture

Body of maxilla

Bony nasal septum

Inferior nasal concha

Anterior nasal spine

Body of mandible

Mental protuberance

4 Skull = Cranium (75%)
Facial aspect (frontal aspect)

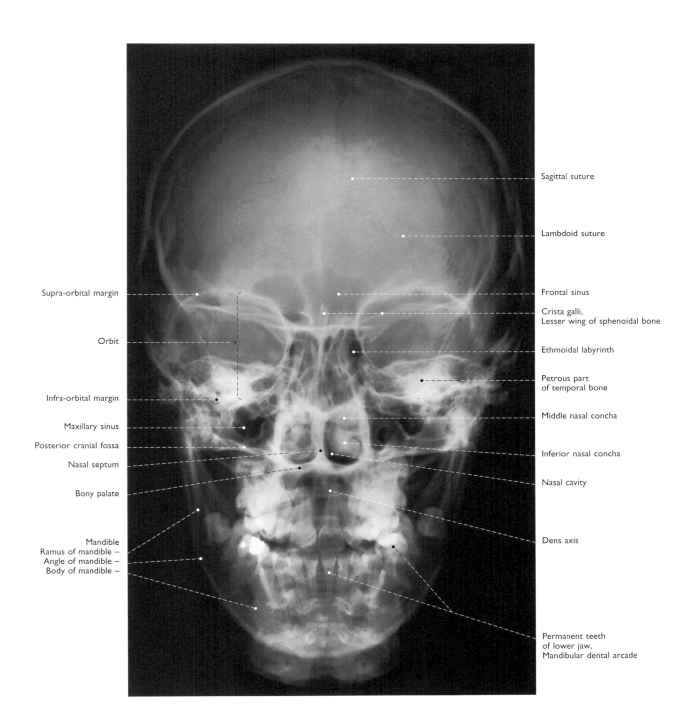

Supra-orbital margin

Orbit

Infra-orbital margin

Maxillary sinus

Posterior cranial fossa

Nasal septum

Bony palate

Mandible
Ramus of mandible –
Angle of mandible –
Body of mandible –

Sagittal suture

Lambdoid suture

Frontal sinus

Crista galli,
Lesser wing of sphenoidal bone

Ethmoidal labyrinth

Petrous part
of temporal bone

Middle nasal concha

Inferior nasal concha

Nasal cavity

Dens axis

Permanent teeth
of lower jaw,
Mandibular dental arcade

5 Skull = Cranium (75%)
Postero-anterior radiograph of the skull of a young female

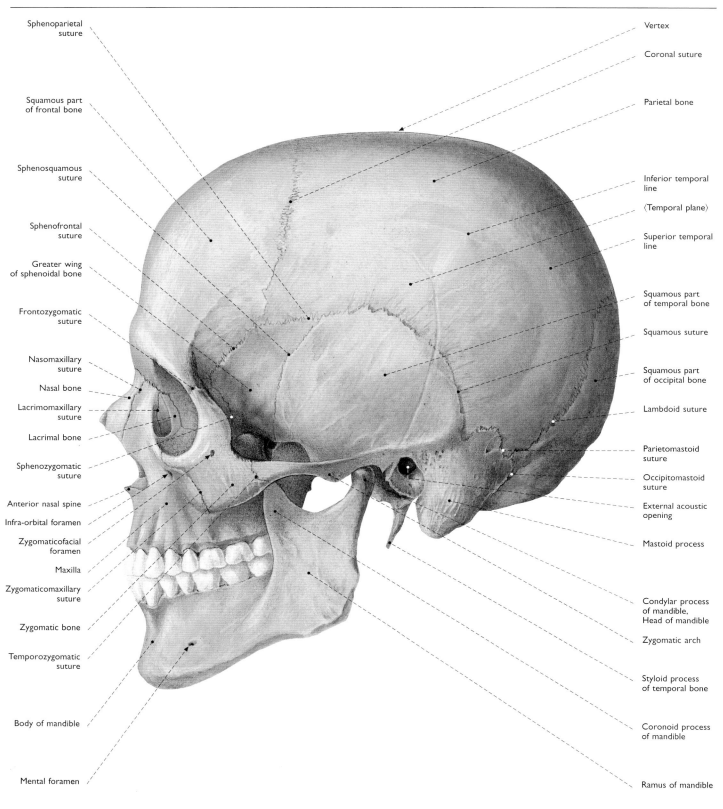

Sphenoparietal suture

Squamous part of frontal bone

Sphenosquamous suture

Sphenofrontal suture

Greater wing of sphenoidal bone

Frontozygomatic suture

Nasomaxillary suture

Nasal bone

Lacrimomaxillary suture

Lacrimal bone

Sphenozygomatic suture

Anterior nasal spine

Infra-orbital foramen

Zygomaticofacial foramen

Maxilla

Zygomaticomaxillary suture

Zygomatic bone

Temporozygomatic suture

Body of mandible

Mental foramen

Vertex

Coronal suture

Parietal bone

Inferior temporal line

⟨Temporal plane⟩

Superior temporal line

Squamous part of temporal bone

Squamous suture

Squamous part of occipital bone

Lambdoid suture

Parietomastoid suture

Occipitomastoid suture

External acoustic opening

Mastoid process

Condylar process of mandible, Head of mandible

Zygomatic arch

Styloid process of temporal bone

Coronoid process of mandible

Ramus of mandible

6 Skull = Cranium (75%)
Left lateral aspect

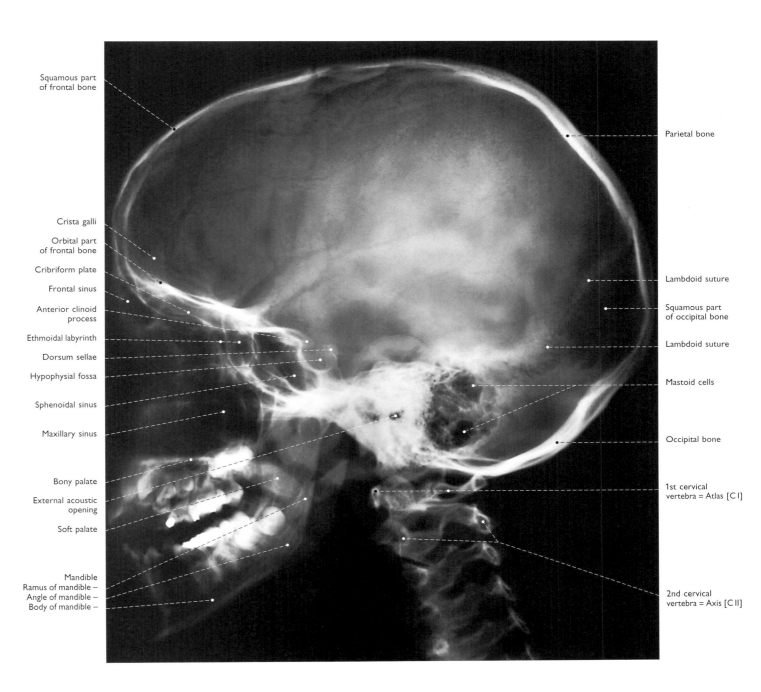

Squamous part
of frontal bone

Crista galli

Orbital part
of frontal bone

Cribriform plate

Frontal sinus

Anterior clinoid
process

Ethmoidal labyrinth

Dorsum sellae

Hypophysial fossa

Sphenoidal sinus

Maxillary sinus

Bony palate

External acoustic
opening

Soft palate

Mandible
Ramus of mandible –
Angle of mandible –
Body of mandible –

Parietal bone

Lambdoid suture

Squamous part
of occipital bone

Lambdoid suture

Mastoid cells

Occipital bone

1st cervical
vertebra = Atlas [C I]

2nd cervical
vertebra = Axis [C II]

7   Skull = Cranium (75%)
Lateral radiograph of the skull of a young female

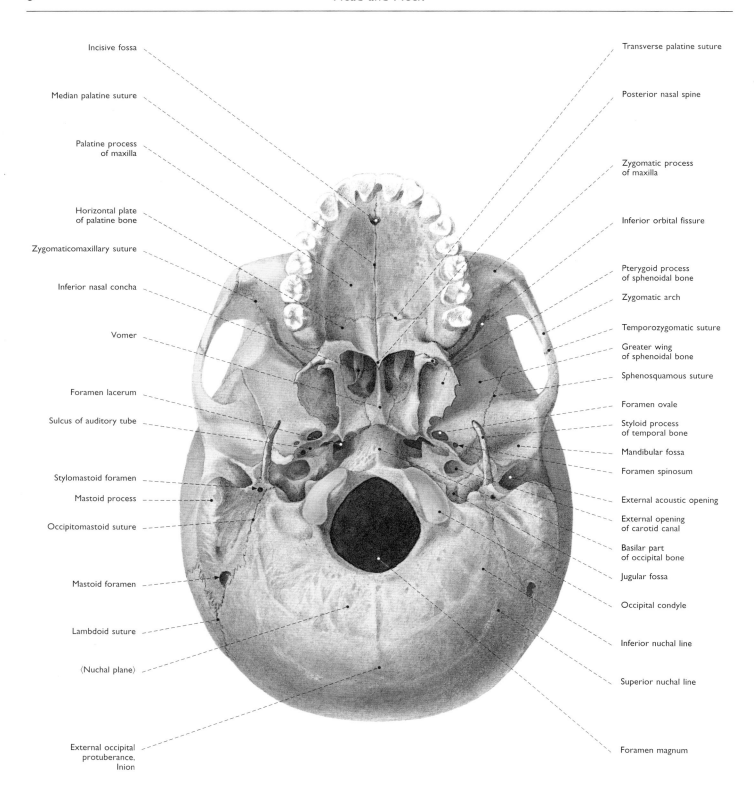

Incisive fossa

Median palatine suture

Palatine process
of maxilla

Horizontal plate
of palatine bone

Zygomaticomaxillary suture

Inferior nasal concha

Vomer

Foramen lacerum

Sulcus of auditory tube

Stylomastoid foramen

Mastoid process

Occipitomastoid suture

Mastoid foramen

Lambdoid suture

⟨Nuchal plane⟩

External occipital
protuberance,
Inion

Transverse palatine suture

Posterior nasal spine

Zygomatic process
of maxilla

Inferior orbital fissure

Pterygoid process
of sphenoidal bone

Zygomatic arch

Temporozygomatic suture

Greater wing
of sphenoidal bone

Sphenosquamous suture

Foramen ovale

Styloid process
of temporal bone

Mandibular fossa

Foramen spinosum

External acoustic opening

External opening
of carotid canal

Basilar part
of occipital bone

Jugular fossa

Occipital condyle

Inferior nuchal line

Superior nuchal line

Foramen magnum

8 External surface of cranial base (75%)
Inferior aspect

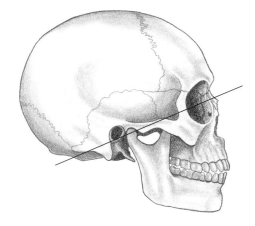

Nasal cavity	Eyeball
Nasal septum	Ethmoidal labyrinth
Temporal fossa	Spheno-ethmoidal recess
	Superior orbital fissure
	Sphenoidal sinus
	Foramen ovale
	Foramen spinosum
Condylar process of mandible	Foramen lacerum
Carotid canal	External acoustic meatus
Jugular fossa	Carotid canal
	Mastoid cells
	Hypoglossal canal
	Foramen magnum

9 Cranial base (100%)
Transverse computed tomogram (CT),
bone window, plane as indicated in the sketch above

Frontal crest

Foramen cecum

Cribriform plate
of ethmoidal bone

Impressions of cerebral gyri

Anterior cranial fossa

Jugum sphenoidale
= Sphenoidal yoke

Sphenoidal bone
Tuberculum sellae –
Hypophysial fossa –

Superior orbital fissure

Dorsum sellae

Foramen rotundum

Foramen lacerum

Sphenoidal lingula

Foramen ovale

Foramen spinosum

Middle cranial fossa

Petrous part
of temporal bone

Petro-occipital fissure

Groove for superior petrosal sinus

Groove for inferior petrosal sinus

Jugular foramen

Condylar canal

Posterior cranial fossa

(Internal occipital crest)

Squamous part
of occipital bone

Squamous part
of frontal bone

Crista galli

Fronto-ethmoidal suture

Spheno-ethmoidal suture

Sphenofrontal suture

Optic canal

(Middle clinoid process)

Lesser wing
of sphenoidal bone

Anterior clinoid process

Posterior clinoid process

Greater wing
of sphenoidal bone

Coronal suture

Sphenoparietal suture

Carotid sulcus

Sphenosquamous suture

Spheno-occipital synchondrosis

Squamous part
of temporal bone

Groove for greater petrosal nerve

Clivus

Arcuate eminence

Internal acoustic opening

Parietomastoid suture

Groove for sigmoid sinus

Hypoglossal canal

Occipitomastoid suture

Foramen magnum

Lambdoid suture

Groove for transverse sinus

Internal occipital protuberance

Groove for superior sagittal sinus

10 Internal surface of cranial base (75%)
Superior aspect (vertical aspect)

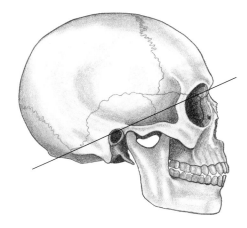

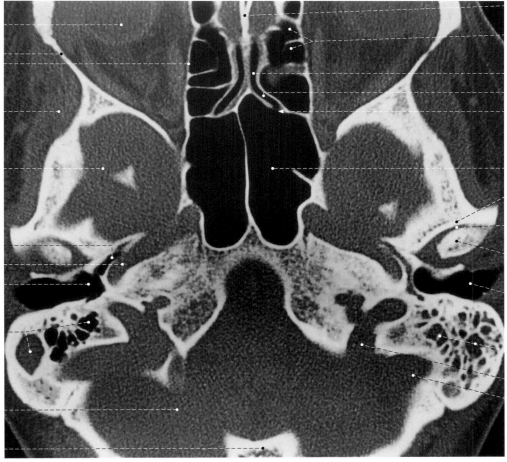

Eyeball

Orbit
Lateral wall –
Medial wall –

Temporal fossa

Middle cranial fossa

Musculotubal canal

Carotid canal

Tympanic cavity

Mastoid cells

Posterior cranial fossa

Internal occipital
protuberance

Nasal septum

Ethmoidal labyrinth

Nasal cavity

Spheno-ethmoidal recess

Opening
of sphenoidal sinus

Sphenoidal sinus

Mandibular fossa
of temporal bone

Temporomandibular
joint

Head of mandible

External acoustic meatus

Mastoid cells

Jugular fossa

Groove for sigmoid sinus

11   Cranial base (100%)
Transverse computed tomogram (CT),
bone window, plane as indicated in the sketch above

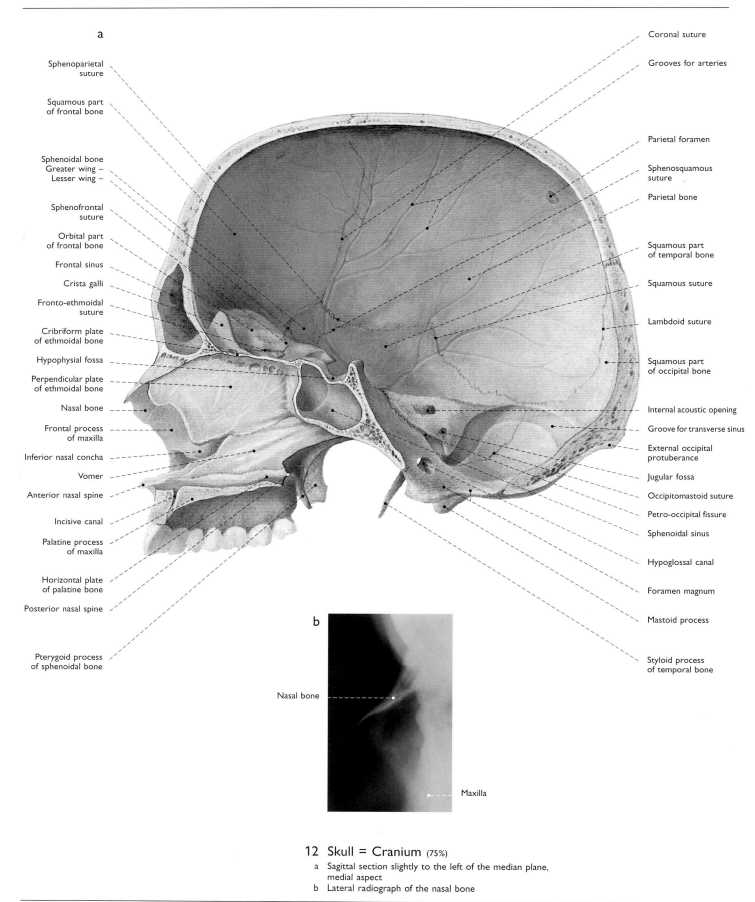

a

Sphenoparietal suture

Squamous part of frontal bone

Sphenoidal bone
Greater wing –
Lesser wing –

Sphenofrontal suture

Orbital part of frontal bone

Frontal sinus

Crista galli

Fronto-ethmoidal suture

Cribriform plate of ethmoidal bone

Hypophysial fossa

Perpendicular plate of ethmoidal bone

Nasal bone

Frontal process of maxilla

Inferior nasal concha

Vomer

Anterior nasal spine

Incisive canal

Palatine process of maxilla

Horizontal plate of palatine bone

Posterior nasal spine

Pterygoid process of sphenoidal bone

Coronal suture

Grooves for arteries

Parietal foramen

Sphenosquamous suture

Parietal bone

Squamous part of temporal bone

Squamous suture

Lambdoid suture

Squamous part of occipital bone

Internal acoustic opening

Groove for transverse sinus

External occipital protuberance

Jugular fossa

Occipitomastoid suture

Petro-occipital fissure

Sphenoidal sinus

Hypoglossal canal

Foramen magnum

Mastoid process

Styloid process of temporal bone

b

Nasal bone

Maxilla

12 Skull = Cranium (75%)

a Sagittal section slightly to the left of the median plane, medial aspect
b Lateral radiograph of the nasal bone

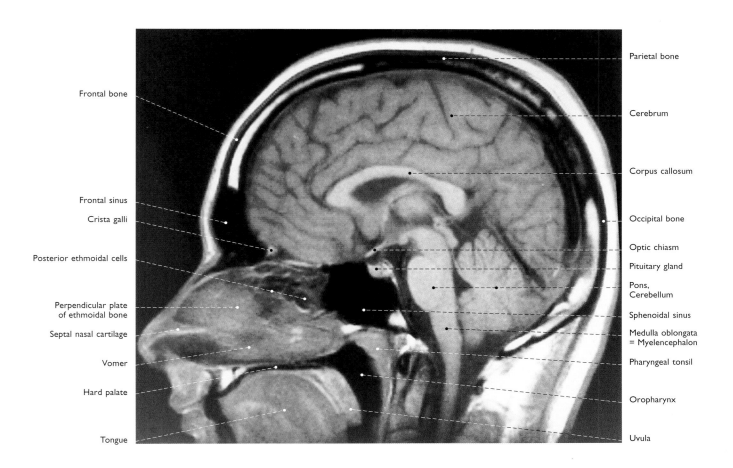

Frontal bone

Frontal sinus

Crista galli

Posterior ethmoidal cells

Perpendicular plate
of ethmoidal bone

Septal nasal cartilage

Vomer

Hard palate

Tongue

Parietal bone

Cerebrum

Corpus callosum

Occipital bone

Optic chiasm

Pituitary gland

Pons,
Cerebellum

Sphenoidal sinus

Medulla oblongata
= Myelencephalon

Pharyngeal tonsil

Oropharynx

Uvula

13 Head (55%)
Sagittal, paramedian magnetic resonance image
(MRI, T_1-weighted)

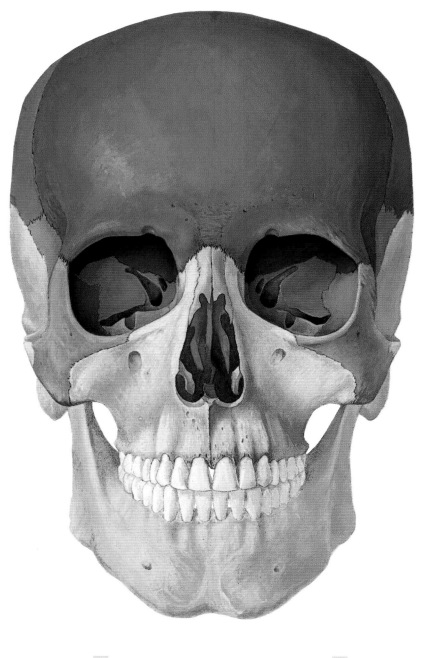

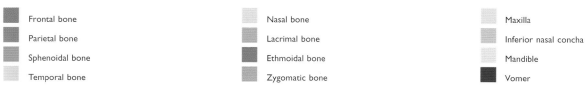

Frontal bone	Nasal bone	Maxilla
Parietal bone	Lacrimal bone	Inferior nasal concha
Sphenoidal bone	Ethmoidal bone	Mandible
Temporal bone	Zygomatic bone	Vomer

14 Skull = Cranium (80%)
The skull bones are marked by different colors.
Facial aspect (frontal aspect)

a

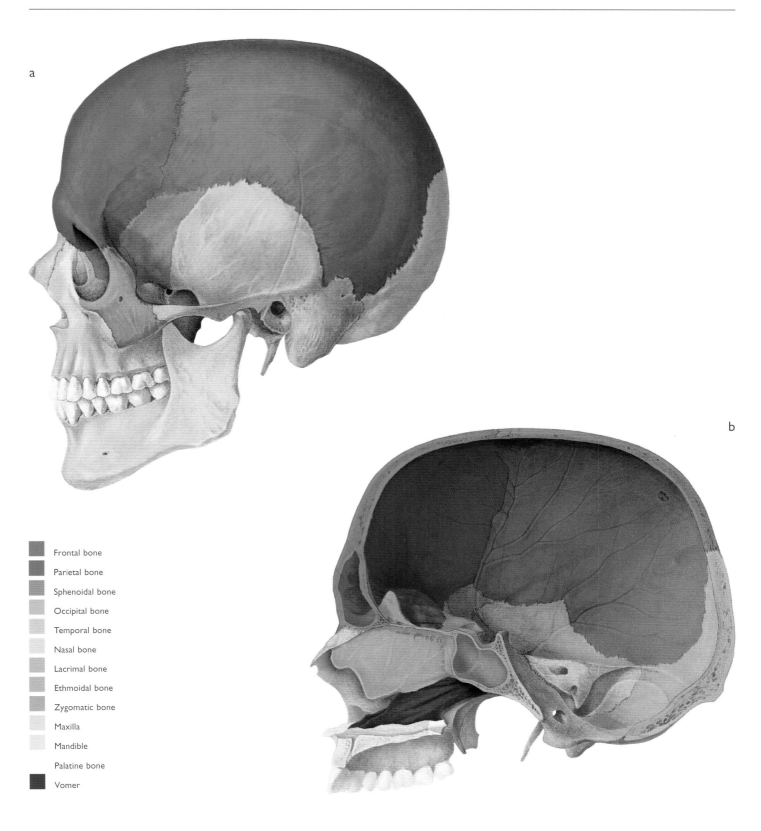

Frontal bone
Parietal bone
Sphenoidal bone
Occipital bone
Temporal bone
Nasal bone
Lacrimal bone
Ethmoidal bone
Zygomatic bone
Maxilla
Mandible
Palatine bone
Vomer

b

15 Skull = Cranium
    The skull bones are marked by different colors.
a   Left lateral aspect
b   Medial aspect of the right half of the skull

a

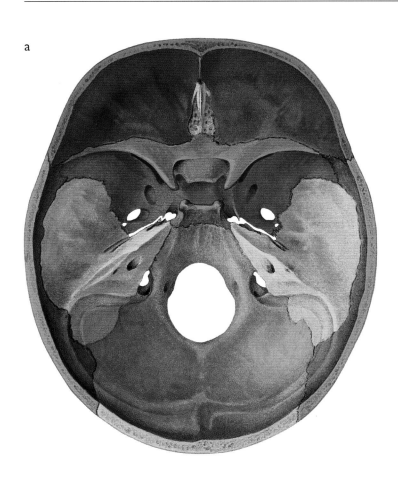

b

Frontal bone

Parietal bone

Sphenoidal bone

Occipital bone

Temporal bone

Ethmoidal bone

Zygomatic bone

Maxilla

Palatine bone

Vomer

16 Cranial base (70%)
   The skull bones are marked by different colors.
   a Internal surface
   b External surface

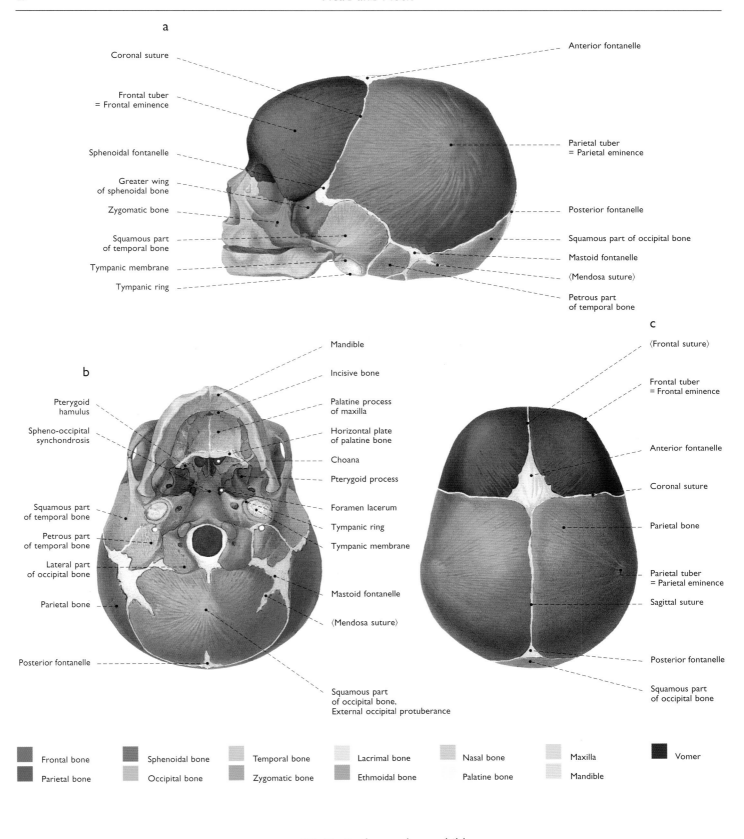

a

Coronal suture

Frontal tuber
= Frontal eminence

Sphenoidal fontanelle

Greater wing
of sphenoidal bone

Zygomatic bone

Squamous part
of temporal bone

Tympanic membrane

Tympanic ring

Anterior fontanelle

Parietal tuber
= Parietal eminence

Posterior fontanelle

Squamous part of occipital bone

Mastoid fontanelle

⟨Mendosa suture⟩

Petrous part
of temporal bone

b

Pterygoid
hamulus

Spheno-occipital
synchondrosis

Squamous part
of temporal bone

Petrous part
of temporal bone

Lateral part
of occipital bone

Parietal bone

Posterior fontanelle

Mandible

Incisive bone

Palatine process
of maxilla

Horizontal plate
of palatine bone

Choana

Pterygoid process

Foramen lacerum

Tympanic ring

Tympanic membrane

Mastoid fontanelle

⟨Mendosa suture⟩

Squamous part
of occipital bone,
External occipital protuberance

c

⟨Frontal suture⟩

Frontal tuber
= Frontal eminence

Anterior fontanelle

Coronal suture

Parietal bone

Parietal tuber
= Parietal eminence

Sagittal suture

Posterior fontanelle

Squamous part
of occipital bone

Frontal bone	Sphenoidal bone	Temporal bone	Lacrimal bone	Nasal bone	Maxilla	Vomer
Parietal bone	Occipital bone	Zygomatic bone	Ethmoidal bone	Palatine bone	Mandible	

17 Skull of a newborn child (80%)
The skull bones are marked by different colors.
a Left lateral aspect
b External surface of cranial base, inferior aspect
c Skull cap = calvaria, superior aspect (vertical aspect)

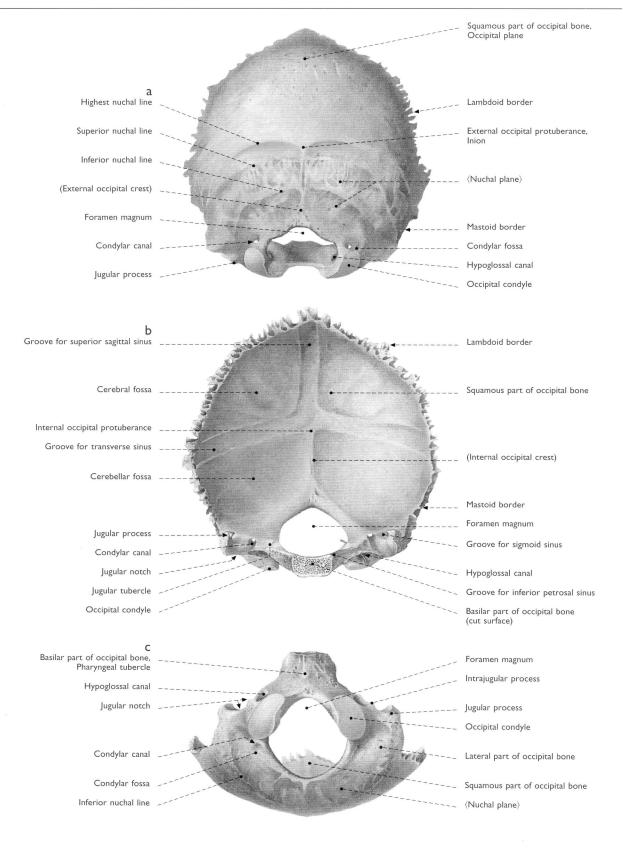

a
Highest nuchal line
Superior nuchal line
Inferior nuchal line
(External occipital crest)
Foramen magnum
Condylar canal
Jugular process

Squamous part of occipital bone, Occipital plane
Lambdoid border
External occipital protuberance, Inion
⟨Nuchal plane⟩
Mastoid border
Condylar fossa
Hypoglossal canal
Occipital condyle

b
Groove for superior sagittal sinus
Cerebral fossa
Internal occipital protuberance
Groove for transverse sinus
Cerebellar fossa
Jugular process
Condylar canal
Jugular notch
Jugular tubercle
Occipital condyle

Lambdoid border
Squamous part of occipital bone
(Internal occipital crest)
Mastoid border
Foramen magnum
Groove for sigmoid sinus
Hypoglossal canal
Groove for inferior petrosal sinus
Basilar part of occipital bone (cut surface)

c
Basilar part of occipital bone, Pharyngeal tubercle
Hypoglossal canal
Jugular notch
Condylar canal
Condylar fossa
Inferior nuchal line

Foramen magnum
Intrajugular process
Jugular process
Occipital condyle
Lateral part of occipital bone
Squamous part of occipital bone
⟨Nuchal plane⟩

18 Occipital bone (70%)
a External surface, occipital aspect
b Internal surface, frontal aspect
c External surface, inferior aspect

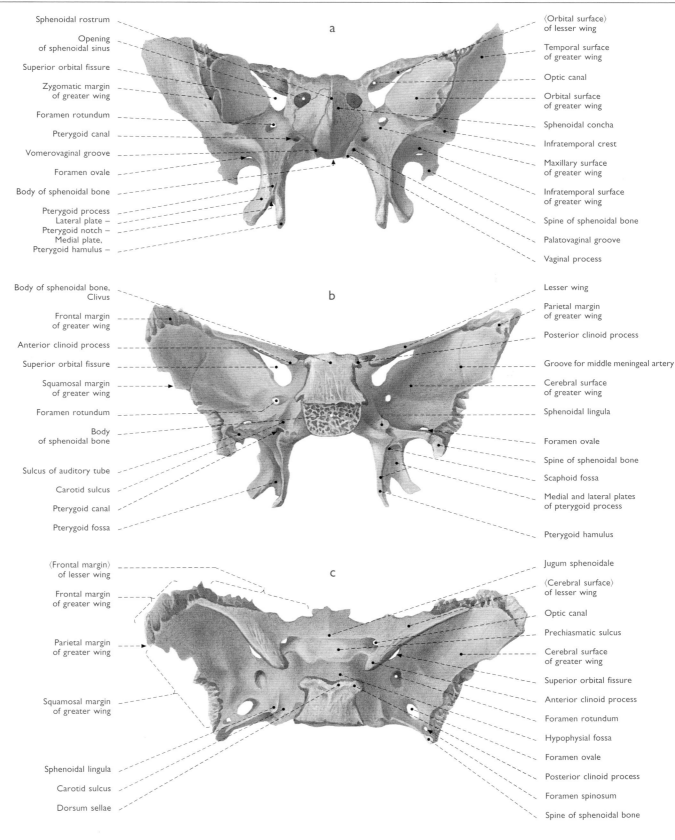

Sphenoidal rostrum

Opening
of sphenoidal sinus

Superior orbital fissure

Zygomatic margin
of greater wing

Foramen rotundum

Pterygoid canal

Vomerovaginal groove

Foramen ovale

Body of sphenoidal bone

Pterygoid process
Lateral plate –
Pterygoid notch –
Medial plate,
Pterygoid hamulus –

a

⟨Orbital surface⟩
of lesser wing

Temporal surface
of greater wing

Optic canal

Orbital surface
of greater wing

Sphenoidal concha

Infratemporal crest

Maxillary surface
of greater wing

Infratemporal surface
of greater wing

Spine of sphenoidal bone

Palatovaginal groove

Vaginal process

Body of sphenoidal bone,
Clivus

Frontal margin
of greater wing

Anterior clinoid process

Superior orbital fissure

Squamosal margin
of greater wing

Foramen rotundum

Body
of sphenoidal bone

Sulcus of auditory tube

Carotid sulcus

Pterygoid canal

Pterygoid fossa

b

Lesser wing

Parietal margin
of greater wing

Posterior clinoid process

Groove for middle meningeal artery

Cerebral surface
of greater wing

Sphenoidal lingula

Foramen ovale

Spine of sphenoidal bone

Scaphoid fossa

Medial and lateral plates
of pterygoid process

Pterygoid hamulus

⟨Frontal margin⟩
of lesser wing

Frontal margin
of greater wing

Parietal margin
of greater wing

Squamosal margin
of greater wing

Sphenoidal lingula

Carotid sulcus

Dorsum sellae

c

Jugum sphenoidale

⟨Cerebral surface⟩
of lesser wing

Optic canal

Prechiasmatic sulcus

Cerebral surface
of greater wing

Superior orbital fissure

Anterior clinoid process

Foramen rotundum

Hypophysial fossa

Foramen ovale

Posterior clinoid process

Foramen spinosum

Spine of sphenoidal bone

19 Sphenoidal bone (70%)
a Frontal aspect
b Occipital aspect
c Superior aspect

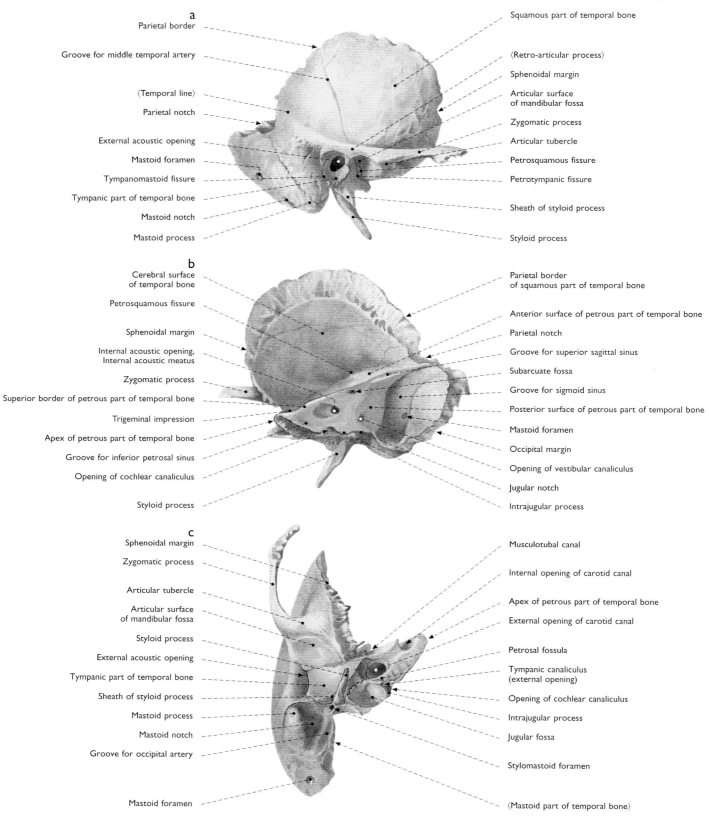

a
Parietal border
Groove for middle temporal artery
⟨Temporal line⟩
Parietal notch
External acoustic opening
Mastoid foramen
Tympanomastoid fissure
Tympanic part of temporal bone
Mastoid notch
Mastoid process

Squamous part of temporal bone
⟨Retro-articular process⟩
Sphenoidal margin
Articular surface of mandibular fossa
Zygomatic process
Articular tubercle
Petrosquamous fissure
Petrotympanic fissure
Sheath of styloid process
Styloid process

b
Cerebral surface of temporal bone
Petrosquamous fissure
Sphenoidal margin
Internal acoustic opening, Internal acoustic meatus
Zygomatic process
Superior border of petrous part of temporal bone
Trigeminal impression
Apex of petrous part of temporal bone
Groove for inferior petrosal sinus
Opening of cochlear canaliculus
Styloid process

Parietal border of squamous part of temporal bone
Anterior surface of petrous part of temporal bone
Parietal notch
Groove for superior sagittal sinus
Subarcuate fossa
Groove for sigmoid sinus
Posterior surface of petrous part of temporal bone
Mastoid foramen
Occipital margin
Opening of vestibular canaliculus
Jugular notch
Intrajugular process

c
Sphenoidal margin
Zygomatic process
Articular tubercle
Articular surface of mandibular fossa
Styloid process
External acoustic opening
Tympanic part of temporal bone
Sheath of styloid process
Mastoid process
Mastoid notch
Groove for occipital artery
Mastoid foramen

Musculotubal canal
Internal opening of carotid canal
Apex of petrous part of temporal bone
External opening of carotid canal
Petrosal fossula
Tympanic canaliculus (external opening)
Opening of cochlear canaliculus
Intrajugular process
Jugular fossa
Stylomastoid foramen
⟨Mastoid part of temporal bone⟩

20 Right temporal bone (70%)
a Lateral aspect
b Medial aspect
c Inferior aspect

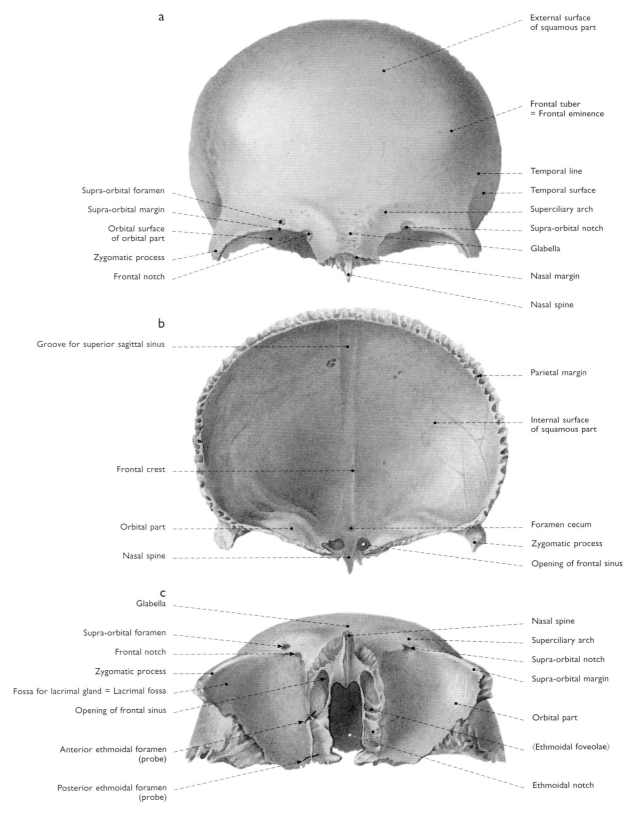

a

External surface
of squamous part

Frontal tuber
= Frontal eminence

Temporal line

Supra-orbital foramen

Temporal surface

Supra-orbital margin

Superciliary arch

Orbital surface
of orbital part

Supra-orbital notch

Zygomatic process

Glabella

Frontal notch

Nasal margin

Nasal spine

b

Groove for superior sagittal sinus

Parietal margin

Internal surface
of squamous part

Frontal crest

Orbital part

Foramen cecum

Zygomatic process

Nasal spine

Opening of frontal sinus

c

Glabella

Nasal spine

Supra-orbital foramen

Superciliary arch

Frontal notch

Supra-orbital notch

Zygomatic process

Supra-orbital margin

Fossa for lacrimal gland = Lacrimal fossa

Opening of frontal sinus

Orbital part

Anterior ethmoidal foramen
(probe)

〈Ethmoidal foveolae〉

Posterior ethmoidal foramen
(probe)

Ethmoidal notch

21 Frontal bone (90%)
  a External surface, frontal aspect
  b Internal surface, occipital aspect
  c Orbital part, inferior aspect

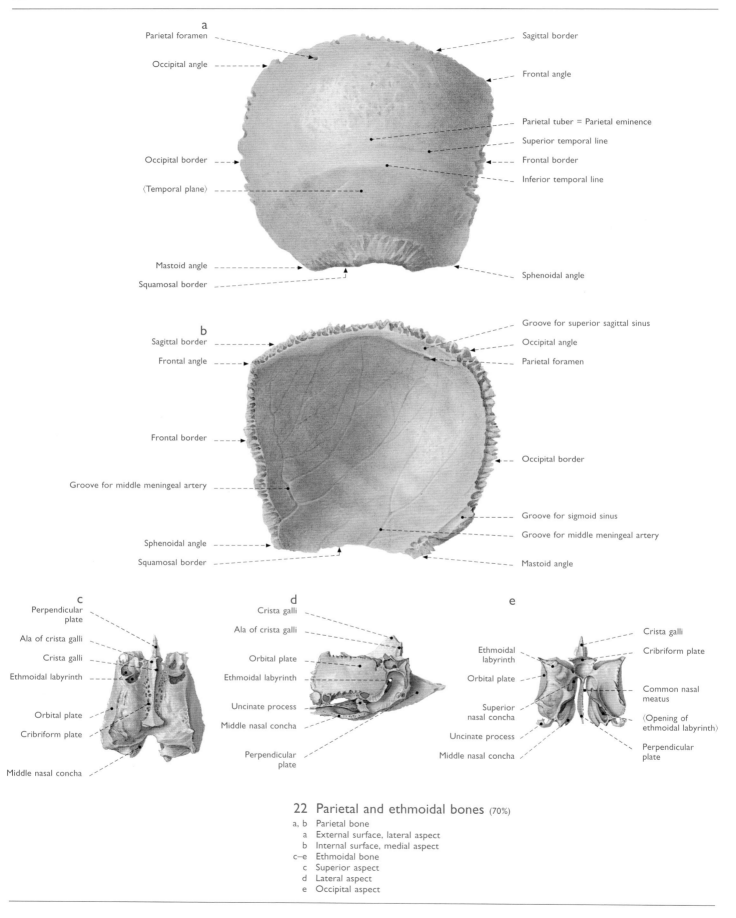

a

Parietal foramen

Occipital angle

Sagittal border

Frontal angle

Parietal tuber = Parietal eminence
Superior temporal line
Frontal border
Inferior temporal line

Occipital border

(Temporal plane)

Mastoid angle
Squamosal border

Sphenoidal angle

b

Sagittal border
Frontal angle

Groove for superior sagittal sinus
Occipital angle
Parietal foramen

Frontal border

Groove for middle meningeal artery

Occipital border

Groove for sigmoid sinus
Groove for middle meningeal artery

Sphenoidal angle
Squamosal border

Mastoid angle

c

Perpendicular plate
Ala of crista galli
Crista galli
Ethmoidal labyrinth

Orbital plate
Cribriform plate

Middle nasal concha

d

Crista galli
Ala of crista galli

Orbital plate

Ethmoidal labyrinth

Uncinate process

Middle nasal concha

Perpendicular plate

e

Crista galli
Cribriform plate

Ethmoidal labyrinth

Orbital plate

Superior nasal concha

Uncinate process

Middle nasal concha

Common nasal meatus

⟨Opening of ethmoidal labyrinth⟩

Perpendicular plate

22 Parietal and ethmoidal bones (70%)

a, b Parietal bone
   a External surface, lateral aspect
   b Internal surface, medial aspect
c–e Ethmoidal bone
   c Superior aspect
   d Lateral aspect
   e Occipital aspect

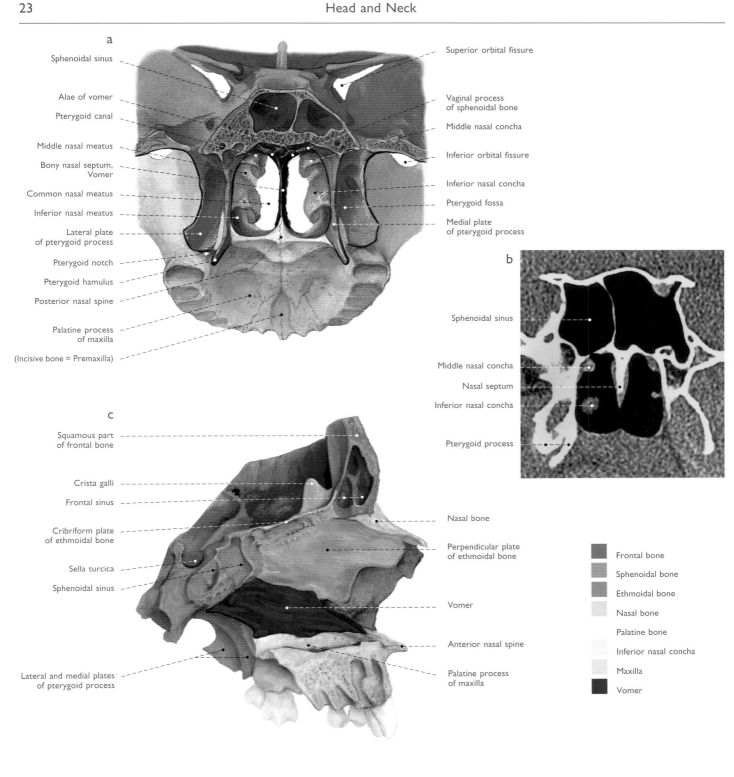

a

Sphenoidal sinus

Alae of vomer

Pterygoid canal

Middle nasal meatus

Bony nasal septum, Vomer

Common nasal meatus

Inferior nasal meatus

Lateral plate of pterygoid process

Pterygoid notch

Pterygoid hamulus

Posterior nasal spine

Palatine process of maxilla

(Incisive bone = Premaxilla)

Superior orbital fissure

Vaginal process of sphenoidal bone

Middle nasal concha

Inferior orbital fissure

Inferior nasal concha

Pterygoid fossa

Medial plate of pterygoid process

b

Sphenoidal sinus

Middle nasal concha

Nasal septum

Inferior nasal concha

Pterygoid process

c

Squamous part of frontal bone

Crista galli

Frontal sinus

Cribriform plate of ethmoidal bone

Sella turcica

Sphenoidal sinus

Lateral and medial plates of pterygoid process

Nasal bone

Perpendicular plate of ethmoidal bone

Vomer

Anterior nasal spine

Palatine process of maxilla

Frontal bone

Sphenoidal bone

Ethmoidal bone

Nasal bone

Palatine bone

Inferior nasal concha

Maxilla

Vomer

23   Skeleton of the nose (100%)

a, c   The different bones are marked by various colors.
    a   Posterior nasal apertures = choanae, occipital aspect
    b   Coronal computed tomogram (CT)
        through the choanae and the sphenoidal sinuses
    c   Bony nasal septum. Medial aspect of the left half of the skull,
        sagittal section slightly to the right of the median plane

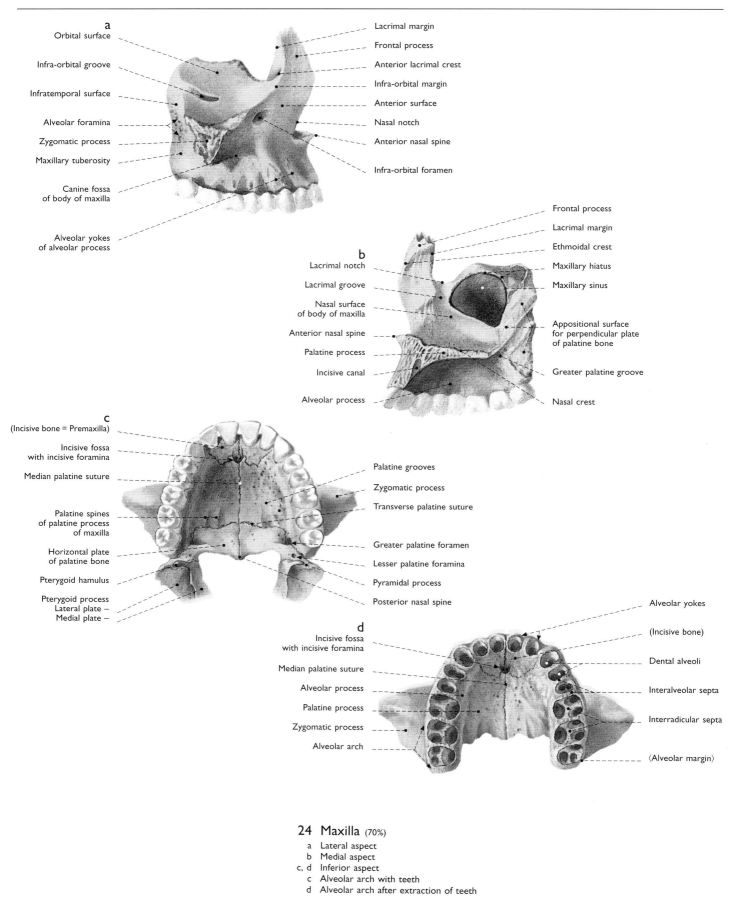

a

Orbital surface

Infra-orbital groove

Infratemporal surface

Alveolar foramina

Zygomatic process

Maxillary tuberosity

Canine fossa
of body of maxilla

Alveolar yokes
of alveolar process

Lacrimal margin

Frontal process

Anterior lacrimal crest

Infra-orbital margin

Anterior surface

Nasal notch

Anterior nasal spine

Infra-orbital foramen

b

Lacrimal notch

Lacrimal groove

Nasal surface
of body of maxilla

Anterior nasal spine

Palatine process

Incisive canal

Alveolar process

Frontal process

Lacrimal margin

Ethmoidal crest

Maxillary hiatus

Maxillary sinus

Appositional surface
for perpendicular plate
of palatine bone

Greater palatine groove

Nasal crest

c

(Incisive bone = Premaxilla)

Incisive fossa
with incisive foramina

Median palatine suture

Palatine spines
of palatine process
of maxilla

Horizontal plate
of palatine bone

Pterygoid hamulus

Pterygoid process
Lateral plate –
Medial plate –

Palatine grooves

Zygomatic process

Transverse palatine suture

Greater palatine foramen

Lesser palatine foramina

Pyramidal process

Posterior nasal spine

d

Incisive fossa
with incisive foramina

Median palatine suture

Alveolar process

Palatine process

Zygomatic process

Alveolar arch

Alveolar yokes

(Incisive bone)

Dental alveoli

Interalveolar septa

Interradicular septa

⟨Alveolar margin⟩

24 Maxilla (70%)
a   Lateral aspect
b   Medial aspect
c, d Inferior aspect
c   Alveolar arch with teeth
d   Alveolar arch after extraction of teeth

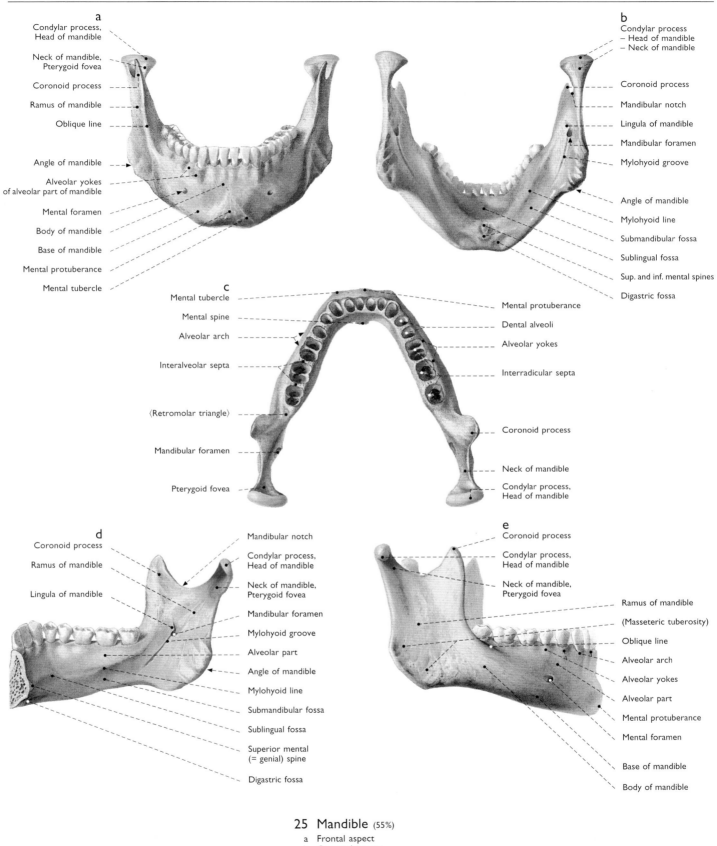

a

Condylar process, Head of mandible

Neck of mandible, Pterygoid fovea

Coronoid process

Ramus of mandible

Oblique line

Angle of mandible

Alveolar yokes of alveolar part of mandible

Mental foramen

Body of mandible

Base of mandible

Mental protuberance

Mental tubercle

b

Condylar process – Head of mandible – Neck of mandible

Coronoid process

Mandibular notch

Lingula of mandible

Mandibular foramen

Mylohyoid groove

Angle of mandible

Mylohyoid line

Submandibular fossa

Sublingual fossa

Sup. and inf. mental spines

Digastric fossa

c

Mental tubercle

Mental spine

Alveolar arch

Interalveolar septa

〈Retromolar triangle〉

Mandibular foramen

Pterygoid fovea

Mental protuberance

Dental alveoli

Alveolar yokes

Interradicular septa

Coronoid process

Neck of mandible

Condylar process, Head of mandible

d

Coronoid process

Ramus of mandible

Lingula of mandible

Mandibular notch

Condylar process, Head of mandible

Neck of mandible, Pterygoid fovea

Mandibular foramen

Mylohyoid groove

Alveolar part

Angle of mandible

Mylohyoid line

Submandibular fossa

Sublingual fossa

Superior mental (= genial) spine

Digastric fossa

e

Coronoid process

Condylar process, Head of mandible

Neck of mandible, Pterygoid fovea

Ramus of mandible

(Masseteric tuberosity)

Oblique line

Alveolar arch

Alveolar yokes

Alveolar part

Mental protuberance

Mental foramen

Base of mandible

Body of mandible

25   Mandible (55%)

a   Frontal aspect
b   Occipital aspect
c   Superior aspect, alveolar arch after extraction of teeth
d   Medial aspect of the right half of the mandible
e   Right lateral aspect

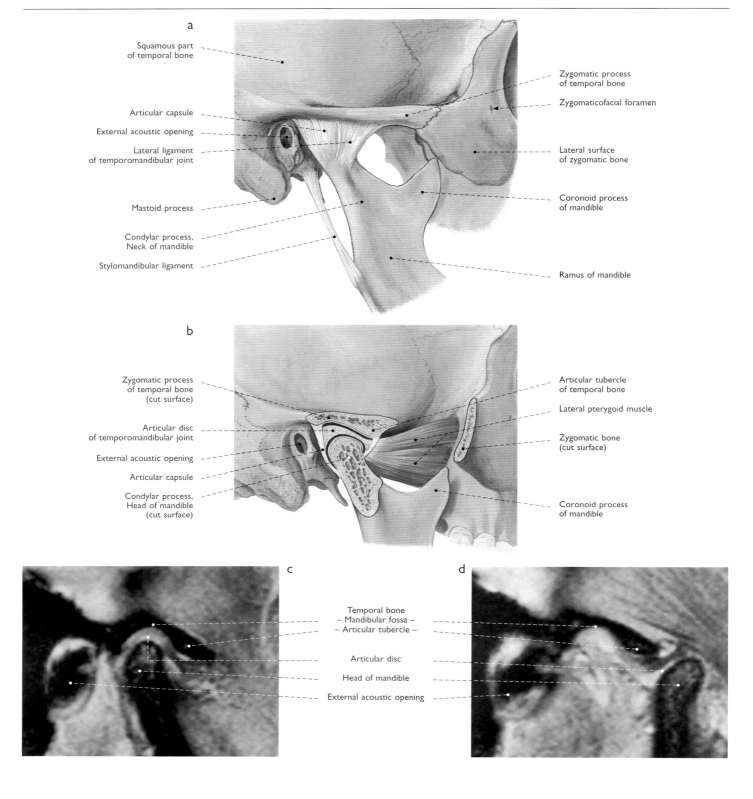

a

Squamous part of temporal bone

Articular capsule

External acoustic opening

Lateral ligament of temporomandibular joint

Mastoid process

Condylar process, Neck of mandible

Stylomandibular ligament

Zygomatic process of temporal bone

Zygomaticofacial foramen

Lateral surface of zygomatic bone

Coronoid process of mandible

Ramus of mandible

b

Zygomatic process of temporal bone (cut surface)

Articular disc of temporomandibular joint

External acoustic opening

Articular capsule

Condylar process, Head of mandible (cut surface)

Articular tubercle of temporal bone

Lateral pterygoid muscle

Zygomatic bone (cut surface)

Coronoid process of mandible

c   d

Temporal bone
– Mandibular fossa –
– Articular tubercle –

Articular disc

Head of mandible

External acoustic opening

26   Temporomandibular joint

a, b   Right lateral aspect (80%)
     a   Capsule and ligaments
     b   Sagittal section, the lateral pterygoid muscle is left in position
c, d   Sagittal magnetic resonance image (MRI, T_2-weighted)
        through the temporomandibular joint
     c   when mouth closed
     d   when mouth opened

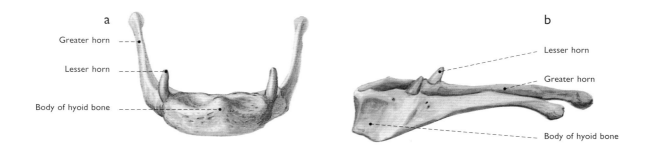

a

Greater horn

Lesser horn

Body of hyoid bone

b

Lesser horn

Greater horn

Body of hyoid bone

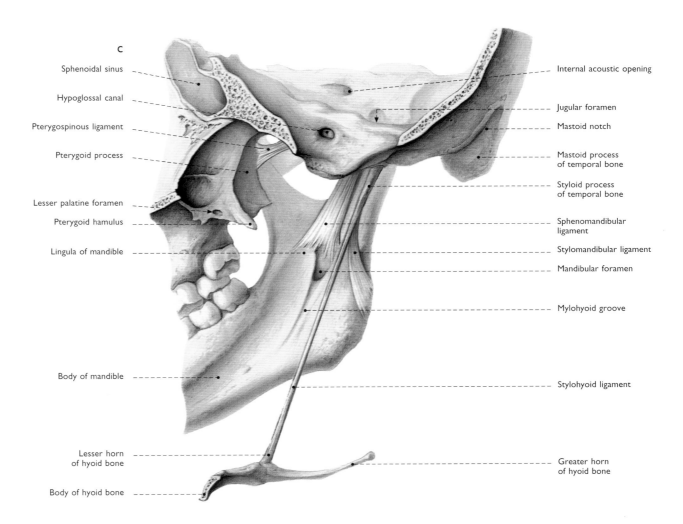

c

Sphenoidal sinus

Hypoglossal canal

Pterygospinous ligament

Pterygoid process

Lesser palatine foramen

Pterygoid hamulus

Lingula of mandible

Body of mandible

Lesser horn
of hyoid bone

Body of hyoid bone

Internal acoustic opening

Jugular foramen

Mastoid notch

Mastoid process
of temporal bone

Styloid process
of temporal bone

Sphenomandibular
ligament

Stylomandibular ligament

Mandibular foramen

Mylohyoid groove

Stylohyoid ligament

Greater horn
of hyoid bone

27 Hyoid bone and ligaments
of the temporomandibular joint

a, b Hyoid bone (80%)
  a Ventral aspect
  b Left lateral aspect
  c Ligaments of the right temporomandibular joint (100%),
    medial aspect

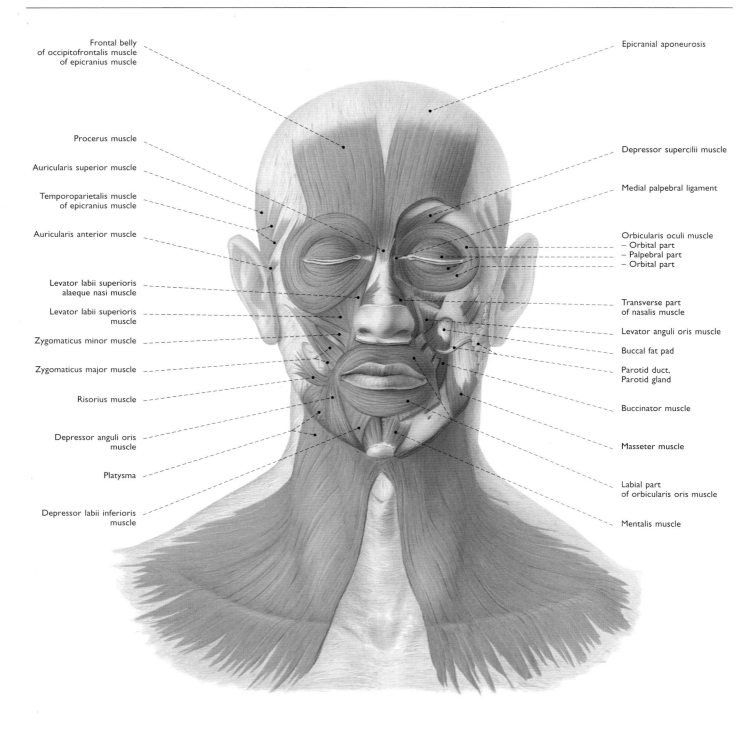

Frontal belly
of occipitofrontalis muscle
of epicranius muscle

Procerus muscle

Auricularis superior muscle

Temporoparietalis muscle
of epicranius muscle

Auricularis anterior muscle

Levator labii superioris
alaeque nasi muscle

Levator labii superioris
muscle

Zygomaticus minor muscle

Zygomaticus major muscle

Risorius muscle

Depressor anguli oris
muscle

Platysma

Depressor labii inferioris
muscle

Epicranial aponeurosis

Depressor supercilii muscle

Medial palpebral ligament

Orbicularis oculi muscle
– Orbital part
– Palpebral part
– Orbital part

Transverse part
of nasalis muscle

Levator anguli oris muscle

Buccal fat pad

Parotid duct,
Parotid gland

Buccinator muscle

Masseter muscle

Labial part
of orbicularis oris muscle

Mentalis muscle

28 Muscles of the scalp and face (50%)
On the right side of the face, the superficial layer of
the facial musculature is demonstrated, the deep layer and
the masseter muscle are shown on the left side. Frontal aspect

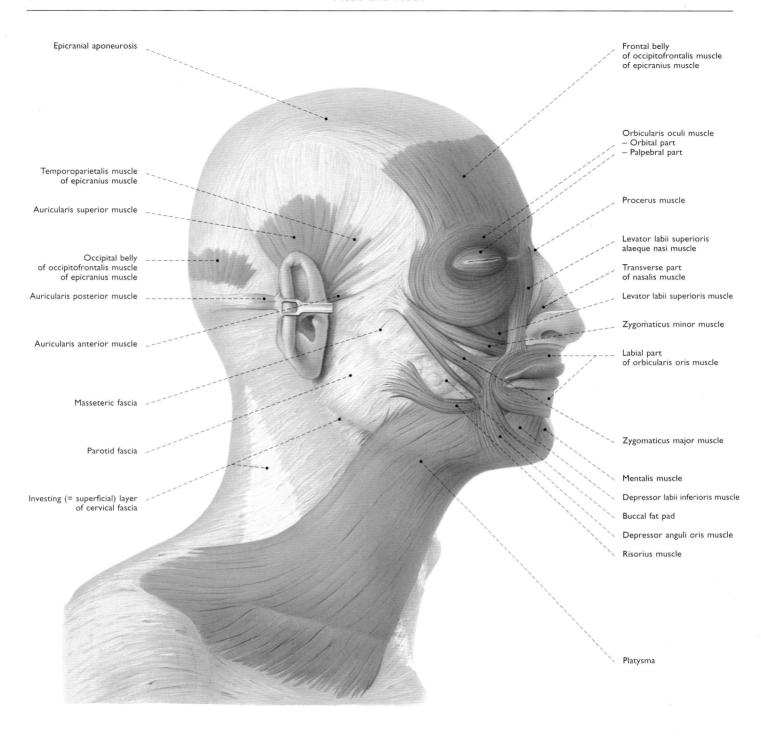

Epicranial aponeurosis

Frontal belly
of occipitofrontalis muscle
of epicranius muscle

Temporoparietalis muscle
of epicranius muscle

Auricularis superior muscle

Orbicularis oculi muscle
– Orbital part
– Palpebral part

Procerus muscle

Occipital belly
of occipitofrontalis muscle
of epicranius muscle

Levator labii superioris
alaeque nasi muscle

Auricularis posterior muscle

Transverse part
of nasalis muscle

Levator labii superioris muscle

Auricularis anterior muscle

Zygomaticus minor muscle

Labial part
of orbicularis oris muscle

Masseteric fascia

Zygomaticus major muscle

Parotid fascia

Mentalis muscle

Depressor labii inferioris muscle

Buccal fat pad

Investing (= superficial) layer
of cervical fascia

Depressor anguli oris muscle

Risorius muscle

Platysma

29 Muscles of the scalp and face (50%)
Superficial layer, right lateral aspect

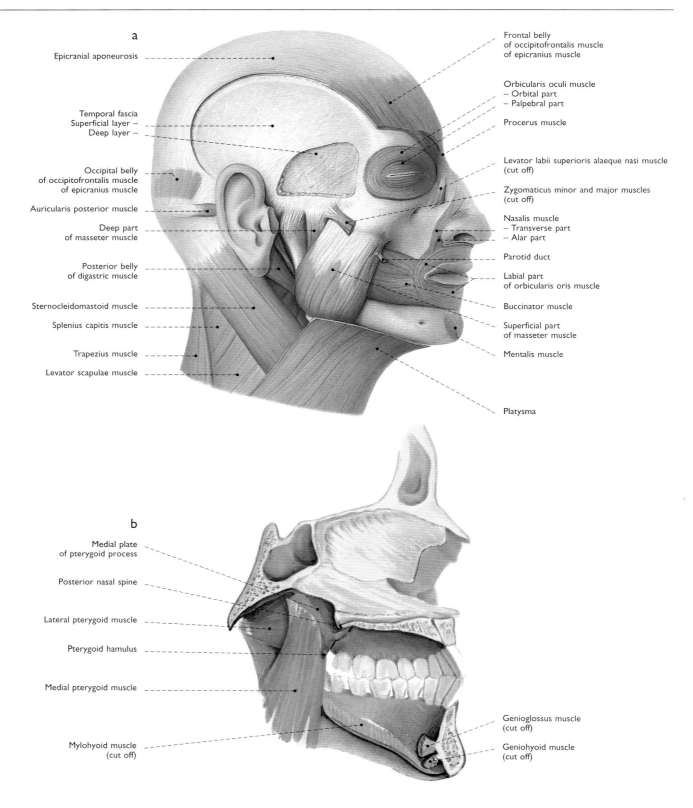

a

Epicranial aponeurosis

Temporal fascia
Superficial layer –
Deep layer –

Occipital belly
of occipitofrontalis muscle
of epicranius muscle

Auricularis posterior muscle

Deep part
of masseter muscle

Posterior belly
of digastric muscle

Sternocleidomastoid muscle

Splenius capitis muscle

Trapezius muscle

Levator scapulae muscle

Frontal belly
of occipitofrontalis muscle
of epicranius muscle

Orbicularis oculi muscle
– Orbital part
– Palpebral part

Procerus muscle

Levator labii superioris alaeque nasi muscle
(cut off)

Zygomaticus minor and major muscles
(cut off)

Nasalis muscle
– Transverse part
– Alar part

Parotid duct

Labial part
of orbicularis oris muscle

Buccinator muscle

Superficial part
of masseter muscle

Mentalis muscle

Platysma

b

Medial plate
of pterygoid process

Posterior nasal spine

Lateral pterygoid muscle

Pterygoid hamulus

Medial pterygoid muscle

Mylohyoid muscle
(cut off)

Genioglossus muscle
(cut off)

Geniohyoid muscle
(cut off)

30 Deep muscles of the face,
    masseter and pterygoid muscles (50%)
    a Deep muscles of the face and masseter muscle after
       removal of the parotid gland and the superficial muscles
       of the face, right lateral aspect
    b Pterygoid muscles, medial aspect

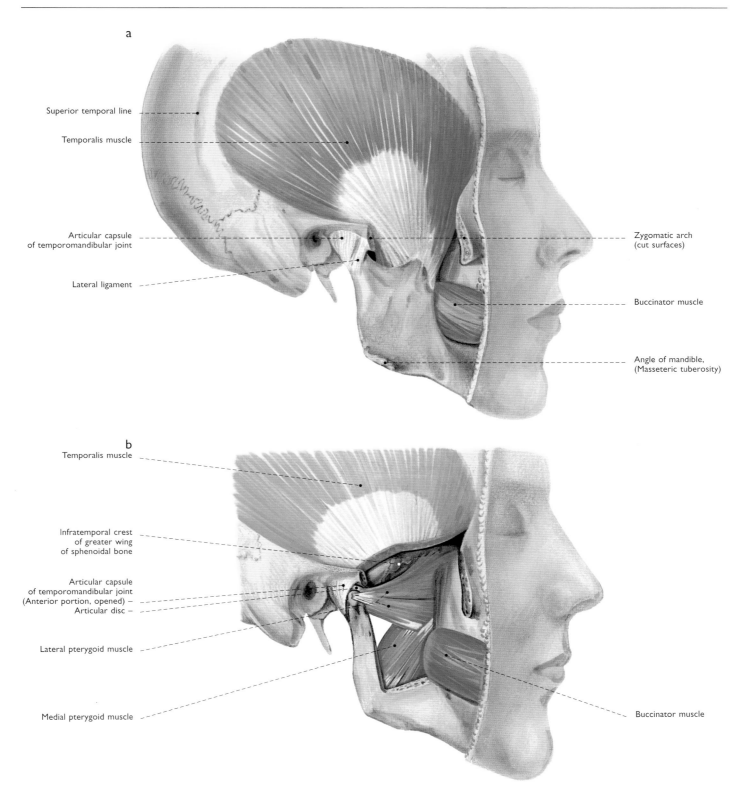

a

Superior temporal line

Temporalis muscle

Articular capsule
of temporomandibular joint

Lateral ligament

Zygomatic arch
(cut surfaces)

Buccinator muscle

Angle of mandible,
(Masseteric tuberosity)

b

Temporalis muscle

Infratemporal crest
of greater wing
of sphenoidal bone

Articular capsule
of temporomandibular joint
(Anterior portion, opened) –
Articular disc –

Lateral pterygoid muscle

Medial pterygoid muscle

Buccinator muscle

31 Buccinator, temporalis, and
    pterygoid muscles (60%)
    Right lateral aspect
  a The zygomatic arch and the masseter muscle were removed.
  b The ramus of the mandible and the temporalis muscle were
     additionally excised partially.

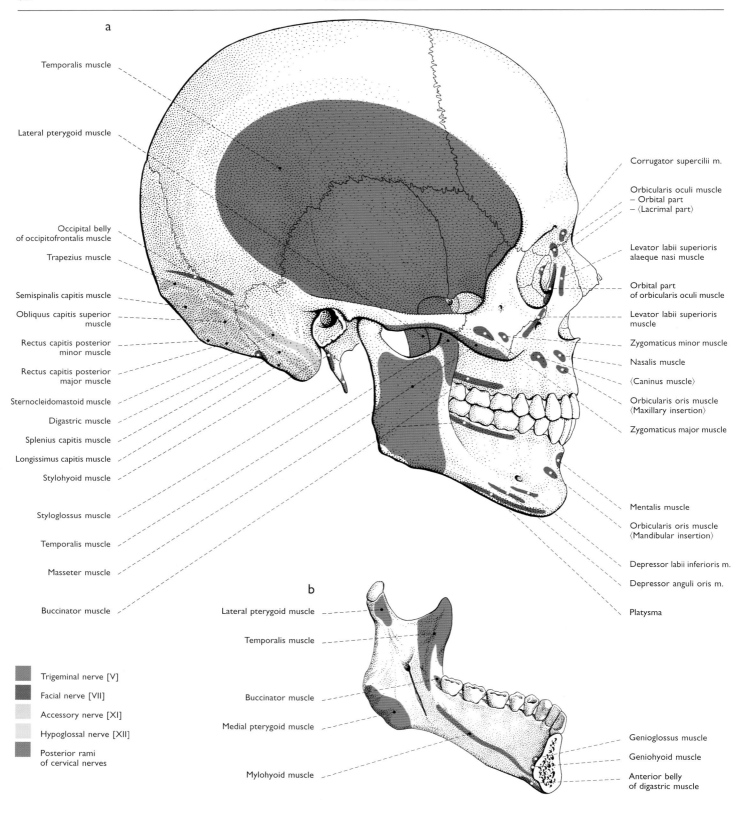

a

Temporalis muscle

Lateral pterygoid muscle

Corrugator supercilii m.

Orbicularis oculi muscle
– Orbital part
– ⟨Lacrimal part⟩

Occipital belly
of occipitofrontalis muscle

Levator labii superioris
alaeque nasi muscle

Trapezius muscle

Orbital part
of orbicularis oculi muscle

Semispinalis capitis muscle

Levator labii superioris
muscle

Obliquus capitis superior
muscle

Zygomaticus minor muscle

Rectus capitis posterior
minor muscle

Nasalis muscle

⟨Caninus muscle⟩

Rectus capitis posterior
major muscle

Orbicularis oris muscle
⟨Maxillary insertion⟩

Sternocleidomastoid muscle

Zygomaticus major muscle

Digastric muscle

Splenius capitis muscle

Longissimus capitis muscle

Stylohyoid muscle

Styloglossus muscle

Mentalis muscle

Temporalis muscle

Orbicularis oris muscle
⟨Mandibular insertion⟩

Masseter muscle

Depressor labii inferioris m.

Depressor anguli oris m.

Buccinator muscle

Platysma

b

Trigeminal nerve [V]

Facial nerve [VII]

Accessory nerve [XI]

Hypoglossal nerve [XII]

Posterior rami
of cervical nerves

Lateral pterygoid muscle

Temporalis muscle

Buccinator muscle

Medial pterygoid muscle

Genioglossus muscle

Geniohyoid muscle

Anterior belly
of digastric muscle

Mylohyoid muscle

32 Muscle attachments on the skull

Attachments on the
a right surface of the skull
b inner side of the mandible

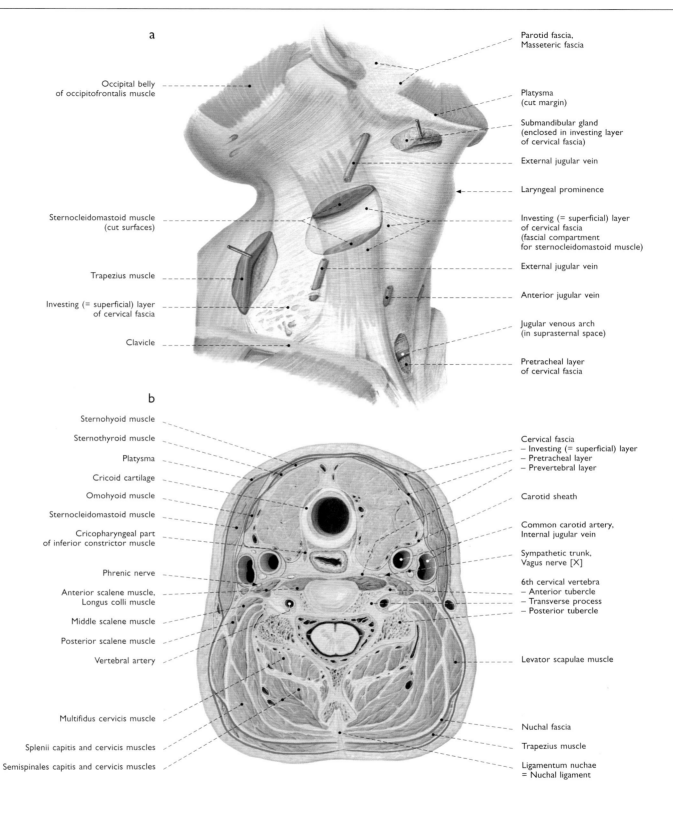

a

Occipital belly
of occipitofrontalis muscle

Sternocleidomastoid muscle
(cut surfaces)

Trapezius muscle

Investing (= superficial) layer
of cervical fascia

Clavicle

Parotid fascia,
Masseteric fascia

Platysma
(cut margin)

Submandibular gland
(enclosed in investing layer
of cervical fascia)

External jugular vein

Laryngeal prominence

Investing (= superficial) layer
of cervical fascia
(fascial compartment
for sternocleidomastoid muscle)

External jugular vein

Anterior jugular vein

Jugular venous arch
(in suprasternal space)

Pretracheal layer
of cervical fascia

b

Sternohyoid muscle

Sternothyroid muscle

Platysma

Cricoid cartilage

Omohyoid muscle

Sternocleidomastoid muscle

Cricopharyngeal part
of inferior constrictor muscle

Phrenic nerve

Anterior scalene muscle,
Longus colli muscle

Middle scalene muscle

Posterior scalene muscle

Vertebral artery

Multifidus cervicis muscle

Splenii capitis and cervicis muscles

Semispinales capitis and cervicis muscles

Cervical fascia
– Investing (= superficial) layer
– Pretracheal layer
– Prevertebral layer

Carotid sheath

Common carotid artery,
Internal jugular vein

Sympathetic trunk,
Vagus nerve [X]

6th cervical vertebra
– Anterior tubercle
– Transverse process
– Posterior tubercle

Levator scapulae muscle

Nuchal fascia

Trapezius muscle

Ligamentum nuchae
= Nuchal ligament

33 Cervical fascia

a Investing layer of the cervical fascia (45%), lateral aspect.
   Several fascial compartments were opened.
b Transverse section through the neck at the level of the sixth
   cervical vertebra (70%), schematic representation of the cervical
   fascia. The diverse laminae are indicated by different colors.

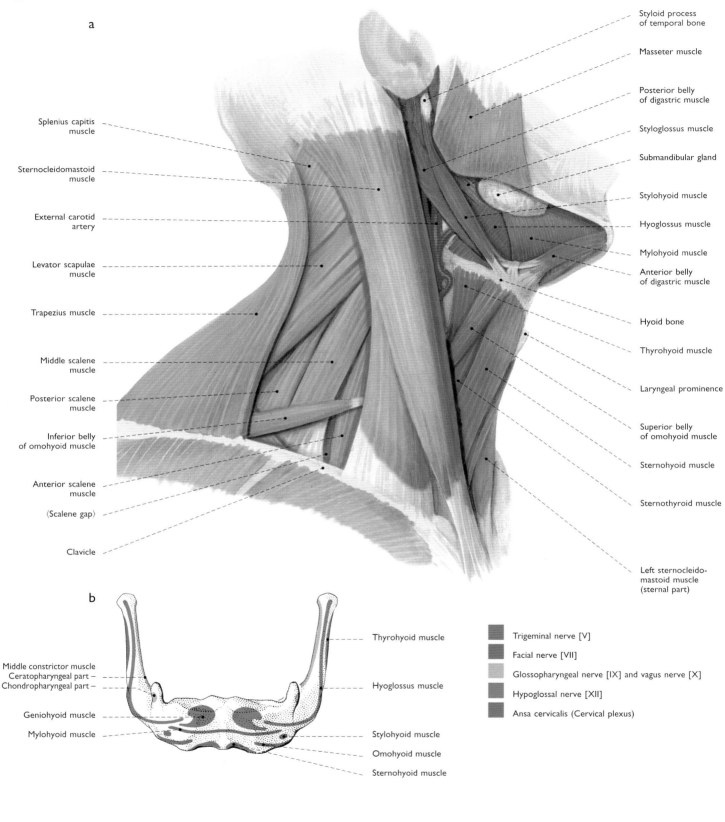

a

Styloid process
of temporal bone

Masseter muscle

Posterior belly
of digastric muscle

Styloglossus muscle

Submandibular gland

Stylohyoid muscle

Hyoglossus muscle

Mylohyoid muscle

Anterior belly
of digastric muscle

Hyoid bone

Thyrohyoid muscle

Laryngeal prominence

Superior belly
of omohyoid muscle

Sternohyoid muscle

Sternothyroid muscle

Left sternocleido-
mastoid muscle
(sternal part)

Splenius capitis
muscle

Sternocleidomastoid
muscle

External carotid
artery

Levator scapulae
muscle

Trapezius muscle

Middle scalene
muscle

Posterior scalene
muscle

Inferior belly
of omohyoid muscle

Anterior scalene
muscle

⟨Scalene gap⟩

Clavicle

b

Middle constrictor muscle
Ceratopharyngeal part –
Chondropharyngeal part –

Geniohyoid muscle

Mylohyoid muscle

Thyrohyoid muscle

Hyoglossus muscle

Stylohyoid muscle

Omohyoid muscle

Sternohyoid muscle

Trigeminal nerve [V]

Facial nerve [VII]

Glossopharyngeal nerve [IX] and vagus nerve [X]

Hypoglossal nerve [XII]

Ansa cervicalis (Cervical plexus)

34 Muscles of the neck
a The platysma and the cervical fascia were removed (60%).
Right lateral aspect
b Muscle attachments on the ventral and superior surfaces
of hyoid bone

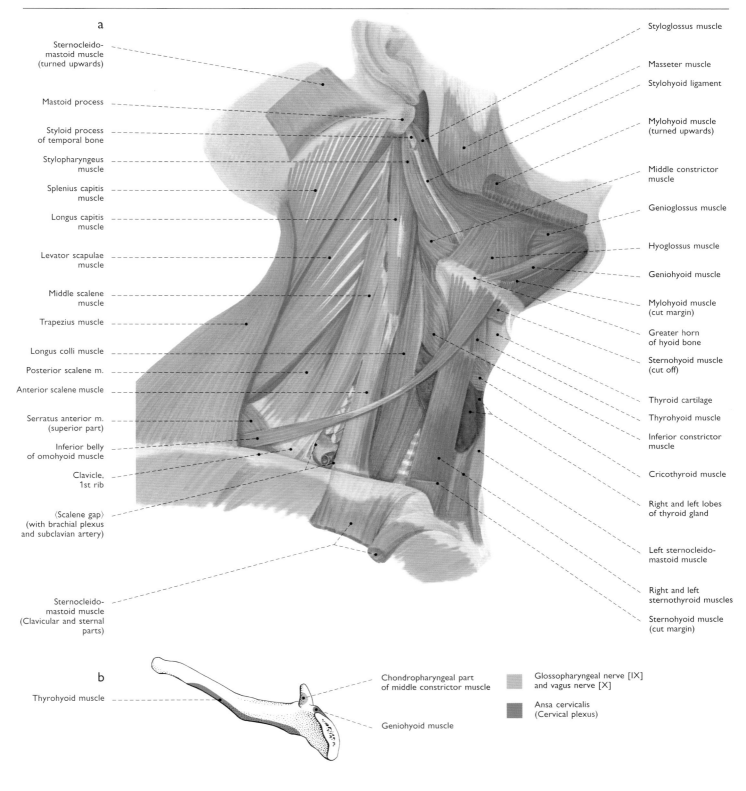

a

Sternocleido-mastoid muscle (turned upwards)

Mastoid process

Styloid process of temporal bone

Stylopharyngeus muscle

Splenius capitis muscle

Longus capitis muscle

Levator scapulae muscle

Middle scalene muscle

Trapezius muscle

Longus colli muscle

Posterior scalene m.

Anterior scalene muscle

Serratus anterior m. (superior part)

Inferior belly of omohyoid muscle

Clavicle, 1st rib

⟨Scalene gap⟩ (with brachial plexus and subclavian artery)

Sternocleido-mastoid muscle (Clavicular and sternal parts)

Styloglossus muscle

Masseter muscle

Stylohyoid ligament

Mylohyoid muscle (turned upwards)

Middle constrictor muscle

Genioglossus muscle

Hyoglossus muscle

Geniohyoid muscle

Mylohyoid muscle (cut margin)

Greater horn of hyoid bone

Sternohyoid muscle (cut off)

Thyroid cartilage

Thyrohyoid muscle

Inferior constrictor muscle

Cricothyroid muscle

Right and left lobes of thyroid gland

Left sternocleido-mastoid muscle

Right and left sternothyroid muscles

Sternohyoid muscle (cut margin)

b

Thyrohyoid muscle

Chondropharyngeal part of middle constrictor muscle

Geniohyoid muscle

Glossopharyngeal nerve [IX] and vagus nerve [X]

Ansa cervicalis (Cervical plexus)

35 Muscles of the neck

a In addition to the platysma and the cervical fascia, the sternocleidomastoid muscle was severed and partially removed (60%). Right lateral aspect

b Muscle attachments on the dorsal surface of hyoid bone

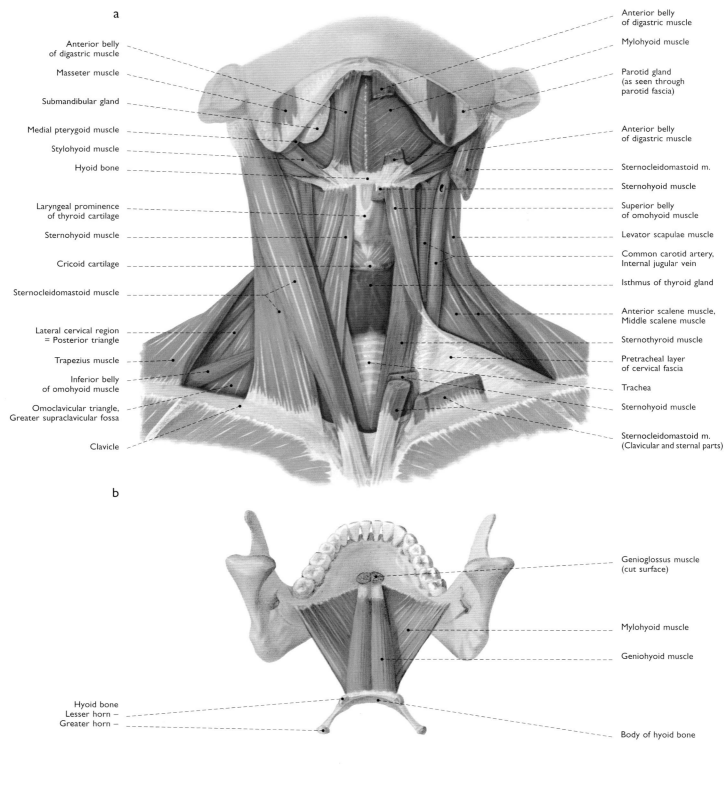

a

Anterior belly
of digastric muscle

Masseter muscle

Submandibular gland

Medial pterygoid muscle

Stylohyoid muscle

Hyoid bone

Laryngeal prominence
of thyroid cartilage

Sternohyoid muscle

Cricoid cartilage

Sternocleidomastoid muscle

Lateral cervical region
= Posterior triangle

Trapezius muscle

Inferior belly
of omohyoid muscle

Omoclavicular triangle,
Greater supraclavicular fossa

Clavicle

Anterior belly
of digastric muscle

Mylohyoid muscle

Parotid gland
(as seen through
parotid fascia)

Anterior belly
of digastric muscle

Sternocleidomastoid m.

Sternohyoid muscle

Superior belly
of omohyoid muscle

Levator scapulae muscle

Common carotid artery,
Internal jugular vein

Isthmus of thyroid gland

Anterior scalene muscle,
Middle scalene muscle

Sternothyroid muscle

Pretracheal layer
of cervical fascia

Trachea

Sternohyoid muscle

Sternocleidomastoid m.
(Clavicular and sternal parts)

b

Genioglossus muscle
(cut surface)

Mylohyoid muscle

Geniohyoid muscle

Hyoid bone
Lesser horn –
Greater horn –

Body of hyoid bone

36 Muscles of the neck
and suprahyoid muscles (60%)

a   On the right side of the body, the platysma was removed.
On the left side, parts of the sternocleidomastoid and
sternohyoid muscles were excised additionally.
Ventral aspect

b   Muscles of the floor of the oral cavity, occipital aspect

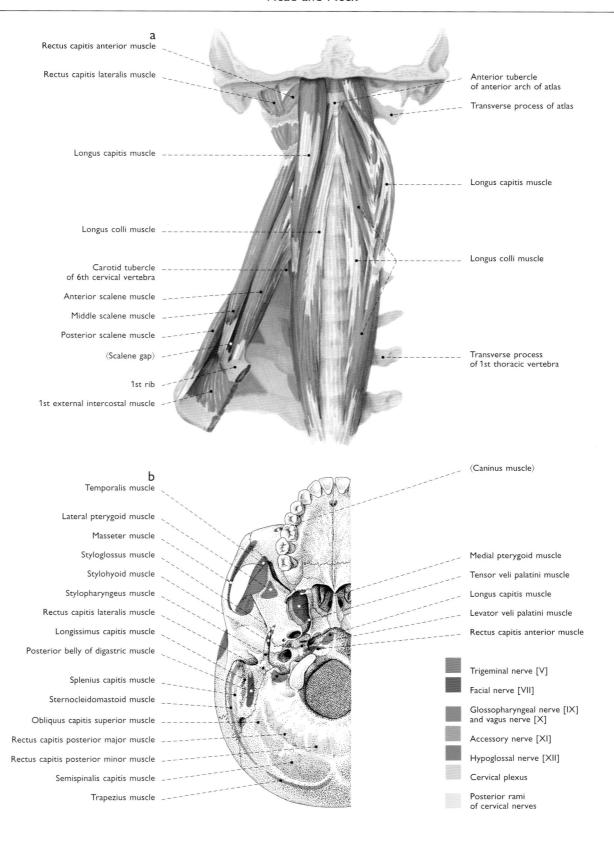

Rectus capitis anterior muscle

Rectus capitis lateralis muscle

Anterior tubercle
of anterior arch of atlas

Transverse process of atlas

Longus capitis muscle

Longus capitis muscle

Longus colli muscle

Longus colli muscle

Carotid tubercle
of 6th cervical vertebra

Anterior scalene muscle

Middle scalene muscle

Posterior scalene muscle

⟨Scalene gap⟩

Transverse process
of 1st thoracic vertebra

1st rib

1st external intercostal muscle

⟨Caninus muscle⟩

Temporalis muscle

Lateral pterygoid muscle

Masseter muscle

Styloglossus muscle

Stylohyoid muscle

Stylopharyngeus muscle

Rectus capitis lateralis muscle

Longissimus capitis muscle

Posterior belly of digastric muscle

Splenius capitis muscle

Sternocleidomastoid muscle

Obliquus capitis superior muscle

Rectus capitis posterior major muscle

Rectus capitis posterior minor muscle

Semispinalis capitis muscle

Trapezius muscle

Medial pterygoid muscle

Tensor veli palatini muscle

Longus capitis muscle

Levator veli palatini muscle

Rectus capitis anterior muscle

Trigeminal nerve [V]

Facial nerve [VII]

Glossopharyngeal nerve [IX]
and vagus nerve [X]

Accessory nerve [XI]

Hypoglossal nerve [XII]

Cervical plexus

Posterior rami
of cervical nerves

37 Muscles of the neck, face, and back

a Anterior and lateral vertebral muscles (55%), ventral aspect
b Muscle attachments on the external surface of cranial base

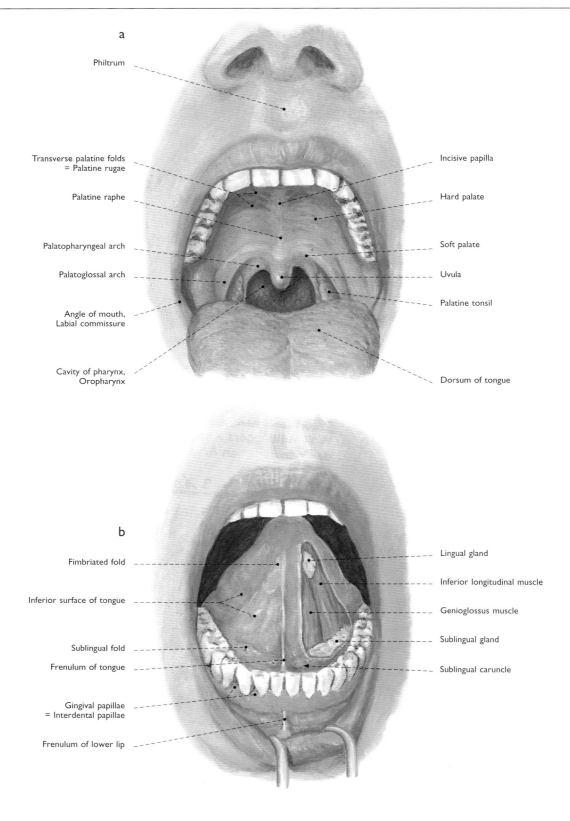

a

Philtrum

Transverse palatine folds
= Palatine rugae

Palatine raphe

Palatopharyngeal arch

Palatoglossal arch

Angle of mouth,
Labial commissure

Cavity of pharynx,
Oropharynx

Incisive papilla

Hard palate

Soft palate

Uvula

Palatine tonsil

Dorsum of tongue

b

Fimbriated fold

Inferior surface of tongue

Sublingual fold

Frenulum of tongue

Gingival papillae
= Interdental papillae

Frenulum of lower lip

Lingual gland

Inferior longitudinal muscle

Genioglossus muscle

Sublingual gland

Sublingual caruncle

38 Oral cavity (100%)

Frontal aspect

a The mouth is wide open and the tongue extended.
b The apex of tongue is turned upwards. Fenestration of the mucosa
on the left side exposes the tongue muscles and the glands.

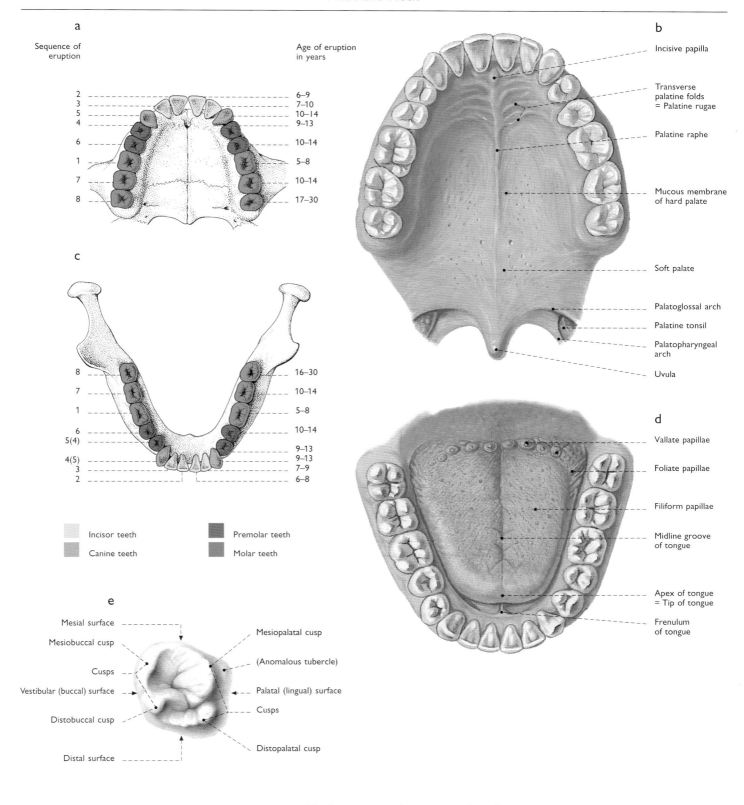

a

Sequence of eruption

Age of eruption in years

2	6–9
3	7–10
5	10–14
4	9–13
6	10–14
1	5–8
7	10–14
8	17–30

c

8	16–30
7	10–14
1	5–8
6	10–14
5(4)	9–13
4(5)	9–13
3	7–9
2	6–8

Incisor teeth
Canine teeth
Premolar teeth
Molar teeth

b

Incisive papilla
Transverse palatine folds = Palatine rugae
Palatine raphe
Mucous membrane of hard palate
Soft palate
Palatoglossal arch
Palatine tonsil
Palatopharyngeal arch
Uvula

d

Vallate papillae
Foliate papillae
Filiform papillae
Midline groove of tongue
Apex of tongue = Tip of tongue
Frenulum of tongue

e

Mesial surface
Mesiobuccal cusp
Cusps
Vestibular (buccal) surface
Distobuccal cusp
Distal surface
Mesiopalatal cusp
(Anomalous tubercle)
Palatal (lingual) surface
Cusps
Distopalatal cusp

39 Permanent dentition and oral cavity

a, c Permanent teeth
  a Upper jaw, inferior aspect
  c Lower jaw, superior aspect
b, d Oral cavity proper (100%)
  b Roof of the oral cavity proper, inferior aspect
  d Floor of the oral cavity proper, superior aspect
  e Occlusal surface of the first upper molar (400%)

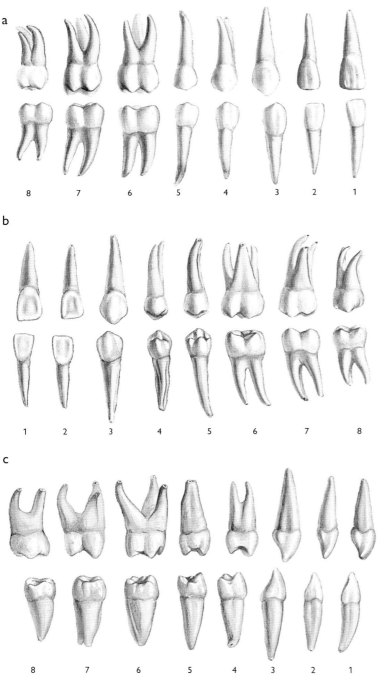

a

8   7   6   5   4   3   2   1

b

1   2   3   4   5   6   7   8

c

8   7   6   5   4   3   2   1

d

Enamel
Dentine
Odontoblast layer
Gingiva = Gum, Gingival margin
Pulp cavity, Dental pulp
Cement
Periodontium
Root canal
Apical foramen
Root apex

Clinical crown
Crown
Neck = Cervix
Clinical root
Root
Mandible

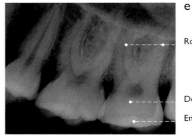

e

Roots
Dentine
Enamel

f

Enamel
Dentine
Neck = Cervix
Root canal = Pulp canal
Root apex

1 Medial upper and lower incisor teeth
2 Lateral upper and lower incisor teeth
3 Upper and lower canine teeth
4 Upper and lower 1st premolar teeth

5 Upper and lower 2nd premolar teeth
6 Upper and lower 1st molar teeth
7 Upper and lower 2nd molar teeth
8 Upper and lower 3rd molar teeth
   = Upper and lower wisdom teeth

40 Permanent teeth

a–c Teeth of the upper and lower jaws (90%)
  a Vestibular surface (labial and buccal surfaces)
  b Palatal surface (lingual surface)
  c Distal surface
  d Lower incisor tooth in situ (400%),
     lateral cut surface, schematized sagittal section
e, f Lateral radiographs of the first two molars (140%)
  e in the upper jaw
  f in the lower jaw

a

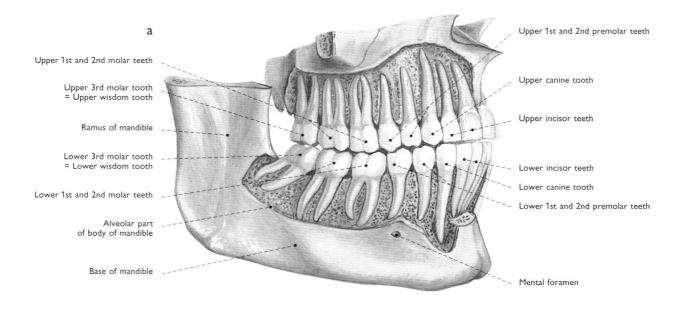

Upper 1st and 2nd molar teeth

Upper 3rd molar tooth = Upper wisdom tooth

Ramus of mandible

Lower 3rd molar tooth = Lower wisdom tooth

Lower 1st and 2nd molar teeth

Alveolar part of body of mandible

Base of mandible

Upper 1st and 2nd premolar teeth

Upper canine tooth

Upper incisor teeth

Lower incisor teeth

Lower canine tooth

Lower 1st and 2nd premolar teeth

Mental foramen

b

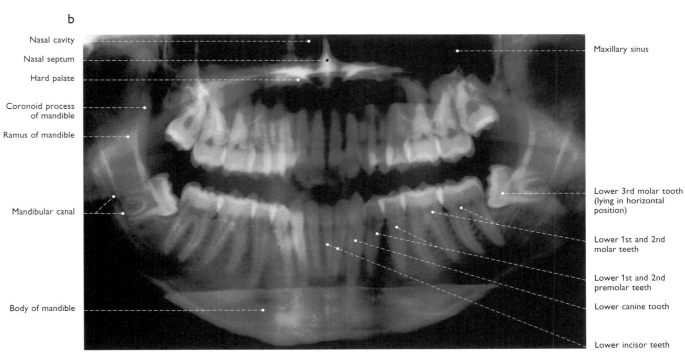

Nasal cavity

Nasal septum

Hard palate

Coronoid process of mandible

Ramus of mandible

Mandibular canal

Body of mandible

Maxillary sinus

Lower 3rd molar tooth (lying in horizontal position)

Lower 1st and 2nd molar teeth

Lower 1st and 2nd premolar teeth

Lower canine tooth

Lower incisor teeth

41 Permanent teeth (90%)

a Teeth of the upper and lower jaws, right lateral aspect. The vestibular roots were exposed by removal of the external alveolar walls.

b Panoral radiograph of the whole dentition of the upper and lower jaws of an adult. As a variation, one of the lower incisor teeth is missing.

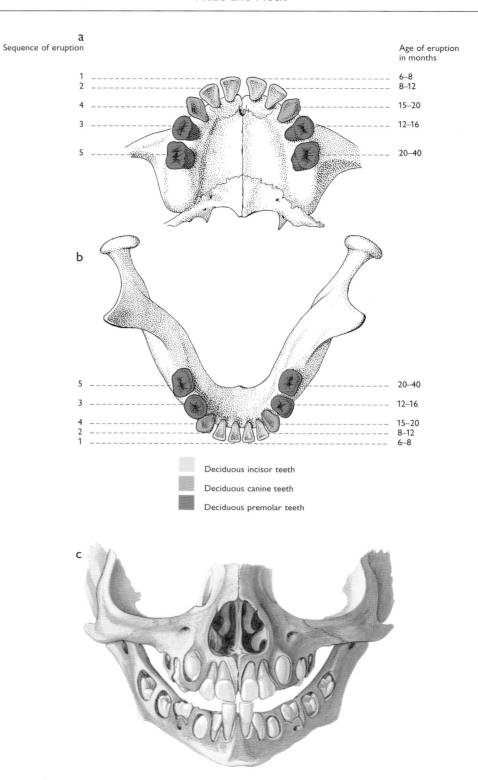

a   Sequence of eruption

Age of eruption
in months

1	6–8
2	8–12
4	15–20
3	12–16
5	20–40

b

5	20–40
3	12–16
4	15–20
2	8–12
1	6–8

Deciduous incisor teeth

Deciduous canine teeth

Deciduous premolar teeth

c

42   Deciduous dentition

a   Upper jaw, inferior aspect
b   Lower jaw, superior aspect
c   Partially erupted deciduous dentition
    of a 1-year-old child (100%), frontal aspect

a

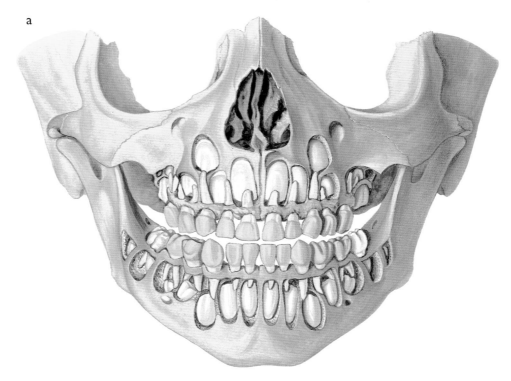

b

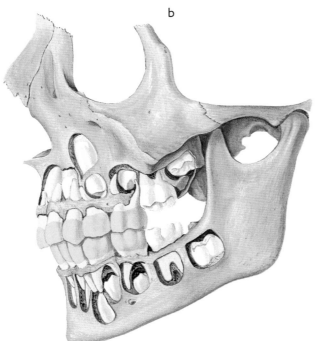

c

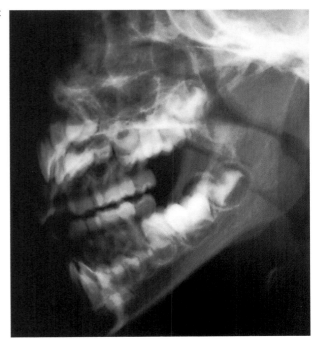

**43 Deciduous dentition and precursors
of the permanent teeth of a 5¹/₂-year-old boy** (100%)
The first molar (the 6th-year molar) has erupted in the lower jaw,
and is erupting in the upper jaw.
a Frontal aspect
b Left lateral aspect
c Lateral radiograph

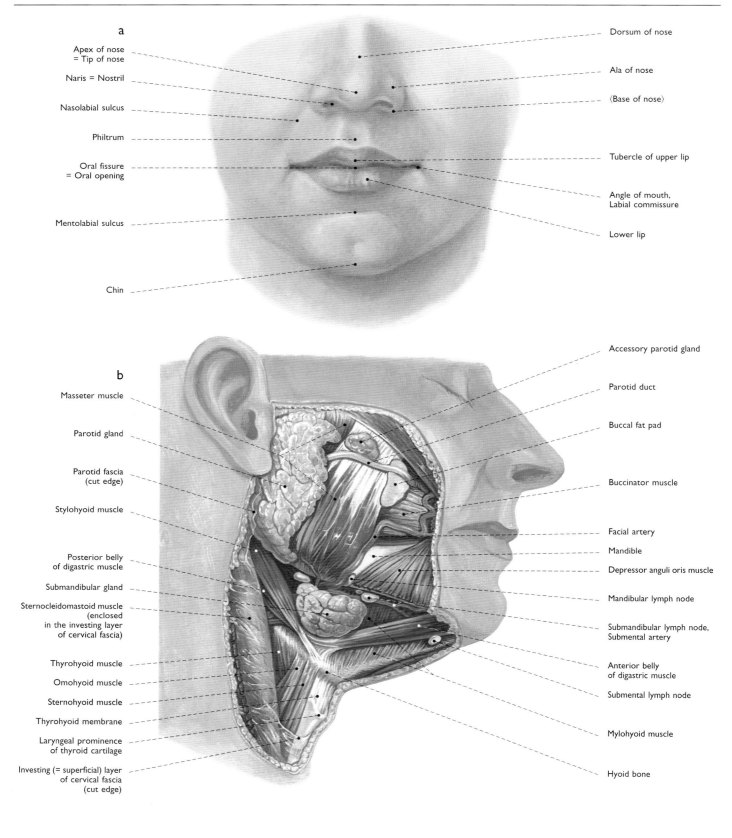

a

Apex of nose = Tip of nose

Naris = Nostril

Nasolabial sulcus

Philtrum

Oral fissure = Oral opening

Mentolabial sulcus

Chin

Dorsum of nose

Ala of nose

⟨Base of nose⟩

Tubercle of upper lip

Angle of mouth, Labial commissure

Lower lip

b

Masseter muscle

Parotid gland

Parotid fascia (cut edge)

Stylohyoid muscle

Posterior belly of digastric muscle

Submandibular gland

Sternocleidomastoid muscle (enclosed in the investing layer of cervical fascia)

Thyrohyoid muscle

Omohyoid muscle

Sternohyoid muscle

Thyrohyoid membrane

Laryngeal prominence of thyroid cartilage

Investing (= superficial) layer of cervical fascia (cut edge)

Accessory parotid gland

Parotid duct

Buccal fat pad

Buccinator muscle

Facial artery

Mandible

Depressor anguli oris muscle

Mandibular lymph node

Submandibular lymph node, Submental artery

Anterior belly of digastric muscle

Submental lymph node

Mylohyoid muscle

Hyoid bone

44 Lower part of the face, parotid and submandibular glands (70%)
a   Lower part of the face, frontal aspect
b   Parotid and submandibular glands, right lateral aspect

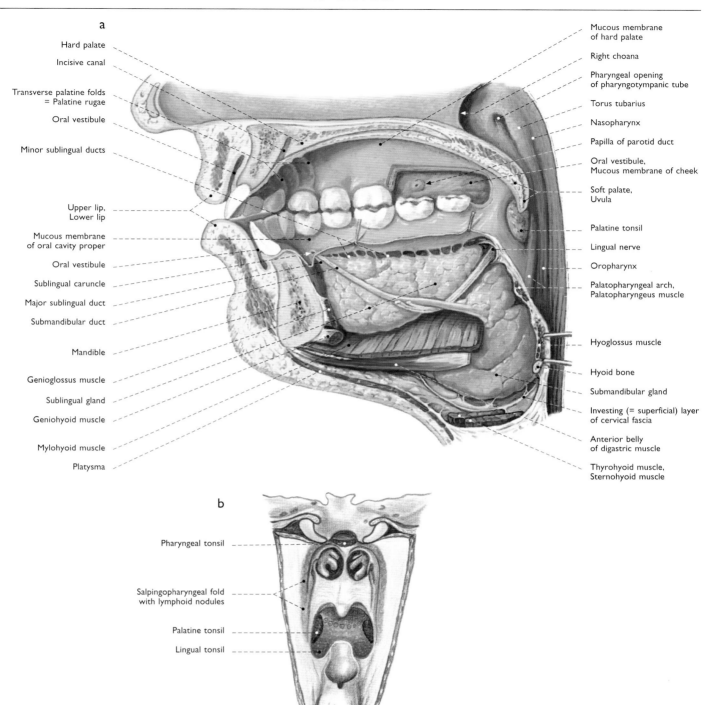

a

Hard palate

Incisive canal

Transverse palatine folds
= Palatine rugae

Oral vestibule

Minor sublingual ducts

Upper lip,
Lower lip

Mucous membrane
of oral cavity proper

Oral vestibule

Sublingual caruncle

Major sublingual duct

Submandibular duct

Mandible

Genioglossus muscle

Sublingual gland

Geniohyoid muscle

Mylohyoid muscle

Platysma

Mucous membrane
of hard palate

Right choana

Pharyngeal opening
of pharyngotympanic tube

Torus tubarius

Nasopharynx

Papilla of parotid duct

Oral vestibule,
Mucous membrane of cheek

Soft palate,
Uvula

Palatine tonsil

Lingual nerve

Oropharynx

Palatopharyngeal arch,
Palatopharyngeus muscle

Hyoglossus muscle

Hyoid bone

Submandibular gland

Investing (= superficial) layer
of cervical fascia

Anterior belly
of digastric muscle

Thyrohyoid muscle,
Sternohyoid muscle

b

Pharyngeal tonsil

Salpingopharyngeal fold
with lymphoid nodules

Palatine tonsil

Lingual tonsil

45　Parotid, submandibular, and sublingual glands

a　Medial aspect of the right half of a head, bisected in the median
plane (100%). A window was cut into the posterior part
of the lateral wall of the palate in order to demonstrate
the papilla of the parotid duct. The ventrolateral wall
of the pharynx together with the posterior part of the hyoid bone
are retracted dorsomedially with hooks in order to expose
the submandibular and sublingual glands.

b　Pharyngeal lymphoid ring (Waldeyer's ring), consisting of the lingual,
palatine, and pharyngeal tonsils and minor lymphoid masses,
dorsal aspect

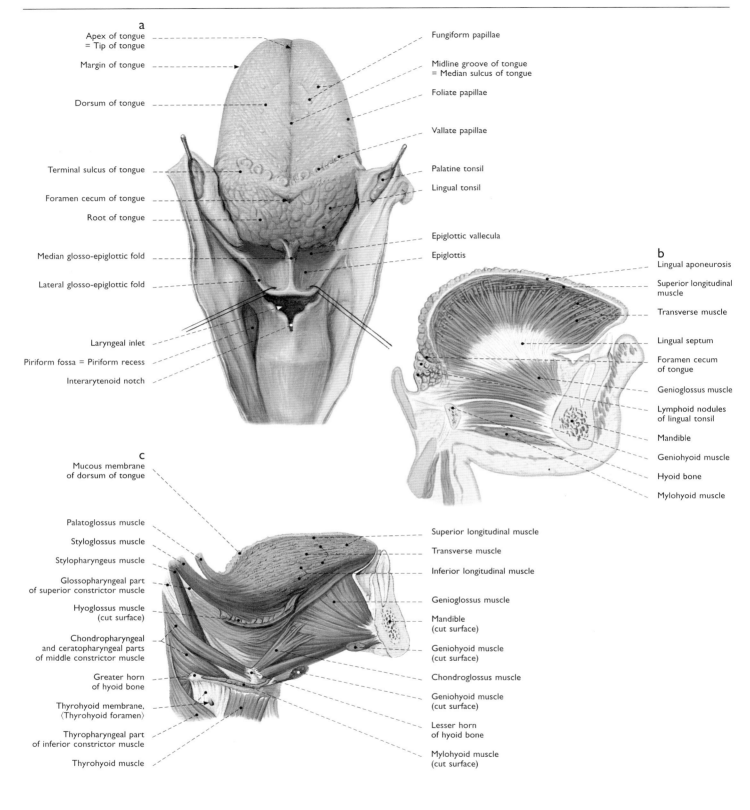

a

Apex of tongue = Tip of tongue

Margin of tongue

Dorsum of tongue

Terminal sulcus of tongue

Foramen cecum of tongue

Root of tongue

Median glosso-epiglottic fold

Lateral glosso-epiglottic fold

Laryngeal inlet

Piriform fossa = Piriform recess

Interarytenoid notch

Fungiform papillae

Midline groove of tongue = Median sulcus of tongue

Foliate papillae

Vallate papillae

Palatine tonsil

Lingual tonsil

Epiglottic vallecula

Epiglottis

b

Lingual aponeurosis

Superior longitudinal muscle

Transverse muscle

Lingual septum

Foramen cecum of tongue

Genioglossus muscle

Lymphoid nodules of lingual tonsil

Mandible

Geniohyoid muscle

Hyoid bone

Mylohyoid muscle

c

Mucous membrane of dorsum of tongue

Palatoglossus muscle

Styloglossus muscle

Stylopharyngeus muscle

Glossopharyngeal part of superior constrictor muscle

Hyoglossus muscle (cut surface)

Chondropharyngeal and ceratopharyngeal parts of middle constrictor muscle

Greater horn of hyoid bone

Thyrohyoid membrane, ⟨Thyrohyoid foramen⟩

Thyropharyngeal part of inferior constrictor muscle

Thyrohyoid muscle

Superior longitudinal muscle

Transverse muscle

Inferior longitudinal muscle

Genioglossus muscle

Mandible (cut surface)

Geniohyoid muscle (cut surface)

Chondroglossus muscle

Geniohyoid muscle (cut surface)

Lesser horn of hyoid bone

Mylohyoid muscle (cut surface)

46 Dorsum and muscles of the tongue (70%)

a Dorsal aspect of the tongue and the ventral wall of pharynx, opened along the mid-dorsal line

b Medial aspect of the tongue sectioned in the sagittal plane

c Lateral aspect of the tongue after removal of the mucous membrane and the lingual aponeurosis

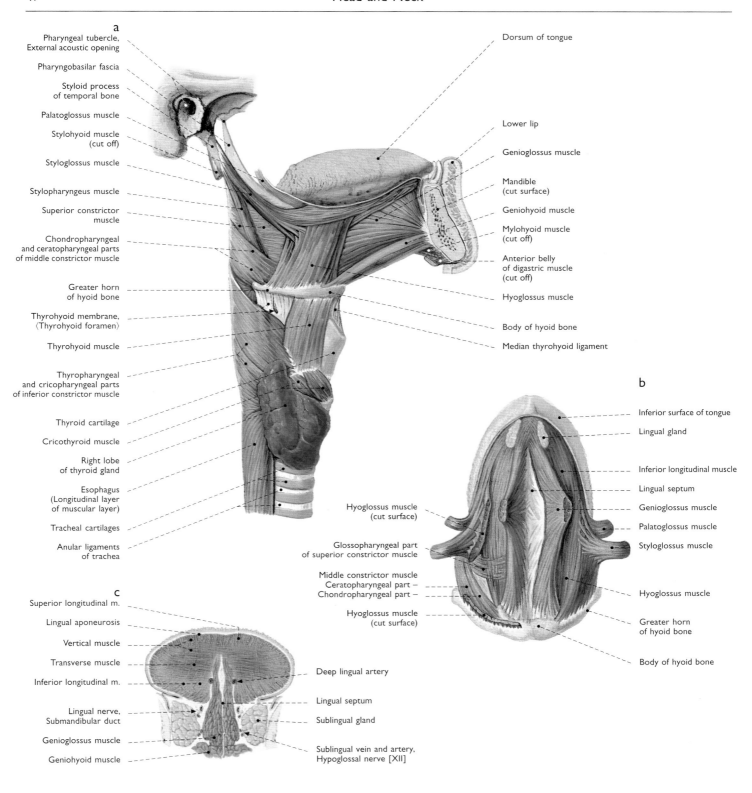

a

Pharyngeal tubercle, External acoustic opening

Pharyngobasilar fascia

Styloid process of temporal bone

Palatoglossus muscle

Stylohyoid muscle (cut off)

Styloglossus muscle

Stylopharyngeus muscle

Superior constrictor muscle

Chondropharyngeal and ceratopharyngeal parts of middle constrictor muscle

Greater horn of hyoid bone

Thyrohyoid membrane, (Thyrohyoid foramen)

Thyrohyoid muscle

Thyropharyngeal and cricopharyngeal parts of inferior constrictor muscle

Thyroid cartilage

Cricothyroid muscle

Right lobe of thyroid gland

Esophagus (Longitudinal layer of muscular layer)

Tracheal cartilages

Anular ligaments of trachea

Dorsum of tongue

Lower lip

Genioglossus muscle

Mandible (cut surface)

Geniohyoid muscle

Mylohyoid muscle (cut off)

Anterior belly of digastric muscle (cut off)

Hyoglossus muscle

Body of hyoid bone

Median thyrohyoid ligament

b

Inferior surface of tongue

Lingual gland

Inferior longitudinal muscle

Lingual septum

Genioglossus muscle

Palatoglossus muscle

Styloglossus muscle

Hyoglossus muscle

Greater horn of hyoid bone

Body of hyoid bone

Hyoglossus muscle (cut surface)

Glossopharyngeal part of superior constrictor muscle

Middle constrictor muscle
Ceratopharyngeal part —
Chondropharyngeal part —

Hyoglossus muscle (cut surface)

c

Superior longitudinal m.

Lingual aponeurosis

Vertical muscle

Transverse muscle

Inferior longitudinal m.

Lingual nerve, Submandibular duct

Genioglossus muscle

Geniohyoid muscle

Deep lingual artery

Lingual septum

Sublingual gland

Sublingual vein and artery, Hypoglossal nerve [XII]

47 Muscles of the tongue, pharynx, and larynx (70%)

a Tongue, mouth floor, and neck, lateral aspect
b The tongue attached to the hyoid bone, inferior aspect
c The tongue and the sublingual region, coronal section

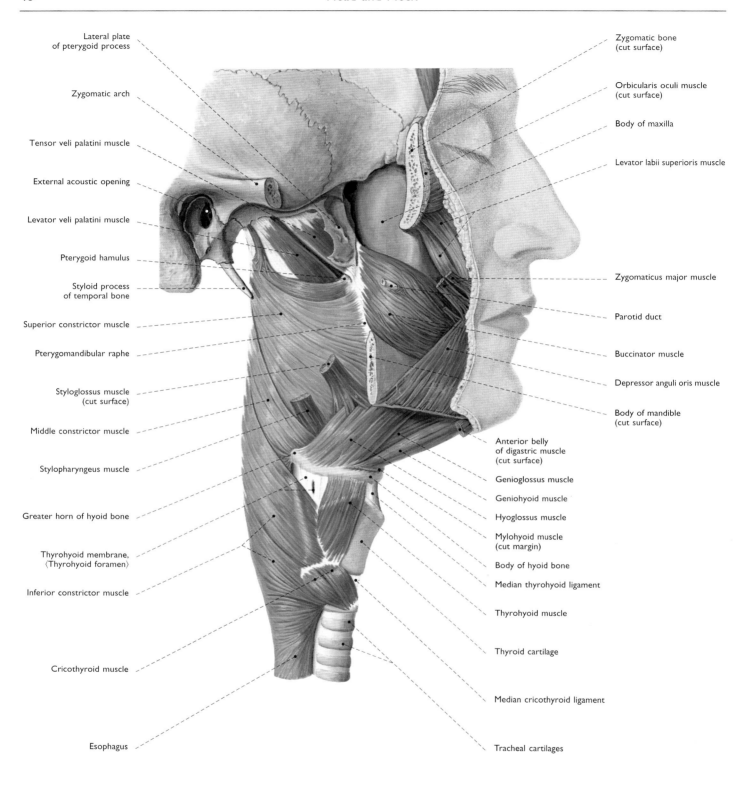

Lateral plate
of pterygoid process

Zygomatic arch

Tensor veli palatini muscle

External acoustic opening

Levator veli palatini muscle

Pterygoid hamulus

Styloid process
of temporal bone

Superior constrictor muscle

Pterygomandibular raphe

Styloglossus muscle
(cut surface)

Middle constrictor muscle

Stylopharyngeus muscle

Greater horn of hyoid bone

Thyrohyoid membrane,
⟨Thyrohyoid foramen⟩

Inferior constrictor muscle

Cricothyroid muscle

Esophagus

Zygomatic bone
(cut surface)

Orbicularis oculi muscle
(cut surface)

Body of maxilla

Levator labii superioris muscle

Zygomaticus major muscle

Parotid duct

Buccinator muscle

Depressor anguli oris muscle

Body of mandible
(cut surface)

Anterior belly
of digastric muscle
(cut surface)

Genioglossus muscle

Geniohyoid muscle

Hyoglossus muscle

Mylohyoid muscle
(cut margin)

Body of hyoid bone

Median thyrohyoid ligament

Thyrohyoid muscle

Thyroid cartilage

Median cricothyroid ligament

Tracheal cartilages

48 Muscles of the pharynx (75%)
Right lateral aspect

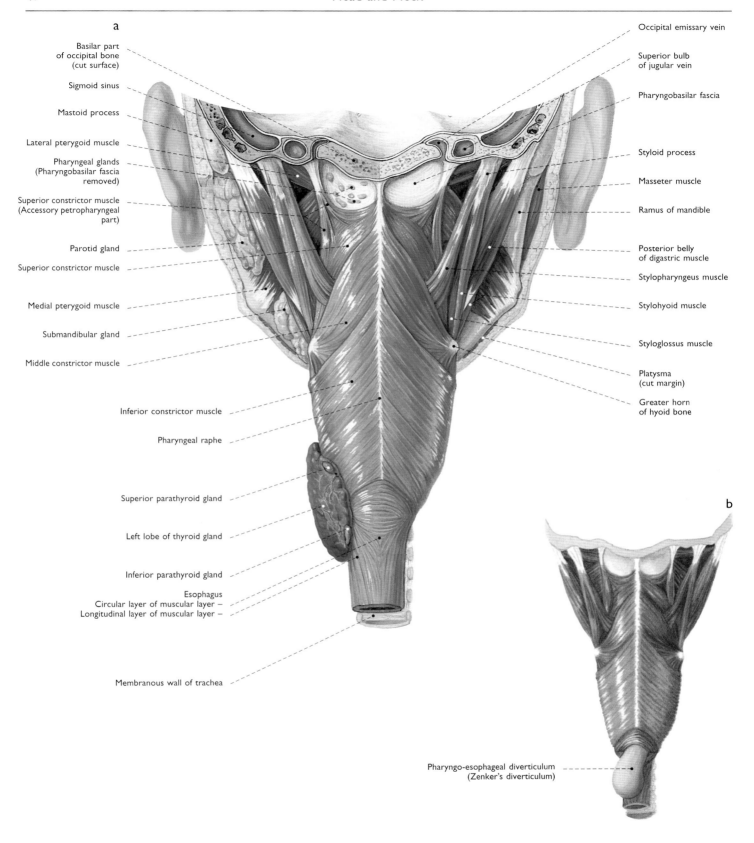

a

Basilar part
of occipital bone
(cut surface)

Sigmoid sinus

Mastoid process

Lateral pterygoid muscle

Pharyngeal glands
(Pharyngobasilar fascia
removed)

Superior constrictor muscle
(Accessory petropharyngeal
part)

Parotid gland

Superior constrictor muscle

Medial pterygoid muscle

Submandibular gland

Middle constrictor muscle

Inferior constrictor muscle

Pharyngeal raphe

Superior parathyroid gland

Left lobe of thyroid gland

Inferior parathyroid gland

Esophagus
Circular layer of muscular layer –
Longitudinal layer of muscular layer –

Membranous wall of trachea

Occipital emissary vein

Superior bulb
of jugular vein

Pharyngobasilar fascia

Styloid process

Masseter muscle

Ramus of mandible

Posterior belly
of digastric muscle

Stylopharyngeus muscle

Stylohyoid muscle

Styloglossus muscle

Platysma
(cut margin)

Greater horn
of hyoid bone

b

Pharyngo-esophageal diverticulum
(Zenker's diverticulum)

49   Muscles of the pharynx

a   Dorsal aspect (70%)
b   Representation of a pharyngeal diverticulum
in the Laimer's triangle, dorsal aspect

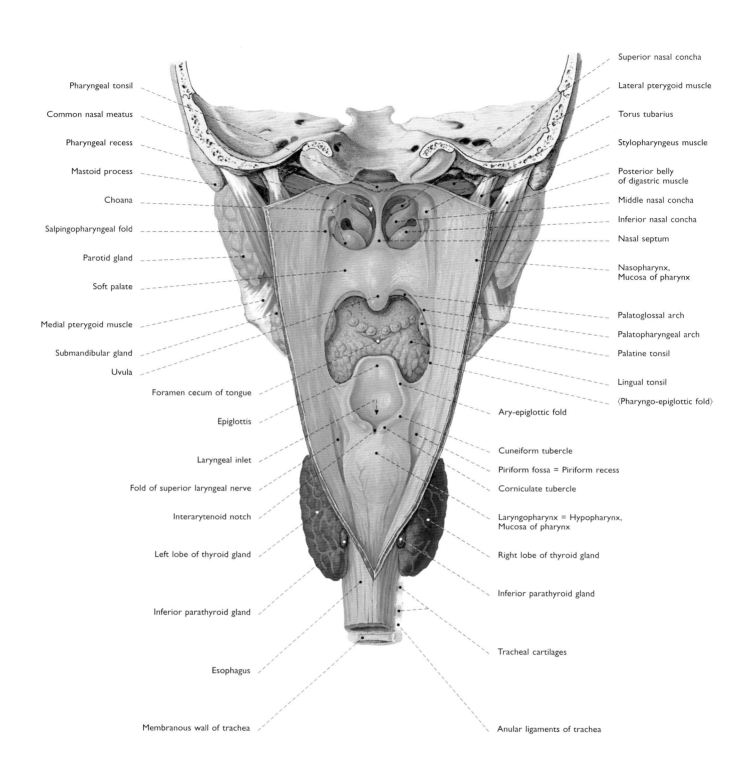

Pharyngeal tonsil

Common nasal meatus

Pharyngeal recess

Mastoid process

Choana

Salpingopharyngeal fold

Parotid gland

Soft palate

Medial pterygoid muscle

Submandibular gland

Uvula

Foramen cecum of tongue

Epiglottis

Laryngeal inlet

Fold of superior laryngeal nerve

Interarytenoid notch

Left lobe of thyroid gland

Inferior parathyroid gland

Esophagus

Membranous wall of trachea

Superior nasal concha

Lateral pterygoid muscle

Torus tubarius

Stylopharyngeus muscle

Posterior belly
of digastric muscle

Middle nasal concha

Inferior nasal concha

Nasal septum

Nasopharynx,
Mucosa of pharynx

Palatoglossal arch

Palatopharyngeal arch

Palatine tonsil

Lingual tonsil

⟨Pharyngo-epiglottic fold⟩

Ary-epiglottic fold

Cuneiform tubercle

Piriform fossa = Piriform recess

Corniculate tubercle

Laryngopharynx = Hypopharynx,
Mucosa of pharynx

Right lobe of thyroid gland

Inferior parathyroid gland

Tracheal cartilages

Anular ligaments of trachea

50 Cavity of the pharynx (70%)
The dorsal wall of the pharynx was cut along
the mid-dorsal line and opened. Dorsal aspect

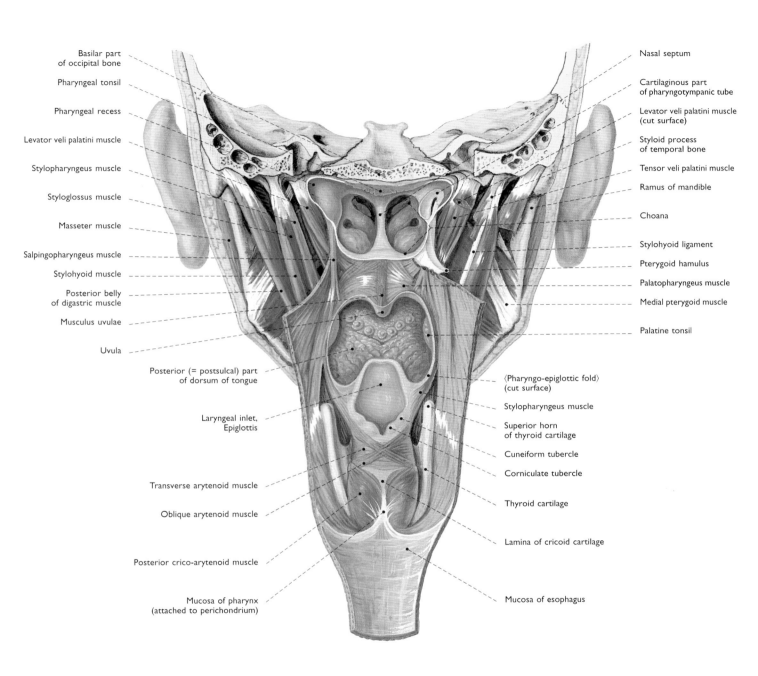

Basilar part
of occipital bone

Pharyngeal tonsil

Pharyngeal recess

Levator veli palatini muscle

Stylopharyngeus muscle

Styloglossus muscle

Masseter muscle

Salpingopharyngeus muscle

Stylohyoid muscle

Posterior belly
of digastric muscle

Musculus uvulae

Uvula

Posterior (= postsulcal) part
of dorsum of tongue

Laryngeal inlet,
Epiglottis

Transverse arytenoid muscle

Oblique arytenoid muscle

Posterior crico-arytenoid muscle

Mucosa of pharynx
(attached to perichondrium)

Nasal septum

Cartilaginous part
of pharyngotympanic tube

Levator veli palatini muscle
(cut surface)

Styloid process
of temporal bone

Tensor veli palatini muscle

Ramus of mandible

Choana

Stylohyoid ligament

Pterygoid hamulus

Palatopharyngeus muscle

Medial pterygoid muscle

Palatine tonsil

⟨Pharyngo-epiglottic fold⟩
(cut surface)

Stylopharyngeus muscle

Superior horn
of thyroid cartilage

Cuneiform tubercle

Corniculate tubercle

Thyroid cartilage

Lamina of cricoid cartilage

Mucosa of esophagus

51 Cavity of the pharynx (70%)
The dorsal wall of the pharynx was cut along the mid-dorsal line
and opened. The mucous membrane and the superior constrictor
muscle were partially removed in order to expose the different muscles.
Dorsal aspect

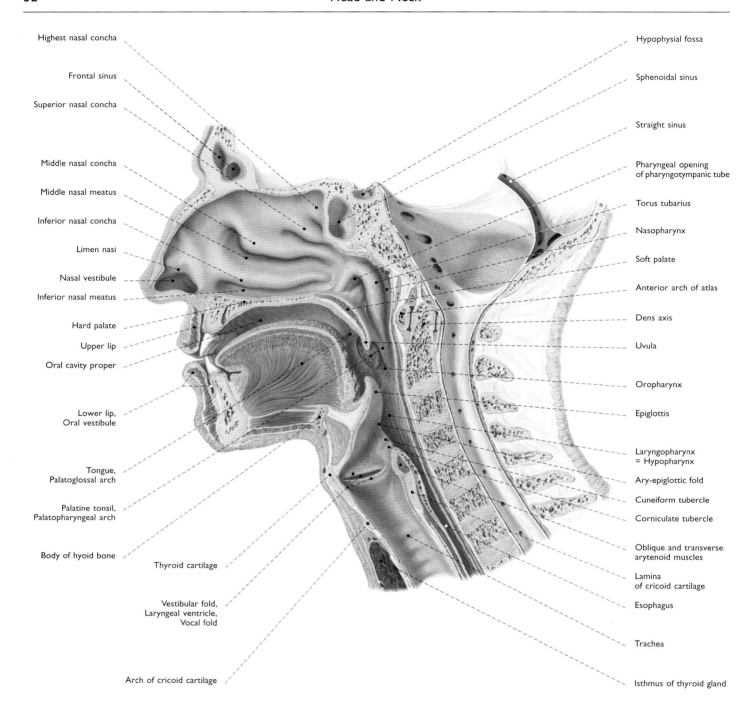

Highest nasal concha

Frontal sinus

Superior nasal concha

Middle nasal concha

Middle nasal meatus

Inferior nasal concha

Limen nasi

Nasal vestibule

Inferior nasal meatus

Hard palate

Upper lip

Oral cavity proper

Lower lip, Oral vestibule

Tongue, Palatoglossal arch

Palatine tonsil, Palatopharyngeal arch

Body of hyoid bone

Thyroid cartilage

Vestibular fold, Laryngeal ventricle, Vocal fold

Arch of cricoid cartilage

Hypophysial fossa

Sphenoidal sinus

Straight sinus

Pharyngeal opening of pharyngotympanic tube

Torus tubarius

Nasopharynx

Soft palate

Anterior arch of atlas

Dens axis

Uvula

Oropharynx

Epiglottis

Laryngopharynx = Hypopharynx

Ary-epiglottic fold

Cuneiform tubercle

Corniculate tubercle

Oblique and transverse arytenoid muscles

Lamina of cricoid cartilage

Esophagus

Trachea

Isthmus of thyroid gland

52 Alimentary and respiratory systems in the head and neck (70%)

Median sagittal section through the head and neck, medial aspect of the right half

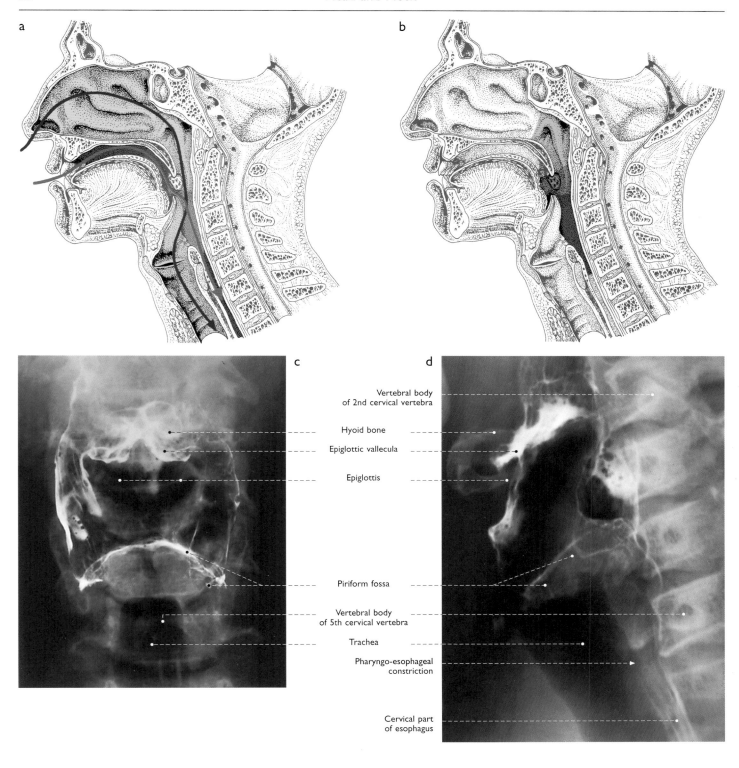

Vertebral body
of 2nd cervical vertebra

Hyoid bone

Epiglottic vallecula

Epiglottis

Piriform fossa

Vertebral body
of 5th cervical vertebra

Trachea

Pharyngo-esophageal
constriction

Cervical part
of esophagus

53 Alimentary and respiratory systems in the head and neck

a, b Midsagittal sections through the head and neck
  a Crossing of the alimentary and respiratory systems in the pharynx
  b Nasopharynx, oropharynx, and laryngopharynx = hypopharynx,
    shown by different colors
c, d Radiographs of the pharynx after oral application of contrast medium
  c Postero-anterior radiograph
  d Lateral radiograph

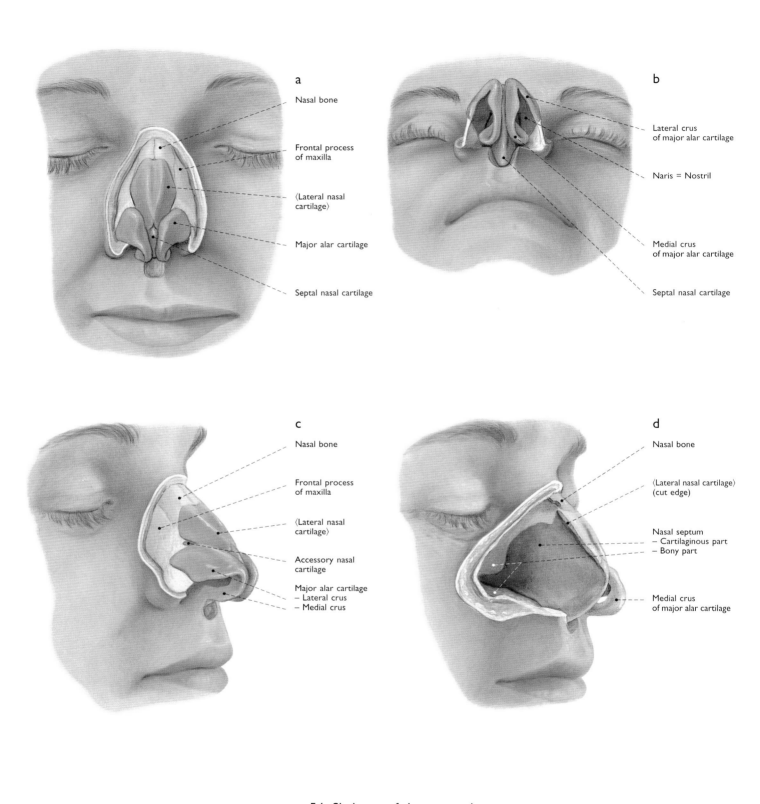

a
Nasal bone

Frontal process
of maxilla

⟨Lateral nasal
cartilage⟩

Major alar cartilage

Septal nasal cartilage

b
Lateral crus
of major alar cartilage

Naris = Nostril

Medial crus
of major alar cartilage

Septal nasal cartilage

c
Nasal bone

Frontal process
of maxilla

⟨Lateral nasal
cartilage⟩

Accessory nasal
cartilage

Major alar cartilage
– Lateral crus
– Medial crus

d
Nasal bone

⟨Lateral nasal cartilage⟩
(cut edge)

Nasal septum
– Cartilaginous part
– Bony part

Medial crus
of major alar cartilage

54 Skeleton of the external nose (80%)

a   Frontal aspect
b   Inferior aspect
c   Lateral aspect
d   The nasal septum. The right lateral wall
    of the external nose was removed. Lateral aspect

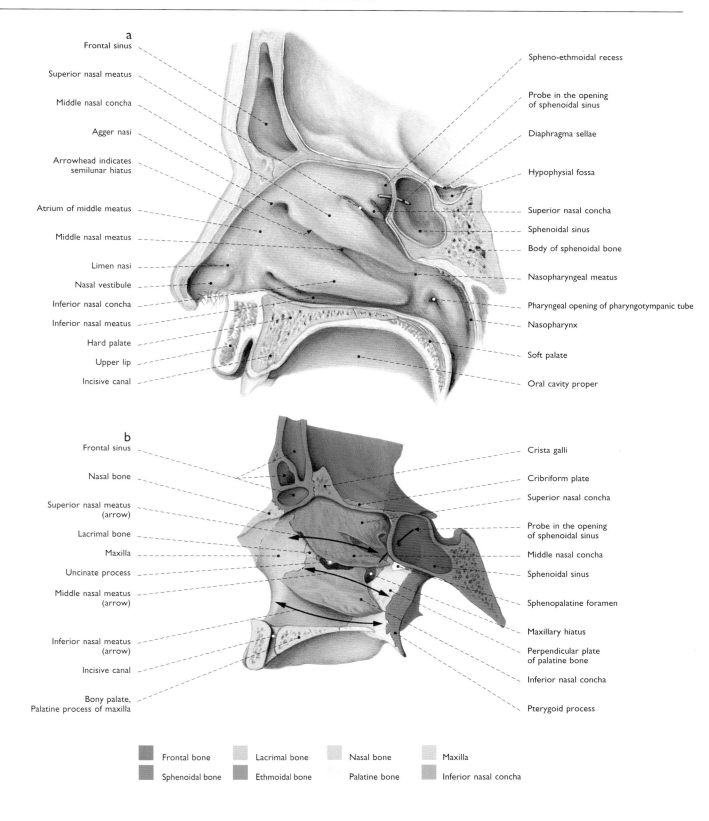

a

Frontal sinus
Superior nasal meatus
Middle nasal concha
Agger nasi
Arrowhead indicates semilunar hiatus
Atrium of middle meatus
Middle nasal meatus
Limen nasi
Nasal vestibule
Inferior nasal concha
Inferior nasal meatus
Hard palate
Upper lip
Incisive canal

Spheno-ethmoidal recess
Probe in the opening of sphenoidal sinus
Diaphragma sellae
Hypophysial fossa
Superior nasal concha
Sphenoidal sinus
Body of sphenoidal bone
Nasopharyngeal meatus
Pharyngeal opening of pharyngotympanic tube
Nasopharynx
Soft palate
Oral cavity proper

b

Frontal sinus
Nasal bone
Superior nasal meatus (arrow)
Lacrimal bone
Maxilla
Uncinate process
Middle nasal meatus (arrow)
Inferior nasal meatus (arrow)
Incisive canal
Bony palate, Palatine process of maxilla

Crista galli
Cribriform plate
Superior nasal concha
Probe in the opening of sphenoidal sinus
Middle nasal concha
Sphenoidal sinus
Sphenopalatine foramen
Maxillary hiatus
Perpendicular plate of palatine bone
Inferior nasal concha
Pterygoid process

Frontal bone   Lacrimal bone   Nasal bone   Maxilla
Sphenoidal bone   Ethmoidal bone   Palatine bone   Inferior nasal concha

55 Lateral wall of the nasal cavity (75%)
Paramedian section to the right of the nasal septum, medial aspect
a Nasal vestibule and mucosa of nasal cavity
b Bony lateral wall of the nasal cavity.
The individual bones are indicated by different colors.

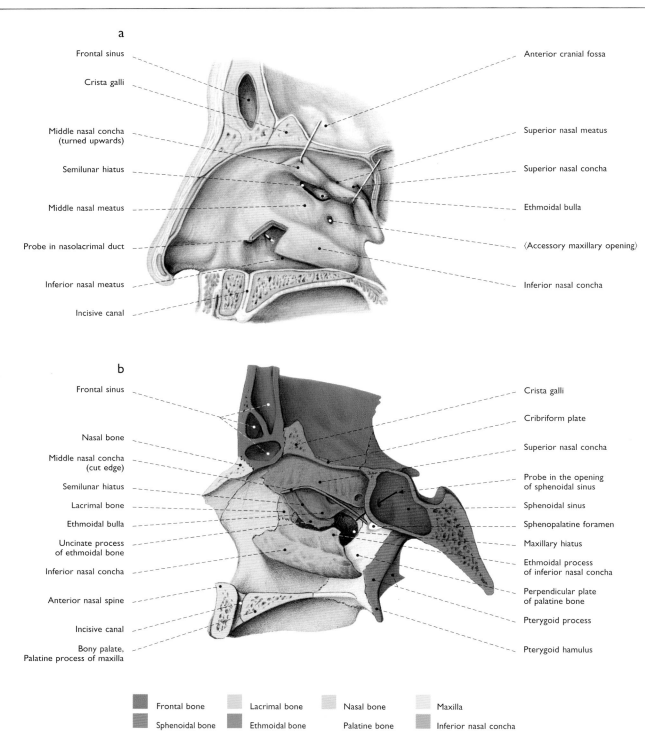

a

Frontal sinus

Crista galli

Middle nasal concha
(turned upwards)

Semilunar hiatus

Middle nasal meatus

Probe in nasolacrimal duct

Inferior nasal meatus

Incisive canal

Anterior cranial fossa

Superior nasal meatus

Superior nasal concha

Ethmoidal bulla

⟨Accessory maxillary opening⟩

Inferior nasal concha

b

Frontal sinus

Nasal bone

Middle nasal concha
(cut edge)

Semilunar hiatus

Lacrimal bone

Ethmoidal bulla

Uncinate process
of ethmoidal bone

Inferior nasal concha

Anterior nasal spine

Incisive canal

Bony palate,
Palatine process of maxilla

Crista galli

Cribriform plate

Superior nasal concha

Probe in the opening
of sphenoidal sinus

Sphenoidal sinus

Sphenopalatine foramen

Maxillary hiatus

Ethmoidal process
of inferior nasal concha

Perpendicular plate
of palatine bone

Pterygoid process

Pterygoid hamulus

Frontal bone	Lacrimal bone	Nasal bone	Maxilla
Sphenoidal bone	Ethmoidal bone	Palatine bone	Inferior nasal concha

56 Lateral wall of the nasal cavity (75%)

Paramedian section to the right of the nasal septum, medial aspect
a Nasal vestibule and mucosa of nasal cavity.
A quadrangular segment was excised from the anterior part
of the inferior nasal concha, the middle nasal concha is turned
upwards by two hooks.
b Bony lateral wall of the nasal cavity. The middle nasal concha
was removed, the incisive canal opened.
The individual bones are indicated by different colors.

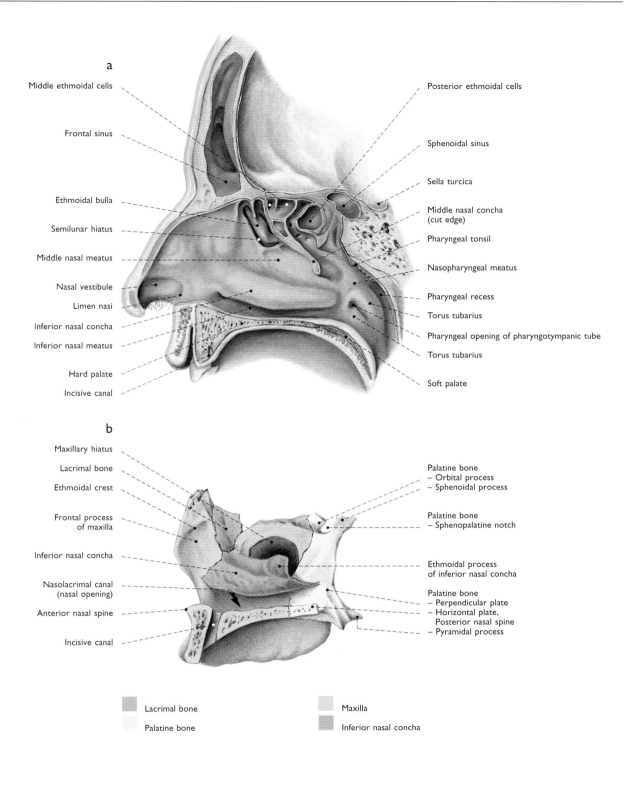

a

Middle ethmoidal cells

Frontal sinus

Ethmoidal bulla

Semilunar hiatus

Middle nasal meatus

Nasal vestibule

Limen nasi

Inferior nasal concha

Inferior nasal meatus

Hard palate

Incisive canal

Posterior ethmoidal cells

Sphenoidal sinus

Sella turcica

Middle nasal concha
(cut edge)

Pharyngeal tonsil

Nasopharyngeal meatus

Pharyngeal recess

Torus tubarius

Pharyngeal opening of pharyngotympanic tube

Torus tubarius

Soft palate

b

Maxillary hiatus

Lacrimal bone

Ethmoidal crest

Frontal process
of maxilla

Inferior nasal concha

Nasolacrimal canal
(nasal opening)

Anterior nasal spine

Incisive canal

Palatine bone
– Orbital process
– Sphenoidal process

Palatine bone
– Sphenopalatine notch

Ethmoidal process
of inferior nasal concha

Palatine bone
– Perpendicular plate
– Horizontal plate,
  Posterior nasal spine
– Pyramidal process

Lacrimal bone

Palatine bone

Maxilla

Inferior nasal concha

57 Lateral wall of the nasal cavity (75%)

Paramedian section to the right of the nasal septum, medial aspect
a Nasal vestibule and mucosa of nasal cavity. The middle nasal concha
was partially removed, the posterior ethmoidal cells were opened.
b Bony lateral wall of the nasal cavity. The nasal, frontal, ethmoidal,
and sphenoidal bones were removed. The individual bones are indicated
by different colors.

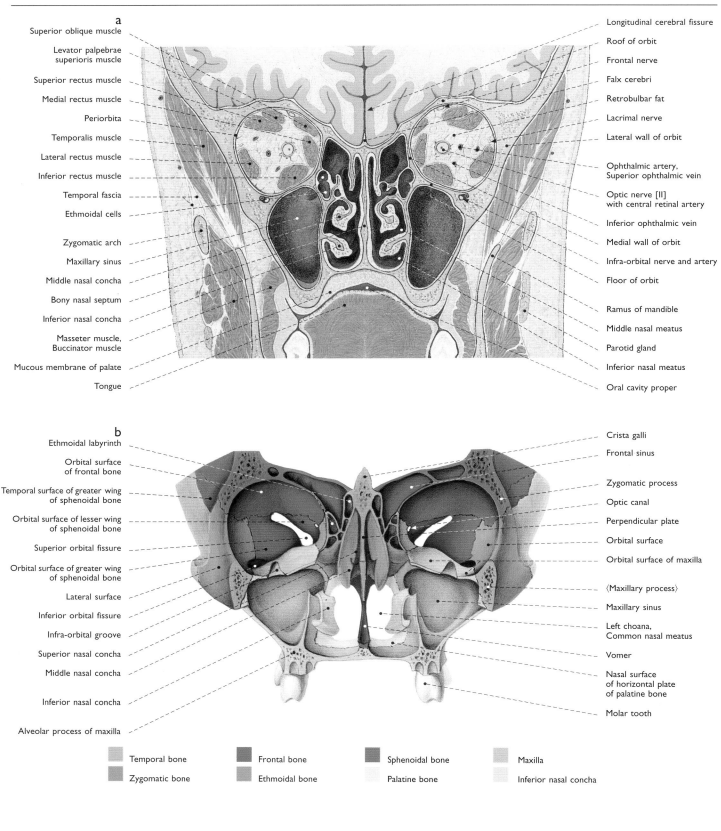

a

Superior oblique muscle
Levator palpebrae superioris muscle
Superior rectus muscle
Medial rectus muscle
Periorbita
Temporalis muscle
Lateral rectus muscle
Inferior rectus muscle
Temporal fascia
Ethmoidal cells
Zygomatic arch
Maxillary sinus
Middle nasal concha
Bony nasal septum
Inferior nasal concha
Masseter muscle, Buccinator muscle
Mucous membrane of palate
Tongue

Longitudinal cerebral fissure
Roof of orbit
Frontal nerve
Falx cerebri
Retrobulbar fat
Lacrimal nerve
Lateral wall of orbit
Ophthalmic artery, Superior ophthalmic vein
Optic nerve [II] with central retinal artery
Inferior ophthalmic vein
Medial wall of orbit
Infra-orbital nerve and artery
Floor of orbit
Ramus of mandible
Middle nasal meatus
Parotid gland
Inferior nasal meatus
Oral cavity proper

b

Ethmoidal labyrinth
Orbital surface of frontal bone
Temporal surface of greater wing of sphenoidal bone
Orbital surface of lesser wing of sphenoidal bone
Superior orbital fissure
Orbital surface of greater wing of sphenoidal bone
Lateral surface
Inferior orbital fissure
Infra-orbital groove
Superior nasal concha
Middle nasal concha
Inferior nasal concha
Alveolar process of maxilla

Crista galli
Frontal sinus
Zygomatic process
Optic canal
Perpendicular plate
Orbital surface
Orbital surface of maxilla
⟨Maxillary process⟩
Maxillary sinus
Left choana, Common nasal meatus
Vomer
Nasal surface of horizontal plate of palatine bone
Molar tooth

Temporal bone
Zygomatic bone
Frontal bone
Ethmoidal bone
Sphenoidal bone
Palatine bone
Maxilla
Inferior nasal concha

58 Nasal and orbital cavities (75%)

Coronal sections, posterior portions, ventral aspect
a Section of the head of an adult male behind the crista galli
b Section of the skull (= cranium) passing the crista galli.
   The individual bones are indicated by different colors.

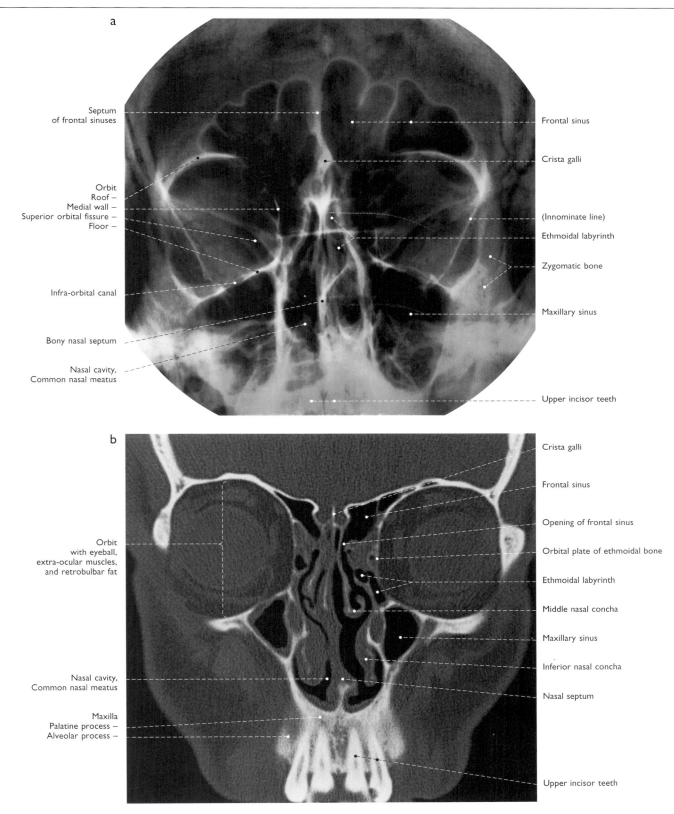

a

Septum
of frontal sinuses

Orbit
Roof –
Medial wall –
Superior orbital fissure –
Floor –

Infra-orbital canal

Bony nasal septum

Nasal cavity,
Common nasal meatus

Frontal sinus

Crista galli

(Innominate line)

Ethmoidal labyrinth

Zygomatic bone

Maxillary sinus

Upper incisor teeth

b

Orbit
with eyeball,
extra-ocular muscles,
and retrobulbar fat

Nasal cavity,
Common nasal meatus

Maxilla
Palatine process –
Alveolar process –

Crista galli

Frontal sinus

Opening of frontal sinus

Orbital plate of ethmoidal bone

Ethmoidal labyrinth

Middle nasal concha

Maxillary sinus

Inferior nasal concha

Nasal septum

Upper incisor teeth

59 Nasal cavity and paranasal sinuses (90%)

a   Postero-anterior radiograph of the skull
b   Coronal computed tomogram (CT) through the viscerocranium

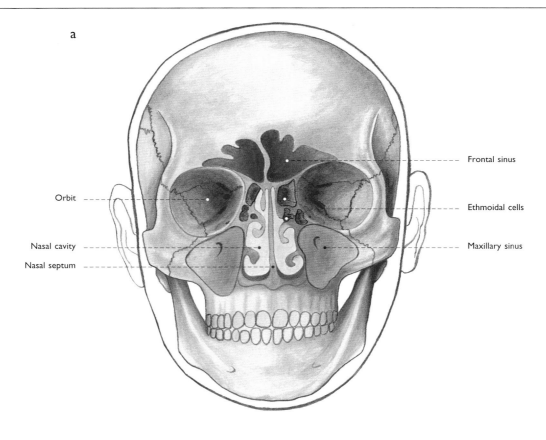

a

Frontal sinus

Orbit

Ethmoidal cells

Nasal cavity

Maxillary sinus

Nasal septum

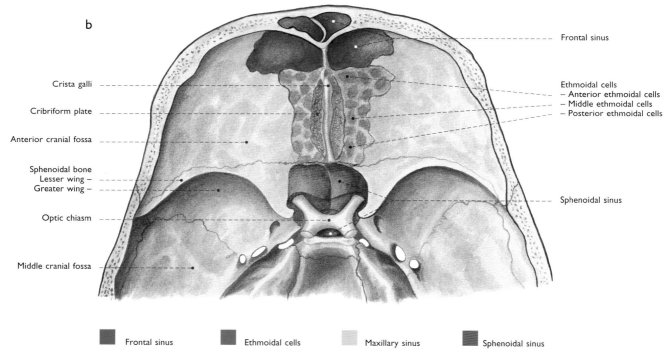

b

Frontal sinus

Crista galli

Ethmoidal cells
– Anterior ethmoidal cells
– Middle ethmoidal cells
– Posterior ethmoidal cells

Cribriform plate

Anterior cranial fossa

Sphenoidal bone
Lesser wing –
Greater wing –

Sphenoidal sinus

Optic chiasm

Middle cranial fossa

▨ Frontal sinus	▨ Ethmoidal cells	▨ Maxillary sinus	▨ Sphenoidal sinus

60 Nasal cavity and paranasal sinuses

Projections of the paranasal sinuses
a   onto the face
b   onto the anterior cranial fossa

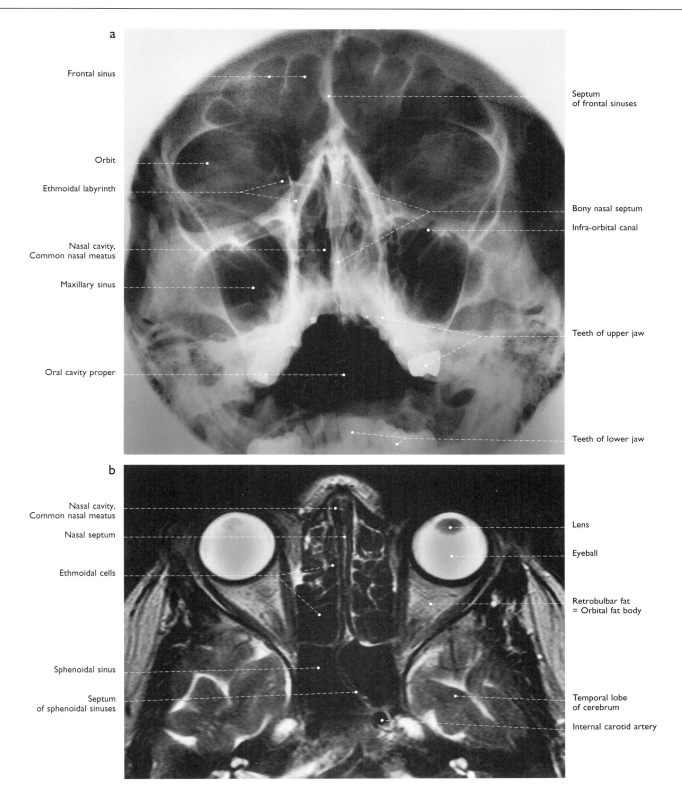

a

Frontal sinus

Orbit

Ethmoidal labyrinth

Nasal cavity,
Common nasal meatus

Maxillary sinus

Oral cavity proper

Septum
of frontal sinuses

Bony nasal septum

Infra-orbital canal

Teeth of upper jaw

Teeth of lower jaw

b

Nasal cavity,
Common nasal meatus

Nasal septum

Ethmoidal cells

Sphenoidal sinus

Septum
of sphenoidal sinuses

Lens

Eyeball

Retrobulbar fat
= Orbital fat body

Temporal lobe
of cerebrum

Internal carotid artery

61 Nasal cavity and paranasal sinuses (90%)
   a Occipitomental radiograph of the skull with the mouth wide open
   b Transverse magnetic resonance image (MRI, T$_2$-weighted) through
      the orbits, the ethmoidal cells, and the sphenoidal sinuses,
      inferior aspect

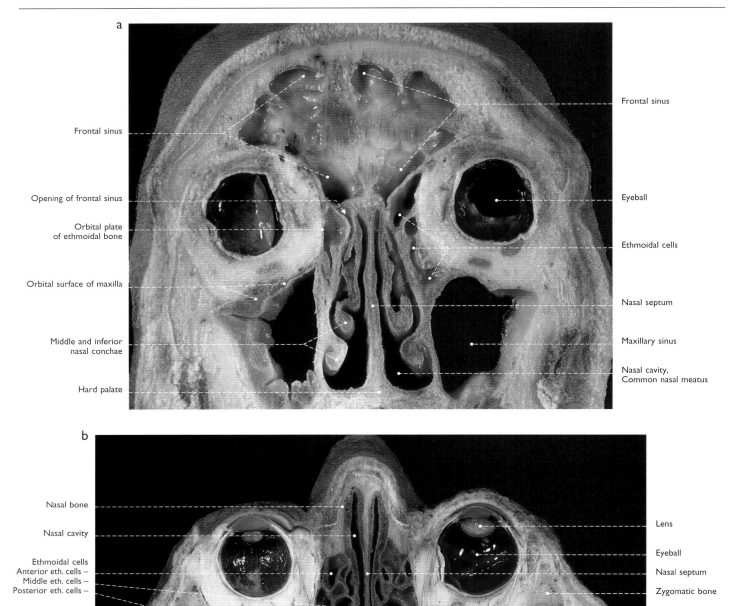

a

Frontal sinus

Opening of frontal sinus

Orbital plate
of ethmoidal bone

Orbital surface of maxilla

Middle and inferior
nasal conchae

Hard palate

Frontal sinus

Eyeball

Ethmoidal cells

Nasal septum

Maxillary sinus

Nasal cavity,
Common nasal meatus

b

Nasal bone

Nasal cavity

Ethmoidal cells
Anterior eth. cells –
Middle eth. cells –
Posterior eth. cells –

Spheno-ethmoidal
recess

Sphenoidal sinus

Internal carotid artery

Lens

Eyeball

Nasal septum

Zygomatic bone

Orbital plate
of ethmoidal bone

Temporalis muscle

Temporal lobe
of cerebrum

Cavernous sinus

62   Nasal cavity and paranasal sinuses (100%)

Anatomical sections
a   Coronal section through both eyeballs and the frontal,
ethmoidal, and maxillary sinuses, ventral aspect
b   Transverse section through both eyeballs, the ethmoidal cells,
and the sphenoidal sinuses, superior aspect

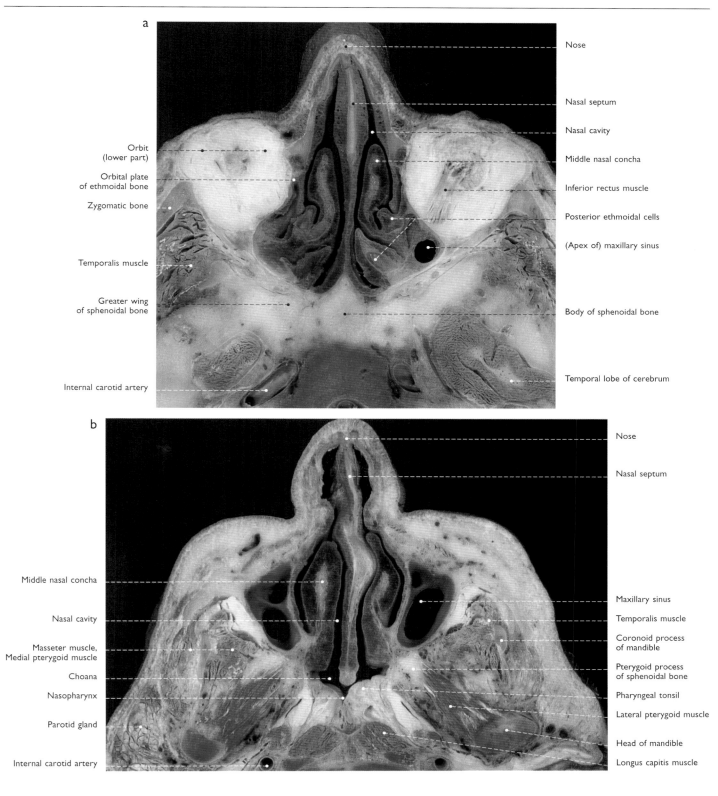

a

Nose

Nasal septum

Nasal cavity

Middle nasal concha

Inferior rectus muscle

Posterior ethmoidal cells

(Apex of) maxillary sinus

Body of sphenoidal bone

Temporal lobe of cerebrum

Orbit (lower part)

Orbital plate of ethmoidal bone

Zygomatic bone

Temporalis muscle

Greater wing of sphenoidal bone

Internal carotid artery

b

Nose

Nasal septum

Middle nasal concha

Nasal cavity

Masseter muscle, Medial pterygoid muscle

Choana

Nasopharynx

Parotid gland

Internal carotid artery

Maxillary sinus

Temporalis muscle

Coronoid process of mandible

Pterygoid process of sphenoidal bone

Pharyngeal tonsil

Lateral pterygoid muscle

Head of mandible

Longus capitis muscle

63 Nasal cavity and paranasal sinuses (100%)

Transverse anatomical sections
a through the caudal part of the orbits and the apex of the maxillary sinus
b through the middle part of the nasal cavity and the maxillary sinuses
a, b Superior aspect

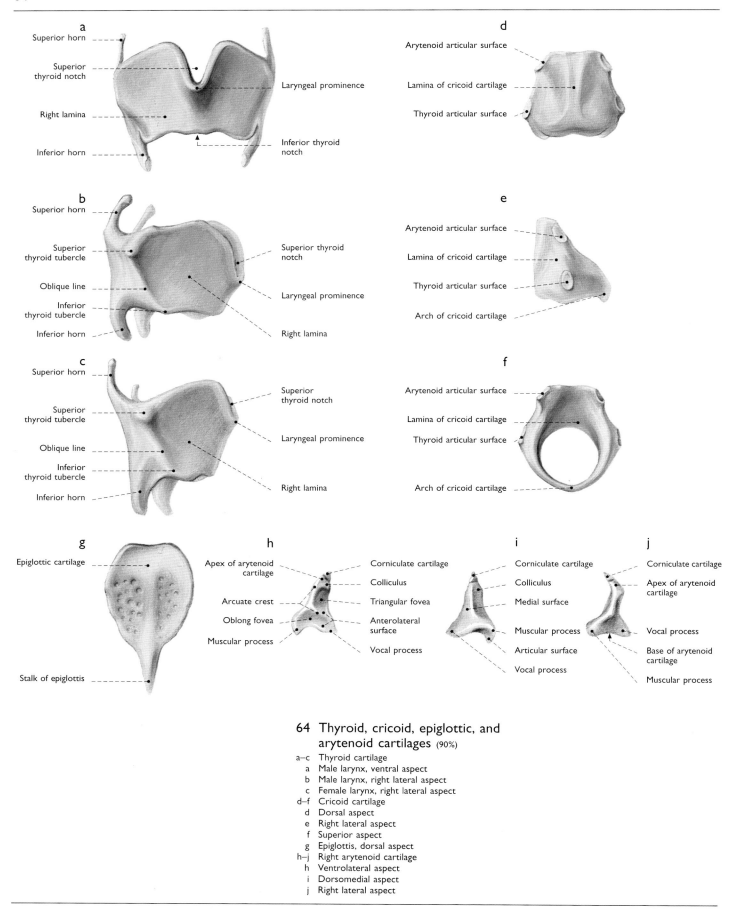

a
Superior horn
Superior thyroid notch
Right lamina
Inferior horn
Laryngeal prominence
Inferior thyroid notch

b
Superior horn
Superior thyroid tubercle
Oblique line
Inferior thyroid tubercle
Inferior horn
Superior thyroid notch
Laryngeal prominence
Right lamina

c
Superior horn
Superior thyroid tubercle
Oblique line
Inferior thyroid tubercle
Inferior horn
Superior thyroid notch
Laryngeal prominence
Right lamina

d
Arytenoid articular surface
Lamina of cricoid cartilage
Thyroid articular surface

e
Arytenoid articular surface
Lamina of cricoid cartilage
Thyroid articular surface
Arch of cricoid cartilage

f
Arytenoid articular surface
Lamina of cricoid cartilage
Thyroid articular surface
Arch of cricoid cartilage

g
Epiglottic cartilage
Stalk of epiglottis

h
Apex of arytenoid cartilage
Arcuate crest
Oblong fovea
Muscular process
Corniculate cartilage
Colliculus
Triangular fovea
Anterolateral surface
Vocal process

i
Corniculate cartilage
Colliculus
Medial surface
Muscular process
Articular surface
Vocal process

j
Corniculate cartilage
Apex of arytenoid cartilage
Vocal process
Base of arytenoid cartilage
Muscular process

64 Thyroid, cricoid, epiglottic, and arytenoid cartilages (90%)

a–c Thyroid cartilage
 a   Male larynx, ventral aspect
 b   Male larynx, right lateral aspect
 c   Female larynx, right lateral aspect
d–f Cricoid cartilage
 d   Dorsal aspect
 e   Right lateral aspect
 f   Superior aspect
 g   Epiglottis, dorsal aspect
h–j Right arytenoid cartilage
 h   Ventrolateral aspect
 i   Dorsomedial aspect
 j   Right lateral aspect

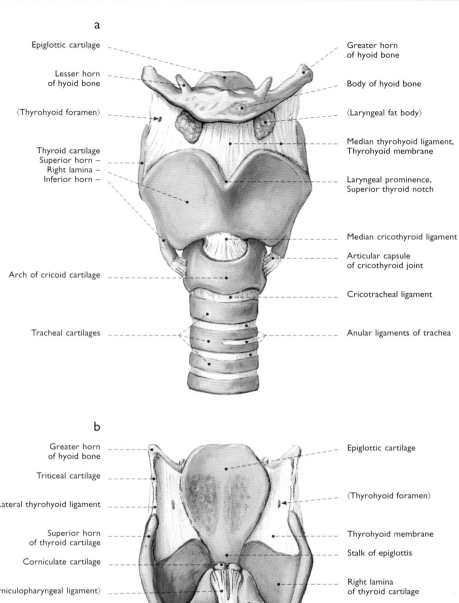

a

Epiglottic cartilage

Lesser horn
of hyoid bone

⟨Thyrohyoid foramen⟩

Thyroid cartilage
Superior horn —
Right lamina —
Inferior horn —

Arch of cricoid cartilage

Tracheal cartilages

Greater horn
of hyoid bone

Body of hyoid bone

⟨Laryngeal fat body⟩

Median thyrohyoid ligament,
Thyrohyoid membrane

Laryngeal prominence,
Superior thyroid notch

Median cricothyroid ligament

Articular capsule
of cricothyroid joint

Cricotracheal ligament

Anular ligaments of trachea

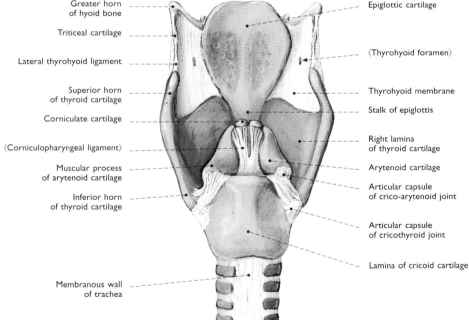

b

Greater horn
of hyoid bone

Triticeal cartilage

Lateral thyrohyoid ligament

Superior horn
of thyroid cartilage

Corniculate cartilage

⟨Corniculopharyngeal ligament⟩

Muscular process
of arytenoid cartilage

Inferior horn
of thyroid cartilage

Membranous wall
of trachea

Epiglottic cartilage

⟨Thyrohyoid foramen⟩

Thyrohyoid membrane

Stalk of epiglottis

Right lamina
of thyroid cartilage

Arytenoid cartilage

Articular capsule
of crico-arytenoid joint

Articular capsule
of cricothyroid joint

Lamina of cricoid cartilage

65 Laryngeal cartilages and joints (100%)
   a Ventral aspect
   b Dorsal aspect

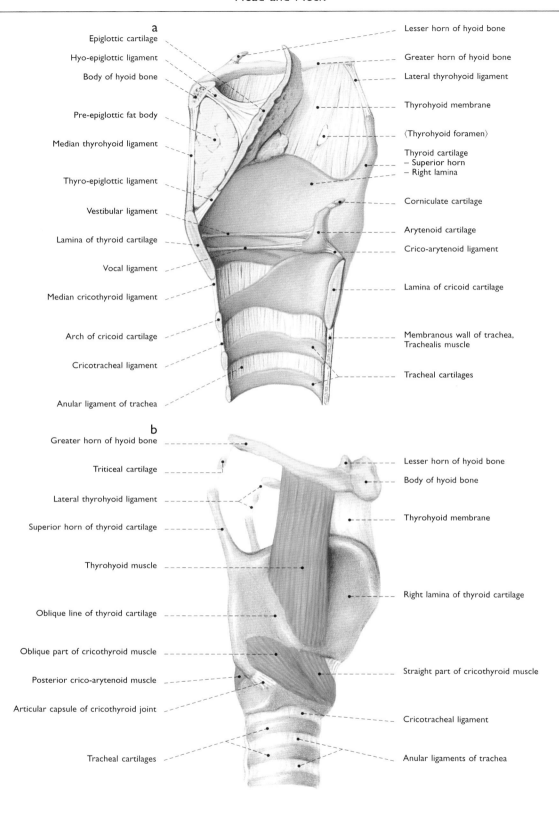

a

Epiglottic cartilage

Hyo-epiglottic ligament

Body of hyoid bone

Pre-epiglottic fat body

Median thyrohyoid ligament

Thyro-epiglottic ligament

Vestibular ligament

Lamina of thyroid cartilage

Vocal ligament

Median cricothyroid ligament

Arch of cricoid cartilage

Cricotracheal ligament

Anular ligament of trachea

Lesser horn of hyoid bone

Greater horn of hyoid bone

Lateral thyrohyoid ligament

Thyrohyoid membrane

⟨Thyrohyoid foramen⟩

Thyroid cartilage
– Superior horn
– Right lamina

Corniculate cartilage

Arytenoid cartilage

Crico-arytenoid ligament

Lamina of cricoid cartilage

Membranous wall of trachea,
Trachealis muscle

Tracheal cartilages

b

Greater horn of hyoid bone

Triticeal cartilage

Lateral thyrohyoid ligament

Superior horn of thyroid cartilage

Thyrohyoid muscle

Oblique line of thyroid cartilage

Oblique part of cricothyroid muscle

Posterior crico-arytenoid muscle

Articular capsule of cricothyroid joint

Tracheal cartilages

Lesser horn of hyoid bone

Body of hyoid bone

Thyrohyoid membrane

Right lamina of thyroid cartilage

Straight part of cricothyroid muscle

Cricotracheal ligament

Anular ligaments of trachea

66 Ligaments and muscles of the larynx (100%)
a Median section through the hyoid bone and the skeleton
   of the larynx, medial aspect
b Thyrohyoid and cricothyroid muscles, right lateral aspect

a

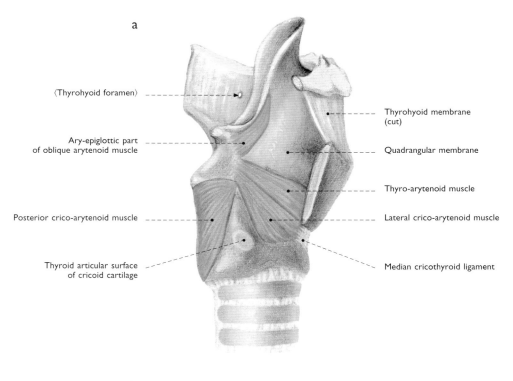

⟨Thyrohyoid foramen⟩

Ary-epiglottic part
of oblique arytenoid muscle

Posterior crico-arytenoid muscle

Thyroid articular surface
of cricoid cartilage

Thyrohyoid membrane
(cut)

Quadrangular membrane

Thyro-arytenoid muscle

Lateral crico-arytenoid muscle

Median cricothyroid ligament

b

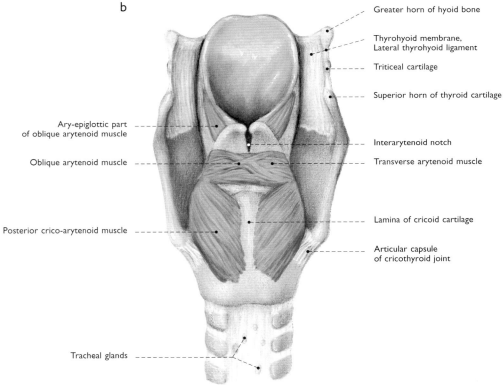

Ary-epiglottic part
of oblique arytenoid muscle

Oblique arytenoid muscle

Posterior crico-arytenoid muscle

Tracheal glands

Greater horn of hyoid bone

Thyrohyoid membrane,
Lateral thyrohyoid ligament

Triticeal cartilage

Superior horn of thyroid cartilage

Interarytenoid notch

Transverse arytenoid muscle

Lamina of cricoid cartilage

Articular capsule
of cricothyroid joint

67 Inner muscles of the larynx (100%)

a The right lamina of the thyroid cartilage was partially removed,
the oblique and transverse arytenoid muscles are omitted.
Right lateral aspect
b The pharyngeal mucosa was completely removed. Dorsal aspect

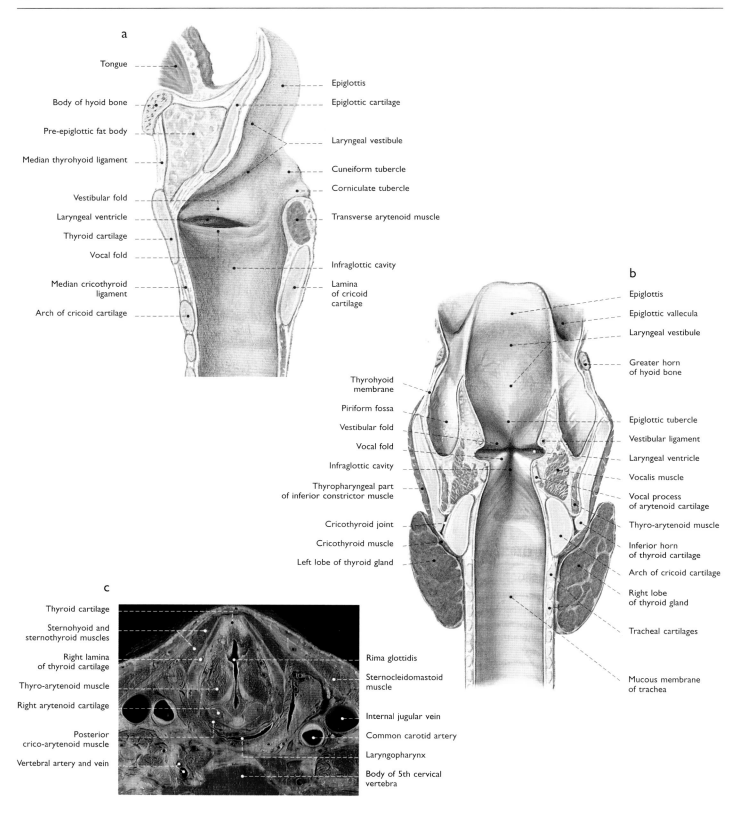

a
Tongue
Body of hyoid bone
Pre-epiglottic fat body
Median thyrohyoid ligament
Vestibular fold
Laryngeal ventricle
Thyroid cartilage
Vocal fold
Median cricothyroid ligament
Arch of cricoid cartilage

Epiglottis
Epiglottic cartilage
Laryngeal vestibule
Cuneiform tubercle
Corniculate tubercle
Transverse arytenoid muscle
Infraglottic cavity
Lamina of cricoid cartilage

b
Thyrohyoid membrane
Piriform fossa
Vestibular fold
Vocal fold
Infraglottic cavity
Thyropharyngeal part of inferior constrictor muscle
Cricothyroid joint
Cricothyroid muscle
Left lobe of thyroid gland

Epiglottis
Epiglottic vallecula
Laryngeal vestibule
Greater horn of hyoid bone
Epiglottic tubercle
Vestibular ligament
Laryngeal ventricle
Vocalis muscle
Vocal process of arytenoid cartilage
Thyro-arytenoid muscle
Inferior horn of thyroid cartilage
Arch of cricoid cartilage
Right lobe of thyroid gland
Tracheal cartilages
Mucous membrane of trachea

c
Thyroid cartilage
Sternohyoid and sternothyroid muscles
Right lamina of thyroid cartilage
Thyro-arytenoid muscle
Right arytenoid cartilage
Posterior crico-arytenoid muscle
Vertebral artery and vein

Rima glottidis
Sternocleidomastoid muscle
Internal jugular vein
Common carotid artery
Laryngopharynx
Body of 5th cervical vertebra

68 Larynx
a Median section through the larynx (100%), medial aspect
b Frontal (coronal) section through the larynx (100%), dorsal aspect of the anterior part
c Transverse anatomical section through the glottis (75%), inferior aspect

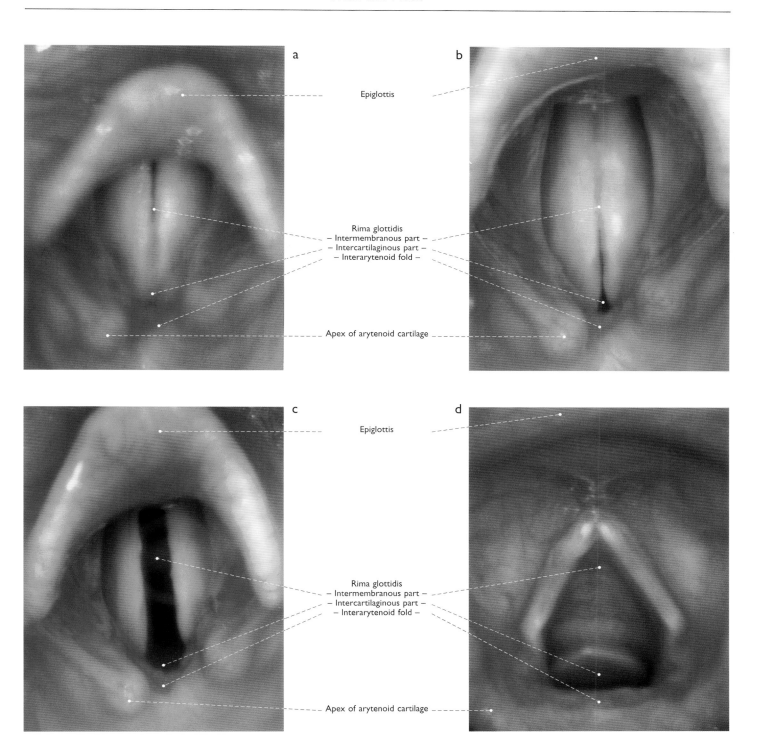

a

b

Epiglottis

Rima glottidis
– Intermembranous part –
– Intercartilaginous part –
– Interarytenoid fold –

Apex of arytenoid cartilage

c   d

Epiglottis

Rima glottidis
– Intermembranous part –
– Intercartilaginous part –
– Interarytenoid fold –

Apex of arytenoid cartilage

69 Laryngoscopic view of the interior of the larynx in a living adult (100%)

a   During loud phonation
b   During whispering
c   During quiet respiration
d   During forced inspiration

a

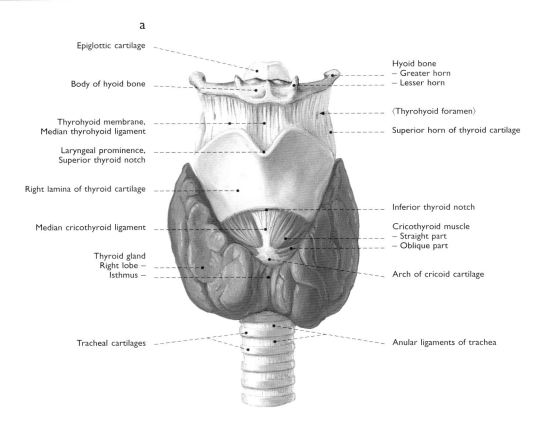

Epiglottic cartilage

Body of hyoid bone

Thyrohyoid membrane,
Median thyrohyoid ligament

Laryngeal prominence,
Superior thyroid notch

Right lamina of thyroid cartilage

Median cricothyroid ligament

Thyroid gland
Right lobe –
Isthmus –

Tracheal cartilages

Hyoid bone
– Greater horn
– Lesser horn

⟨Thyrohyoid foramen⟩

Superior horn of thyroid cartilage

Inferior thyroid notch

Cricothyroid muscle
– Straight part
– Oblique part

Arch of cricoid cartilage

Anular ligaments of trachea

b

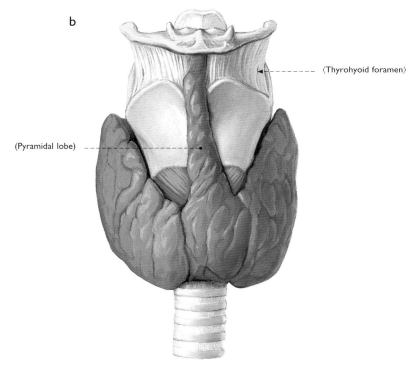

(Pyramidal lobe)

⟨Thyrohyoid foramen⟩

70 Thyroid gland and larynx (80%)
        Ventral aspect
    a Normal situation
    b Pyramidal lobe as a variation

a

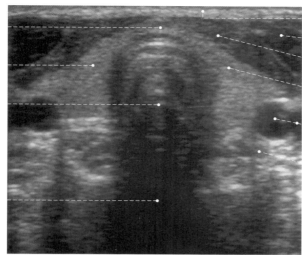

Isthmus
of thyroid gland

Right lobe
of thyroid gland

Trachea

Vertebral body

Skin

Sternocleidomastoid muscle

Sternothyroid and
sternohyoid muscles

Left lobe
of thyroid gland

Common carotid artery,
Internal jugular vein

Longus colli muscle

b

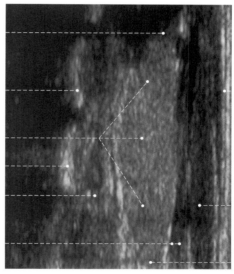

Superior pole
of thyroid gland

Body of 3rd cervical
vertebra

Right/left lobe
of thyroid gland

Body of 4th cervical
vertebra

Longus colli muscle

Sternothyroid and
sternohyoid muscles

Skin

Sternocleido-
mastoid muscle

Inferior pole
of thyroid gland

c

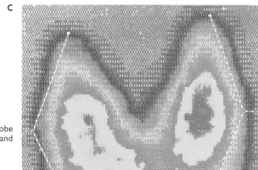

Right lobe
of thyroid gland

Left lobe
of thyroid gland

71 Thyroid gland (100%)
  a Transverse ultrasound image
  b Longitudinal ultrasound image through one of the two thyroid lobes
  c Scan of a thyroid gland with normal function after application of ^{99m}Tc

a

Occipital bone

1st cervical vertebra = Atlas,
Lateral mass of atlas

2nd cervical vertebra = Axis
Dens –
Vertebral body –

Intervertebral disc

1st thoracic vertebra
Transverse process –
Vertebral body –

Parotid gland

Sternocleidomastoid muscle

Anterior scalene muscle

Middle scalene muscle

Brachial plexus

Left subclavian artery

Apex of lung

b

Atlanto-occipital joint

Lateral atlanto-axial joint

Parotid gland

Right internal carotid artery

Intervertebral disc

Sternocleidomastoid muscle

Foramen magnum

Occipital condyle
of occipital bone

1st cervical vertebra = Atlas [C I]
– Transverse process
– Lateral mass of atlas

2nd cervical vertebra = Axis [C II]
– Dens
– Superior articular process
– Vertebral body

Cervical part
of left vertebral artery

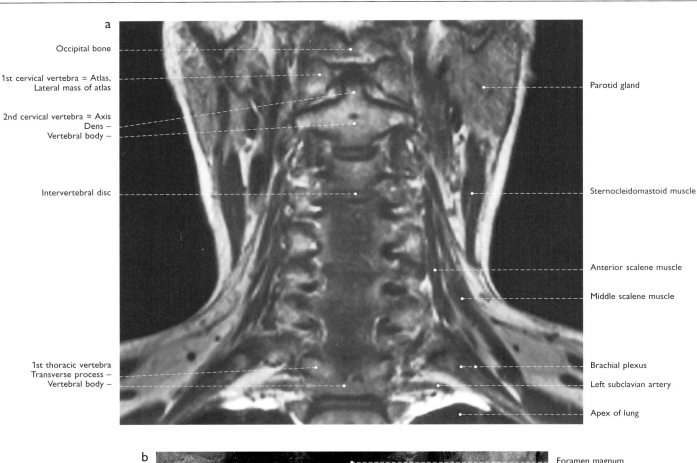

72 Neck (80%)
     Coronal sections through the neck in the plane
     of vertebral bodies
   a Magnetic resonance image (MRI, T$_1$-weighted)
   b Anatomical section, ventral aspect

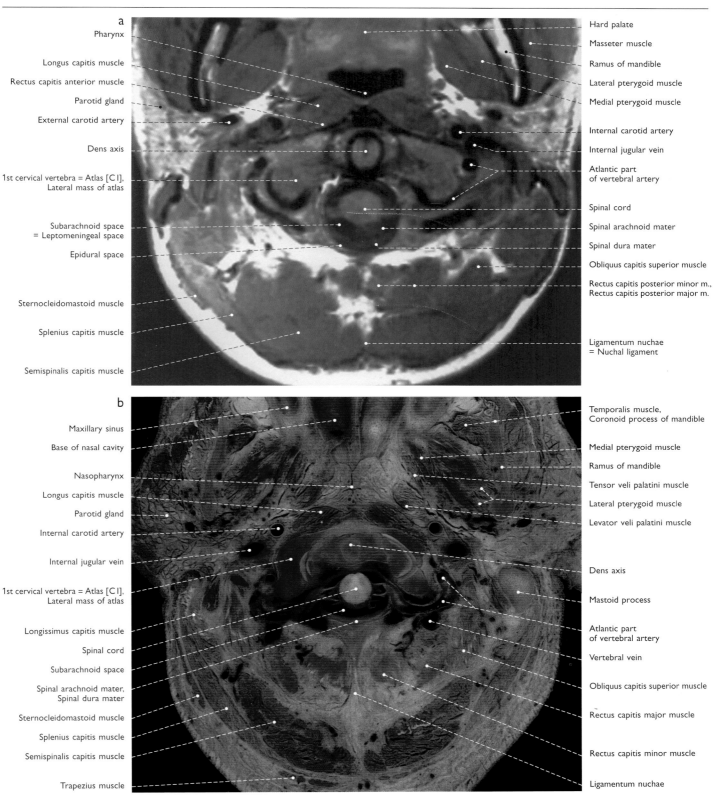

a

Pharynx

Longus capitis muscle

Rectus capitis anterior muscle

Parotid gland

External carotid artery

Dens axis

1st cervical vertebra = Atlas [C I],
Lateral mass of atlas

Subarachnoid space
= Leptomeningeal space

Epidural space

Sternocleidomastoid muscle

Splenius capitis muscle

Semispinalis capitis muscle

Hard palate

Masseter muscle

Ramus of mandible

Lateral pterygoid muscle

Medial pterygoid muscle

Internal carotid artery

Internal jugular vein

Atlantic part
of vertebral artery

Spinal cord

Spinal arachnoid mater

Spinal dura mater

Obliquus capitis superior muscle

Rectus capitis posterior minor m.,
Rectus capitis posterior major m.

Ligamentum nuchae
= Nuchal ligament

b

Maxillary sinus

Base of nasal cavity

Nasopharynx

Longus capitis muscle

Parotid gland

Internal carotid artery

Internal jugular vein

1st cervical vertebra = Atlas [C I],
Lateral mass of atlas

Longissimus capitis muscle

Spinal cord

Subarachnoid space

Spinal arachnoid mater,
Spinal dura mater

Sternocleidomastoid muscle

Splenius capitis muscle

Semispinalis capitis muscle

Trapezius muscle

Temporalis muscle,
Coronoid process of mandible

Medial pterygoid muscle

Ramus of mandible

Tensor veli palatini muscle

Lateral pterygoid muscle

Levator veli palatini muscle

Dens axis

Mastoid process

Atlantic part
of vertebral artery

Vertebral vein

Obliquus capitis superior muscle

Rectus capitis major muscle

Rectus capitis minor muscle

Ligamentum nuchae

73 Neck (90%)
Transverse sections through the neck at the level
of the first cervical vertebra (C I, atlas)
a Magnetic resonance image (MRI, T₁-weighted), inferior aspect
b Anatomical section, superior aspect

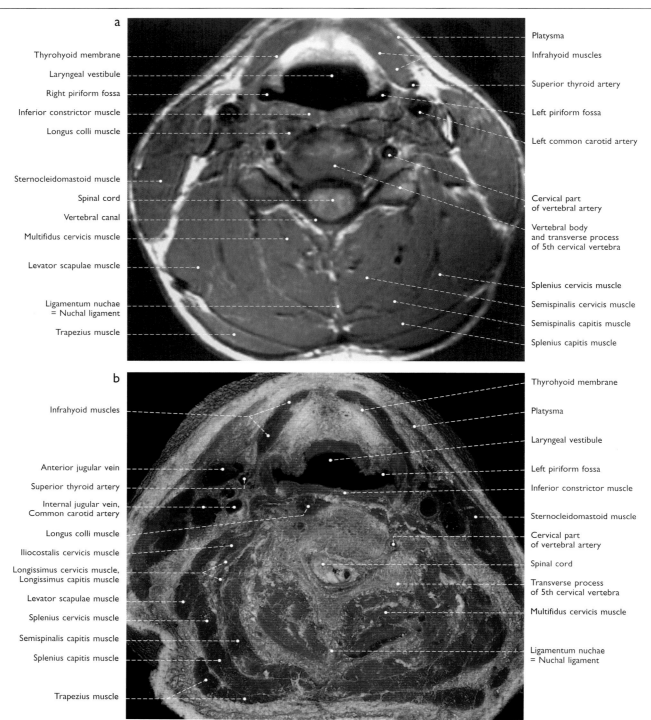

a

Thyrohyoid membrane
Laryngeal vestibule
Right piriform fossa
Inferior constrictor muscle
Longus colli muscle

Sternocleidomastoid muscle
Spinal cord
Vertebral canal
Multifidus cervicis muscle

Levator scapulae muscle

Ligamentum nuchae
= Nuchal ligament
Trapezius muscle

Platysma
Infrahyoid muscles
Superior thyroid artery
Left piriform fossa
Left common carotid artery

Cervical part
of vertebral artery
Vertebral body
and transverse process
of 5th cervical vertebra

Splenius cervicis muscle
Semispinalis cervicis muscle
Semispinalis capitis muscle
Splenius capitis muscle

b

Infrahyoid muscles

Anterior jugular vein
Superior thyroid artery
Internal jugular vein,
Common carotid artery
Longus colli muscle
Iliocostalis cervicis muscle
Longissimus cervicis muscle,
Longissimus capitis muscle
Levator scapulae muscle
Splenius cervicis muscle
Semispinalis capitis muscle
Splenius capitis muscle

Trapezius muscle

Thyrohyoid membrane
Platysma
Laryngeal vestibule
Left piriform fossa
Inferior constrictor muscle
Sternocleidomastoid muscle
Cervical part
of vertebral artery
Spinal cord
Transverse process
of 5th cervical vertebra
Multifidus cervicis muscle

Ligamentum nuchae
= Nuchal ligament

74 Neck (90%)

Transverse sections through the neck at the level
of the fifth cervical vertebra (C V), inferior aspect
a Magnetic resonance image (MRI, T$_1$-weighted)
b Anatomical section

a

Right and left lobes of thyroid gland

Trachea

Sternocleidomastoid muscle

Esophagus

Vertebral body of 7th cervical vertebra

Cerebrospinal fluid in subarachnoid space

Spinal cord

Ligamentum flavum

Spinous process

Nuchal fascia

Common carotid artery

Internal jugular vein

Vagus nerve [X]

Longus colli muscle

Anterior scalene muscle

Middle scalene muscle

Posterior scalene muscle

Levator scapulae muscle

Multifidus cervicis muscle

Semispinalis capitis muscle

Splenius capitis muscle

Trapezius muscle

b

Anterior jugular vein (extended)

Right lobe of thyroid gland

Sternocleidomastoid muscle

Internal jugular vein, Common carotid artery

Vagus nerve [X]

Anterior scalene muscle, Brachial plexus

Middle scalene muscle

Posterior scalene muscle

Tubercle of 1st rib

Costotransverse joint

1st thoracic vertebra Transverse process – Spinous process –

Trapezius muscle

Sternohyoid muscle, Sternothyroid muscle

Trachea

Left lobe of thyroid gland

Esophagus

Longus colli muscle

Vertebral vein and artery

Vertebral body

Zygapophysial joint

Spinal cord

Subarachnoid space

Spinal dura mater

Levator scapulae muscle

Splenius capitis muscle

Semispinalis capitis muscle

Multifidus cervicis muscle

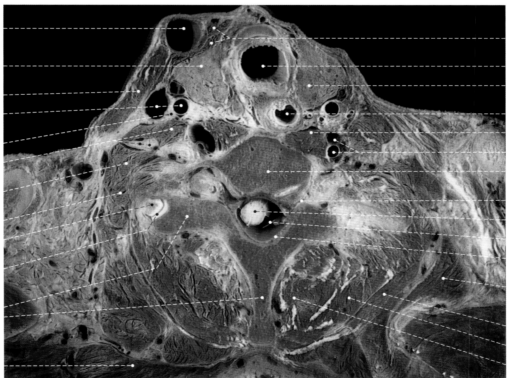

75   Neck (90%)

Transverse sections through the neck at the level
of the seventh cervical vertebra (C VII, a)
or the first thoracic vertebra (Th I, b), respectively,
inferior aspect
a   Magnetic resonance image (MRI, T$_2$-weighted)
b   Anatomical section

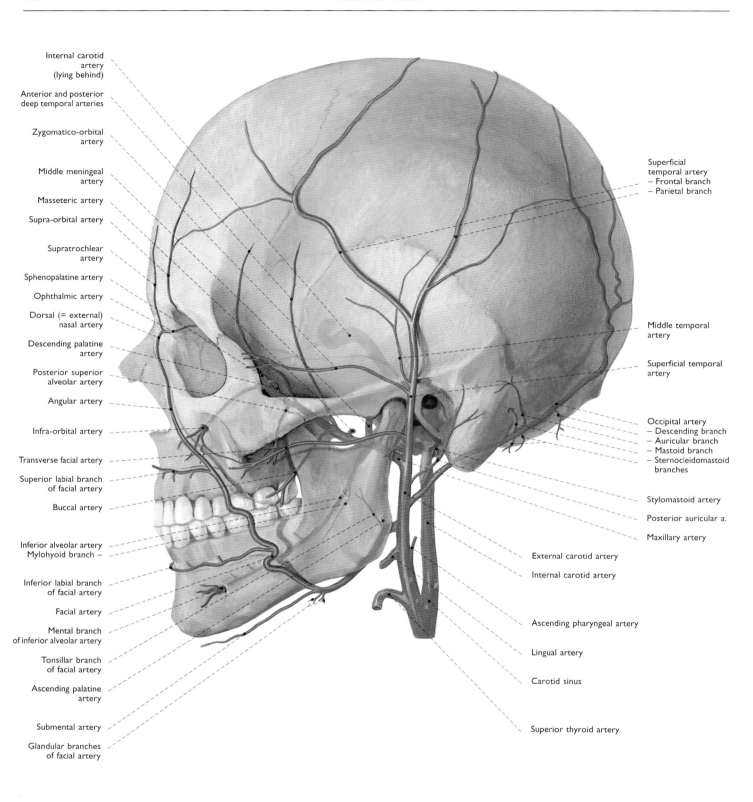

Internal carotid artery (lying behind)

Anterior and posterior deep temporal arteries

Zygomatico-orbital artery

Middle meningeal artery

Masseteric artery

Supra-orbital artery

Supratrochlear artery

Sphenopalatine artery

Ophthalmic artery

Dorsal (= external) nasal artery

Descending palatine artery

Posterior superior alveolar artery

Angular artery

Infra-orbital artery

Transverse facial artery

Superior labial branch of facial artery

Buccal artery

Inferior alveolar artery Mylohyoid branch

Inferior labial branch of facial artery

Facial artery

Mental branch of inferior alveolar artery

Tonsillar branch of facial artery

Ascending palatine artery

Submental artery

Glandular branches of facial artery

Superficial temporal artery
– Frontal branch
– Parietal branch

Middle temporal artery

Superficial temporal artery

Occipital artery
– Descending branch
– Auricular branch
– Mastoid branch
– Sternocleidomastoid branches

Stylomastoid artery

Posterior auricular a.

Maxillary artery

External carotid artery

Internal carotid artery

Ascending pharyngeal artery

Lingual artery

Carotid sinus

Superior thyroid artery

76 Arteries of the skull (75%)
Schematic representation, left lateral aspect

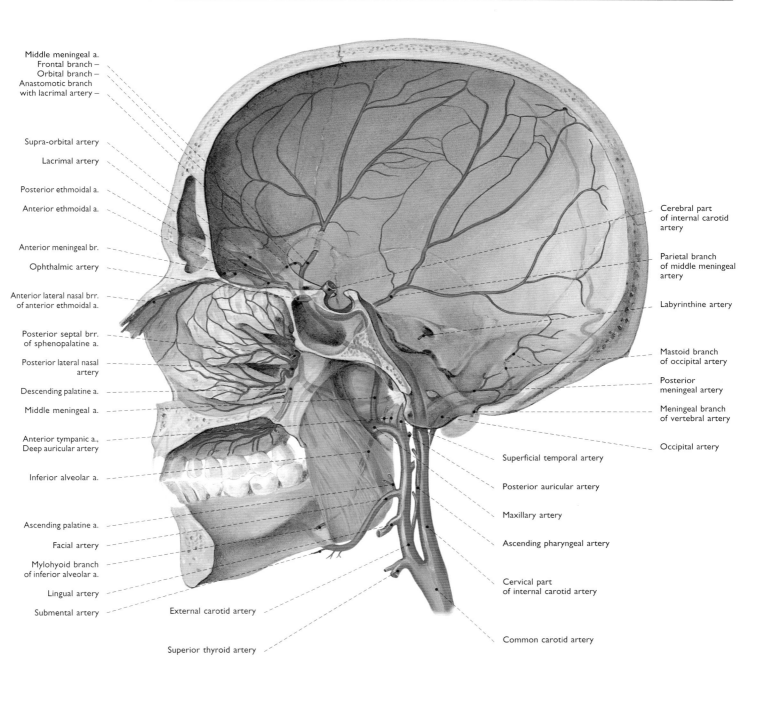

Middle meningeal a.
Frontal branch –
Orbital branch –
Anastomotic branch
with lacrimal artery –

Supra-orbital artery

Lacrimal artery

Posterior ethmoidal a.

Anterior ethmoidal a.

Anterior meningeal br.

Ophthalmic artery

Anterior lateral nasal brr.
of anterior ethmoidal a.

Posterior septal brr.
of sphenopalatine a.

Posterior lateral nasal
artery

Descending palatine a.

Middle meningeal a.

Anterior tympanic a.,
Deep auricular artery

Inferior alveolar a.

Ascending palatine a.

Facial artery

Mylohyoid branch
of inferior alveolar a.

Lingual artery

Submental artery

External carotid artery

Superior thyroid artery

Cerebral part
of internal carotid
artery

Parietal branch
of middle meningeal
artery

Labyrinthine artery

Mastoid branch
of occipital artery

Posterior
meningeal artery

Meningeal branch
of vertebral artery

Occipital artery

Superficial temporal artery

Posterior auricular artery

Maxillary artery

Ascending pharyngeal artery

Cervical part
of internal carotid artery

Common carotid artery

77 Arteries of the skull (75%)
Schematic representation, median section,
medial aspect of the right half of the skull

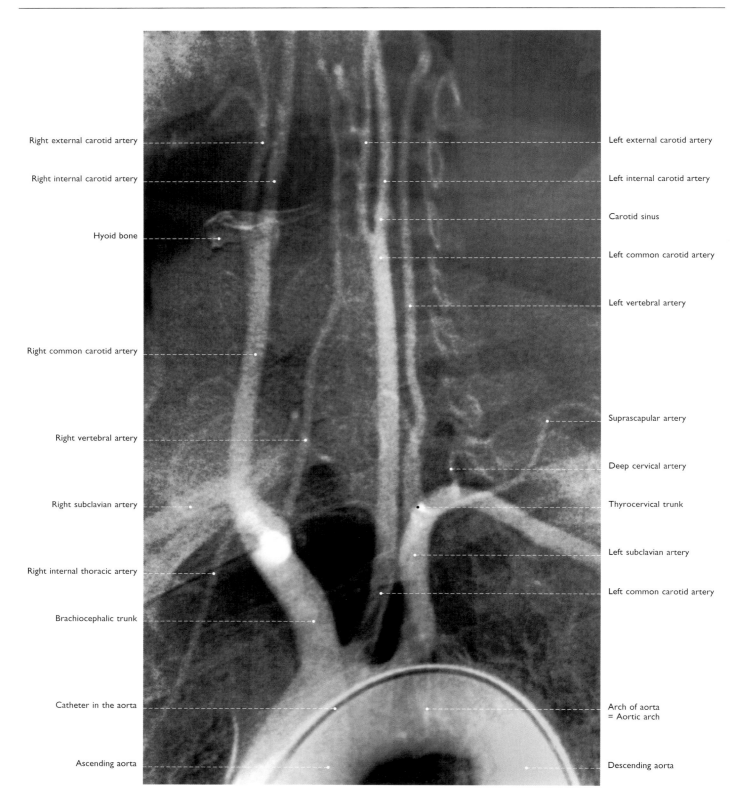

Right external carotid artery

Right internal carotid artery

Hyoid bone

Right common carotid artery

Right vertebral artery

Right subclavian artery

Right internal thoracic artery

Brachiocephalic trunk

Catheter in the aorta

Ascending aorta

Left external carotid artery

Left internal carotid artery

Carotid sinus

Left common carotid artery

Left vertebral artery

Suprascapular artery

Deep cervical artery

Thyrocervical trunk

Left subclavian artery

Left common carotid artery

Arch of aorta
= Aortic arch

Descending aorta

78 Arteries of the neck and head (90%)
Arteriogram, left anterior oblique view (LAO projection)

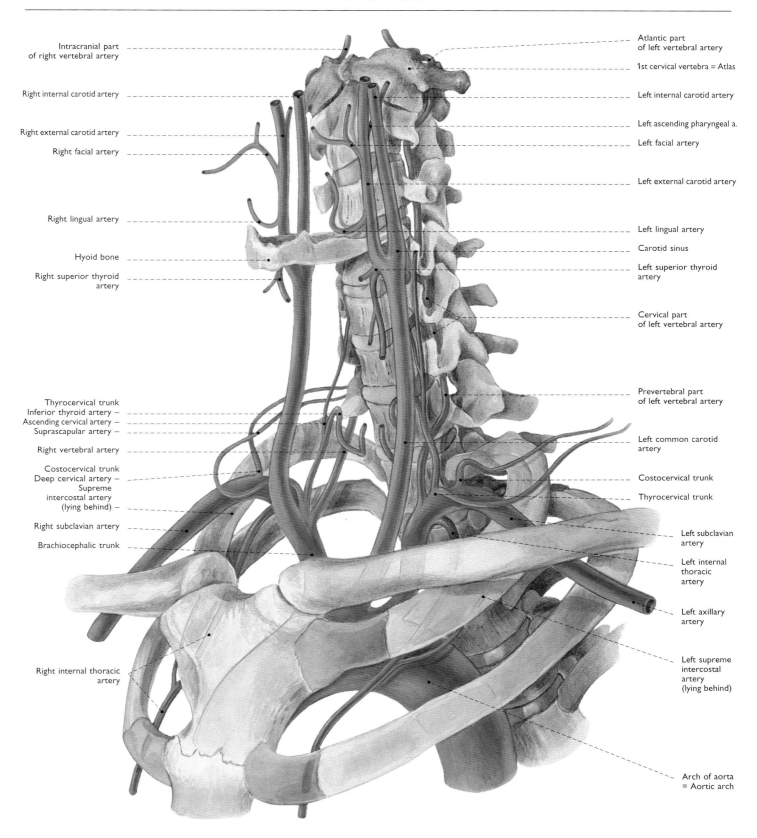

Intracranial part
of right vertebral artery

Right internal carotid artery

Right external carotid artery

Right facial artery

Right lingual artery

Hyoid bone

Right superior thyroid
artery

Thyrocervical trunk
Inferior thyroid artery –
Ascending cervical artery –
Suprascapular artery –

Right vertebral artery

Costocervical trunk
Deep cervical artery –
Supreme
intercostal artery
(lying behind) –

Right subclavian artery

Brachiocephalic trunk

Right internal thoracic
artery

Atlantic part
of left vertebral artery

1st cervical vertebra = Atlas

Left internal carotid artery

Left ascending pharyngeal a.

Left facial artery

Left external carotid artery

Left lingual artery

Carotid sinus

Left superior thyroid
artery

Cervical part
of left vertebral artery

Prevertebral part
of left vertebral artery

Left common carotid
artery

Costocervical trunk

Thyrocervical trunk

Left subclavian
artery

Left internal
thoracic
artery

Left axillary
artery

Left supreme
intercostal
artery
(lying behind)

Arch of aorta
= Aortic arch

79 Arteries of the neck and head (90%)
Left anterior oblique view (LAO projection)

a

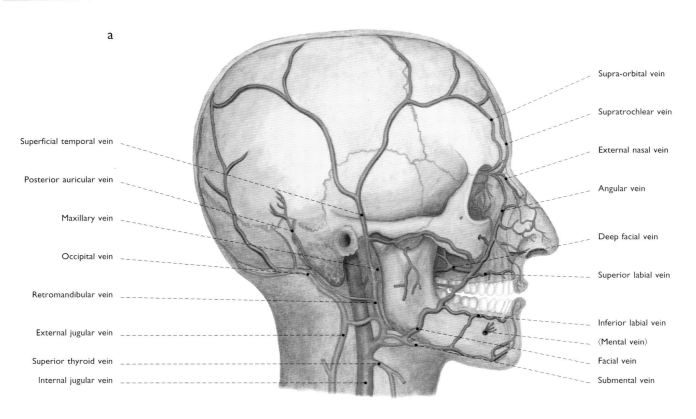

Superficial temporal vein
Posterior auricular vein
Maxillary vein
Occipital vein
Retromandibular vein
External jugular vein
Superior thyroid vein
Internal jugular vein

Supra-orbital vein
Supratrochlear vein
External nasal vein
Angular vein
Deep facial vein
Superior labial vein
Inferior labial vein
⟨Mental vein⟩
Facial vein
Submental vein

b

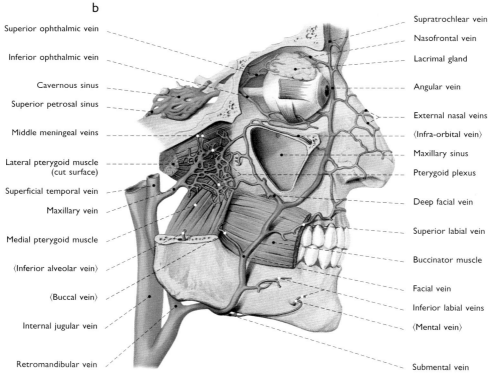

Superior ophthalmic vein
Inferior ophthalmic vein
Cavernous sinus
Superior petrosal sinus
Middle meningeal veins
Lateral pterygoid muscle (cut surface)
Superficial temporal vein
Maxillary vein
Medial pterygoid muscle
⟨Inferior alveolar vein⟩
⟨Buccal vein⟩
Internal jugular vein
Retromandibular vein

Supratrochlear vein
Nasofrontal vein
Lacrimal gland
Angular vein
External nasal veins
⟨Infra-orbital vein⟩
Maxillary sinus
Pterygoid plexus
Deep facial vein
Superior labial vein
Buccinator muscle
Facial vein
Inferior labial veins
⟨Mental vein⟩
Submental vein

80 Veins of the head
Right lateral aspect
a Superficial veins (50%)
b Deep veins (65%)

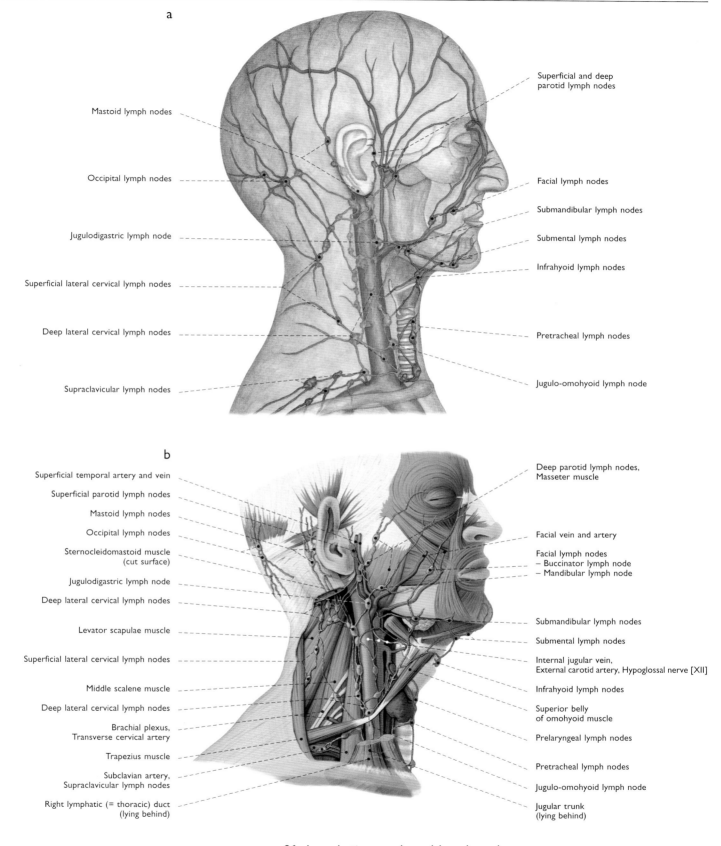

a

Mastoid lymph nodes

Occipital lymph nodes

Jugulodigastric lymph node

Superficial lateral cervical lymph nodes

Deep lateral cervical lymph nodes

Supraclavicular lymph nodes

Superficial and deep
parotid lymph nodes

Facial lymph nodes

Submandibular lymph nodes

Submental lymph nodes

Infrahyoid lymph nodes

Pretracheal lymph nodes

Jugulo-omohyoid lymph node

b

Superficial temporal artery and vein

Superficial parotid lymph nodes

Mastoid lymph nodes

Occipital lymph nodes

Sternocleidomastoid muscle
(cut surface)

Jugulodigastric lymph node

Deep lateral cervical lymph nodes

Levator scapulae muscle

Superficial lateral cervical lymph nodes

Middle scalene muscle

Deep lateral cervical lymph nodes

Brachial plexus,
Transverse cervical artery

Trapezius muscle

Subclavian artery,
Supraclavicular lymph nodes

Right lymphatic (= thoracic) duct
(lying behind)

Deep parotid lymph nodes,
Masseter muscle

Facial vein and artery

Facial lymph nodes
– Buccinator lymph node
– Mandibular lymph node

Submandibular lymph nodes

Submental lymph nodes

Internal jugular vein,
External carotid artery, Hypoglossal nerve [XII]

Infrahyoid lymph nodes

Superior belly
of omohyoid muscle

Prelaryngeal lymph nodes

Pretracheal lymph nodes

Jugulo-omohyoid lymph node

Jugular trunk
(lying behind)

81 Lymphatic vessels and lymph nodes
of the head and neck (40%)
Schematic representations, right lateral aspect

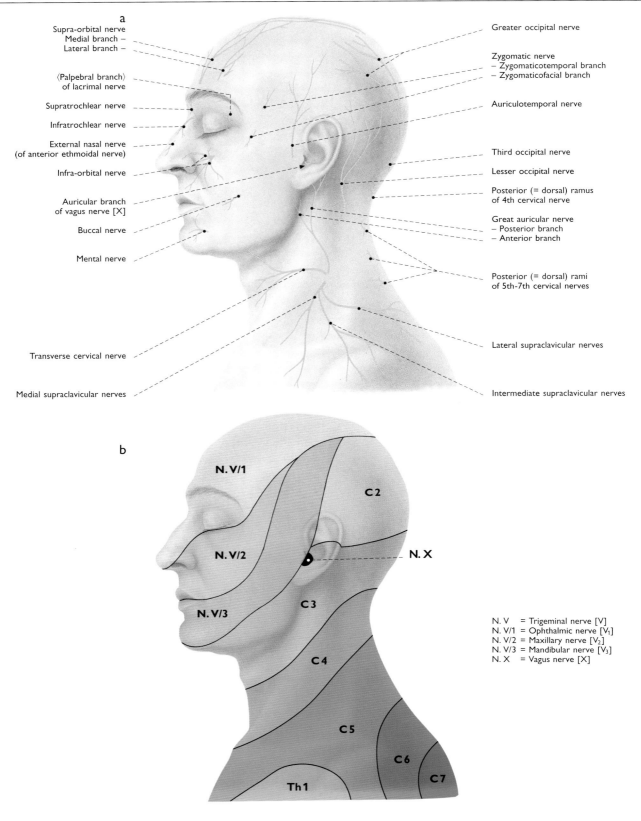

a

Supra-orbital nerve
Medial branch –
Lateral branch –

⟨Palpebral branch⟩
of lacrimal nerve

Supratrochlear nerve

Infratrochlear nerve

External nasal nerve
(of anterior ethmoidal nerve)

Infra-orbital nerve

Auricular branch
of vagus nerve [X]

Buccal nerve

Mental nerve

Transverse cervical nerve

Medial supraclavicular nerves

Greater occipital nerve

Zygomatic nerve
– Zygomaticotemporal branch
– Zygomaticofacial branch

Auriculotemporal nerve

Third occipital nerve

Lesser occipital nerve

Posterior (= dorsal) ramus
of 4th cervical nerve

Great auricular nerve
– Posterior branch
– Anterior branch

Posterior (= dorsal) rami
of 5th-7th cervical nerves

Lateral supraclavicular nerves

Intermediate supraclavicular nerves

b

N. V/1

C 2

N. V/2

N. X

N. V/3

C 3

C 4

C 5

C 6

C 7

Th 1

N. V   = Trigeminal nerve [V]
N. V/1 = Ophthalmic nerve [V₁]
N. V/2 = Maxillary nerve [V₂]
N. V/3 = Mandibular nerve [V₃]
N. X   = Vagus nerve [X]

82 Cutaneous and segmental innervation
of the head and neck (30%)
Schematic representations, left lateral aspect
a Cutaneous nerves
b Segmental innervation

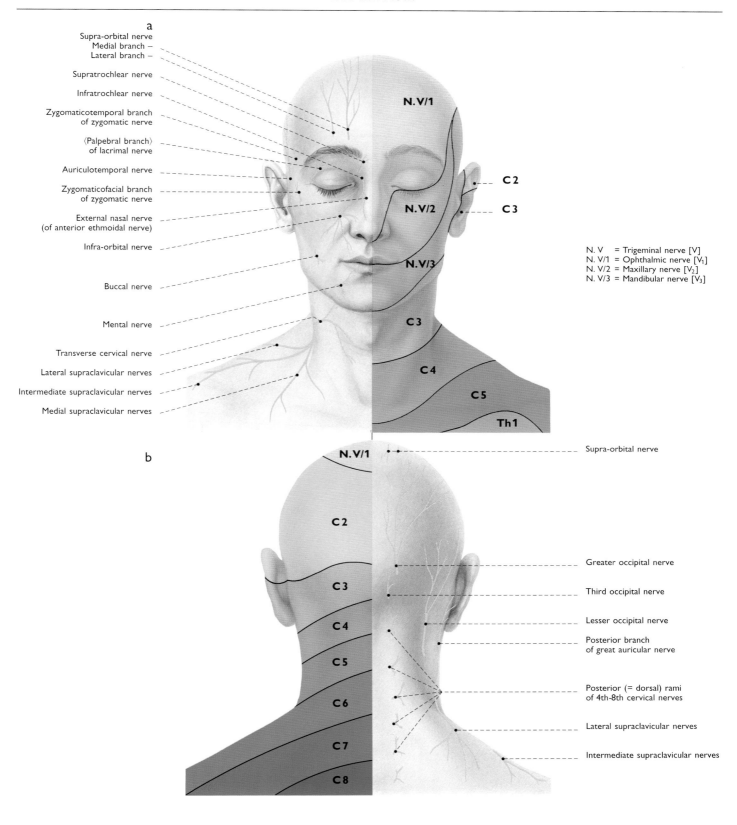

a

Supra-orbital nerve
Medial branch –
Lateral branch –

Supratrochlear nerve

Infratrochlear nerve

Zygomaticotemporal branch
of zygomatic nerve

⟨Palpebral branch⟩
of lacrimal nerve

Auriculotemporal nerve

Zygomaticofacial branch
of zygomatic nerve

External nasal nerve
(of anterior ethmoidal nerve)

Infra-orbital nerve

Buccal nerve

Mental nerve

Transverse cervical nerve

Lateral supraclavicular nerves

Intermediate supraclavicular nerves

Medial supraclavicular nerves

N.V/1

N.V/2

N.V/3

C 2

C 3

C 3

C 4

C 5

Th 1

N. V   = Trigeminal nerve [V]
N. V/1 = Ophthalmic nerve [V₁]
N. V/2 = Maxillary nerve [V₂]
N. V/3 = Mandibular nerve [V₃]

b

N.V/1

C 2

C 3

C 4

C 5

C 6

C 7

C 8

Supra-orbital nerve

Greater occipital nerve

Third occipital nerve

Lesser occipital nerve

Posterior branch
of great auricular nerve

Posterior (= dorsal) rami
of 4th-8th cervical nerves

Lateral supraclavicular nerves

Intermediate supraclavicular nerves

83 Cutaneous and segmental innervation
    of the head and neck (30%)
    Schematic representations
    a Anterior aspect
    b Posterior aspect

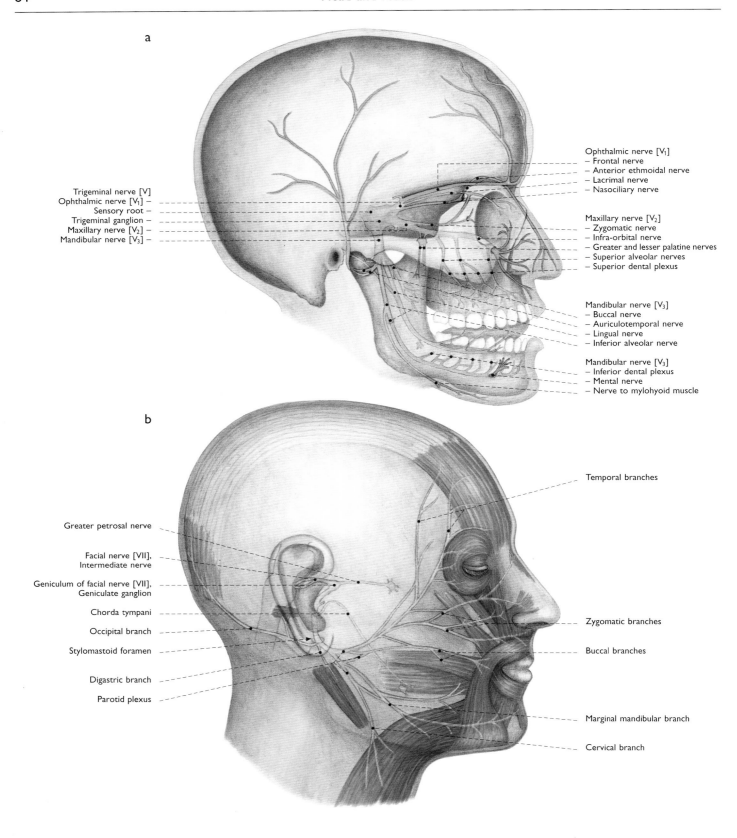

a

Ophthalmic nerve [V₁]
– Frontal nerve
– Anterior ethmoidal nerve
– Lacrimal nerve
– Nasociliary nerve

Trigeminal nerve [V]
Ophthalmic nerve [V₁] –
Sensory root –
Trigeminal ganglion –
Maxillary nerve [V₂] –
Mandibular nerve [V₃] –

Maxillary nerve [V₂]
– Zygomatic nerve
– Infra-orbital nerve
– Greater and lesser palatine nerves
– Superior alveolar nerves
– Superior dental plexus

Mandibular nerve [V₃]
– Buccal nerve
– Auriculotemporal nerve
– Lingual nerve
– Inferior alveolar nerve

Mandibular nerve [V₃]
– Inferior dental plexus
– Mental nerve
– Nerve to mylohyoid muscle

b

Temporal branches

Greater petrosal nerve

Facial nerve [VII],
Intermediate nerve

Geniculum of facial nerve [VII],
Geniculate ganglion

Chorda tympani

Occipital branch

Stylomastoid foramen

Digastric branch

Parotid plexus

Zygomatic branches

Buccal branches

Marginal mandibular branch

Cervical branch

84 Nerves of the head (50%)
Schematic representations, right lateral aspect
a Ramification of the trigeminal nerve (N. V) in the deep facial region
b Ramification of the facial nerve (N. VII) in the superficial facial region

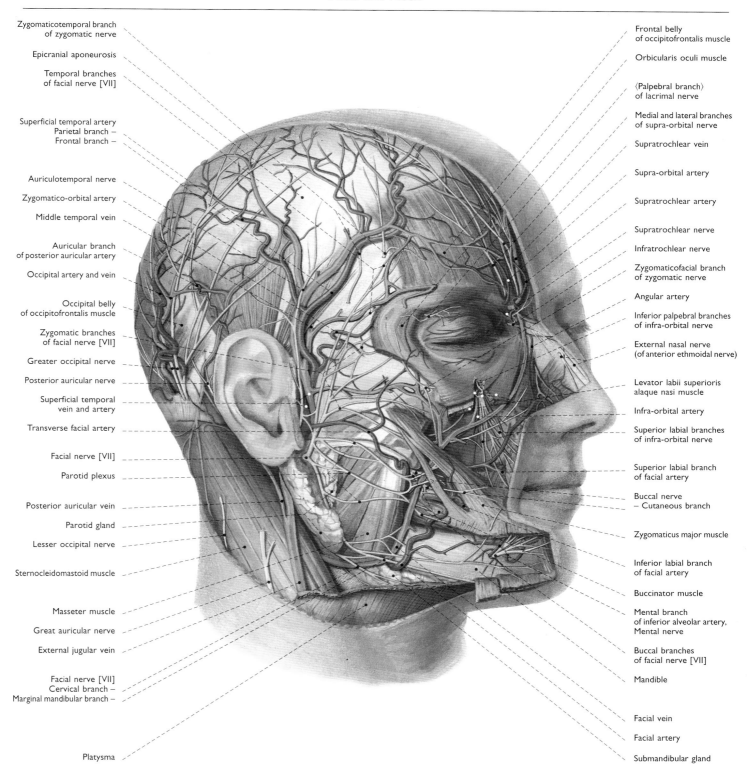

Zygomaticotemporal branch
of zygomatic nerve

Epicranial aponeurosis

Temporal branches
of facial nerve [VII]

Superficial temporal artery
Parietal branch —
Frontal branch —

Auriculotemporal nerve

Zygomatico-orbital artery

Middle temporal vein

Auricular branch
of posterior auricular artery

Occipital artery and vein

Occipital belly
of occipitofrontalis muscle

Zygomatic branches
of facial nerve [VII]

Greater occipital nerve

Posterior auricular nerve

Superficial temporal
vein and artery

Transverse facial artery

Facial nerve [VII]

Parotid plexus

Posterior auricular vein

Parotid gland

Lesser occipital nerve

Sternocleidomastoid muscle

Masseter muscle

Great auricular nerve

External jugular vein

Facial nerve [VII]
Cervical branch —
Marginal mandibular branch —

Platysma

Frontal belly
of occipitofrontalis muscle

Orbicularis oculi muscle

⟨Palpebral branch⟩
of lacrimal nerve

Medial and lateral branches
of supra-orbital nerve

Supratrochlear vein

Supra-orbital artery

Supratrochlear artery

Supratrochlear nerve

Infratrochlear nerve

Zygomaticofacial branch
of zygomatic nerve

Angular artery

Inferior palpebral branches
of infra-orbital nerve

External nasal nerve
(of anterior ethmoidal nerve)

Levator labii superioris
alaque nasi muscle

Infra-orbital artery

Superior labial branches
of infra-orbital nerve

Superior labial branch
of facial artery

Buccal nerve
– Cutaneous branch

Zygomaticus major muscle

Inferior labial branch
of facial artery

Buccinator muscle

Mental branch
of inferior alveolar artery,
Mental nerve

Buccal branches
of facial nerve [VII]

Mandible

Facial vein

Facial artery

Submandibular gland

**85 Superficial blood vessels and nerves
of the head** (60%)
Right lateral aspect

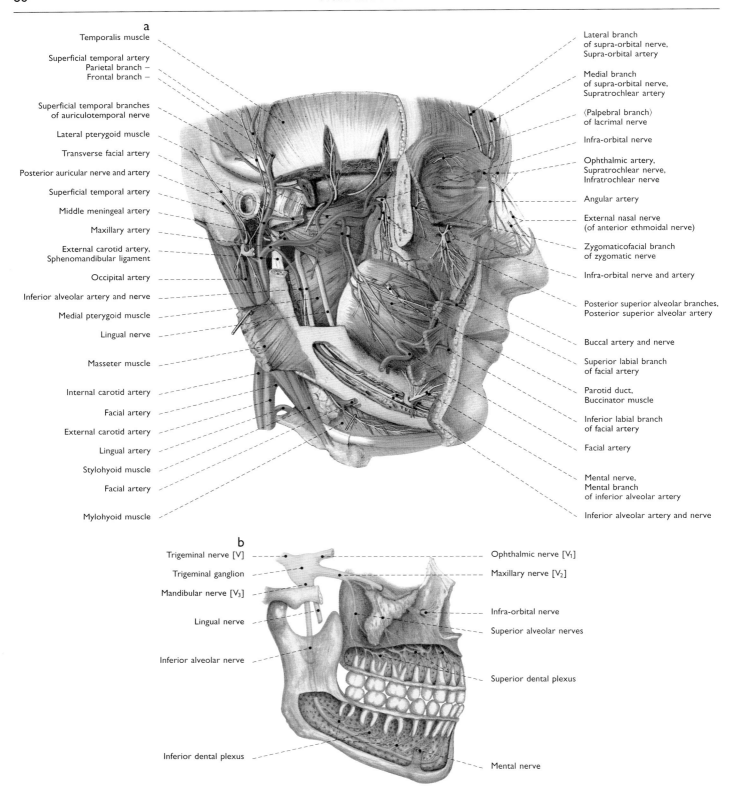

a

Temporalis muscle

Superficial temporal artery
Parietal branch –
Frontal branch –

Superficial temporal branches
of auriculotemporal nerve

Lateral pterygoid muscle

Transverse facial artery

Posterior auricular nerve and artery

Superficial temporal artery

Middle meningeal artery

Maxillary artery

External carotid artery,
Sphenomandibular ligament

Occipital artery

Inferior alveolar artery and nerve

Medial pterygoid muscle

Lingual nerve

Masseter muscle

Internal carotid artery

Facial artery

External carotid artery

Lingual artery

Stylohyoid muscle

Facial artery

Mylohyoid muscle

Lateral branch
of supra-orbital nerve,
Supra-orbital artery

Medial branch
of supra-orbital nerve,
Supratrochlear artery

⟨Palpebral branch⟩
of lacrimal nerve

Infra-orbital nerve

Ophthalmic artery,
Supratrochlear nerve,
Infratrochlear nerve

Angular artery

External nasal nerve
(of anterior ethmoidal nerve)

Zygomaticofacial branch
of zygomatic nerve

Infra-orbital nerve and artery

Posterior superior alveolar branches,
Posterior superior alveolar artery

Buccal artery and nerve

Superior labial branch
of facial artery

Parotid duct,
Buccinator muscle

Inferior labial branch
of facial artery

Facial artery

Mental nerve,
Mental branch
of inferior alveolar artery

Inferior alveolar artery and nerve

b

Trigeminal nerve [V]

Trigeminal ganglion

Mandibular nerve [V₃]

Lingual nerve

Inferior alveolar nerve

Inferior dental plexus

Ophthalmic nerve [V₁]

Maxillary nerve [V₂]

Infra-orbital nerve

Superior alveolar nerves

Superior dental plexus

Mental nerve

**86 Arteries and nerves
of the deep lateral facial region** (65%)

Right lateral aspect
a The zygomatic arch and the ramus of the mandible were removed,
the mandibular canal was opened.
b Innervation of the teeth in the upper and lower jaws by branches
of the trigeminal nerve (N. V), schematic representation

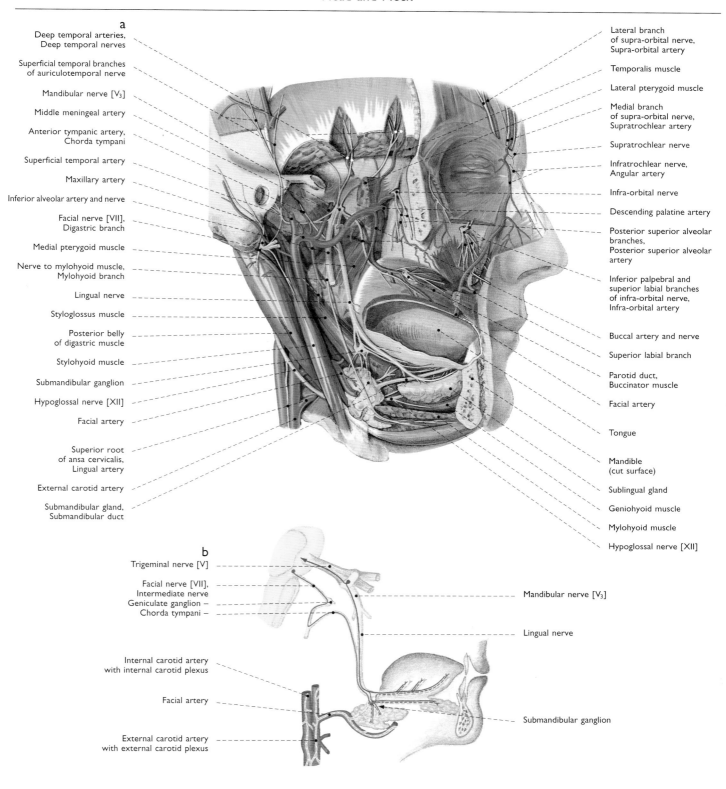

a
Deep temporal arteries,
Deep temporal nerves

Superficial temporal branches
of auriculotemporal nerve

Mandibular nerve [V₃]

Middle meningeal artery

Anterior tympanic artery,
Chorda tympani

Superficial temporal artery

Maxillary artery

Inferior alveolar artery and nerve

Facial nerve [VII],
Digastric branch

Medial pterygoid muscle

Nerve to mylohyoid muscle,
Mylohyoid branch

Lingual nerve

Styloglossus muscle

Posterior belly
of digastric muscle

Stylohyoid muscle

Submandibular ganglion

Hypoglossal nerve [XII]

Facial artery

Superior root
of ansa cervicalis,
Lingual artery

External carotid artery

Submandibular gland,
Submandibular duct

Lateral branch
of supra-orbital nerve,
Supra-orbital artery

Temporalis muscle

Lateral pterygoid muscle

Medial branch
of supra-orbital nerve,
Supratrochlear artery

Supratrochlear nerve

Infratrochlear nerve,
Angular artery

Infra-orbital nerve

Descending palatine artery

Posterior superior alveolar
branches,
Posterior superior alveolar
artery

Inferior palpebral and
superior labial branches
of infra-orbital nerve,
Infra-orbital artery

Buccal artery and nerve

Superior labial branch

Parotid duct,
Buccinator muscle

Facial artery

Tongue

Mandible
(cut surface)

Sublingual gland

Geniohyoid muscle

Mylohyoid muscle

Hypoglossal nerve [XII]

b
Trigeminal nerve [V]

Facial nerve [VII],
Intermediate nerve
Geniculate ganglion
Chorda tympani

Internal carotid artery
with internal carotid plexus

Facial artery

External carotid artery
with external carotid plexus

Mandibular nerve [V₃]

Lingual nerve

Submandibular ganglion

87 Arteries and nerves
of the deep lateral facial region
Right lateral aspect
a The zygomatic arch, the right half of the mandible and parts
of the lateral pterygoid muscle were removed (65%).
b Submandibular ganglion and innervation
of the submandibular and sublingual glands (50%),
schematic representation

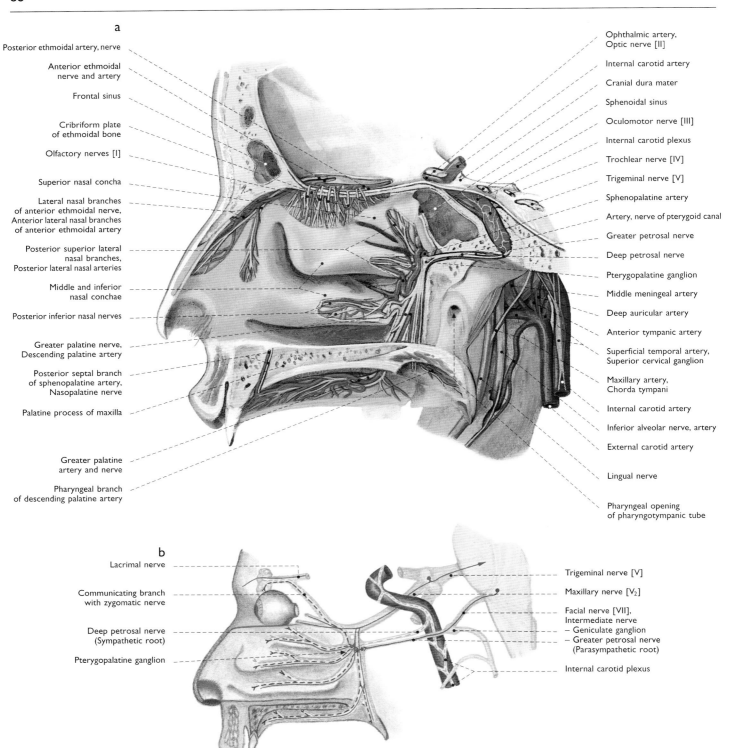

a

Posterior ethmoidal artery, nerve

Anterior ethmoidal nerve and artery

Frontal sinus

Cribriform plate of ethmoidal bone

Olfactory nerves [I]

Superior nasal concha

Lateral nasal branches of anterior ethmoidal nerve, Anterior lateral nasal branches of anterior ethmoidal artery

Posterior superior lateral nasal branches, Posterior lateral nasal arteries

Middle and inferior nasal conchae

Posterior inferior nasal nerves

Greater palatine nerve, Descending palatine artery

Posterior septal branch of sphenopalatine artery, Nasopalatine nerve

Palatine process of maxilla

Greater palatine artery and nerve

Pharyngeal branch of descending palatine artery

Ophthalmic artery, Optic nerve [II]

Internal carotid artery

Cranial dura mater

Sphenoidal sinus

Oculomotor nerve [III]

Internal carotid plexus

Trochlear nerve [IV]

Trigeminal nerve [V]

Sphenopalatine artery

Artery, nerve of pterygoid canal

Greater petrosal nerve

Deep petrosal nerve

Pterygopalatine ganglion

Middle meningeal artery

Deep auricular artery

Anterior tympanic artery

Superficial temporal artery, Superior cervical ganglion

Maxillary artery, Chorda tympani

Internal carotid artery

Inferior alveolar nerve, artery

External carotid artery

Lingual nerve

Pharyngeal opening of pharyngotympanic tube

b

Lacrimal nerve

Communicating branch with zygomatic nerve

Deep petrosal nerve (Sympathetic root)

Pterygopalatine ganglion

Trigeminal nerve [V]

Maxillary nerve [V₂]

Facial nerve [VII], Intermediate nerve
– Geniculate ganglion
– Greater petrosal nerve (Parasympathetic root)

Internal carotid plexus

88   Arteries and nerves of the deep medial facial region

Medial aspect
a   Lateral wall of the nasal cavity, palate, infratemporal, and pterygopalatine fossae (90%)
b   Pterygopalatine ganglion and innervation of the lacrimal gland and the mucous membranes of nasal cavity and palate (50%), schematic representation

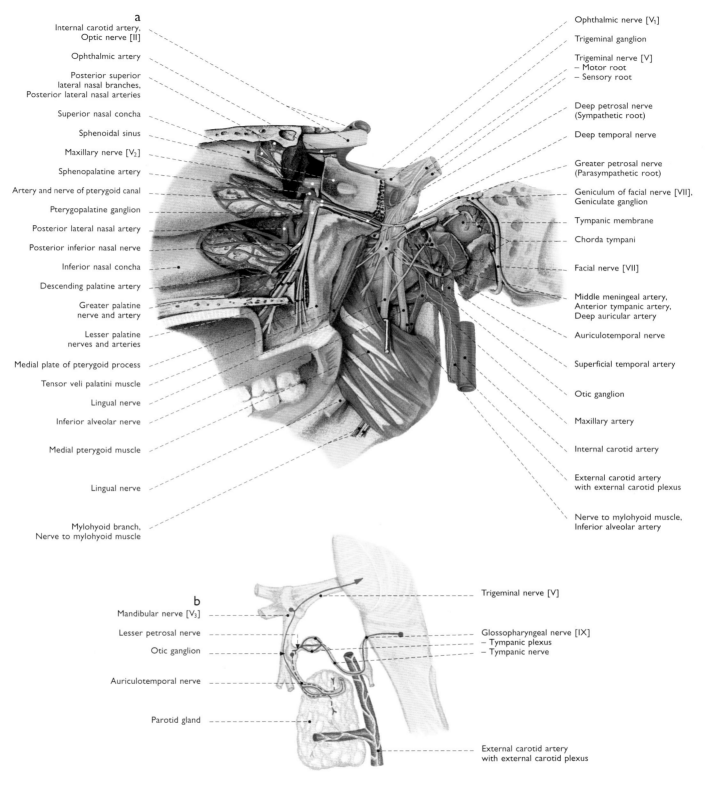

a
Internal carotid artery,
Optic nerve [II]

Ophthalmic artery

Posterior superior
lateral nasal branches,
Posterior lateral nasal arteries

Superior nasal concha

Sphenoidal sinus

Maxillary nerve [V₂]

Sphenopalatine artery

Artery and nerve of pterygoid canal

Pterygopalatine ganglion

Posterior lateral nasal artery

Posterior inferior nasal nerve

Inferior nasal concha

Descending palatine artery

Greater palatine
nerve and artery

Lesser palatine
nerves and arteries

Medial plate of pterygoid process

Tensor veli palatini muscle

Lingual nerve

Inferior alveolar nerve

Medial pterygoid muscle

Lingual nerve

Mylohyoid branch,
Nerve to mylohyoid muscle

Ophthalmic nerve [V₁]

Trigeminal ganglion

Trigeminal nerve [V]
– Motor root
– Sensory root

Deep petrosal nerve
(Sympathetic root)

Deep temporal nerve

Greater petrosal nerve
(Parasympathetic root)

Geniculum of facial nerve [VII],
Geniculate ganglion

Tympanic membrane

Chorda tympani

Facial nerve [VII]

Middle meningeal artery,
Anterior tympanic artery,
Deep auricular artery

Auriculotemporal nerve

Superficial temporal artery

Otic ganglion

Maxillary artery

Internal carotid artery

External carotid artery
with external carotid plexus

Nerve to mylohyoid muscle,
Inferior alveolar artery

b

Mandibular nerve [V₃]

Lesser petrosal nerve

Otic ganglion

Auriculotemporal nerve

Parotid gland

Trigeminal nerve [V]

Glossopharyngeal nerve [IX]
– Tympanic plexus
– Tympanic nerve

External carotid artery
with external carotid plexus

**89 Arteries and nerves
of the deep medial facial region**

Medial aspect
a Lateral wall of the nasal cavity, infratemporal and pterygopalatine
   fossae. The facial canal was opened (90%).
b Otic ganglion and innervation of the parotid gland (50%),
   schematic representation

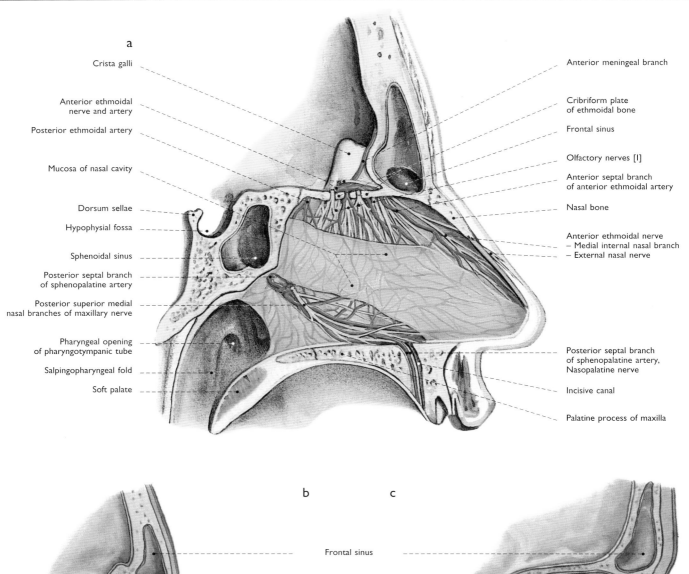

a

Crista galli

Anterior ethmoidal
nerve and artery

Posterior ethmoidal artery

Mucosa of nasal cavity

Dorsum sellae

Hypophysial fossa

Sphenoidal sinus

Posterior septal branch
of sphenopalatine artery

Posterior superior medial
nasal branches of maxillary nerve

Pharyngeal opening
of pharyngotympanic tube

Salpingopharyngeal fold

Soft palate

Anterior meningeal branch

Cribriform plate
of ethmoidal bone

Frontal sinus

Olfactory nerves [I]

Anterior septal branch
of anterior ethmoidal artery

Nasal bone

Anterior ethmoidal nerve
– Medial internal nasal branch
– External nasal nerve

Posterior septal branch
of sphenopalatine artery,
Nasopalatine nerve

Incisive canal

Palatine process of maxilla

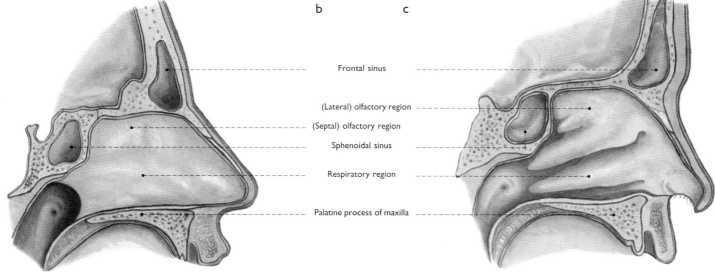

b   c

Frontal sinus

(Lateral) olfactory region

(Septal) olfactory region

Sphenoidal sinus

Respiratory region

Palatine process of maxilla

90   Arteries and nerves
      of the deep medial facial region
       Medial aspect
    a   Nasal septum, sagittal section slightly to the right of the median
       plane. The nasal mucous membrane was partially removed (90%).
  b, c   Olfactory regions (50%), marked by yellow color,
    b   at the nasal septum
    c   at the lateral wall of the nasal cavity

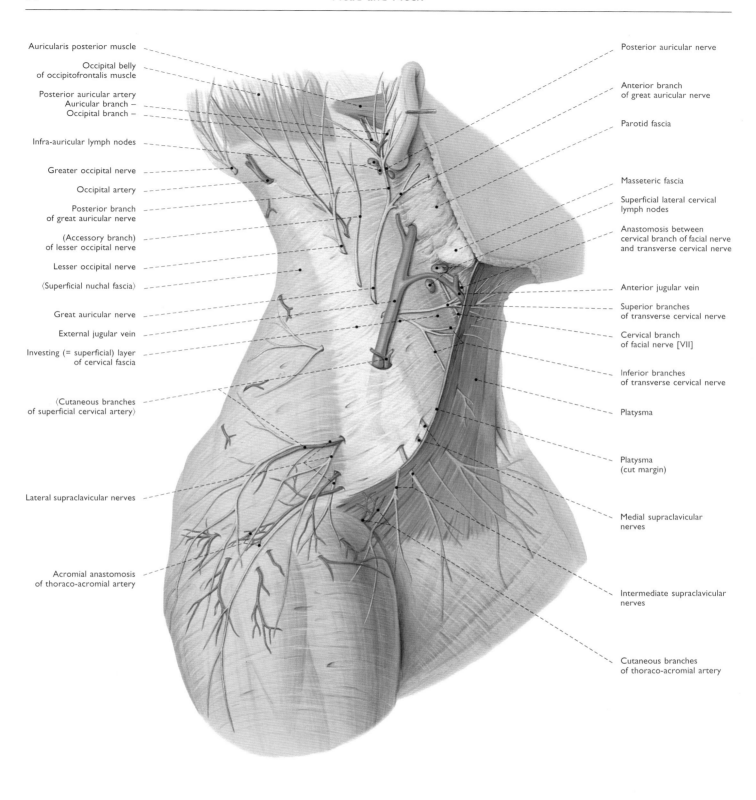

Auricularis posterior muscle

Occipital belly
of occipitofrontalis muscle

Posterior auricular artery
Auricular branch –
Occipital branch –

Infra-auricular lymph nodes

Greater occipital nerve

Occipital artery

Posterior branch
of great auricular nerve

(Accessory branch)
of lesser occipital nerve

Lesser occipital nerve

⟨Superficial nuchal fascia⟩

Great auricular nerve

External jugular vein

Investing (= superficial) layer
of cervical fascia

⟨Cutaneous branches
of superficial cervical artery⟩

Lateral supraclavicular nerves

Acromial anastomosis
of thoraco-acromial artery

Posterior auricular nerve

Anterior branch
of great auricular nerve

Parotid fascia

Masseteric fascia

Superficial lateral cervical
lymph nodes

Anastomosis between
cervical branch of facial nerve
and transverse cervical nerve

Anterior jugular vein

Superior branches
of transverse cervical nerve

Cervical branch
of facial nerve [VII]

Inferior branches
of transverse cervical nerve

Platysma

Platysma
(cut margin)

Medial supraclavicular
nerves

Intermediate supraclavicular
nerves

Cutaneous branches
of thoraco-acromial artery

**91 Subcutaneous blood vessels and nerves
of the neck region** (50%)
Right lateral aspect

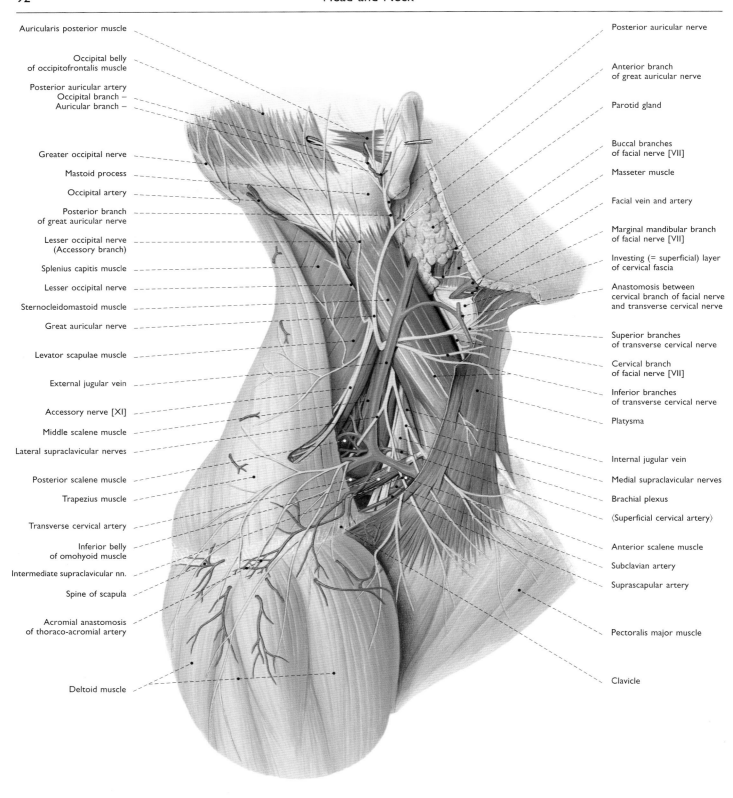

Auricularis posterior muscle

Occipital belly
of occipitofrontalis muscle

Posterior auricular artery
Occipital branch —
Auricular branch —

Greater occipital nerve

Mastoid process

Occipital artery

Posterior branch
of great auricular nerve

Lesser occipital nerve
(Accessory branch)

Splenius capitis muscle

Lesser occipital nerve

Sternocleidomastoid muscle

Great auricular nerve

Levator scapulae muscle

External jugular vein

Accessory nerve [XI]

Middle scalene muscle

Lateral supraclavicular nerves

Posterior scalene muscle

Trapezius muscle

Transverse cervical artery

Inferior belly
of omohyoid muscle

Intermediate supraclavicular nn.

Spine of scapula

Acromial anastomosis
of thoraco-acromial artery

Deltoid muscle

Posterior auricular nerve

Anterior branch
of great auricular nerve

Parotid gland

Buccal branches
of facial nerve [VII]

Masseter muscle

Facial vein and artery

Marginal mandibular branch
of facial nerve [VII]

Investing (= superficial) layer
of cervical fascia

Anastomosis between
cervical branch of facial nerve
and transverse cervical nerve

Superior branches
of transverse cervical nerve

Cervical branch
of facial nerve [VII]

Inferior branches
of transverse cervical nerve

Platysma

Internal jugular vein

Medial supraclavicular nerves

Brachial plexus

⟨Superficial cervical artery⟩

Anterior scalene muscle

Subclavian artery

Suprascapular artery

Pectoralis major muscle

Clavicle

**92 Superficial blood vessels and nerves
of the neck region** (50%)
Right lateral aspect

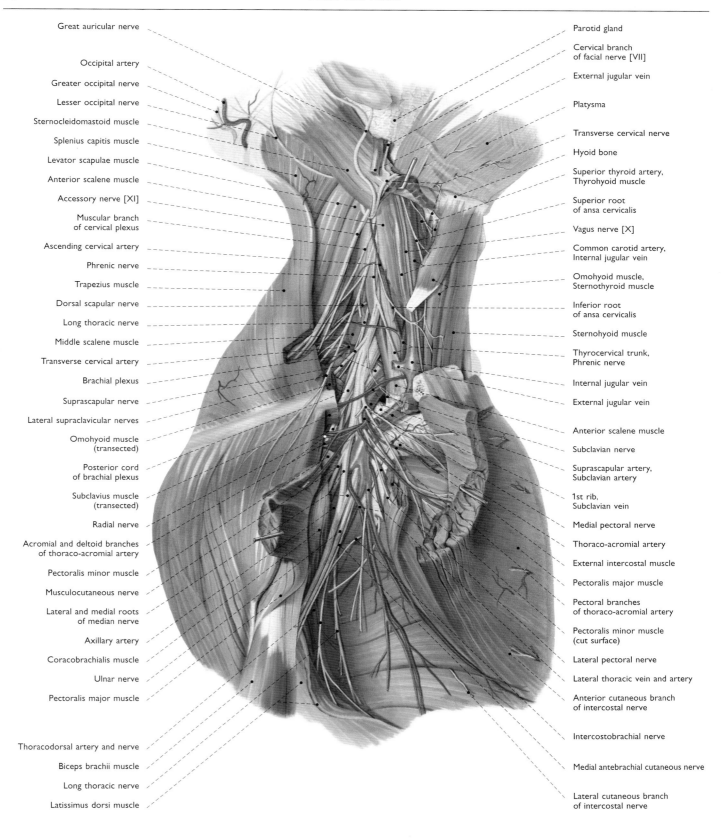

Great auricular nerve

Occipital artery

Greater occipital nerve

Lesser occipital nerve

Sternocleidomastoid muscle

Splenius capitis muscle

Levator scapulae muscle

Anterior scalene muscle

Accessory nerve [XI]

Muscular branch
of cervical plexus

Ascending cervical artery

Phrenic nerve

Trapezius muscle

Dorsal scapular nerve

Long thoracic nerve

Middle scalene muscle

Transverse cervical artery

Brachial plexus

Suprascapular nerve

Lateral supraclavicular nerves

Omohyoid muscle
(transected)

Posterior cord
of brachial plexus

Subclavius muscle
(transected)

Radial nerve

Acromial and deltoid branches
of thoraco-acromial artery

Pectoralis minor muscle

Musculocutaneous nerve

Lateral and medial roots
of median nerve

Axillary artery

Coracobrachialis muscle

Ulnar nerve

Pectoralis major muscle

Thoracodorsal artery and nerve

Biceps brachii muscle

Long thoracic nerve

Latissimus dorsi muscle

Parotid gland

Cervical branch
of facial nerve [VII]

External jugular vein

Platysma

Transverse cervical nerve

Hyoid bone

Superior thyroid artery,
Thyrohyoid muscle

Superior root
of ansa cervicalis

Vagus nerve [X]

Common carotid artery,
Internal jugular vein

Omohyoid muscle,
Sternothyroid muscle

Inferior root
of ansa cervicalis

Sternohyoid muscle

Thyrocervical trunk,
Phrenic nerve

Internal jugular vein

External jugular vein

Anterior scalene muscle

Subclavian nerve

Suprascapular artery,
Subclavian artery

1st rib,
Subclavian vein

Medial pectoral nerve

Thoraco-acromial artery

External intercostal muscle

Pectoralis major muscle

Pectoral branches
of thoraco-acromial artery

Pectoralis minor muscle
(cut surface)

Lateral pectoral nerve

Lateral thoracic vein and artery

Anterior cutaneous branch
of intercostal nerve

Intercostobrachial nerve

Medial antebrachial cutaneous nerve

Lateral cutaneous branch
of intercostal nerve

**93 Blood vessels and nerves
of the neck, axilla, and thorax** (50%)
The platysma and the sternocleidomastoid muscle
were removed. Right lateral aspect

a

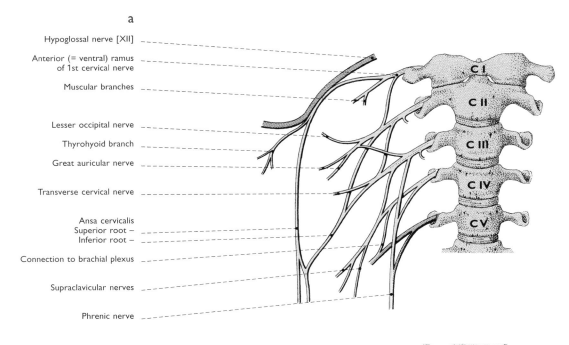

Hypoglossal nerve [XII]

Anterior (= ventral) ramus
of 1st cervical nerve

Muscular branches

Lesser occipital nerve

Thyrohyoid branch

Great auricular nerve

Transverse cervical nerve

Ansa cervicalis
Superior root –
Inferior root –

Connection to brachial plexus

Supraclavicular nerves

Phrenic nerve

b

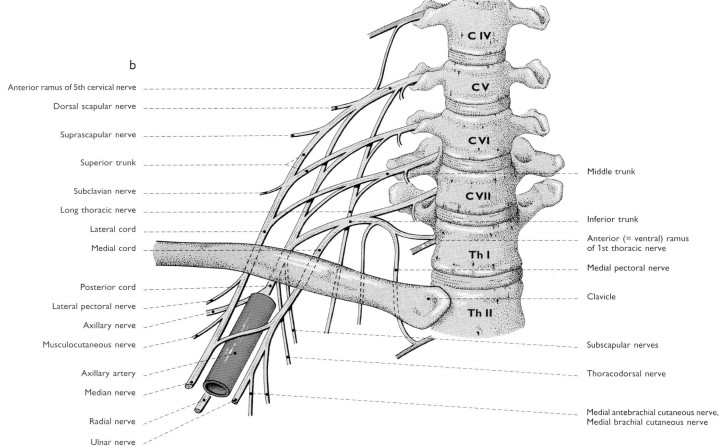

Anterior ramus of 5th cervical nerve

Dorsal scapular nerve

Suprascapular nerve

Superior trunk

Subclavian nerve

Long thoracic nerve

Lateral cord

Medial cord

Posterior cord

Lateral pectoral nerve

Axillary nerve

Musculocutaneous nerve

Axillary artery

Median nerve

Radial nerve

Ulnar nerve

Middle trunk

Inferior trunk

Anterior (= ventral) ramus
of 1st thoracic nerve

Medial pectoral nerve

Clavicle

Subscapular nerves

Thoracodorsal nerve

Medial antebrachial cutaneous nerve,
Medial brachial cutaneous nerve

94 Cervical and brachial plexuses

Schematic representations, ventral aspect
a Cervical plexus
b Brachial plexus

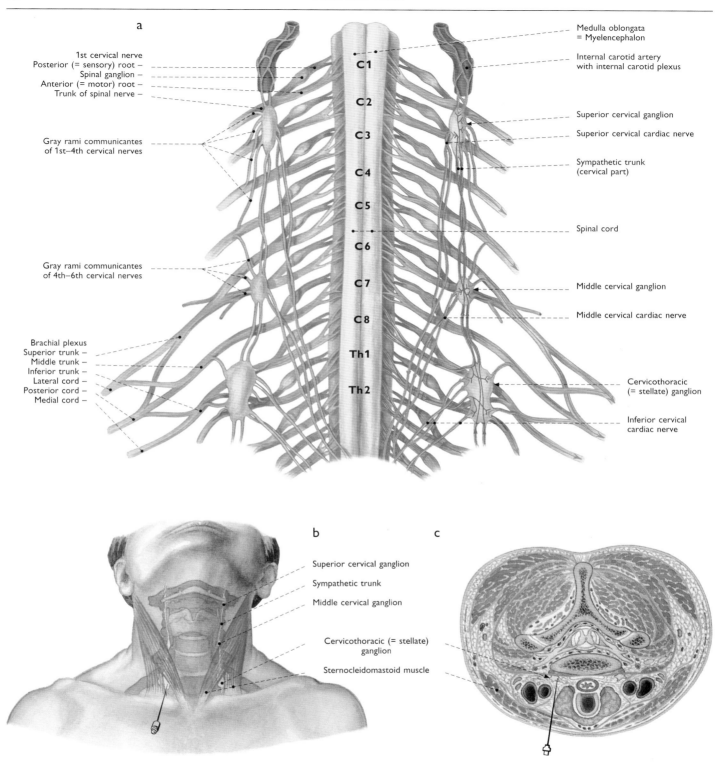

a

1st cervical nerve
Posterior (= sensory) root –
Spinal ganglion –
Anterior (= motor) root –
Trunk of spinal nerve –

Gray rami communicantes
of 1st–4th cervical nerves

Gray rami communicantes
of 4th–6th cervical nerves

Brachial plexus
Superior trunk –
Middle trunk –
Inferior trunk –
Lateral cord –
Posterior cord –
Medial cord –

C1
C2
C3
C4
C5
C6
C7
C8
Th1
Th2

Medulla oblongata
= Myelencephalon

Internal carotid artery
with internal carotid plexus

Superior cervical ganglion
Superior cervical cardiac nerve

Sympathetic trunk
(cervical part)

Spinal cord

Middle cervical ganglion

Middle cervical cardiac nerve

Cervicothoracic
(= stellate) ganglion

Inferior cervical
cardiac nerve

b
Superior cervical ganglion
Sympathetic trunk
Middle cervical ganglion
Cervicothoracic (= stellate)
ganglion
Sternocleidomastoid muscle

c

95 Sympathetic part of the autonomic division
of peripheral nervous system in the neck

a Essential circuitry and origins of the sympathetic nervous system
in the neck and upper thorax. On the right side of the picture,
the preganglionic neurons of the sympathetic efferent nervous system
are indicated by blue lines, the postganglionic neurons by green ones (60%).
Schematic representation, ventral aspect
b, c Puncture of the cervicothoracic (= stellate) ganglion
b Ventral aspect (25%)
c Transverse section at the level of the first thoracic vertebra (Th1) (50%),
superior aspect

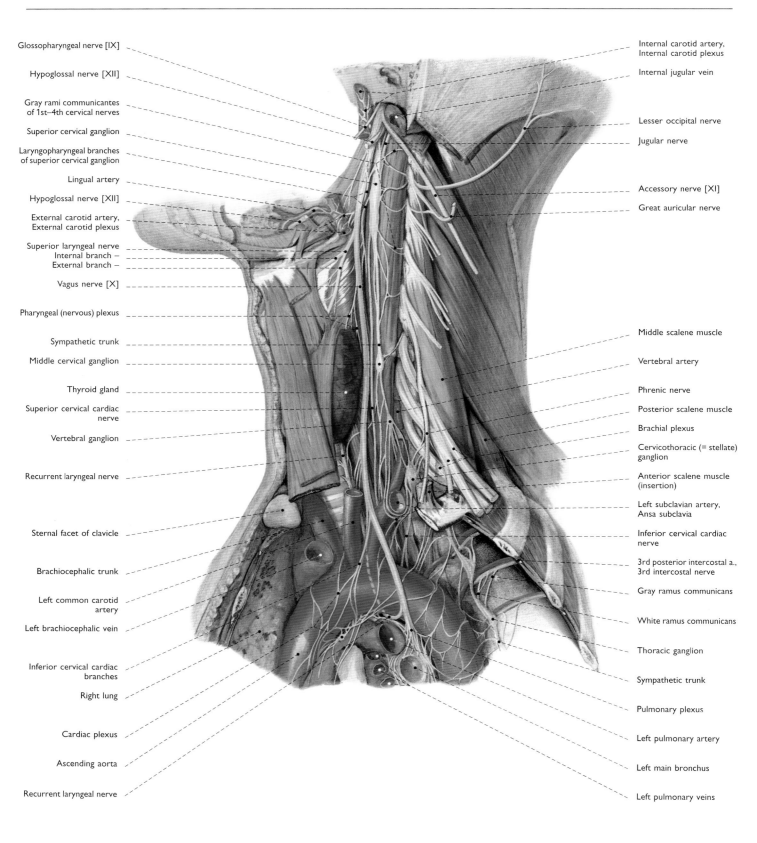

Glossopharyngeal nerve [IX]

Hypoglossal nerve [XII]

Gray rami communicantes
of 1st–4th cervical nerves

Superior cervical ganglion

Laryngopharyngeal branches
of superior cervical ganglion

Lingual artery

Hypoglossal nerve [XII]

External carotid artery,
External carotid plexus

Superior laryngeal nerve
Internal branch –
External branch –

Vagus nerve [X]

Pharyngeal (nervous) plexus

Sympathetic trunk

Middle cervical ganglion

Thyroid gland

Superior cervical cardiac
nerve

Vertebral ganglion

Recurrent laryngeal nerve

Sternal facet of clavicle

Brachiocephalic trunk

Left common carotid
artery

Left brachiocephalic vein

Inferior cervical cardiac
branches

Right lung

Cardiac plexus

Ascending aorta

Recurrent laryngeal nerve

Internal carotid artery,
Internal carotid plexus

Internal jugular vein

Lesser occipital nerve

Jugular nerve

Accessory nerve [XI]

Great auricular nerve

Middle scalene muscle

Vertebral artery

Phrenic nerve

Posterior scalene muscle

Brachial plexus

Cervicothoracic (= stellate)
ganglion

Anterior scalene muscle
(insertion)

Left subclavian artery,
Ansa subclavia

Inferior cervical cardiac
nerve

3rd posterior intercostal a.,
3rd intercostal nerve

Gray ramus communicans

White ramus communicans

Thoracic ganglion

Sympathetic trunk

Pulmonary plexus

Left pulmonary artery

Left main bronchus

Left pulmonary veins

96 Autonomic division of the peripheral nervous system
in the neck and the upper thorax (60%)
Left lateral aspect

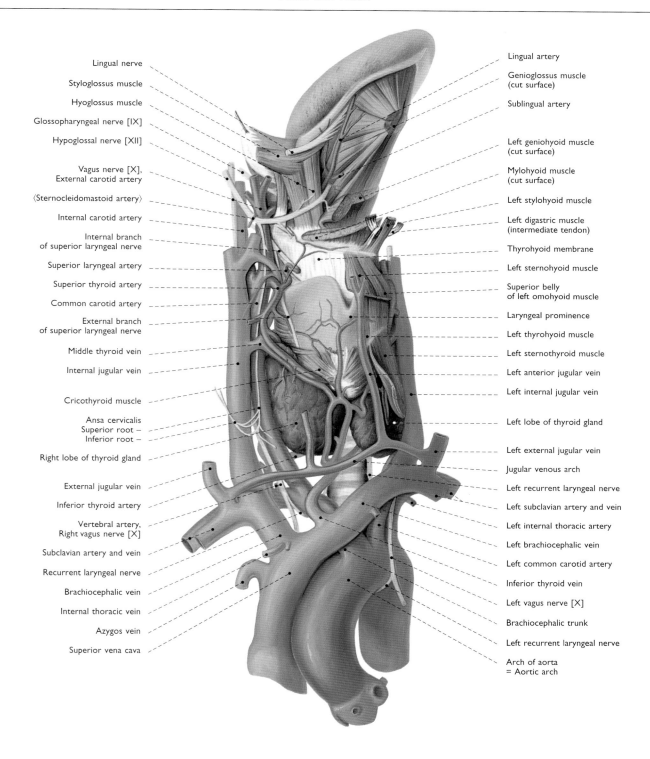

Lingual nerve

Styloglossus muscle

Hyoglossus muscle

Glossopharyngeal nerve [IX]

Hypoglossal nerve [XII]

Vagus nerve [X],
External carotid artery

⟨Sternocleidomastoid artery⟩

Internal carotid artery

Internal branch
of superior laryngeal nerve

Superior laryngeal artery

Superior thyroid artery

Common carotid artery

External branch
of superior laryngeal nerve

Middle thyroid vein

Internal jugular vein

Cricothyroid muscle

Ansa cervicalis
Superior root –
Inferior root –

Right lobe of thyroid gland

External jugular vein

Inferior thyroid artery

Vertebral artery,
Right vagus nerve [X]

Subclavian artery and vein

Recurrent laryngeal nerve

Brachiocephalic vein

Internal thoracic vein

Azygos vein

Superior vena cava

Lingual artery

Genioglossus muscle
(cut surface)

Sublingual artery

Left geniohyoid muscle
(cut surface)

Mylohyoid muscle
(cut surface)

Left stylohyoid muscle

Left digastric muscle
(intermediate tendon)

Thyrohyoid membrane

Left sternohyoid muscle

Superior belly
of left omohyoid muscle

Laryngeal prominence

Left thyrohyoid muscle

Left sternothyroid muscle

Left anterior jugular vein

Left internal jugular vein

Left lobe of thyroid gland

Left external jugular vein

Jugular venous arch

Left recurrent laryngeal nerve

Left subclavian artery and vein

Left internal thoracic artery

Left brachiocephalic vein

Left common carotid artery

Inferior thyroid vein

Left vagus nerve [X]

Brachiocephalic trunk

Left recurrent laryngeal nerve

Arch of aorta
= Aortic arch

97 Blood vessels and nerves
    of the cervical viscera and the tongue (70%)
    Right ventrolateral aspect

Zygomaticus major muscle

Facial nerve [VII]
Zygomatic branches –
Buccal branches –
Temporal branches –

Deep part
of masseter muscle

Transverse facial artery

Auriculotemporal nerve,
Zygomatico-orbital artery

Superficial temporal
artery and vein

Anterior auricular branches

Parotid plexus
of facial nerve [VII]

Parotid gland,
Posterior auricular artery

Marginal mandibular branch
and cervical branch (cut off)
of facial nerve [VII]

Posterior belly
of digastric muscle,
Stylohyoid muscle

Occipital artery,
Facial vein and artery

Accessory nerve [XI],
Retromandibular vein

Great auricular nerve,
Lesser occipital nerve
(cut off)

Trapezius muscle,
Levator scapulae muscle,
Hypoglossal nerve [XII]

Supraclavicular nerves,
External jugular vein

〈Superficial cervical
artery and vein〉

Clavicle,
Inferior belly
of omohyoid muscle

Dorsal scapular nerve,
Long thoracic nerve

Cephalic vein,
Acromial branch
of thoraco-acromial artery

Brachial plexus,
Subclavian nerve

Anterior scalene muscle

Parotid duct

Facial vein

Facial artery

Superficial part
of masseter muscle

Platysma
(turned cranially)

Mylohyoid muscle,
Submental artery

Mylohyoid muscle
(cut off)

Sublingual artery,
Hypoglossal nerve [XII]

Hyoglossus muscle,
Geniohyoid muscle

Submandibular gland,
Anterior belly
of digastric muscle

Hyoid bone

Suprahyoid branch
of lingual artery,
Superior belly
of omohyoid muscle,
Sternohyoid muscle

Infrahyoid branch,
Thyrohyoid branch
of ansa cervicalis

Superior laryngeal artery

Superior laryngeal nerve
– Internal branch
– External branch

Superior thyroid
vein and artery,
Cricothyroid branch

Transverse cervical nerve,
Right lobe of thyroid gland

Internal jugular vein,
Ansa cervicalis
– Inferior root
– Superior root

Suprascapular artery,
Anterior jugular vein

Sternocleidomastoid muscle
(turned caudally)

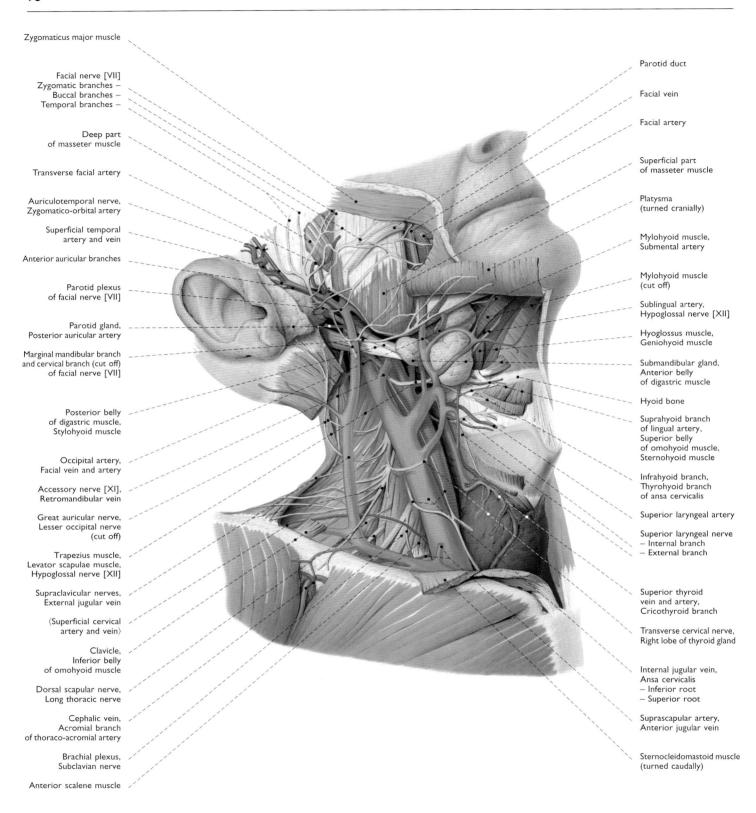

98   Blood vessels and nerves of the neck (60%)
The parotid gland, the sternocleidomastoid muscle,
the supra- and infrahyoid muscles were partially removed.
Right ventrolateral aspect

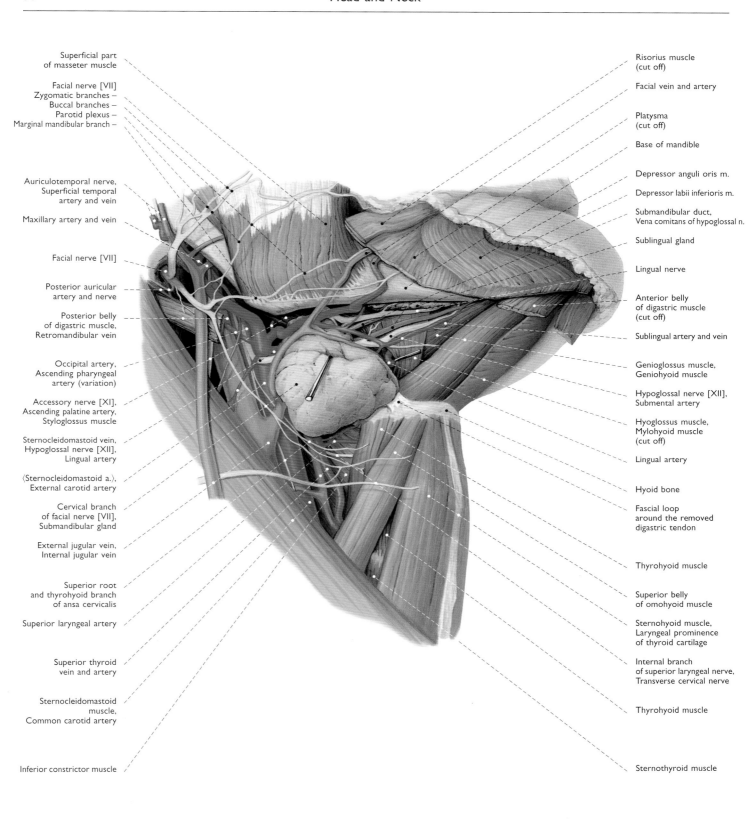

Superficial part
of masseter muscle

Facial nerve [VII]
Zygomatic branches –
Buccal branches –
Parotid plexus –
Marginal mandibular branch –

Auriculotemporal nerve,
Superficial temporal
artery and vein

Maxillary artery and vein

Facial nerve [VII]

Posterior auricular
artery and nerve

Posterior belly
of digastric muscle,
Retromandibular vein

Occipital artery,
Ascending pharyngeal
artery (variation)

Accessory nerve [XI],
Ascending palatine artery,
Styloglossus muscle

Sternocleidomastoid vein,
Hypoglossal nerve [XII],
Lingual artery

⟨Sternocleidomastoid a.⟩,
External carotid artery

Cervical branch
of facial nerve [VII],
Submandibular gland

External jugular vein,
Internal jugular vein

Superior root
and thyrohyoid branch
of ansa cervicalis

Superior laryngeal artery

Superior thyroid
vein and artery

Sternocleidomastoid
muscle,
Common carotid artery

Inferior constrictor muscle

Risorius muscle
(cut off)

Facial vein and artery

Platysma
(cut off)

Base of mandible

Depressor anguli oris m.

Depressor labii inferioris m.

Submandibular duct,
Vena comitans of hypoglossal n.

Sublingual gland

Lingual nerve

Anterior belly
of digastric muscle
(cut off)

Sublingual artery and vein

Genioglossus muscle,
Geniohyoid muscle

Hypoglossal nerve [XII],
Submental artery

Hyoglossus muscle,
Mylohyoid muscle
(cut off)

Lingual artery

Hyoid bone

Fascial loop
around the removed
digastric tendon

Thyrohyoid muscle

Superior belly
of omohyoid muscle

Sternohyoid muscle,
Laryngeal prominence
of thyroid cartilage

Internal branch
of superior laryngeal nerve,
Transverse cervical nerve

Thyrohyoid muscle

Sternothyroid muscle

**99 Blood vessels and nerves
in the anterior cervical region** (100%)
The parotid gland and parts of the mylohyoid muscle
and the platysma were removed. Right lateral aspect

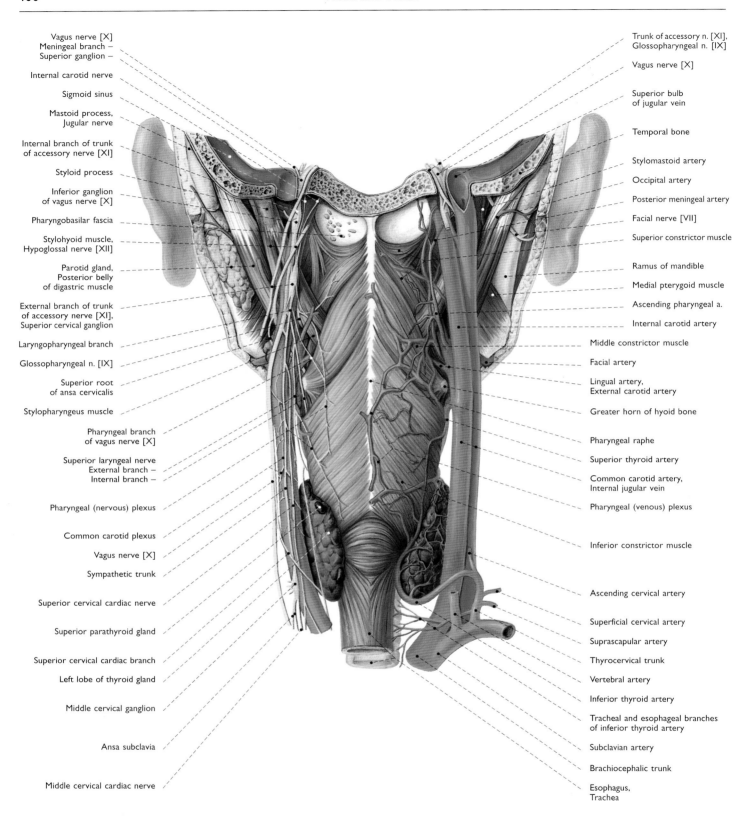

Vagus nerve [X]
Meningeal branch –
Superior ganglion –

Internal carotid nerve

Sigmoid sinus

Mastoid process,
Jugular nerve

Internal branch of trunk
of accessory nerve [XI]

Styloid process

Inferior ganglion
of vagus nerve [X]

Pharyngobasilar fascia

Stylohyoid muscle,
Hypoglossal nerve [XII]

Parotid gland,
Posterior belly
of digastric muscle

External branch of trunk
of accessory nerve [XI],
Superior cervical ganglion

Laryngopharyngeal branch

Glossopharyngeal n. [IX]

Superior root
of ansa cervicalis

Stylopharyngeus muscle

Pharyngeal branch
of vagus nerve [X]

Superior laryngeal nerve
External branch –
Internal branch –

Pharyngeal (nervous) plexus

Common carotid plexus

Vagus nerve [X]

Sympathetic trunk

Superior cervical cardiac nerve

Superior parathyroid gland

Superior cervical cardiac branch

Left lobe of thyroid gland

Middle cervical ganglion

Ansa subclavia

Middle cervical cardiac nerve

Trunk of accessory n. [XI],
Glossopharyngeal n. [IX]

Vagus nerve [X]

Superior bulb
of jugular vein

Temporal bone

Stylomastoid artery

Occipital artery

Posterior meningeal artery

Facial nerve [VII]

Superior constrictor muscle

Ramus of mandible

Medial pterygoid muscle

Ascending pharyngeal a.

Internal carotid artery

Middle constrictor muscle

Facial artery

Lingual artery,
External carotid artery

Greater horn of hyoid bone

Pharyngeal raphe

Superior thyroid artery

Common carotid artery,
Internal jugular vein

Pharyngeal (venous) plexus

Inferior constrictor muscle

Ascending cervical artery

Superficial cervical artery

Suprascapular artery

Thyrocervical trunk

Vertebral artery

Inferior thyroid artery

Tracheal and esophageal branches
of inferior thyroid artery

Subclavian artery

Brachiocephalic trunk

Esophagus,
Trachea

**100   Blood vessels and nerves
on the dorsolateral wall of the pharynx** (70%)
The right side especially emphasizes the blood vessels,
the left side the nerves. Dorsal aspect

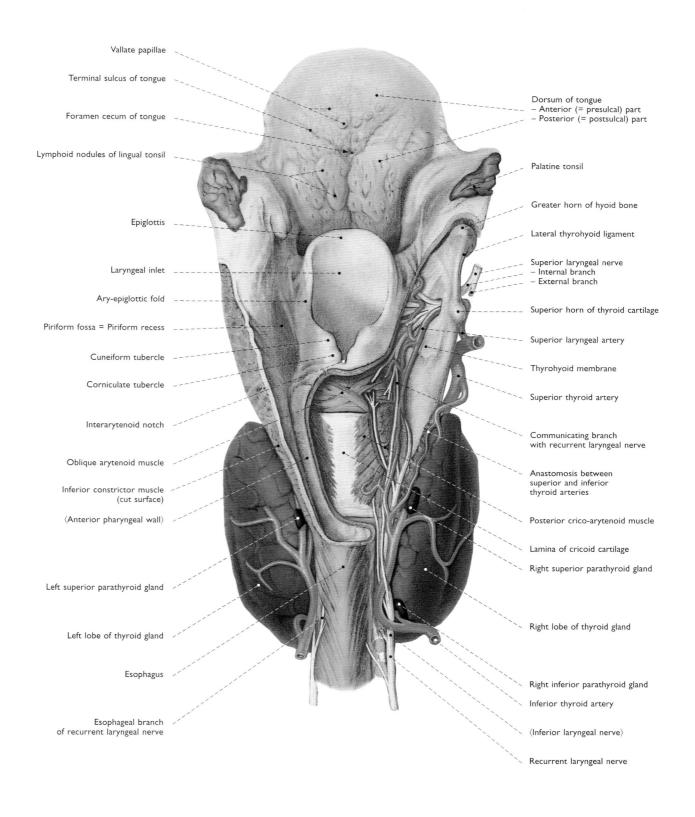

Vallate papillae

Terminal sulcus of tongue

Foramen cecum of tongue

Lymphoid nodules of lingual tonsil

Epiglottis

Laryngeal inlet

Ary-epiglottic fold

Piriform fossa = Piriform recess

Cuneiform tubercle

Corniculate tubercle

Interarytenoid notch

Oblique arytenoid muscle

Inferior constrictor muscle
(cut surface)

⟨Anterior pharyngeal wall⟩

Left superior parathyroid gland

Left lobe of thyroid gland

Esophagus

Esophageal branch
of recurrent laryngeal nerve

Dorsum of tongue
– Anterior (= presulcal) part
– Posterior (= postsulcal) part

Palatine tonsil

Greater horn of hyoid bone

Lateral thyrohyoid ligament

Superior laryngeal nerve
– Internal branch
– External branch

Superior horn of thyroid cartilage

Superior laryngeal artery

Thyrohyoid membrane

Superior thyroid artery

Communicating branch
with recurrent laryngeal nerve

Anastomosis between
superior and inferior
thyroid arteries

Posterior crico-arytenoid muscle

Lamina of cricoid cartilage

Right superior parathyroid gland

Right lobe of thyroid gland

Right inferior parathyroid gland

Inferior thyroid artery

⟨Inferior laryngeal nerve⟩

Recurrent laryngeal nerve

**101 Arteries and nerves
of the larynx and thyroid gland** (100%)
The dorsal wall of the pharynx was removed completely,
the ventral one partially. Dorsal aspect

Thoracic Viscera

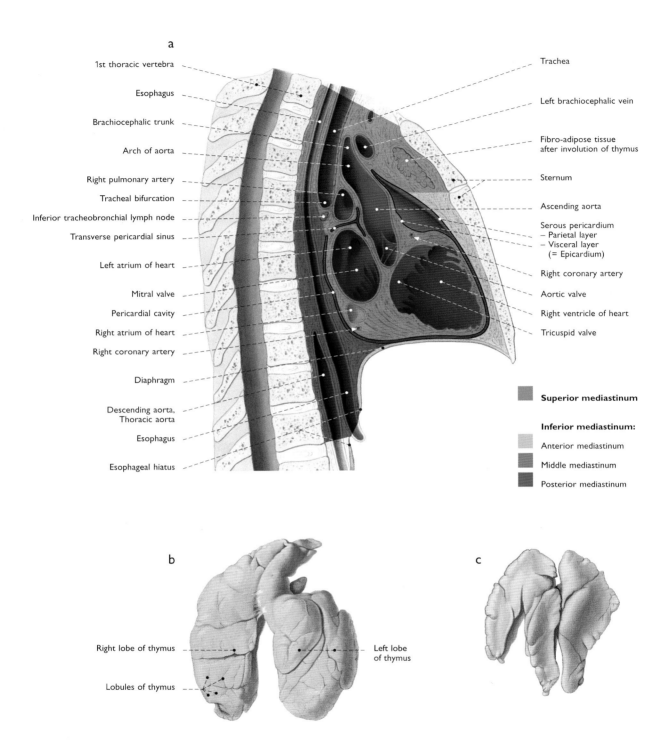

a

1st thoracic vertebra

Esophagus

Brachiocephalic trunk

Arch of aorta

Right pulmonary artery

Tracheal bifurcation

Inferior tracheobronchial lymph node

Transverse pericardial sinus

Left atrium of heart

Mitral valve

Pericardial cavity

Right atrium of heart

Right coronary artery

Diaphragm

Descending aorta,
Thoracic aorta

Esophagus

Esophageal hiatus

Trachea

Left brachiocephalic vein

Fibro-adipose tissue
after involution of thymus

Sternum

Ascending aorta

Serous pericardium
– Parietal layer
– Visceral layer
   (= Epicardium)

Right coronary artery

Aortic valve

Right ventricle of heart

Tricuspid valve

Superior mediastinum

Inferior mediastinum:

Anterior mediastinum

Middle mediastinum

Posterior mediastinum

b

Right lobe of thymus

Lobules of thymus

Left lobe
of thymus

c

104   Mediastinum and thymus

a   Subdivision of the mediastinum, median section (40%),
    medial aspect of the left half
b   Thymus of a 3-year-old child (75%), ventral aspect
c   Thymus of a newborn child (75%), ventral aspect

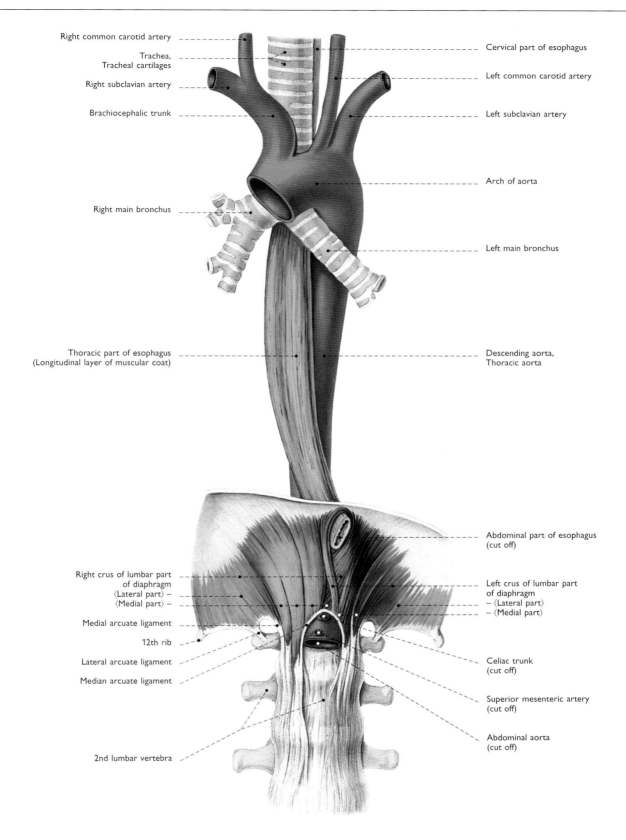

Right common carotid artery

Trachea,
Tracheal cartilages

Right subclavian artery

Brachiocephalic trunk

Right main bronchus

Thoracic part of esophagus
(Longitudinal layer of muscular coat)

Right crus of lumbar part
of diaphragm
⟨Lateral part⟩ –
⟨Medial part⟩ –

Medial arcuate ligament

12th rib

Lateral arcuate ligament

Median arcuate ligament

2nd lumbar vertebra

Cervical part of esophagus

Left common carotid artery

Left subclavian artery

Arch of aorta

Left main bronchus

Descending aorta,
Thoracic aorta

Abdominal part of esophagus
(cut off)

Left crus of lumbar part
of diaphragm
– ⟨Lateral part⟩
– ⟨Medial part⟩

Celiac trunk
(cut off)

Superior mesenteric artery
(cut off)

Abdominal aorta
(cut off)

105 Esophagus and adjacent organs (50%)
Ventral aspect

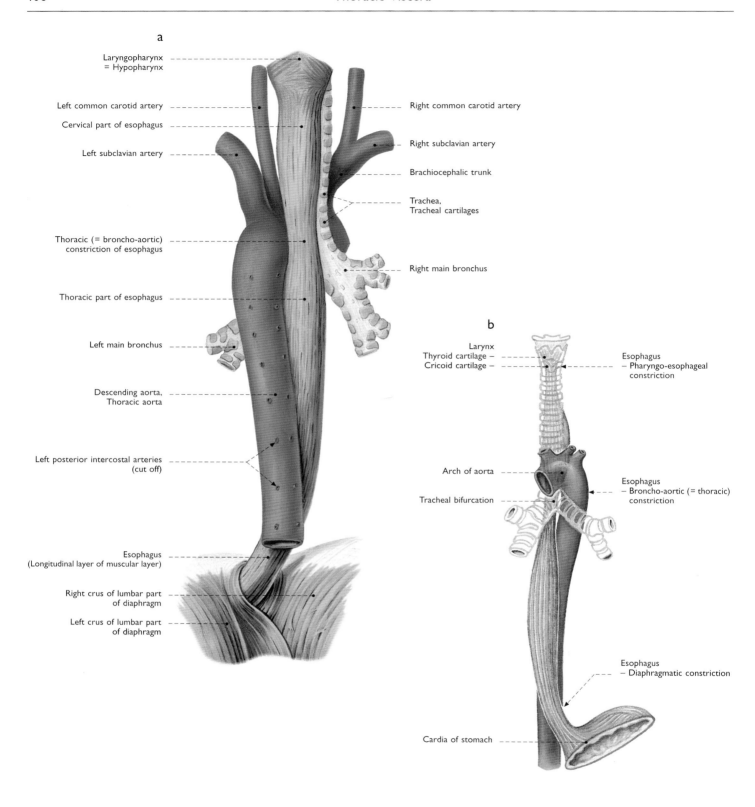

a

Laryngopharynx = Hypopharynx

Left common carotid artery

Cervical part of esophagus

Left subclavian artery

Thoracic (= broncho-aortic) constriction of esophagus

Thoracic part of esophagus

Left main bronchus

Descending aorta, Thoracic aorta

Left posterior intercostal arteries (cut off)

Esophagus (Longitudinal layer of muscular layer)

Right crus of lumbar part of diaphragm

Left crus of lumbar part of diaphragm

Right common carotid artery

Right subclavian artery

Brachiocephalic trunk

Trachea, Tracheal cartilages

Right main bronchus

b

Larynx
Thyroid cartilage –
Cricoid cartilage –

Arch of aorta

Tracheal bifurcation

Cardia of stomach

Esophagus – Pharyngo-esophageal constriction

Esophagus – Broncho-aortic (= thoracic) constriction

Esophagus – Diaphragmatic constriction

106 Esophagus and adjacent organs
a   Dorsal aspect (50%)
b   Typical constrictions of the esophagus (35%), schematic representation, ventral aspect

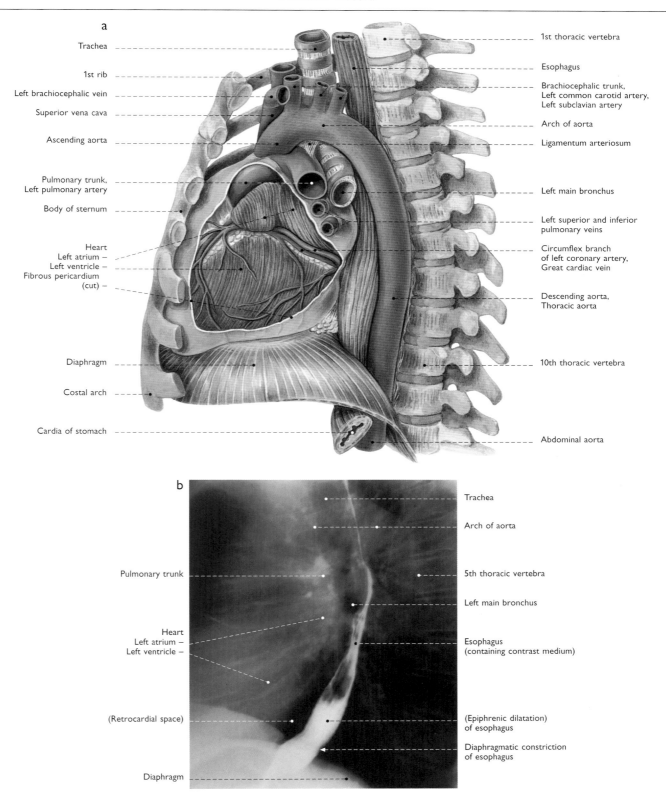

a

Trachea

1st rib

Left brachiocephalic vein

Superior vena cava

Ascending aorta

Pulmonary trunk,
Left pulmonary artery

Body of sternum

Heart
Left atrium —
Left ventricle —
Fibrous pericardium
(cut) —

Diaphragm

Costal arch

Cardia of stomach

1st thoracic vertebra

Esophagus

Brachiocephalic trunk,
Left common carotid artery,
Left subclavian artery

Arch of aorta

Ligamentum arteriosum

Left main bronchus

Left superior and inferior
pulmonary veins

Circumflex branch
of left coronary artery,
Great cardiac vein

Descending aorta,
Thoracic aorta

10th thoracic vertebra

Abdominal aorta

b

Pulmonary trunk

Heart
Left atrium —
Left ventricle —

(Retrocardial space)

Diaphragm

Trachea

Arch of aorta

5th thoracic vertebra

Left main bronchus

Esophagus
(containing contrast medium)

(Epiphrenic dilatation)
of esophagus

Diaphragmatic constriction
of esophagus

107 Esophagus and adjacent organs (35%)

a Left lateral aspect of the mediastinum.
   The pericardium was partially removed.
b Lateral radiograph. The esophagus contains contrast medium.

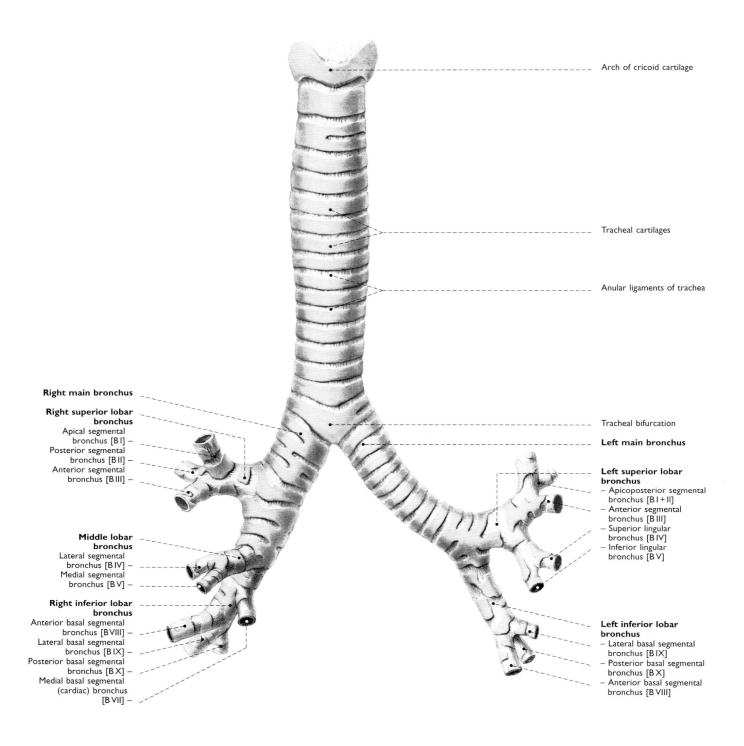

Arch of cricoid cartilage

Tracheal cartilages

Anular ligaments of trachea

Tracheal bifurcation

Left main bronchus

Left superior lobar bronchus
- Apicoposterior segmental bronchus [B I + II]
- Anterior segmental bronchus [B III]
- Superior lingular bronchus [B IV]
- Inferior lingular bronchus [B V]

Left inferior lobar bronchus
- Lateral basal segmental bronchus [B IX]
- Posterior basal segmental bronchus [B X]
- Anterior basal segmental bronchus [B VIII]

Right main bronchus

Right superior lobar bronchus
Apical segmental bronchus [B I] —
Posterior segmental bronchus [B II] —
Anterior segmental bronchus [B III] —

Middle lobar bronchus
Lateral segmental bronchus [B IV] —
Medial segmental bronchus [B V] —

Right inferior lobar bronchus
Anterior basal segmental bronchus [B VIII] —
Lateral basal segmental bronchus [B IX] —
Posterior basal segmental bronchus [B X] —
Medial basal segmental (cardiac) bronchus [B VII] —

108 Trachea and bronchi (90%)
Ventral aspect

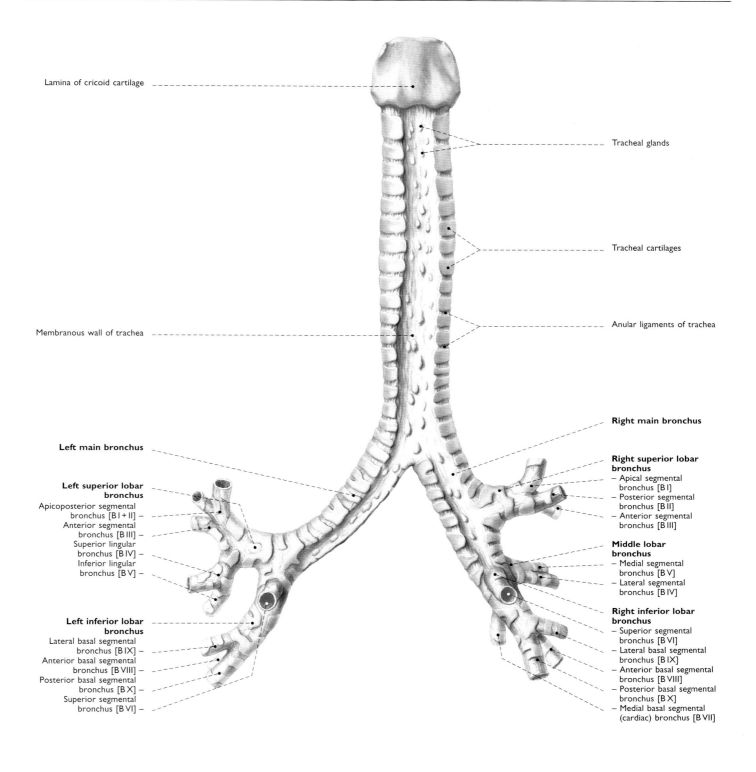

Lamina of cricoid cartilage

Tracheal glands

Tracheal cartilages

Membranous wall of trachea

Anular ligaments of trachea

Right main bronchus

Left main bronchus

Right superior lobar bronchus
– Apical segmental bronchus [B I]
– Posterior segmental bronchus [B II]
– Anterior segmental bronchus [B III]

Left superior lobar bronchus
Apicoposterior segmental bronchus [B I + II] –
Anterior segmental bronchus [B III] –
Superior lingular bronchus [B IV] –
Inferior lingular bronchus [B V] –

Middle lobar bronchus
– Medial segmental bronchus [B V]
– Lateral segmental bronchus [B IV]

Right inferior lobar bronchus
– Superior segmental bronchus [B VI]
– Lateral basal segmental bronchus [B IX]
– Anterior basal segmental bronchus [B VIII]
– Posterior basal segmental bronchus [B X]
– Medial basal segmental (cardiac) bronchus [B VII]

Left inferior lobar bronchus
Lateral basal segmental bronchus [B IX] –
Anterior basal segmental bronchus [B VIII] –
Posterior basal segmental bronchus [B X] –
Superior segmental bronchus [B VI] –

109 Trachea and bronchi (90%)
Dorsal aspect

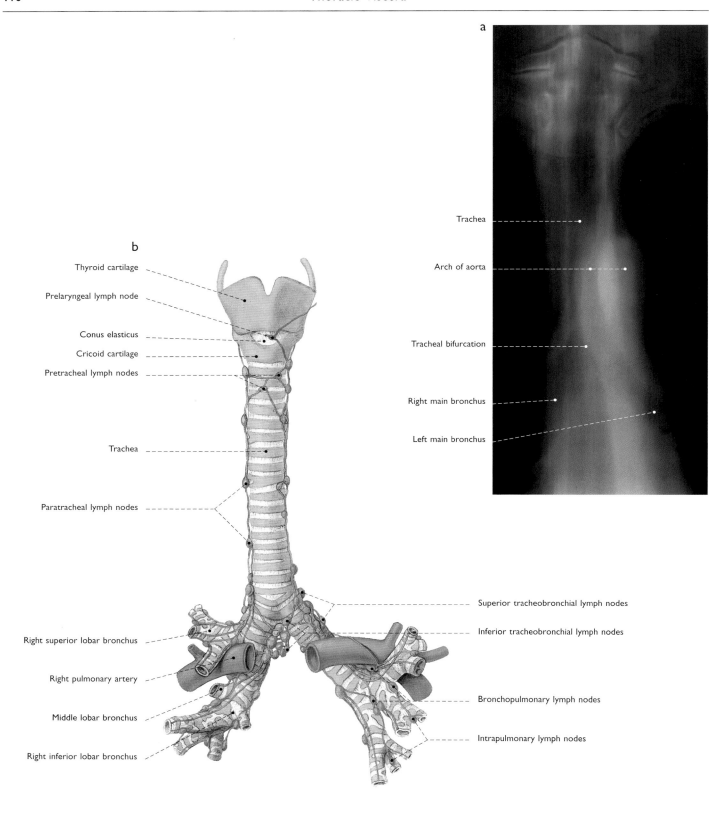

a

Trachea

Arch of aorta

Tracheal bifurcation

Right main bronchus

Left main bronchus

b

Thyroid cartilage

Prelaryngeal lymph node

Conus elasticus

Cricoid cartilage

Pretracheal lymph nodes

Trachea

Paratracheal lymph nodes

Right superior lobar bronchus

Right pulmonary artery

Middle lobar bronchus

Right inferior lobar bronchus

Superior tracheobronchial lymph nodes

Inferior tracheobronchial lymph nodes

Bronchopulmonary lymph nodes

Intrapulmonary lymph nodes

110 Trachea and bronchi
a   Postero-anterior tomogram of the trachea (50%)
b   Lymphatic vessels and lymph nodes of the trachea
    and the bronchi (70%), ventral aspect

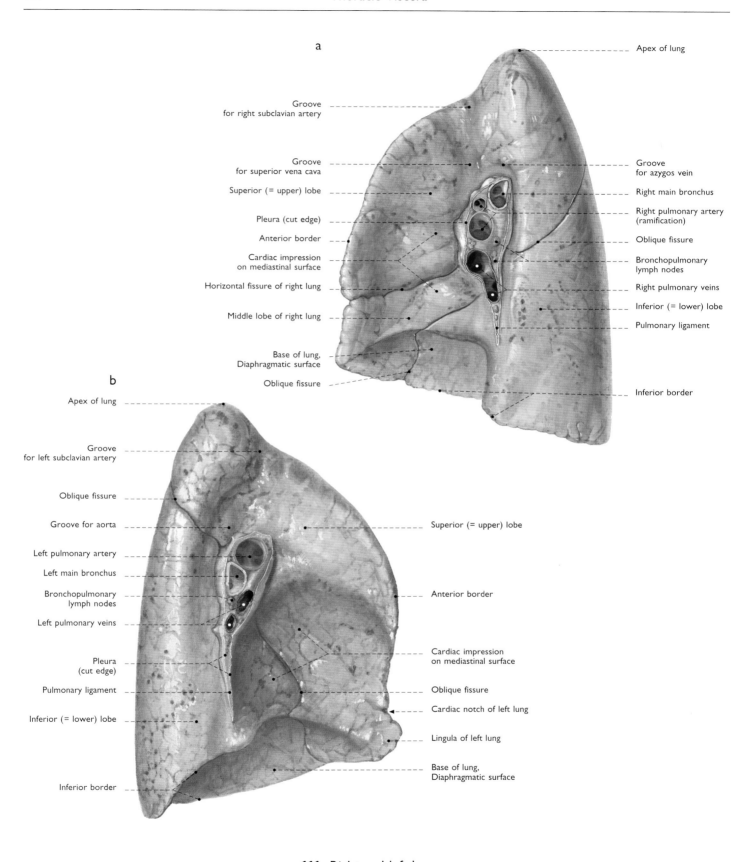

a

Apex of lung

Groove
for right subclavian artery

Groove
for superior vena cava

Groove
for azygos vein

Superior (= upper) lobe

Right main bronchus

Right pulmonary artery
(ramification)

Pleura (cut edge)

Oblique fissure

Anterior border

Cardiac impression
on mediastinal surface

Bronchopulmonary
lymph nodes

Horizontal fissure of right lung

Right pulmonary veins

Middle lobe of right lung

Inferior (= lower) lobe

Pulmonary ligament

Base of lung,
Diaphragmatic surface

Oblique fissure

Inferior border

b

Apex of lung

Groove
for left subclavian artery

Oblique fissure

Groove for aorta

Superior (= upper) lobe

Left pulmonary artery

Left main bronchus

Bronchopulmonary
lymph nodes

Anterior border

Left pulmonary veins

Pleura
(cut edge)

Cardiac impression
on mediastinal surface

Pulmonary ligament

Oblique fissure

Cardiac notch of left lung

Inferior (= lower) lobe

Lingula of left lung

Base of lung,
Diaphragmatic surface

Inferior border

111 Right and left lungs (40%)
a Right lung, mediastinal surface
b Left lung, mediastinal surface

a

Apex of lung - - - - - - - - - - - - - - - - - -

Groove
for right subclavian artery

Superior (= upper) lobe - - - - - -

Anterior border

Costal surface - - - -

Horizontal fissure of right lung

Oblique fissure - - - -

Middle lobe of right lung

Inferior (= lower) lobe - - - - - -

Inferior border - - - -

Base of lung,
Diaphragmatic surface

Apex of lung

Groove
for left subclavian artery

Superior (= upper) lobe - - - - - -

Costal surface

Anterior border - - - -

Cardiac notch of left lung - - - -

Oblique fissure

Lingula of left lung - - - -

Inferior (= lower) lobe

Inferior border - - - - - - - - - - - -

Base of lung,
Diaphragmatic surface

b

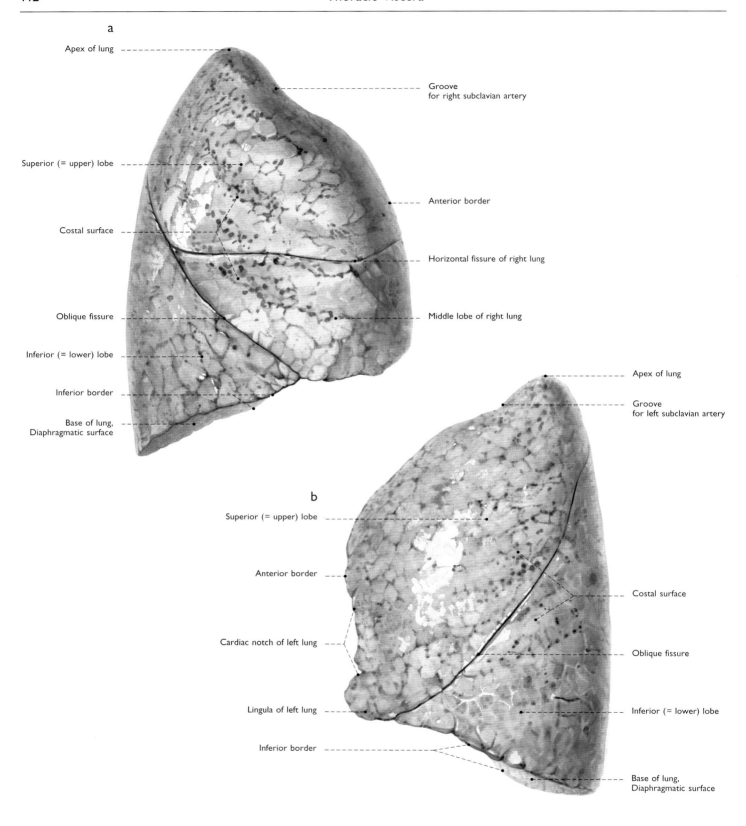

112 Right and left lungs (40%)
a Right lung, costal surface
b Left lung, costal surface

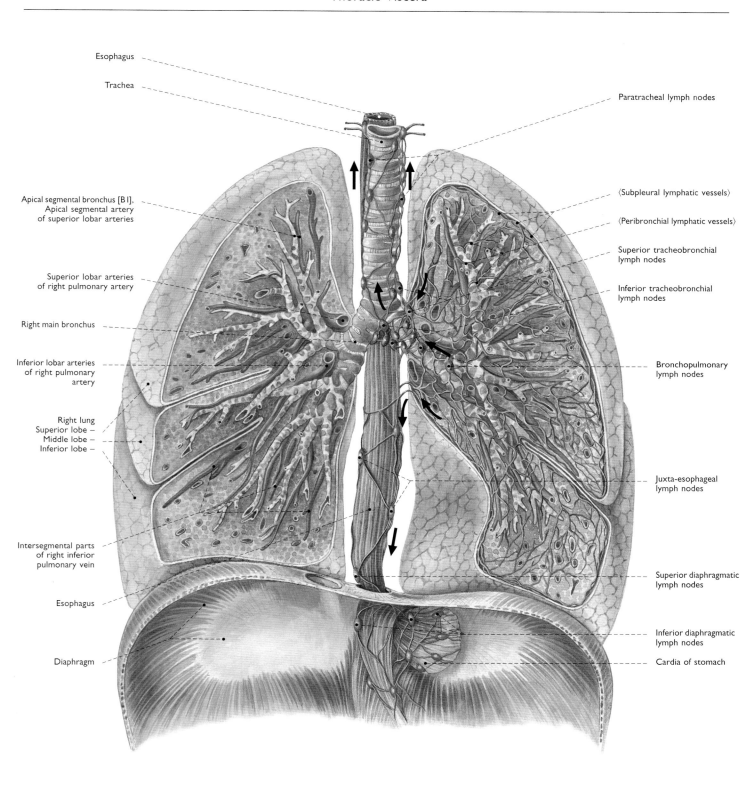

Esophagus

Trachea

Paratracheal lymph nodes

Apical segmental bronchus [B I], Apical segmental artery of superior lobar arteries

⟨Subpleural lymphatic vessels⟩

⟨Peribronchial lymphatic vessels⟩

Superior tracheobronchial lymph nodes

Superior lobar arteries of right pulmonary artery

Inferior tracheobronchial lymph nodes

Right main bronchus

Inferior lobar arteries of right pulmonary artery

Bronchopulmonary lymph nodes

Right lung
Superior lobe –
Middle lobe –
Inferior lobe –

Intersegmental parts of right inferior pulmonary vein

Juxta-esophageal lymph nodes

Esophagus

Superior diaphragmatic lymph nodes

Inferior diaphragmatic lymph nodes

Diaphragm

Cardia of stomach

113 Right and left lungs (80%)
Lymphatic vessels, lymph nodes, and lymphatic drainage
from the left lung, ventral aspect

a

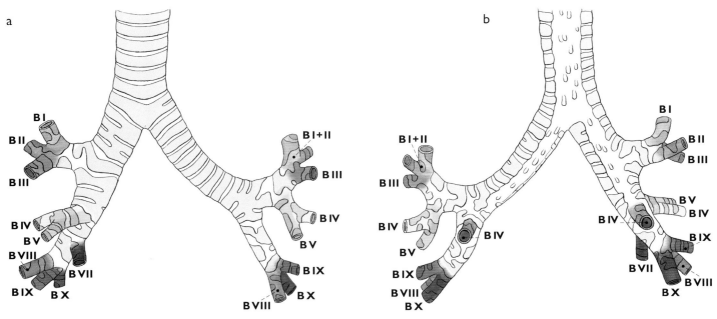

b

Ramification of the two main bronchi

Right main bronchus

Right superior lobar bronchus
B I   Apical segmental bronchus
B II   Posterior segmental bronchus
B III   Anterior segmental bronchus
Middle lobar bronchus
B IV   Lateral segmental bronchus
B V   Medial segmental bronchus

Right inferior lobar bronchus
B VI   Superior segmental bronchus
B VII   Medial basal segmental (cardiac) bronchus
B VIII   Anterior basal segmental bronchus
B IX   Lateral basal segmental bronchus
B X   Posterior basal segmental bronchus

Left main bronchus

Left superior lobar bronchus
B I + II   Apicoposterior segmental bronchus
B III   Anterior segmental bronchus
B IV   Superior lingular bronchus
B V   Inferior lingular bronchus

Left inferior lobar bronchus
B VI   Superior segmental bronchus
B VIII   Anterior basal segmental bronchus
B IX   Lateral basal segmental bronchus
B X   Posterior basal segmental bronchus

c

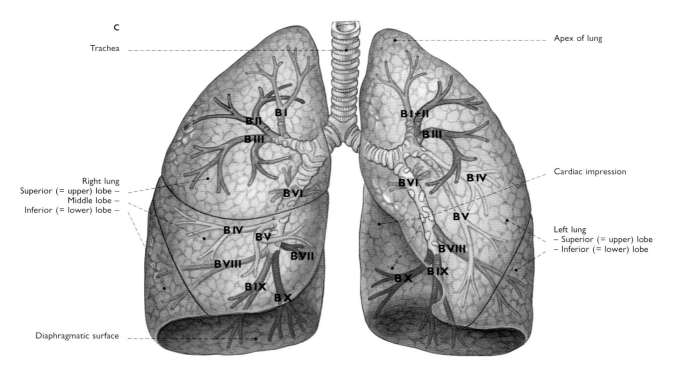

Trachea

Apex of lung

Right lung
Superior (= upper) lobe –
Middle lobe –
Inferior (= lower) lobe –

Cardiac impression

Left lung
– Superior (= upper) lobe
– Inferior (= lower) lobe

Diaphragmatic surface

114   Bronchial tree

Schematic representations
a   Bronchial tree (70%), ventral aspect
b   Bronchial tree (70%), dorsal aspect
c   Subdivision of the bronchial tree
    in the right and left lungs (50%), ventral aspect

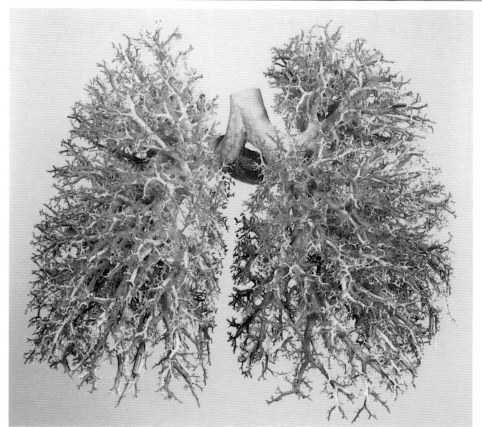

Yellow: Trachea and bronchial tree
Blue: Pulmonary trunk and its ramifications

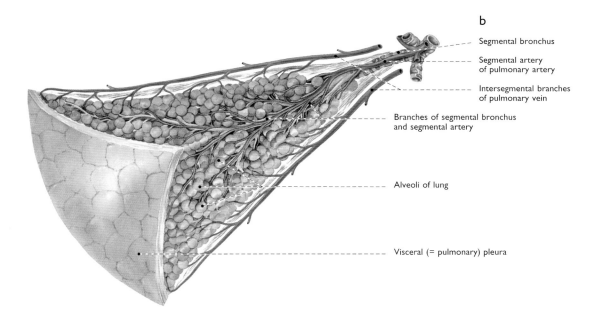

b

Segmental bronchus

Segmental artery of pulmonary artery

Intersegmental branches of pulmonary vein

Branches of segmental bronchus and segmental artery

Alveoli of lung

Visceral (= pulmonary) pleura

115 Bronchial tree and bronchopulmonary segment
a Bronchial tree and branches of the pulmonary arteries, corrosion preparation (70%), dorsal aspect (Anatomical Collection, Basel)
b Bronchopulmonary segment, schematic representation

a

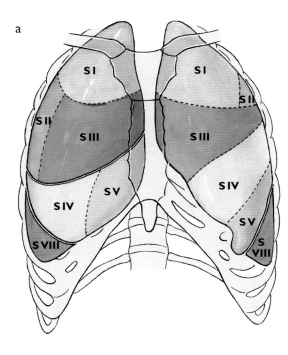

b

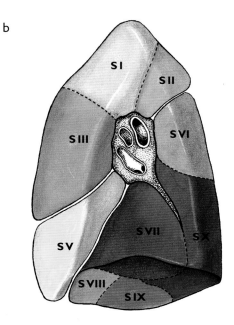

c

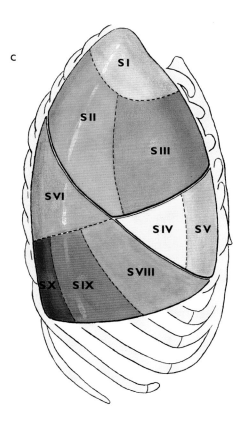

Right lung

Superior (= upper) lobe
S I   Apical segment
S II   Posterior segment
S III   Anterior segment

Middle lobe
S IV   Lateral segment
S V   Medial segment

Inferior (= lower) lobe
S VI   Superior segment
S VII   Medial basal (cardiac) segment
S VIII Anterior basal segment
S IX   Lateral basal segment
S X   Posterior basal segment

Segment borders are represented as dashed lines,
lobe borders as solid lines

116 Bronchopulmonary segments (25%)
      Schematic representations. Diverse segments
      are indicated by different colors.
   a   Right and left lungs, ventral aspect
   b   Right lung, mediastinal surface
   c   Right lung, costal surface

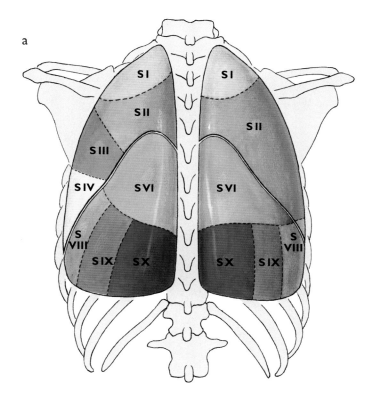

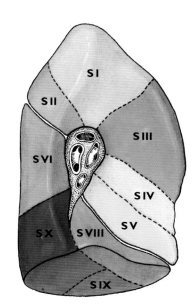

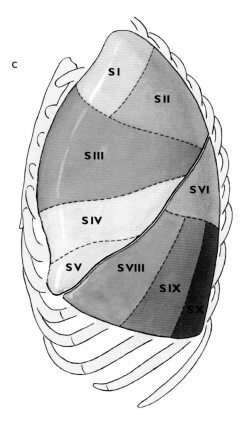

Left lung

Superior (= upper) lobe
S I + II	Apicoposterior segment
S III	Anterior segment
S IV	Superior lingular segment
S V	Inferior lingular segment

Inferior (= lower) lobe
S VI	Superior segment
S VIII	Anterior basal segment
S IX	Lateral basal segment
S X	Posterior basal segment

Segment borders are represented as dashed lines,
lobe borders as solid lines

117 Bronchopulmonary segments (25%)
Schematic representations. Diverse segments
are indicated by different colors.
a   Right and left lungs, dorsal aspect
b   Left lung, mediastinal surface
c   Left lung, costal surface

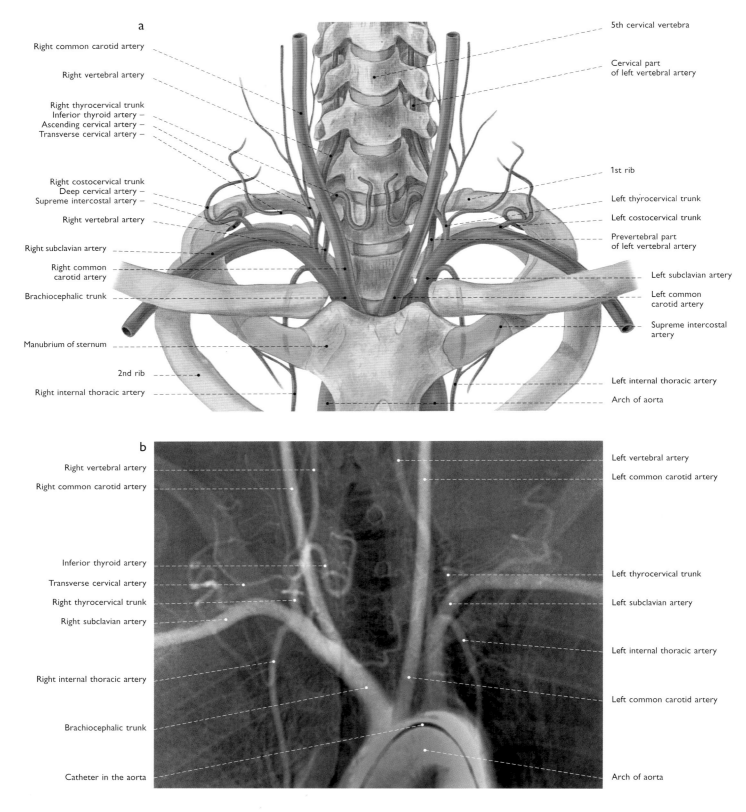

a

Right common carotid artery

Right vertebral artery

Right thyrocervical trunk
Inferior thyroid artery –
Ascending cervical artery –
Transverse cervical artery –

Right costocervical trunk
Deep cervical artery –
Supreme intercostal artery –

Right vertebral artery

Right subclavian artery

Right common
carotid artery

Brachiocephalic trunk

Manubrium of sternum

2nd rib

Right internal thoracic artery

5th cervical vertebra

Cervical part
of left vertebral artery

1st rib

Left thyrocervical trunk

Left costocervical trunk

Prevertebral part
of left vertebral artery

Left subclavian artery

Left common
carotid artery

Supreme intercostal
artery

Left internal thoracic artery

Arch of aorta

b

Right vertebral artery

Right common carotid artery

Inferior thyroid artery

Transverse cervical artery

Right thyrocervical trunk

Right subclavian artery

Right internal thoracic artery

Brachiocephalic trunk

Catheter in the aorta

Left vertebral artery

Left common carotid artery

Left thyrocervical trunk

Left subclavian artery

Left internal thoracic artery

Left common carotid artery

Arch of aorta

**118 Arteries of the upper thorax
and the lower neck** (65%)
a Schematic representation, ventral aspect
b Anteroposterior aortogram

a

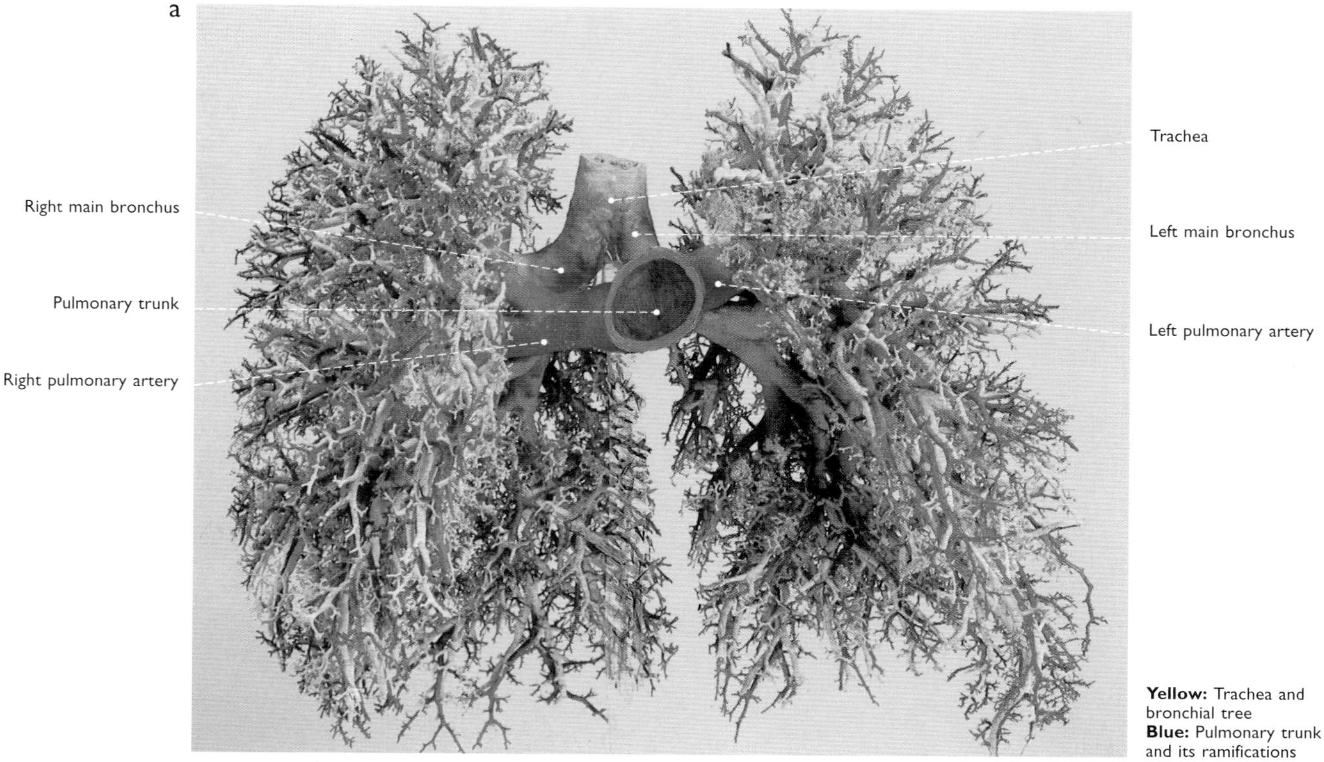

Trachea

Right main bronchus

Left main bronchus

Pulmonary trunk

Left pulmonary artery

Right pulmonary artery

Yellow: Trachea and bronchial tree
Blue: Pulmonary trunk and its ramifications

b

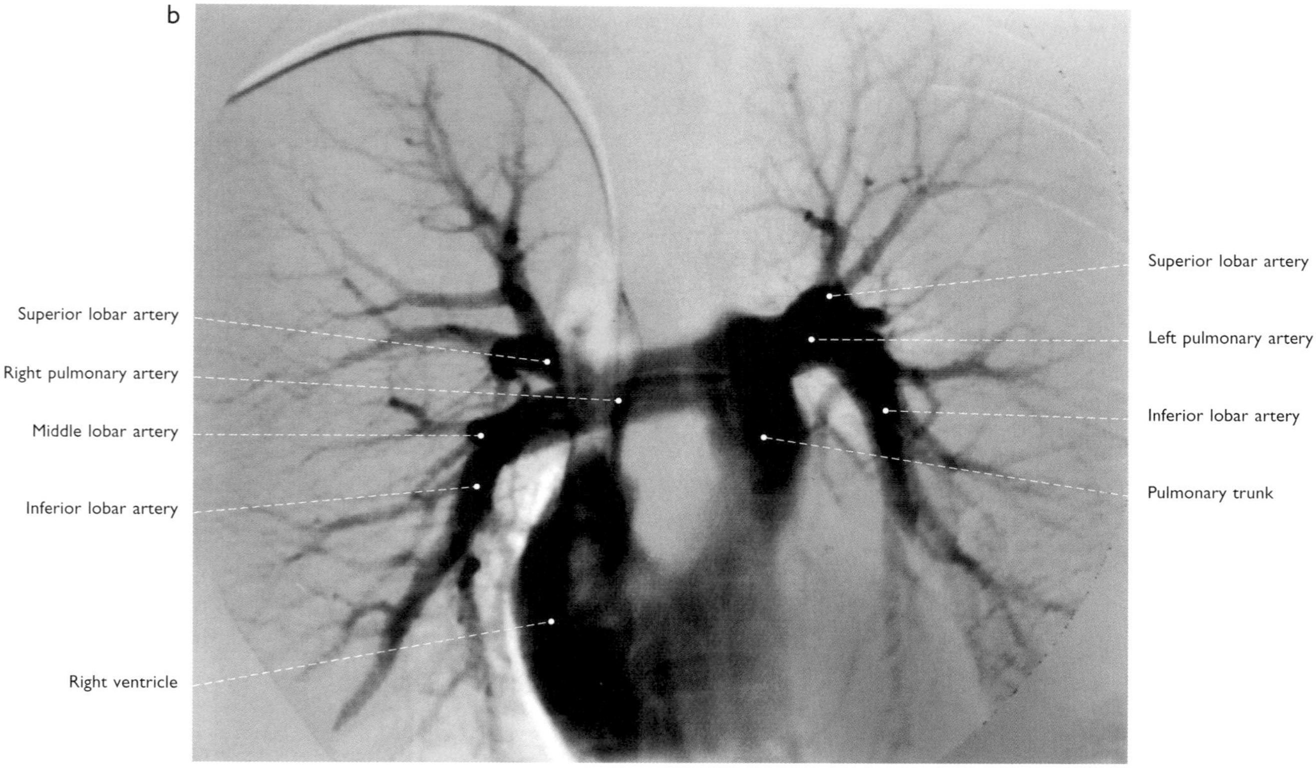

Superior lobar artery

Right pulmonary artery

Superior lobar artery

Middle lobar artery

Left pulmonary artery

Inferior lobar artery

Inferior lobar artery

Pulmonary trunk

Right ventricle

119 Bronchial tree and pulmonary arteries (70%)

a Bronchial tree, pulmonary trunk, and branches of the pulmonary arteries, corrosion preparation, ventral aspect
b Dextrocardiogram and pulmonary arteriogram after injection of contrast medium into the right ventricle of the heart, ventral aspect

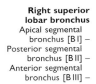

**Right superior
lobar bronchus**
Apical segmental
bronchus [B I] –
Posterior segmental
bronchus [B II] –
Anterior segmental
bronchus [B III] –

**Right inferior
lobar bronchus**
Superior segmental
bronchus [B VI] –

**Middle
lobar bronchus**
Lateral segmental
bronchus [B IV] –
Medial segmental
bronchus [B V] –

**Right inferior
lobar bronchus**
Anterior basal
segmental bronchus [B VIII] –
Lateral basal
segmental bronchus [B IX] –
Medial basal
segmental (cardiac)
bronchus [B VII] –
Posterior basal
segmental bronchus [B X] –

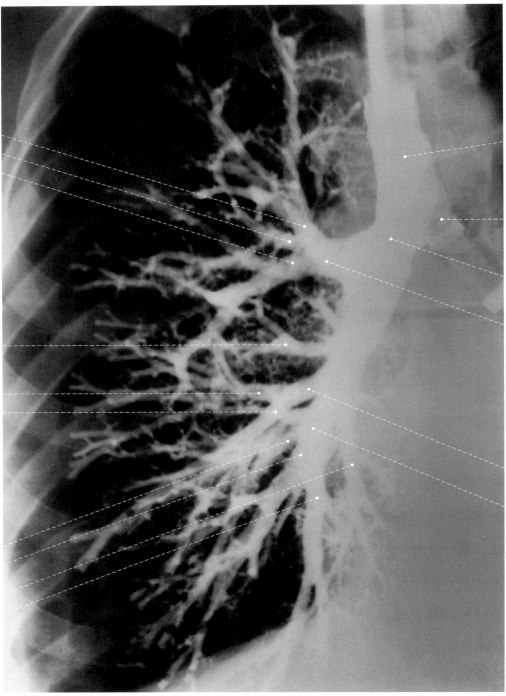

Trachea

Left main bronchus
(blocked)

Right main bronchus

Right superior
lobar bronchus

Middle lobar bronchus

Right inferior
lobar bronchus

120 Right bronchial tree (75%)
Bronchography, anteroposterior radiograph

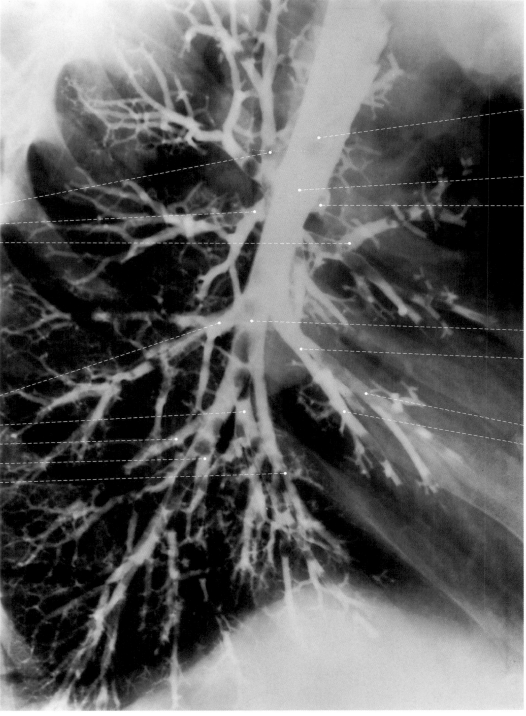

Right superior lobar bronchus
Apical segmental bronchus [B I] –
Posterior segmental bronchus [B II] –
Anterior segmental bronchus [B III] –

Right inferior lobar bronchus
Superior segmental bronchus [B VI] –
Medial basal segmental (cardiac) bronchus [B VII] –
Posterior basal segmental bronchus [B X] –
Lateral basal segmental bronchus [B IX] –
Anterior basal segmental bronchus [B VIII] –

Trachea

Right main bronchus

Left main bronchus (blocked)

Right inferior lobar bronchus

Middle lobar bronchus

Middle lobar bronchus
– Lateral segmental bronchus [B IV]
– Medial segmental bronchus [B V]

121 Right bronchial tree (70%)
Bronchography, lateral radiograph

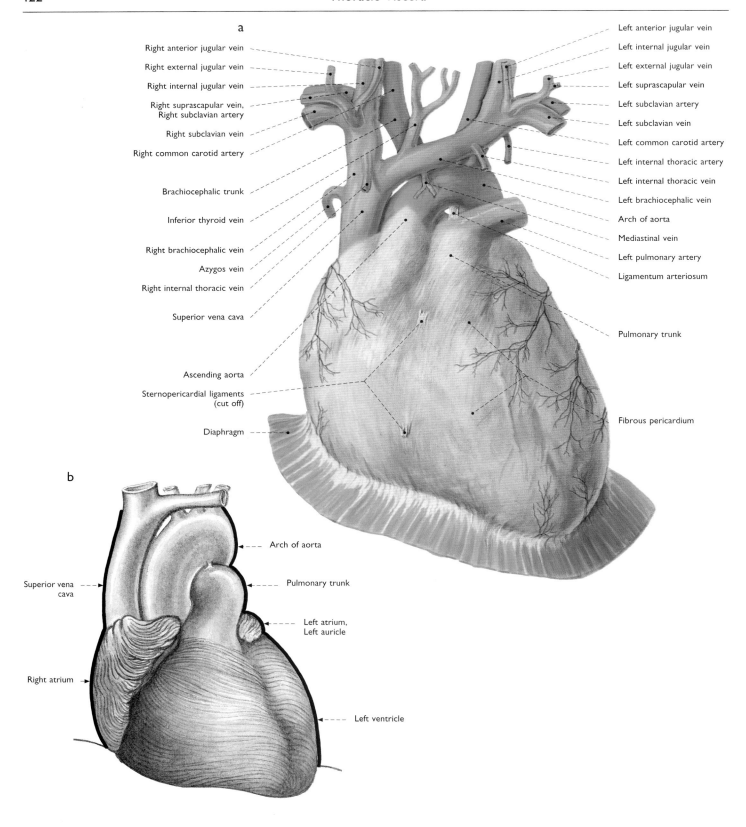

a

Right anterior jugular vein
Right external jugular vein
Right internal jugular vein
Right suprascapular vein,
Right subclavian artery
Right subclavian vein
Right common carotid artery

Brachiocephalic trunk

Inferior thyroid vein

Right brachiocephalic vein
Azygos vein
Right internal thoracic vein

Superior vena cava

Ascending aorta
Sternopericardial ligaments
(cut off)

Diaphragm

Left anterior jugular vein
Left internal jugular vein
Left external jugular vein
Left suprascapular vein
Left subclavian artery
Left subclavian vein
Left common carotid artery
Left internal thoracic artery
Left internal thoracic vein
Left brachiocephalic vein
Arch of aorta
Mediastinal vein
Left pulmonary artery
Ligamentum arteriosum

Pulmonary trunk

Fibrous pericardium

b

Arch of aorta

Pulmonary trunk

Left atrium,
Left auricle

Superior vena
cava

Right atrium

Left ventricle

122 Pericardial sac and silhouette of the heart
Ventral aspect
a Pericardial sac and great blood vessels close to the heart (75%)
b Silhouette of the heart marked by the black marginal line (50%),
   schematic representation

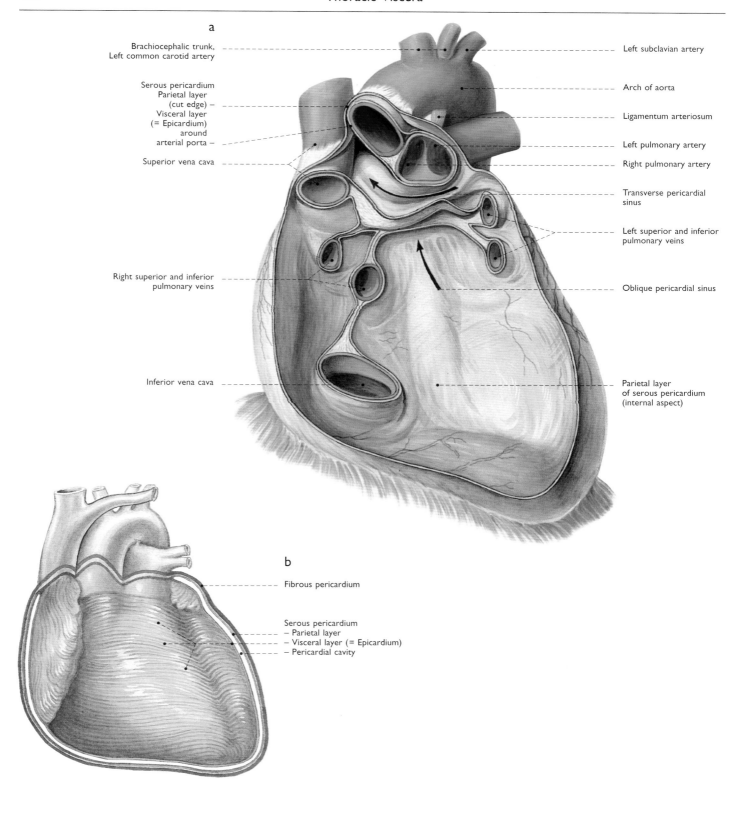

a

Brachiocephalic trunk, Left common carotid artery

Serous pericardium
Parietal layer (cut edge) –
Visceral layer (= Epicardium) around arterial porta –

Superior vena cava

Right superior and inferior pulmonary veins

Inferior vena cava

Left subclavian artery

Arch of aorta

Ligamentum arteriosum

Left pulmonary artery

Right pulmonary artery

Transverse pericardial sinus

Left superior and inferior pulmonary veins

Oblique pericardial sinus

Parietal layer of serous pericardium (internal aspect)

b

Fibrous pericardium

Serous pericardium
– Parietal layer
– Visceral layer (= Epicardium)
– Pericardial cavity

123 Pericardial sac
Ventral aspect
a Posterior wall of the pericardial cavity (75%)
b Construction of the pericardium (50%), schematic representation

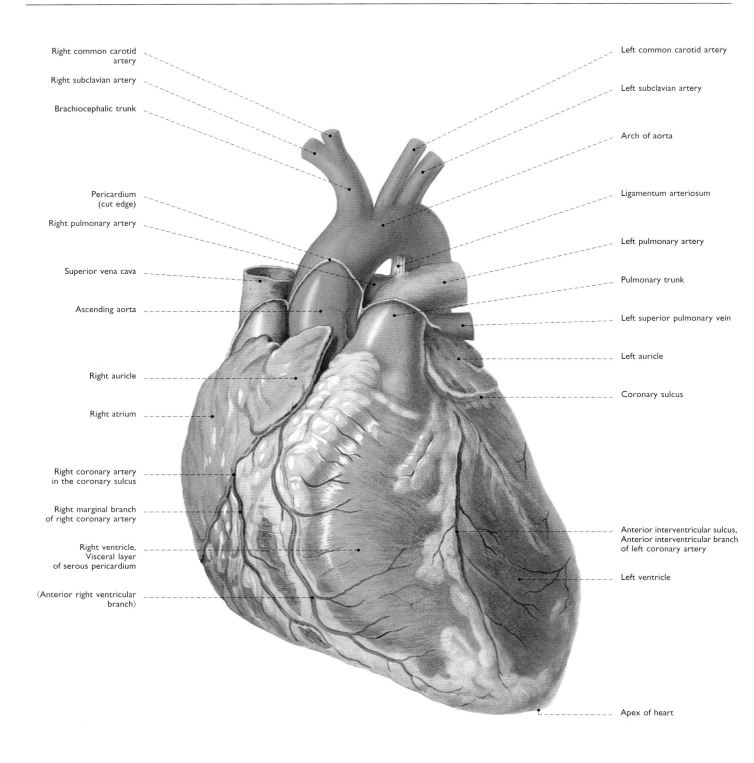

Right common carotid artery

Right subclavian artery

Brachiocephalic trunk

Pericardium (cut edge)

Right pulmonary artery

Superior vena cava

Ascending aorta

Right auricle

Right atrium

Right coronary artery in the coronary sulcus

Right marginal branch of right coronary artery

Right ventricle, Visceral layer of serous pericardium

⟨Anterior right ventricular branch⟩

Left common carotid artery

Left subclavian artery

Arch of aorta

Ligamentum arteriosum

Left pulmonary artery

Pulmonary trunk

Left superior pulmonary vein

Left auricle

Coronary sulcus

Anterior interventricular sulcus, Anterior interventricular branch of left coronary artery

Left ventricle

Apex of heart

124 Heart and great blood vessels (100%)
The fibrous pericardium and the parietal layer
of the serous pericardium were removed. Ventral aspect

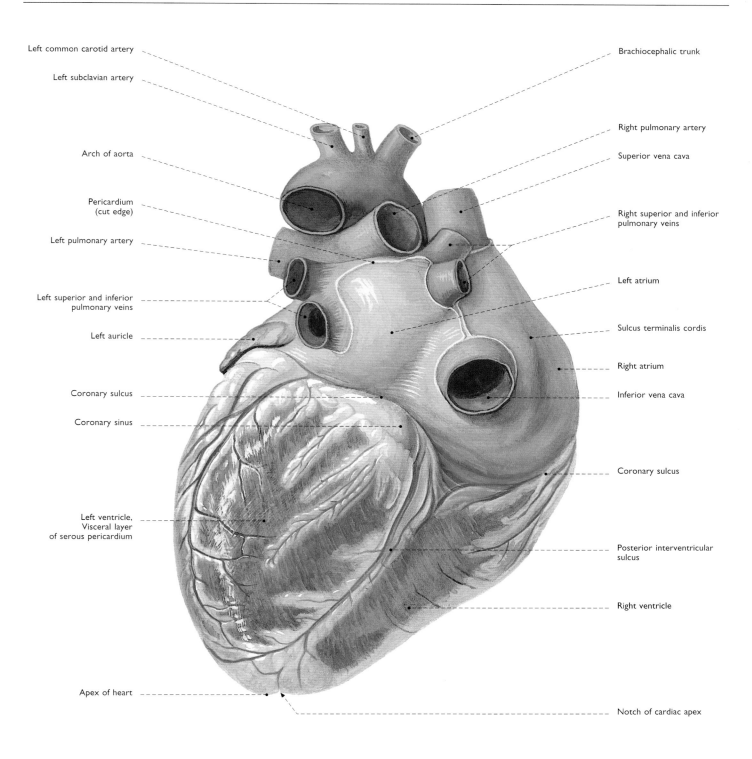

Left common carotid artery

Left subclavian artery

Arch of aorta

Pericardium
(cut edge)

Left pulmonary artery

Left superior and inferior
pulmonary veins

Left auricle

Coronary sulcus

Coronary sinus

Left ventricle,
Visceral layer
of serous pericardium

Apex of heart

Brachiocephalic trunk

Right pulmonary artery

Superior vena cava

Right superior and inferior
pulmonary veins

Left atrium

Sulcus terminalis cordis

Right atrium

Inferior vena cava

Coronary sulcus

Posterior interventricular
sulcus

Right ventricle

Notch of cardiac apex

125　Heart and great blood vessels (100%)
The fibrous pericardium and the parietal layer
of the serous pericardium were removed. Dorsal aspect

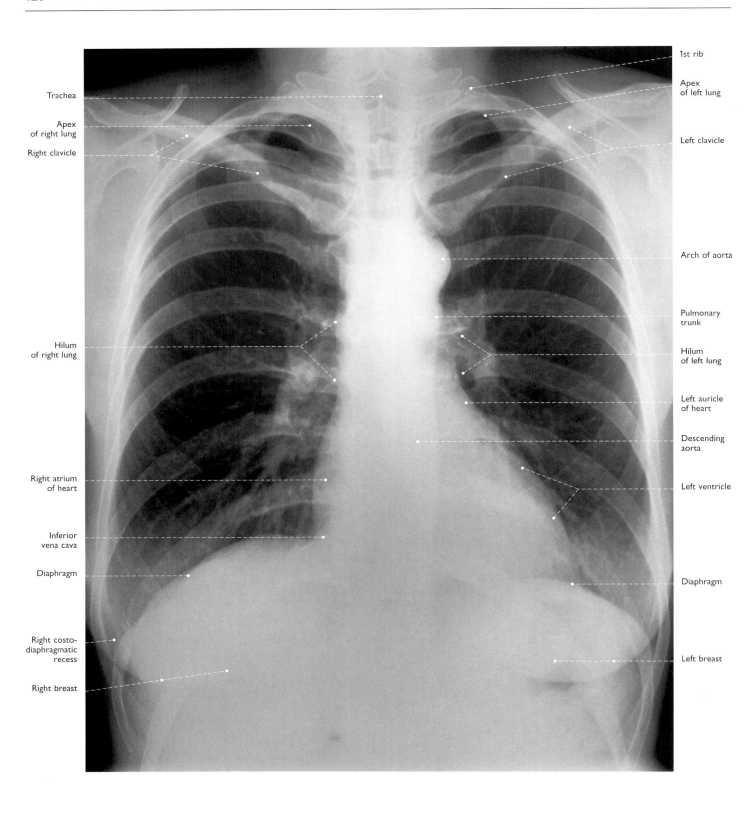

Trachea

Apex
of right lung

Right clavicle

Hilum
of right lung

Right atrium
of heart

Inferior
vena cava

Diaphragm

Right costo-
diaphragmatic
recess

Right breast

1st rib

Apex
of left lung

Left clavicle

Arch of aorta

Pulmonary
trunk

Hilum
of left lung

Left auricle
of heart

Descending
aorta

Left ventricle

Diaphragm

Left breast

126 Thoracic organs (55%)
Postero-anterior radiograph

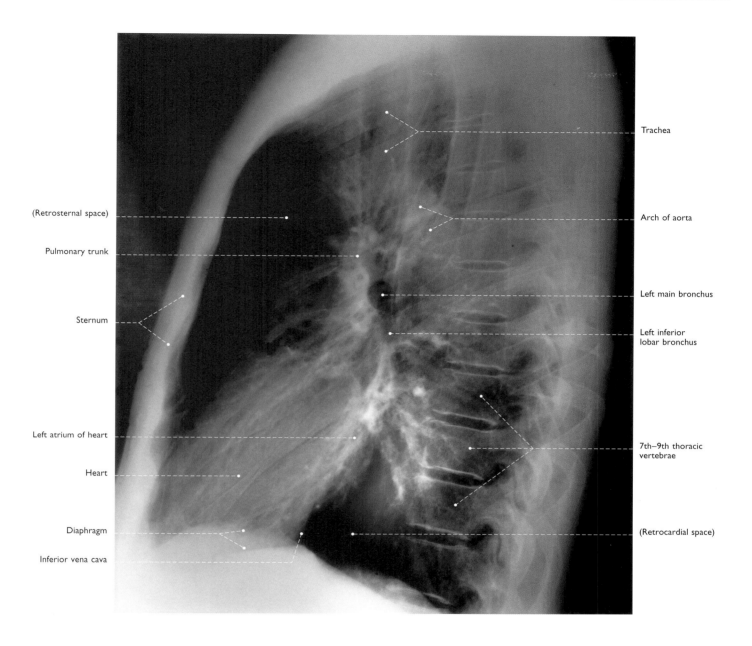

(Retrosternal space)

Pulmonary trunk

Sternum

Left atrium of heart

Heart

Diaphragm

Inferior vena cava

Trachea

Arch of aorta

Left main bronchus

Left inferior
lobar bronchus

7th–9th thoracic
vertebrae

(Retrocardial space)

127 Thoracic organs (55%)
Lateral radiograph

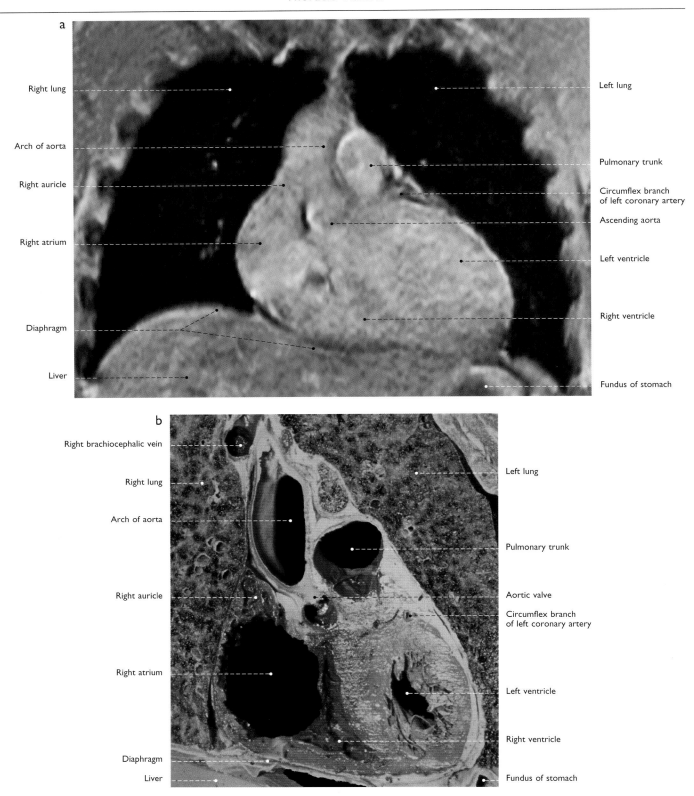

a

Right lung

Arch of aorta

Right auricle

Right atrium

Diaphragm

Liver

Left lung

Pulmonary trunk

Circumflex branch
of left coronary artery

Ascending aorta

Left ventricle

Right ventricle

Fundus of stomach

b

Right brachiocephalic vein

Right lung

Arch of aorta

Right auricle

Right atrium

Diaphragm

Liver

Left lung

Pulmonary trunk

Aortic valve

Circumflex branch
of left coronary artery

Left ventricle

Right ventricle

Fundus of stomach

128 Heart and great blood vessels (55%)
Coronal sections through the thorax in the plane
of ventral parts of the heart, ventral aspect
a Magnetic resonance image (MRI, T$_2$-weighted)
b Anatomical section

a

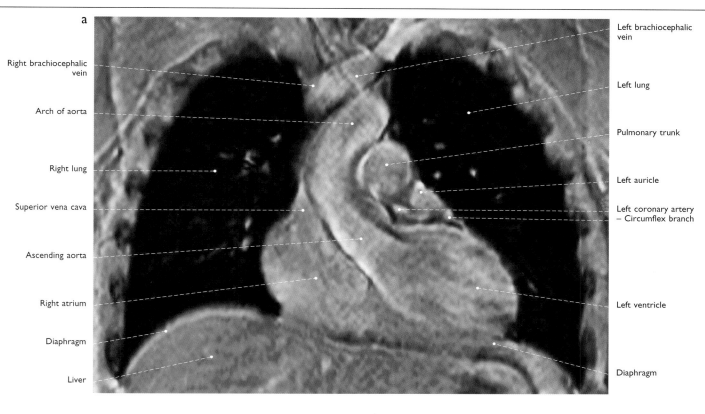

Right brachiocephalic vein

Arch of aorta

Right lung

Superior vena cava

Ascending aorta

Right atrium

Diaphragm

Liver

Left brachiocephalic vein

Left lung

Pulmonary trunk

Left auricle

Left coronary artery – Circumflex branch

Left ventricle

Diaphragm

b

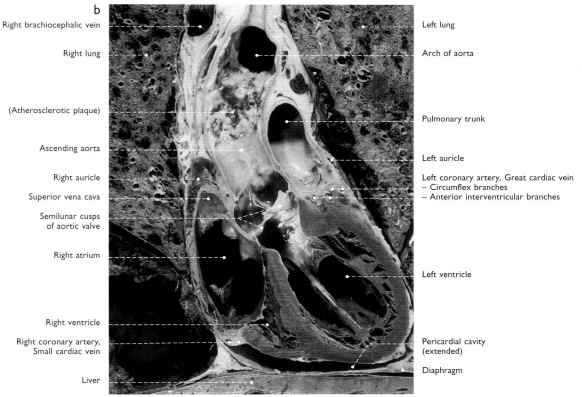

Right brachiocephalic vein

Right lung

(Atherosclerotic plaque)

Ascending aorta

Right auricle

Superior vena cava

Semilunar cusps of aortic valve

Right atrium

Right ventricle

Right coronary artery, Small cardiac vein

Liver

Left lung

Arch of aorta

Pulmonary trunk

Left auricle

Left coronary artery, Great cardiac vein – Circumflex branches – Anterior interventricular branches

Left ventricle

Pericardial cavity (extended)

Diaphragm

129 Heart and great blood vessels (55%)

Coronal sections through the thorax and the heart, cut more dorsally than in fig. 128, ventral aspect

a Magnetic resonance image (MRI, T$_2$-weighted)

b Anatomical section

a

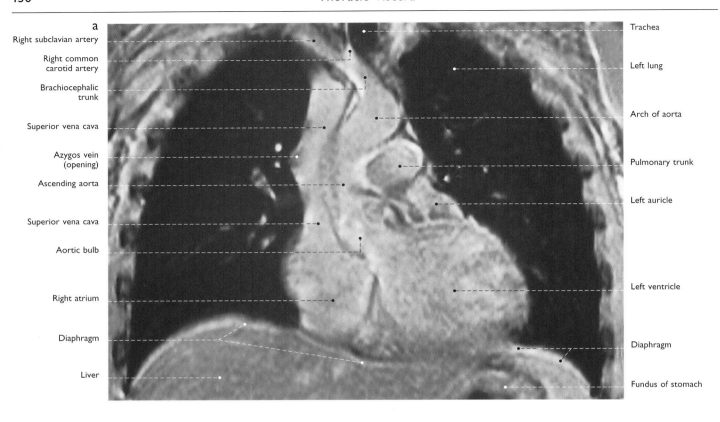

Right subclavian artery

Right common
carotid artery

Brachiocephalic
trunk

Superior vena cava

Azygos vein
(opening)

Ascending aorta

Superior vena cava

Aortic bulb

Right atrium

Diaphragm

Liver

Trachea

Left lung

Arch of aorta

Pulmonary trunk

Left auricle

Left ventricle

Diaphragm

Fundus of stomach

b

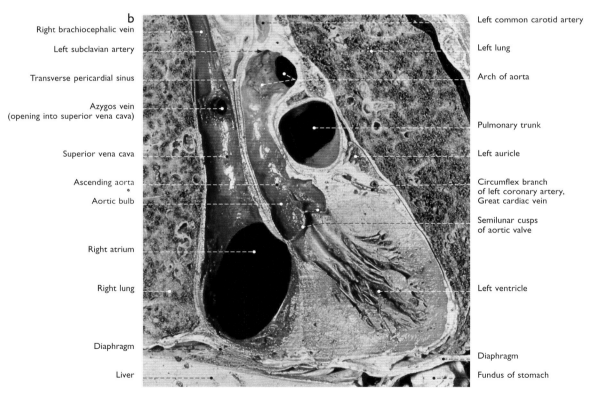

Right brachiocephalic vein

Left subclavian artery

Transverse pericardial sinus

Azygos vein
(opening into superior vena cava)

Superior vena cava

Ascending aorta

Aortic bulb

Right atrium

Right lung

Diaphragm

Liver

Left common carotid artery

Left lung

Arch of aorta

Pulmonary trunk

Left auricle

Circumflex branch
of left coronary artery,
Great cardiac vein

Semilunar cusps
of aortic valve

Left ventricle

Diaphragm

Fundus of stomach

130 Heart and great blood vessels (55%)
Coronal sections through the thorax and the heart,
cut a little more dorsally than in fig. 129, ventral aspect
a Magnetic resonance image (MRI, T$_2$-weighted)
b Anatomical section

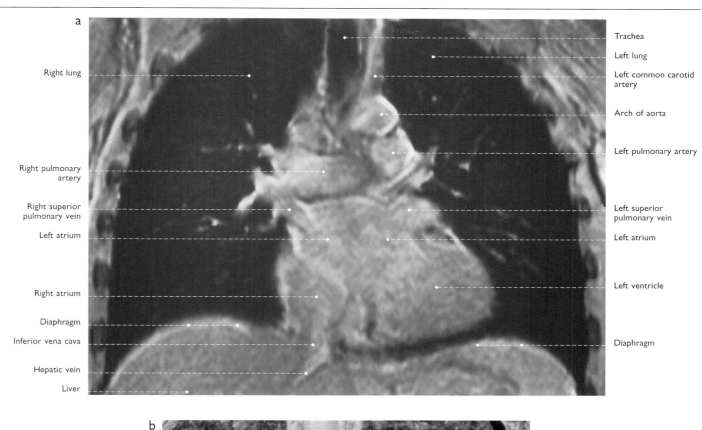

a

Right lung

Right pulmonary
artery

Right superior
pulmonary vein

Left atrium

Right atrium

Diaphragm

Inferior vena cava

Hepatic vein

Liver

Trachea

Left lung

Left common carotid
artery

Arch of aorta

Left pulmonary artery

Left superior
pulmonary vein

Left atrium

Left ventricle

Diaphragm

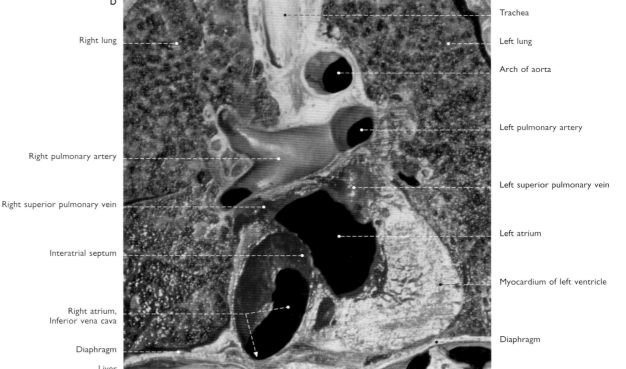

b

Right lung

Right pulmonary artery

Right superior pulmonary vein

Interatrial septum

Right atrium,
Inferior vena cava

Diaphragm

Liver

Trachea

Left lung

Arch of aorta

Left pulmonary artery

Left superior pulmonary vein

Left atrium

Myocardium of left ventricle

Diaphragm

131 Heart and great blood vessels (55%)
      Coronal sections through the thorax in the plane
      of dorsal parts of the heart, ventral aspect
   a Magnetic resonance image (MRI, T$_2$-weighted)
   b Anatomical section

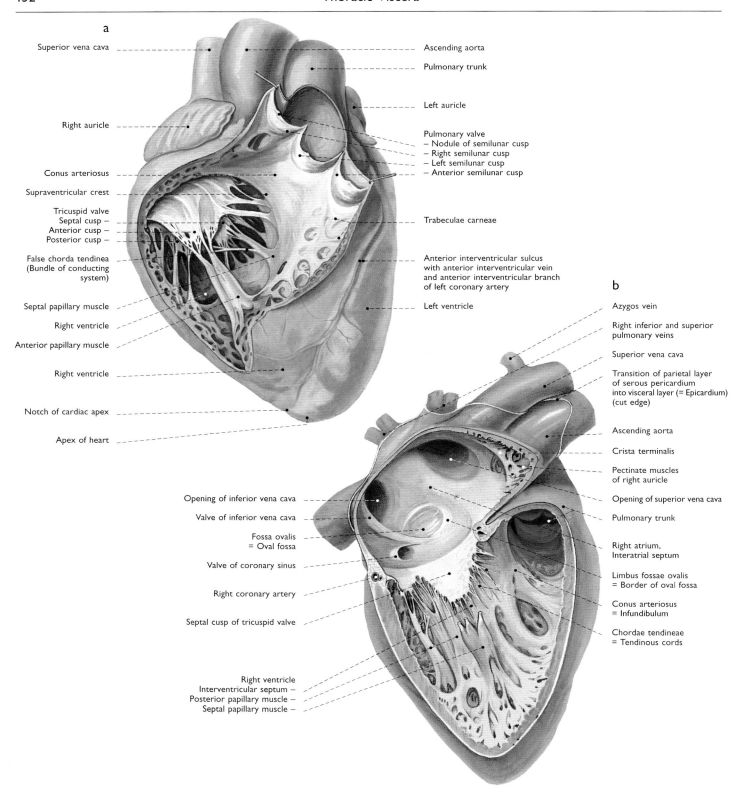

a

Superior vena cava
Right auricle
Conus arteriosus
Supraventricular crest
Tricuspid valve
Septal cusp –
Anterior cusp –
Posterior cusp –
False chorda tendinea
(Bundle of conducting
system)
Septal papillary muscle
Right ventricle
Anterior papillary muscle
Right ventricle
Notch of cardiac apex
Apex of heart

Ascending aorta
Pulmonary trunk
Left auricle
Pulmonary valve
– Nodule of semilunar cusp
– Right semilunar cusp
– Left semilunar cusp
– Anterior semilunar cusp
Trabeculae carneae
Anterior interventricular sulcus
with anterior interventricular vein
and anterior interventricular branch
of left coronary artery
Left ventricle

b

Azygos vein
Right inferior and superior
pulmonary veins
Superior vena cava
Transition of parietal layer
of serous pericardium
into visceral layer (= Epicardium)
(cut edge)
Ascending aorta
Crista terminalis
Pectinate muscles
of right auricle
Opening of superior vena cava
Pulmonary trunk
Right atrium,
Interatrial septum
Limbus fossae ovalis
= Border of oval fossa
Conus arteriosus
= Infundibulum
Chordae tendineae
= Tendinous cords

Opening of inferior vena cava
Valve of inferior vena cava
Fossa ovalis
= Oval fossa
Valve of coronary sinus
Right coronary artery
Septal cusp of tricuspid valve

Right ventricle
Interventricular septum –
Posterior papillary muscle –
Septal papillary muscle –

132 Heart (70%)
a Right ventricle and opening of the pulmonary trunk after
   having cut a window in the anterior walls of the right ventricle
   and the opening of the pulmonary trunk, ventral aspect
b Right atrium and right ventricle of the heart after removal
   of the lateral walls of the right atrium and the right ventricle,
   lateral aspect

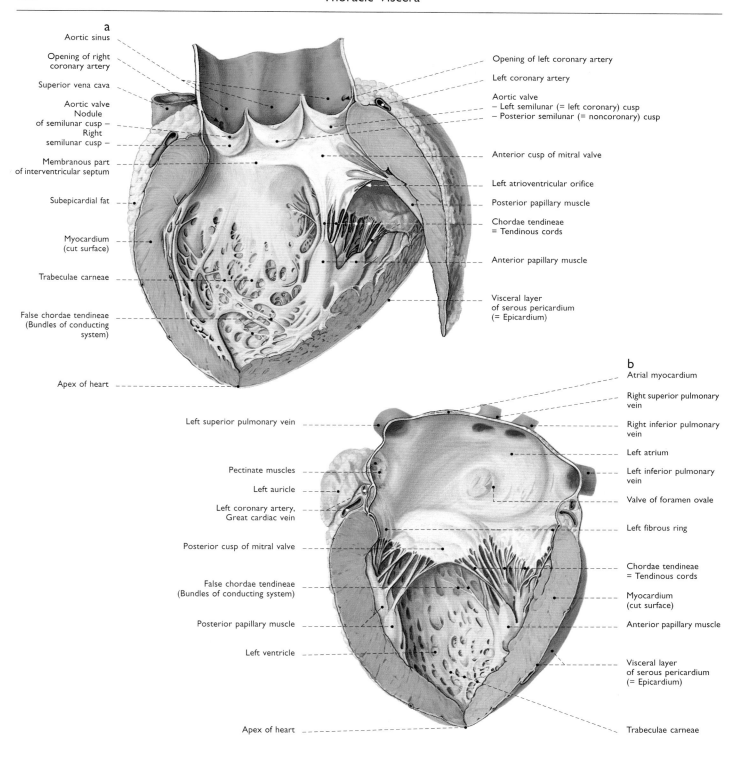

a

Aortic sinus

Opening of right coronary artery

Superior vena cava

Aortic valve
Nodule of semilunar cusp –
Right semilunar cusp –

Membranous part of interventricular septum

Subepicardial fat

Myocardium (cut surface)

Trabeculae carneae

False chordae tendineae (Bundles of conducting system)

Apex of heart

Opening of left coronary artery

Left coronary artery

Aortic valve
– Left semilunar (= left coronary) cusp
– Posterior semilunar (= noncoronary) cusp

Anterior cusp of mitral valve

Left atrioventricular orifice

Posterior papillary muscle

Chordae tendineae = Tendinous cords

Anterior papillary muscle

Visceral layer of serous pericardium (= Epicardium)

b

Left superior pulmonary vein

Pectinate muscles

Left auricle

Left coronary artery, Great cardiac vein

Posterior cusp of mitral valve

False chordae tendineae (Bundles of conducting system)

Posterior papillary muscle

Left ventricle

Apex of heart

Atrial myocardium

Right superior pulmonary vein

Right inferior pulmonary vein

Left atrium

Left inferior pulmonary vein

Valve of foramen ovale

Left fibrous ring

Chordae tendineae = Tendinous cords

Myocardium (cut surface)

Anterior papillary muscle

Visceral layer of serous pericardium (= Epicardium)

Trabeculae carneae

133 Heart (70%)

a   Internal aspect of the left ventricle and the ascending aorta (effluent blood pathway). Incision from the apex of the heart to the point between the right and left semilunar cusps of the aortic valve. A second longitudinal section exposes the affluent blood pathway of the left ventricle.

b   Internal aspect of the left atrium and the affluent blood pathway of the left ventricle. Longitudinal incision along the rounded (left) margin of the heart

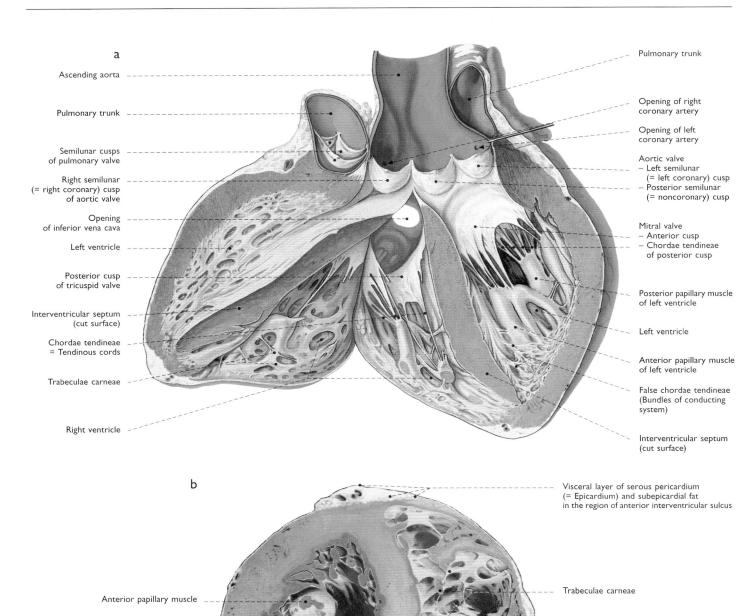

a

Ascending aorta

Pulmonary trunk

Semilunar cusps
of pulmonary valve

Right semilunar
(= right coronary) cusp
of aortic valve

Opening
of inferior vena cava

Left ventricle

Posterior cusp
of tricuspid valve

Interventricular septum
(cut surface)

Chordae tendineae
= Tendinous cords

Trabeculae carneae

Right ventricle

Pulmonary trunk

Opening of right
coronary artery

Opening of left
coronary artery

Aortic valve
– Left semilunar
  (= left coronary) cusp
– Posterior semilunar
  (= noncoronary) cusp

Mitral valve
– Anterior cusp
– Chordae tendineae
  of posterior cusp

Posterior papillary muscle
of left ventricle

Left ventricle

Anterior papillary muscle
of left ventricle

False chordae tendineae
(Bundles of conducting
system)

Interventricular septum
(cut surface)

b

Anterior papillary muscle

Left ventricle

Myocardium

Posterior papillary muscle

Visceral layer of serous pericardium
(= Epicardium) and subepicardial fat
in the region of anterior interventricular sulcus

Trabeculae carneae

Right ventricle

False chordae tendineae
(Bundle of conducting system)

Muscular part
of interventricular septum

134 Heart

a Internal aspect of both ventricles of the heart and
   the left effluent blood pathway. Longitudinal section
   perpendicular to the interventricular septum (70%)
b Superior view into both ventricles of the heart,
   opened by a transverse section (80%)

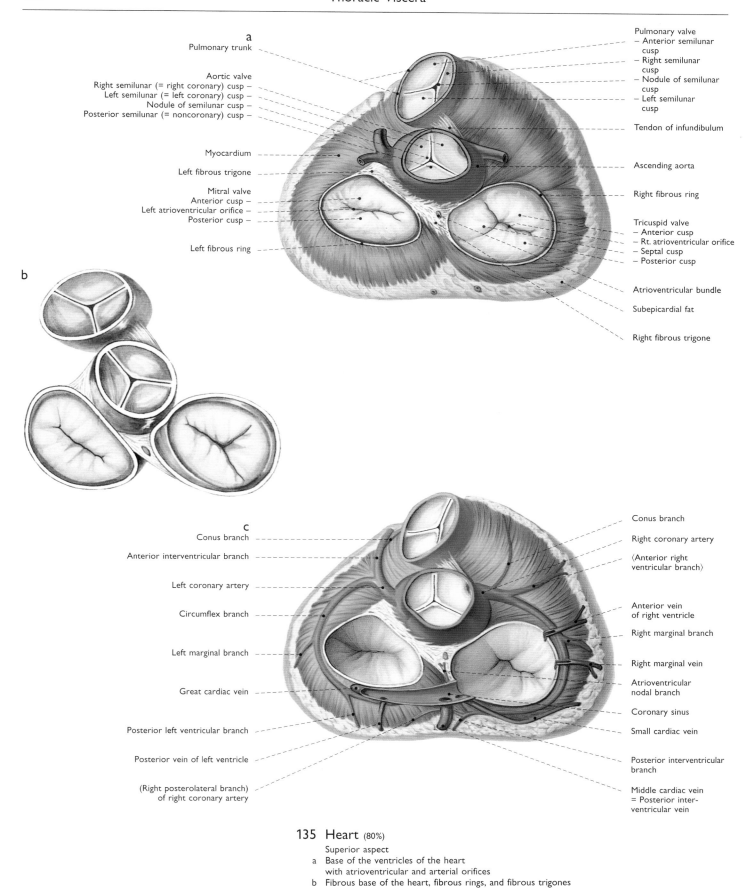

a
Pulmonary trunk

Aortic valve
Right semilunar (= right coronary) cusp –
Left semilunar (= left coronary) cusp –
Nodule of semilunar cusp –
Posterior semilunar (= noncoronary) cusp –

Myocardium

Left fibrous trigone

Mitral valve
Anterior cusp –
Left atrioventricular orifice –
Posterior cusp –

Left fibrous ring

Pulmonary valve
– Anterior semilunar cusp
– Right semilunar cusp
– Nodule of semilunar cusp
– Left semilunar cusp

Tendon of infundibulum

Ascending aorta

Right fibrous ring

Tricuspid valve
– Anterior cusp
– Rt. atrioventricular orifice
– Septal cusp
– Posterior cusp

Atrioventricular bundle

Subepicardial fat

Right fibrous trigone

b

c
Conus branch

Anterior interventricular branch

Left coronary artery

Circumflex branch

Left marginal branch

Great cardiac vein

Posterior left ventricular branch

Posterior vein of left ventricle

(Right posterolateral branch)
of right coronary artery

Conus branch

Right coronary artery

⟨Anterior right ventricular branch⟩

Anterior vein of right ventricle

Right marginal branch

Right marginal vein

Atrioventricular nodal branch

Coronary sinus

Small cardiac vein

Posterior interventricular branch

Middle cardiac vein
= Posterior interventricular vein

135 Heart (80%)
Superior aspect
a Base of the ventricles of the heart
   with atrioventricular and arterial orifices
b Fibrous base of the heart, fibrous rings, and fibrous trigones
c Origin of the coronary vessels

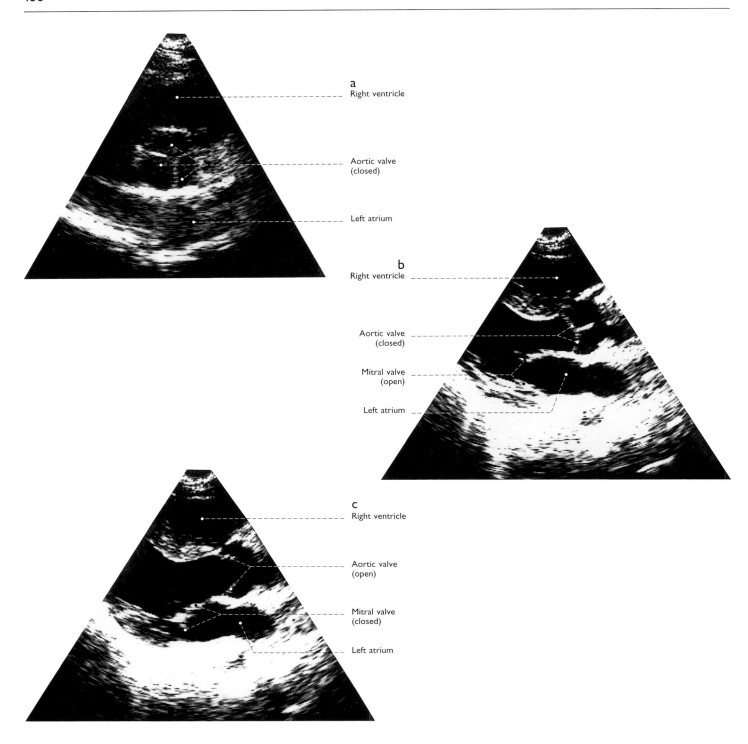

a
Right ventricle

Aortic valve
(closed)

Left atrium

b
Right ventricle

Aortic valve
(closed)

Mitral valve
(open)

Left atrium

c
Right ventricle

Aortic valve
(open)

Mitral valve
(closed)

Left atrium

136 Heart

Ultrasound images (echocardiograms)
a Transverse section through the aortic valve along the short axis.
   The aortic valve is closed. Inferior aspect
b, c Longitudinal section through the heart along the parasternal long axis
   of the left ventricle
b when, during the filling phase of the ventricular diastole,
   the aortic valve is closed and the mitral valve open
c when, during the ejection phase of the ventricular systole,
   the aortic valve is open and the mitral valve closed

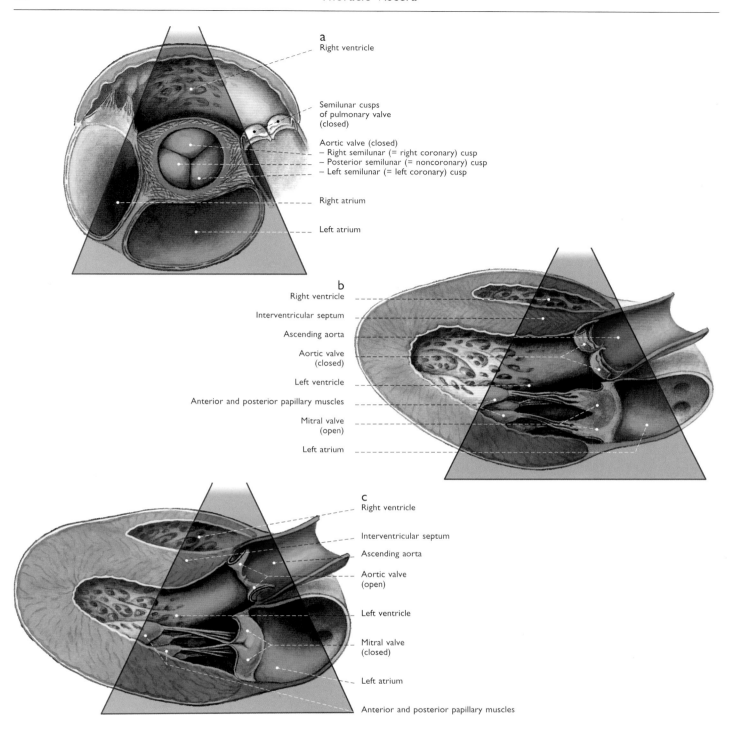

a
Right ventricle

Semilunar cusps
of pulmonary valve
(closed)

Aortic valve (closed)
– Right semilunar (= right coronary) cusp
– Posterior semilunar (= noncoronary) cusp
– Left semilunar (= left coronary) cusp

Right atrium

Left atrium

b
Right ventricle
Interventricular septum
Ascending aorta
Aortic valve
(closed)
Left ventricle
Anterior and posterior papillary muscles
Mitral valve
(open)
Left atrium

c
Right ventricle
Interventricular septum
Ascending aorta
Aortic valve
(open)
Left ventricle
Mitral valve
(closed)
Left atrium
Anterior and posterior papillary muscles

137 Heart
Sections through the heart in analogy to the echocardiograms of fig. 136.
The sectors shown in these echocardiograms are indicated by lines.
a Transverse section just below the aortic valve. The aortic valve is closed.
Inferior aspect
b, c Longitudinal section through the left ventricle
b when, during the filling phase of the ventricular diastole,
the aortic valve is closed and the mitral valve open
c when, during the ejection phase of the ventricular systole,
the aortic valve is open and the mitral valve closed

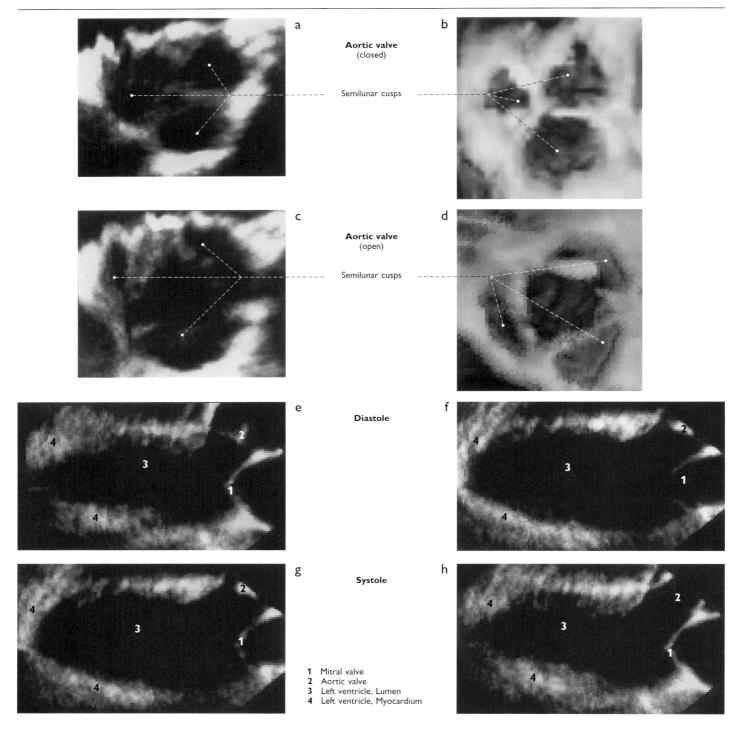

a

Aortic valve
(closed)

Semilunar cusps

b

c

Aortic valve
(open)

Semilunar cusps

d

e

Diastole

f

g

Systole

h

1 Mitral valve
2 Aortic valve
3 Left ventricle, Lumen
4 Left ventricle, Myocardium

138 Heart

Ultrasound images (echocardiograms)
a–d Transverse sections through the aortic valve along the short axis
when the aortic valve is
a, b closed
c, d open
e–h Longitudinal sections through the left ventricle
e during the relaxation phase of diastole when the mitral
and aortic valves are closed
f during the filling phase of diastole when the mitral valve is open
g during the contraction phase of systole when the mitral
and aortic valves are closed
h during the ejection phase of systole when the aortic valve is open

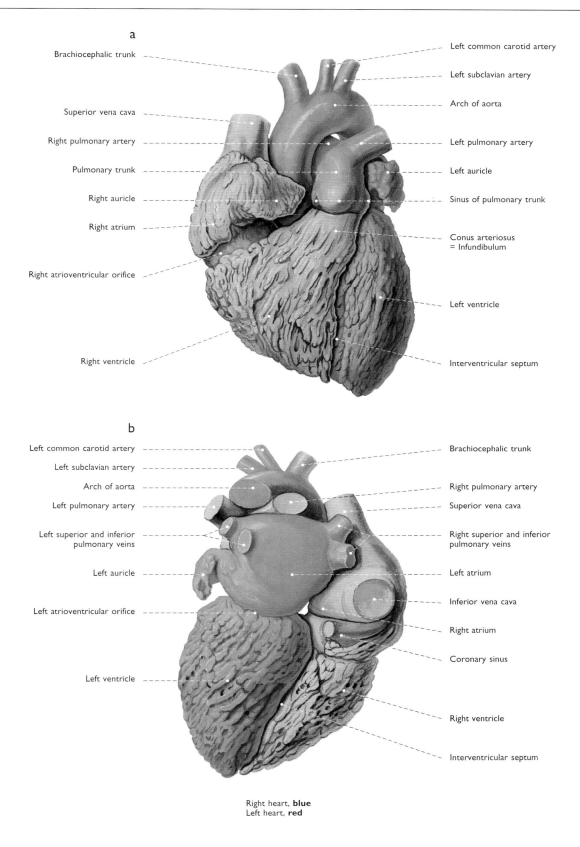

a

Brachiocephalic trunk

Superior vena cava

Right pulmonary artery

Pulmonary trunk

Right auricle

Right atrium

Right atrioventricular orifice

Right ventricle

Left common carotid artery

Left subclavian artery

Arch of aorta

Left pulmonary artery

Left auricle

Sinus of pulmonary trunk

Conus arteriosus
= Infundibulum

Left ventricle

Interventricular septum

b

Left common carotid artery

Left subclavian artery

Arch of aorta

Left pulmonary artery

Left superior and inferior
pulmonary veins

Left auricle

Left atrioventricular orifice

Left ventricle

Brachiocephalic trunk

Right pulmonary artery

Superior vena cava

Right superior and inferior
pulmonary veins

Left atrium

Inferior vena cava

Right atrium

Coronary sinus

Right ventricle

Interventricular septum

Right heart, **blue**
Left heart, **red**

139 Cast of the cavities of heart (80%)
a Ventral aspect
b Dorsal aspect

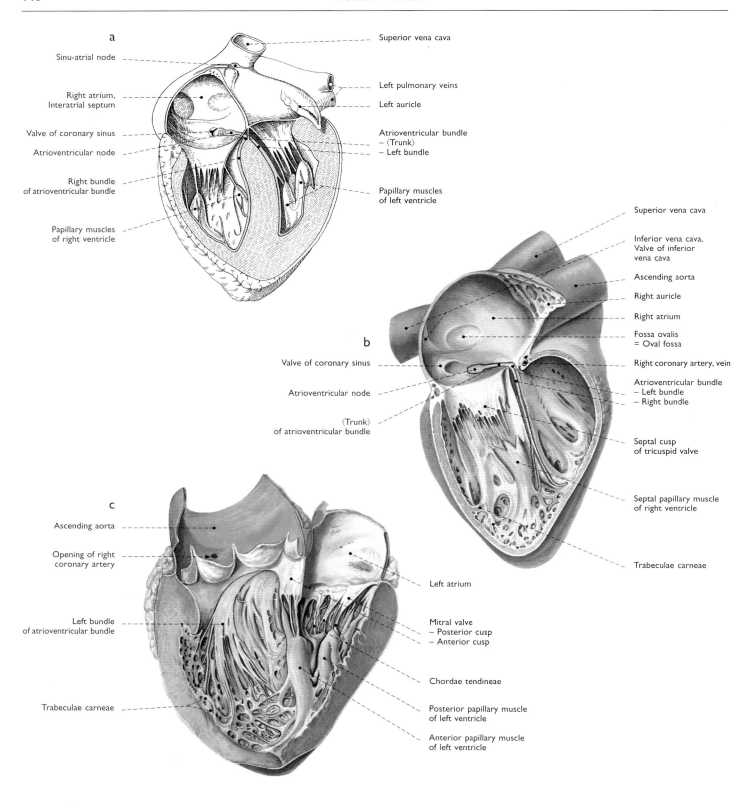

a

Sinu-atrial node

Right atrium,
Interatrial septum

Valve of coronary sinus

Atrioventricular node

Right bundle
of atrioventricular bundle

Papillary muscles
of right ventricle

Superior vena cava

Left pulmonary veins

Left auricle

Atrioventricular bundle
– ⟨Trunk⟩
– Left bundle

Papillary muscles
of left ventricle

b

Valve of coronary sinus

Atrioventricular node

⟨Trunk⟩
of atrioventricular bundle

Superior vena cava

Inferior vena cava,
Valve of inferior
vena cava

Ascending aorta

Right auricle

Right atrium

Fossa ovalis
= Oval fossa

Right coronary artery, vein

Atrioventricular bundle
– Left bundle
– Right bundle

Septal cusp
of tricuspid valve

Septal papillary muscle
of right ventricle

Trabeculae carneae

c

Ascending aorta

Opening of right
coronary artery

Left bundle
of atrioventricular bundle

Trabeculae carneae

Left atrium

Mitral valve
– Posterior cusp
– Anterior cusp

Chordae tendineae

Posterior papillary muscle
of left ventricle

Anterior papillary muscle
of left ventricle

140 Conducting system of the heart (40%)

a The right atrium and both ventricles are opened by a longitudinal
    section perpendicular to the plane of the interventricular septum.
    Ventral aspect, schematic representation

b View from the right to the interventricular septum

c View from the left to the interventricular septum

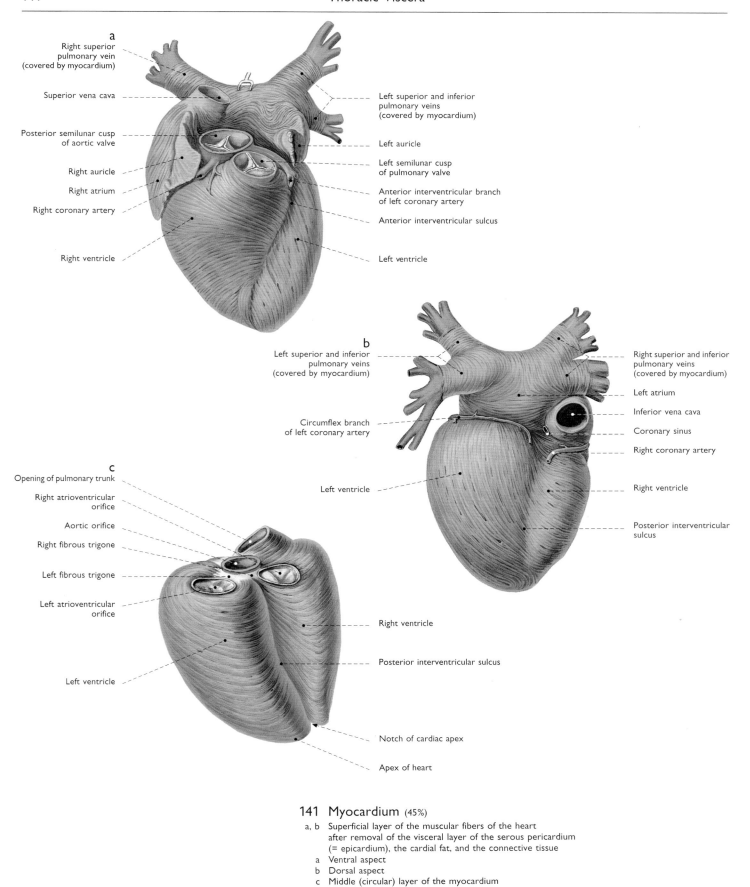

a

Right superior pulmonary vein (covered by myocardium)

Superior vena cava

Posterior semilunar cusp of aortic valve

Right auricle

Right atrium

Right coronary artery

Right ventricle

Left superior and inferior pulmonary veins (covered by myocardium)

Left auricle

Left semilunar cusp of pulmonary valve

Anterior interventricular branch of left coronary artery

Anterior interventricular sulcus

Left ventricle

b

Left superior and inferior pulmonary veins (covered by myocardium)

Circumflex branch of left coronary artery

Left ventricle

Right superior and inferior pulmonary veins (covered by myocardium)

Left atrium

Inferior vena cava

Coronary sinus

Right coronary artery

Right ventricle

Posterior interventricular sulcus

c

Opening of pulmonary trunk

Right atrioventricular orifice

Aortic orifice

Right fibrous trigone

Left fibrous trigone

Left atrioventricular orifice

Left ventricle

Right ventricle

Posterior interventricular sulcus

Notch of cardiac apex

Apex of heart

141 Myocardium (45%)

a, b Superficial layer of the muscular fibers of the heart
after removal of the visceral layer of the serous pericardium
(= epicardium), the cardial fat, and the connective tissue
a Ventral aspect
b Dorsal aspect
c Middle (circular) layer of the myocardium
of both ventricles, dorsal aspect

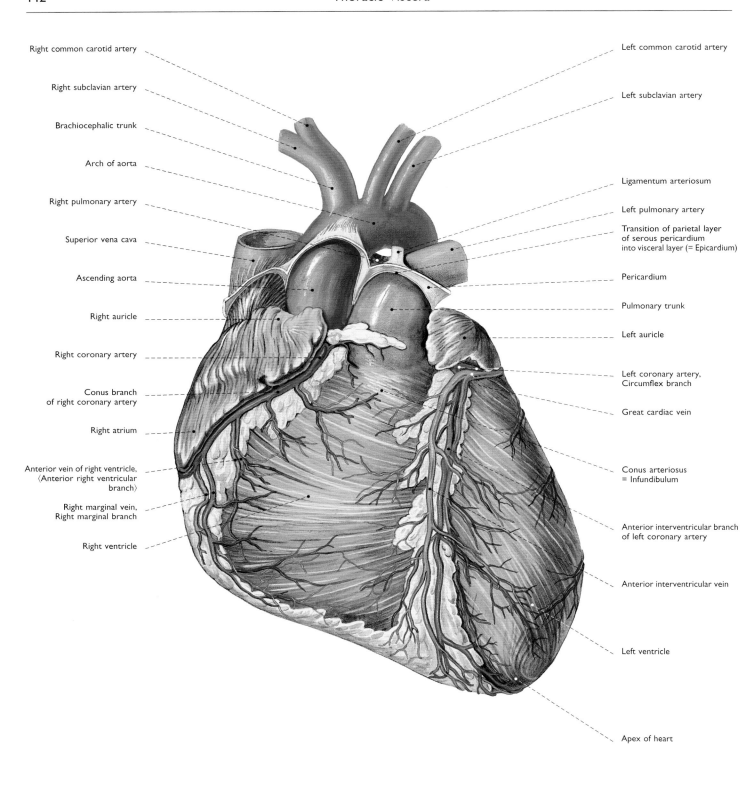

Right common carotid artery

Right subclavian artery

Brachiocephalic trunk

Arch of aorta

Right pulmonary artery

Superior vena cava

Ascending aorta

Right auricle

Right coronary artery

Conus branch
of right coronary artery

Right atrium

Anterior vein of right ventricle,
⟨Anterior right ventricular
branch⟩

Right marginal vein,
Right marginal branch

Right ventricle

Left common carotid artery

Left subclavian artery

Ligamentum arteriosum

Left pulmonary artery

Transition of parietal layer
of serous pericardium
into visceral layer (= Epicardium)

Pericardium

Pulmonary trunk

Left auricle

Left coronary artery,
Circumflex branch

Great cardiac vein

Conus arteriosus
= Infundibulum

Anterior interventricular branch
of left coronary artery

Anterior interventricular vein

Left ventricle

Apex of heart

142 Arteries and veins of the heart (100%)
The epicardium was removed.
Sternocostal (= anterior) surface, ventral aspect

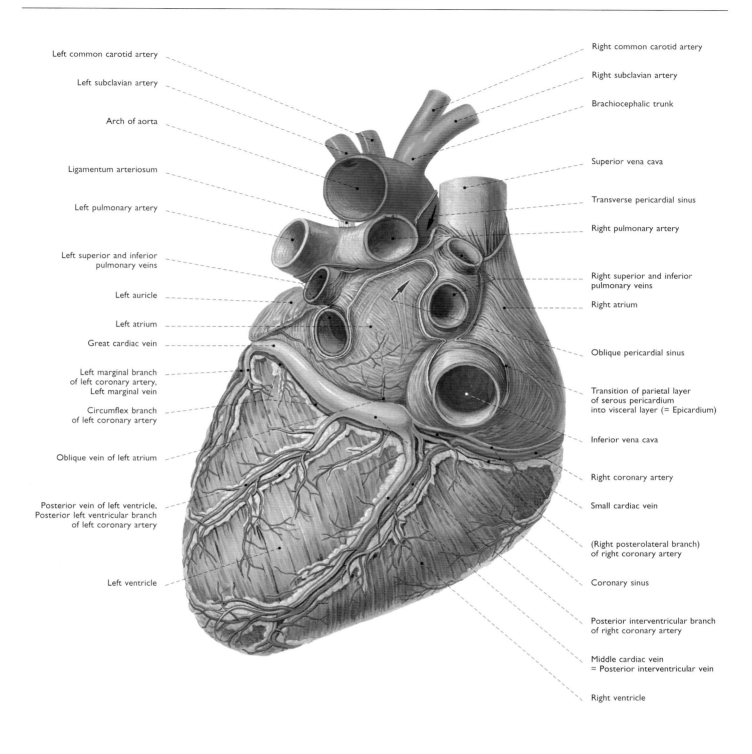

Left common carotid artery

Left subclavian artery

Arch of aorta

Ligamentum arteriosum

Left pulmonary artery

Left superior and inferior pulmonary veins

Left auricle

Left atrium

Great cardiac vein

Left marginal branch of left coronary artery, Left marginal vein

Circumflex branch of left coronary artery

Oblique vein of left atrium

Posterior vein of left ventricle, Posterior left ventricular branch of left coronary artery

Left ventricle

Right common carotid artery

Right subclavian artery

Brachiocephalic trunk

Superior vena cava

Transverse pericardial sinus

Right pulmonary artery

Right superior and inferior pulmonary veins

Right atrium

Oblique pericardial sinus

Transition of parietal layer of serous pericardium into visceral layer (= Epicardium)

Inferior vena cava

Right coronary artery

Small cardiac vein

(Right posterolateral branch) of right coronary artery

Coronary sinus

Posterior interventricular branch of right coronary artery

Middle cardiac vein = Posterior interventricular vein

Right ventricle

143 Arteries and veins of the heart (100%)
The epicardium was removed. Base of the heart and diaphragmatic (= inferior) surface, dorsal aspect

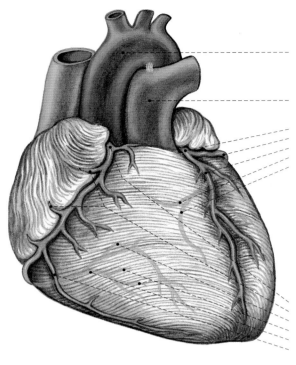

a

Arch of aorta

Pulmonary trunk

Left coronary artery
– Circumflex branch
– Anterior interventricular branch
– Atrial branch
– Posterior left ventricular branch

Right coronary artery
– Atrial branches
– Atrioventricular nodal branch
– Interventricular septal branches
– Posterior interventricular branch
– Right marginal branch

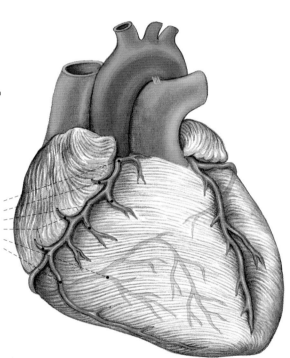

b

Right coronary artery
Sinu-atrial nodal branch –
⟨Anterior right ventricular branches⟩ –
Atrial branches –
Posterior interventricular branch –
Right marginal branch –

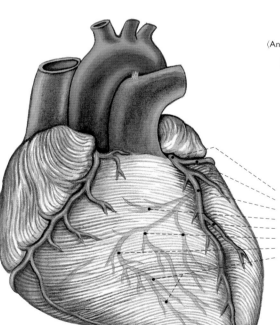

c

Left coronary artery
– Circumflex branch
– Anterior interventricular branch
– Atrial branch
– Lateral branch
– Posterior left ventricular branches
– (Posterior interventricular branch)
– (Interventricular septal branches)

144 Coronary arteries of the heart (70%)
Schematic representations, ventral aspect
a Commonest arrangement
b Right dominance, the right coronary artery
   supplying the posterior walls of both ventricles
c Left dominance, the left coronary artery
   supplying the posterior walls of both ventricles

a

Anterior interventricular sulcus

Muscular part
of interventricular septum

Myocardium
of left ventricle

Posterior interventricular sulcus

b

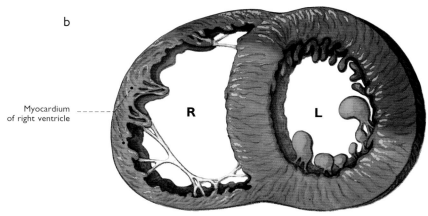

Myocardium
of right ventricle

c

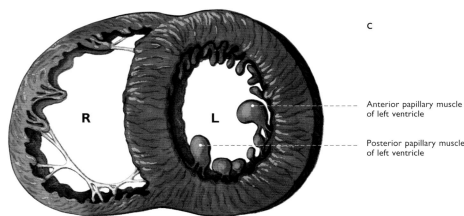

Anterior papillary muscle
of left ventricle

Posterior papillary muscle
of left ventricle

145 Coronary arteries of the heart (80%)
Circulation areas of both coronary arteries in correspondence
to fig. 144, transverse section through both ventricles of the heart
perpendicular to the cardiac axis, schematic representations,
inferior aspect from the apex of heart
(according to Bargmann, 1963, and Töndury, 1970)
a Commonest arrangement
b Right dominance
c Left dominance
The circulation areas of the right coronary artery are marked
by **red**, those of the left coronary artery by **brown** color.

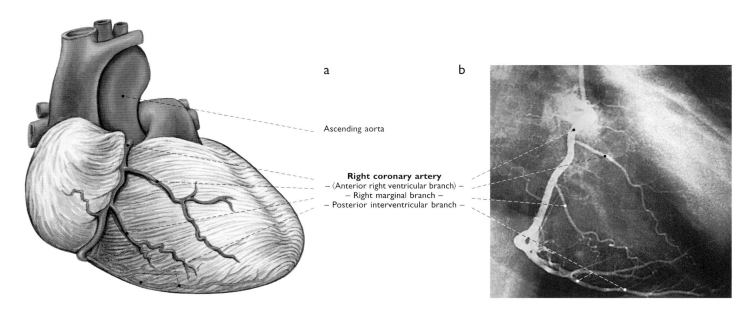

a

Ascending aorta

Right coronary artery
– ⟨Anterior right ventricular branch⟩ –
– Right marginal branch –
– Posterior interventricular branch –

b

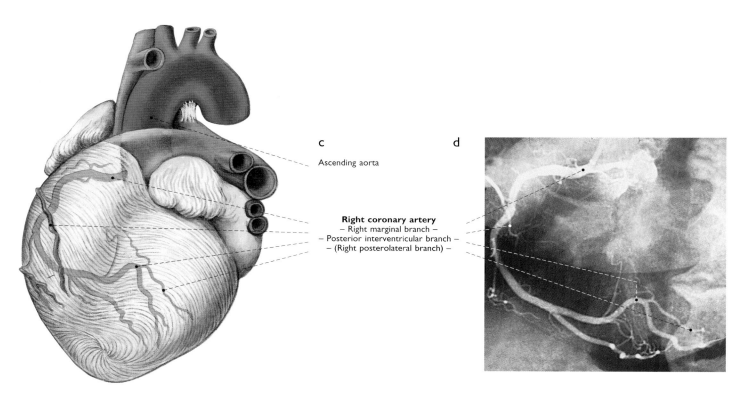

c

Ascending aorta

Right coronary artery
– Right marginal branch –
– Posterior interventricular branch –
– (Right posterolateral branch) –

d

146 Coronary arteries of the heart (50%)
        Right coronary artery
a, b   Right anterior oblique view (RAO projection)
c, d   Left anterior oblique view (LAO projection)
a, c   Schematic representations
b, d   Selective coronary angiograms

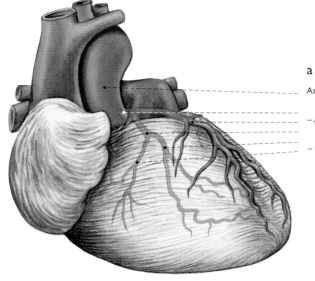

a

Ascending aorta

Left coronary artery
– Anterior interventricular branch –
– Circumflex branch –
– Left marginal branch –
– Posterior left ventricular branch –

b

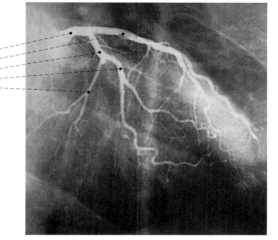

c

Ascending aorta

Left coronary artery
– Anterior interventricular branch –
– Lateral branch –
– Circumflex branch –
– Left marginal branch –
– Posterior left ventricular branch –

d

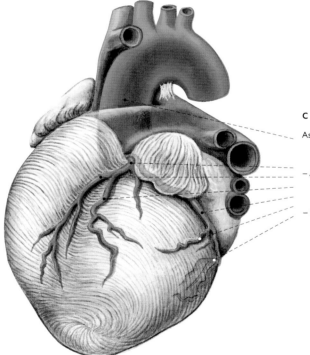

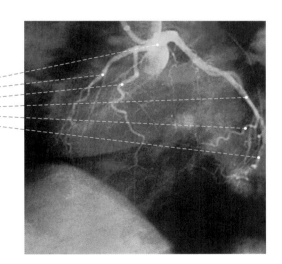

147 Coronary arteries of the heart (50%)

Left coronary artery

a, b   Right anterior oblique view (RAO projection)
c, d   Left anterior oblique view (LAO projection)
a, c   Schematic representations
b, d   Selective coronary angiograms

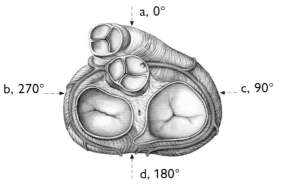

a, 0°

b, 270°

c, 90°

d, 180°

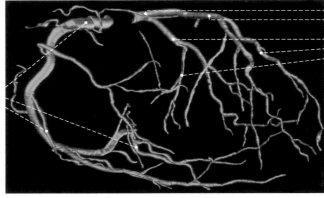

a

Right coronary artery
Posterior interventricular branch –
Right marginal branch –

Left coronary artery
– Anterior interventricular branch
– Circumflex branch
– Lateral branch
– Posterior left ventricular branch

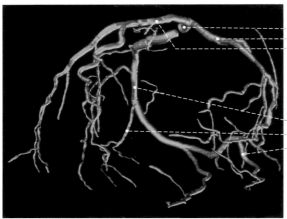

b

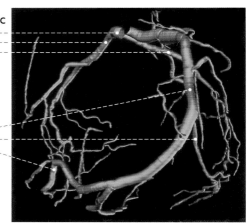

c

Left coronary artery
– Circumflex branch –
– Anterior interventricular branch –

Right coronary artery
– Right marginal branch –
– Posterior interventricular branch –

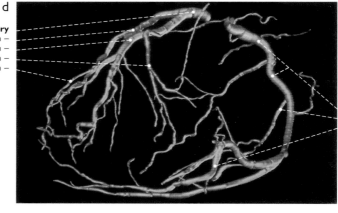

d

Left coronary artery
Anterior interventricular branch –
Circumflex branch –
Posterior left ventricular branch –
Lateral branch –

Right coronary artery
– Right marginal branch
– Posterior interventricular branch

148 Coronary arteries of the heart (50%)
Three-dimensional reconstruction of the course
of the **right** and **left** coronary arteries
a seen from ventral (0°)
b seen from left lateral (270°)
c seen from right lateral (90°)
d seen from dorsal (180°)
   as indicated in the sketch above

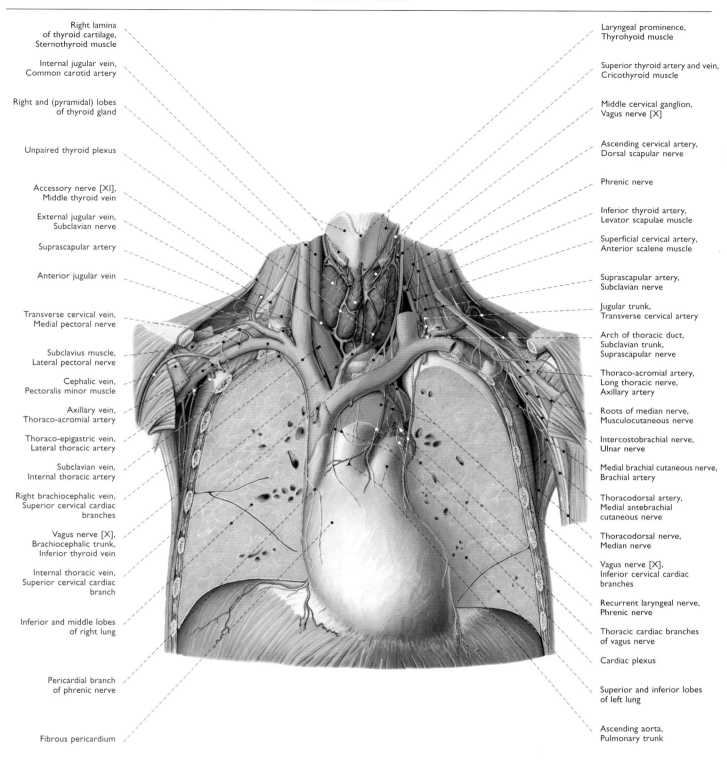

Right lamina of thyroid cartilage, Sternothyroid muscle

Internal jugular vein, Common carotid artery

Right and (pyramidal) lobes of thyroid gland

Unpaired thyroid plexus

Accessory nerve [XI], Middle thyroid vein

External jugular vein, Subclavian nerve

Suprascapular artery

Anterior jugular vein

Transverse cervical vein, Medial pectoral nerve

Subclavius muscle, Lateral pectoral nerve

Cephalic vein, Pectoralis minor muscle

Axillary vein, Thoraco-acromial artery

Thoraco-epigastric vein, Lateral thoracic artery

Subclavian vein, Internal thoracic artery

Right brachiocephalic vein, Superior cervical cardiac branches

Vagus nerve [X], Brachiocephalic trunk, Inferior thyroid vein

Internal thoracic vein, Superior cervical cardiac branch

Inferior and middle lobes of right lung

Pericardial branch of phrenic nerve

Fibrous pericardium

Laryngeal prominence, Thyrohyoid muscle

Superior thyroid artery and vein, Cricothyroid muscle

Middle cervical ganglion, Vagus nerve [X]

Ascending cervical artery, Dorsal scapular nerve

Phrenic nerve

Inferior thyroid artery, Levator scapulae muscle

Superficial cervical artery, Anterior scalene muscle

Suprascapular artery, Subclavian nerve

Jugular trunk, Transverse cervical artery

Arch of thoracic duct, Subclavian trunk, Suprascapular nerve

Thoraco-acromial artery, Long thoracic nerve, Axillary artery

Roots of median nerve, Musculocutaneous nerve

Intercostobrachial nerve, Ulnar nerve

Medial brachial cutaneous nerve, Brachial artery

Thoracodorsal artery, Medial antebrachial cutaneous nerve

Thoracodorsal nerve, Median nerve

Vagus nerve [X], Inferior cervical cardiac branches

Recurrent laryngeal nerve, Phrenic nerve

Thoracic cardiac branches of vagus nerve

Cardiac plexus

Superior and inferior lobes of left lung

Ascending aorta, Pulmonary trunk

149   Blood vessels and nerves of the neck, mediastinum, and axilla (40%)

The sternocleidomastoid and infrahyoid muscles, the anterior thoracic wall, and anterior parts of the lungs were removed. Ventral aspect

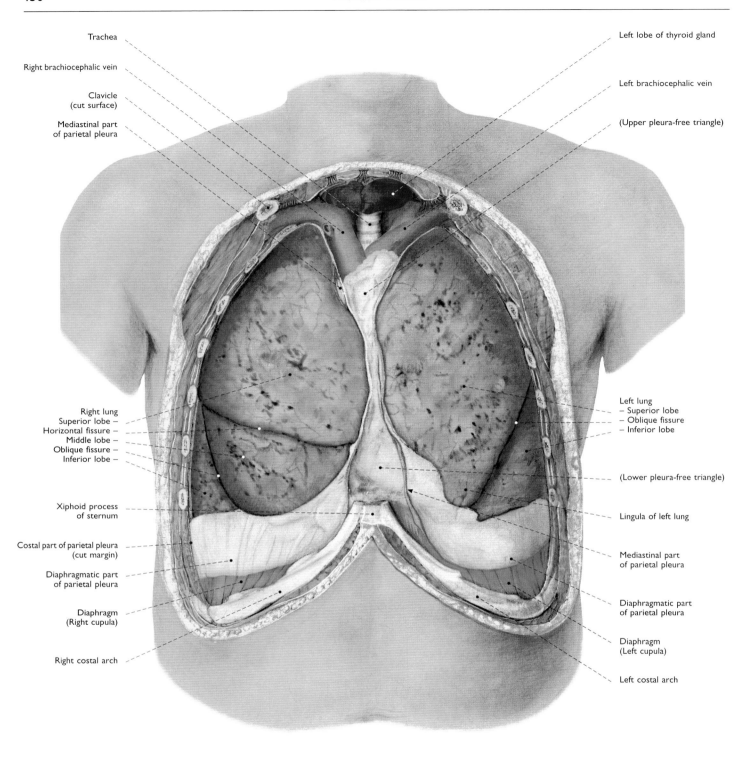

Trachea

Right brachiocephalic vein

Clavicle
(cut surface)

Mediastinal part
of parietal pleura

Left lobe of thyroid gland

Left brachiocephalic vein

(Upper pleura-free triangle)

Right lung
Superior lobe –
Horizontal fissure –
Middle lobe –
Oblique fissure –
Inferior lobe –

Left lung
– Superior lobe
– Oblique fissure
– Inferior lobe

(Lower pleura-free triangle)

Xiphoid process
of sternum

Lingula of left lung

Costal part of parietal pleura
(cut margin)

Mediastinal part
of parietal pleura

Diaphragmatic part
of parietal pleura

Diaphragm
(Right cupula)

Diaphragmatic part
of parietal pleura

Right costal arch

Diaphragm
(Left cupula)

Left costal arch

150   Thoracic viscera in situ (40%)
The anterior thoracic wall was removed.
Ventral aspect

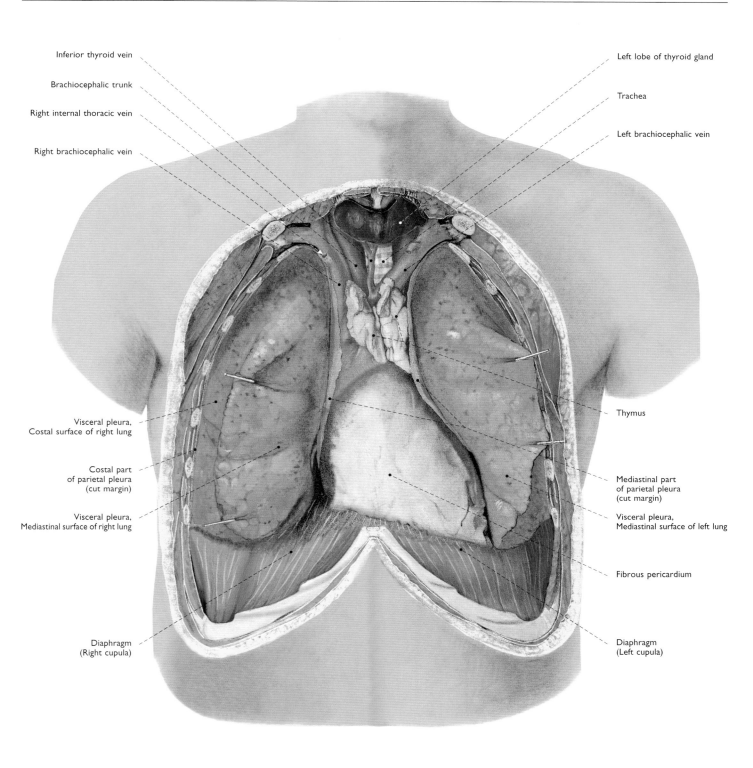

Inferior thyroid vein

Brachiocephalic trunk

Right internal thoracic vein

Right brachiocephalic vein

Left lobe of thyroid gland

Trachea

Left brachiocephalic vein

Visceral pleura,
Costal surface of right lung

Costal part
of parietal pleura
(cut margin)

Visceral pleura,
Mediastinal surface of right lung

Diaphragm
(Right cupula)

Thymus

Mediastinal part
of parietal pleura
(cut margin)

Visceral pleura,
Mediastinal surface of left lung

Fibrous pericardium

Diaphragm
(Left cupula)

151 Thoracic viscera (40%)
From the same preparation used for fig. 150 after removal
of the diaphragmatic part of the parietal pleura. Both lungs were displaced
laterally and rotated by hooks inserted along their anterior margins.
The anterior (= ventral) surface of the fibrous pericardium is revealed,
the thymus and the large vessels are exposed in the upper triangle free of pleura.
Ventral aspect

a
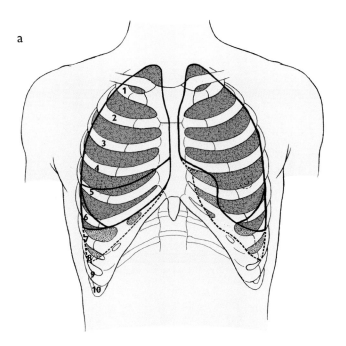

b
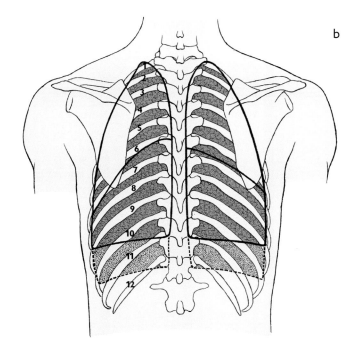

c
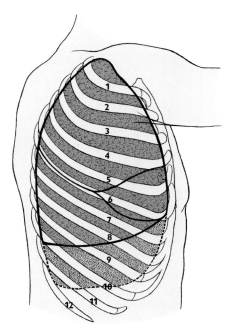

d
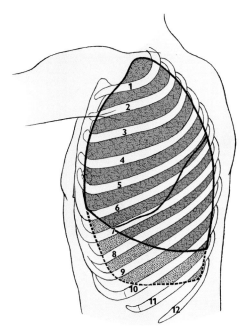

.... Borders of pleura
——— Borders of lungs and lung lobes

152 Borders of the pleura, the lungs, and lung lobes

Schematic representations. The borders of the pleura are
indicated by a dashed line, the lung borders by a continuous line.
a   Ventral aspect
b   Dorsal aspect
c   Right lateral aspect
d   Left lateral aspect

a

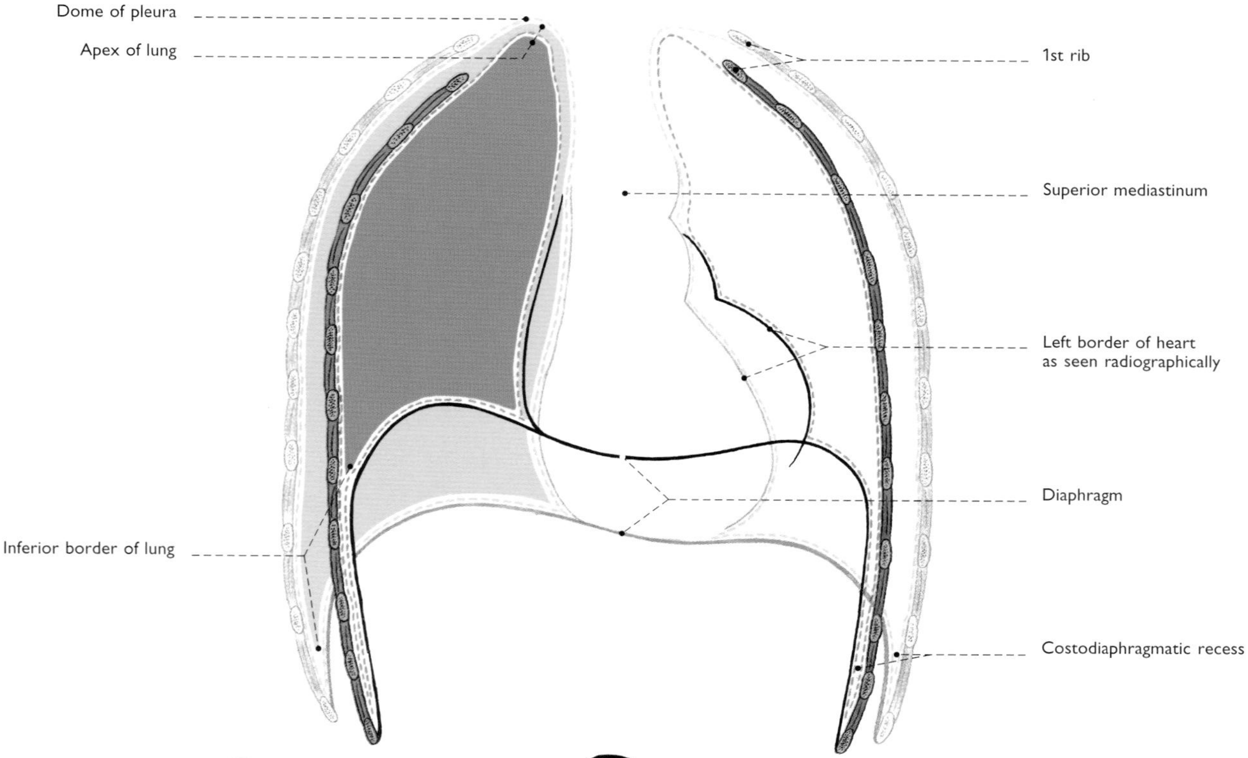

Dome of pleura ----------- •

Apex of lung -----------

1st rib

Superior mediastinum

Left border of heart
as seen radiographically

Diaphragm

Inferior border of lung -----------

Costodiaphragmatic recess

b

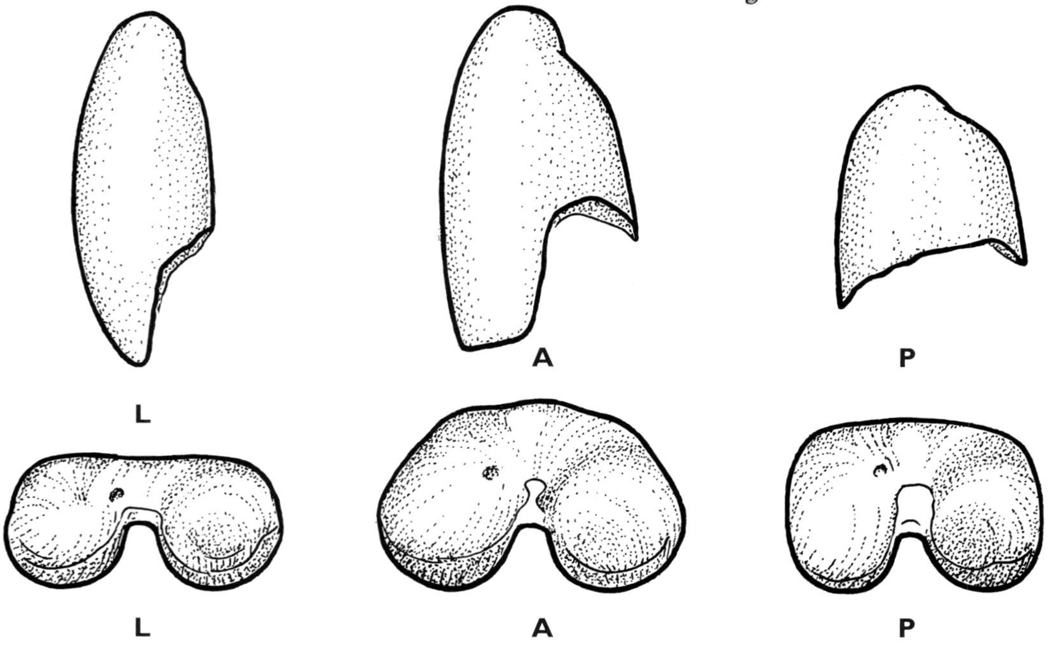

L

A

P

L

A

P

153 Pleural and thoracic cavities

Schematic representations

a Outline of the parietal pleura (dashed line) in the expiratory phase
given in dark blue, in the inspiratory phase in middle blue.
Projection of the right lung during expiration shown in dark blue,
inspiratory increase in middle blue, coronal section of the thorax

b Shapes of the thorax of leptosomatic (L), athletic (A), and pyknic (P) subjects,
schematic outlines, lateral and inferior aspects

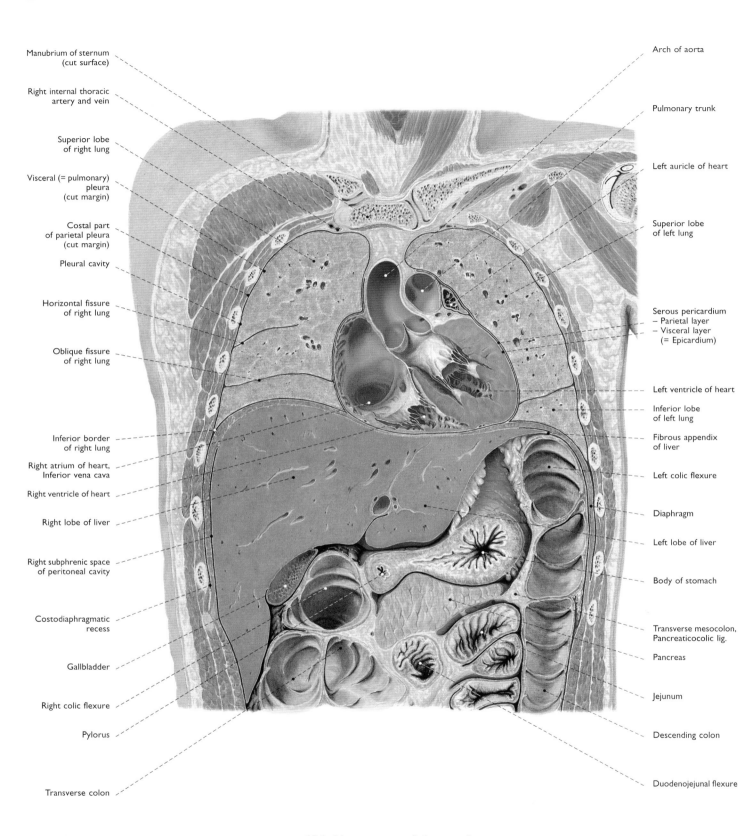

Manubrium of sternum (cut surface)

Right internal thoracic artery and vein

Superior lobe of right lung

Visceral (= pulmonary) pleura (cut margin)

Costal part of parietal pleura (cut margin)

Pleural cavity

Horizontal fissure of right lung

Oblique fissure of right lung

Inferior border of right lung

Right atrium of heart, Inferior vena cava

Right ventricle of heart

Right lobe of liver

Right subphrenic space of peritoneal cavity

Costodiaphragmatic recess

Gallbladder

Right colic flexure

Pylorus

Transverse colon

Arch of aorta

Pulmonary trunk

Left auricle of heart

Superior lobe of left lung

Serous pericardium
– Parietal layer
– Visceral layer (= Epicardium)

Left ventricle of heart

Inferior lobe of left lung

Fibrous appendix of liver

Left colic flexure

Diaphragm

Left lobe of liver

Body of stomach

Transverse mesocolon, Pancreaticocolic lig.

Pancreas

Jejunum

Descending colon

Duodenojejunal flexure

154   Upper part of the trunk (40%)
Coronal section through the trunk in the plane of the two sternoclavicular joints, drawing of an anatomical section, ventral aspect

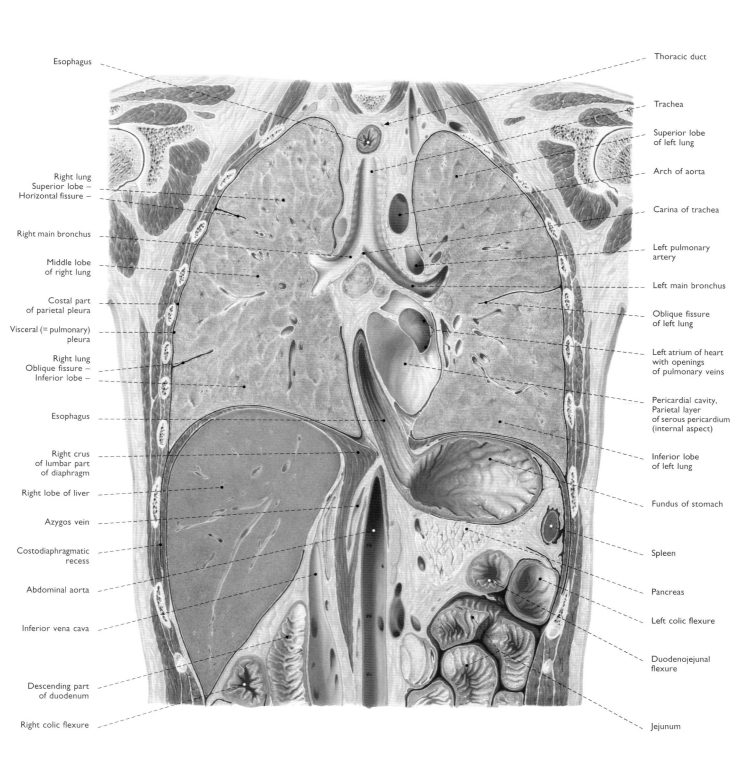

Esophagus

Right lung
Superior lobe –
Horizontal fissure –

Right main bronchus

Middle lobe
of right lung

Costal part
of parietal pleura

Visceral (= pulmonary)
pleura

Right lung
Oblique fissure –
Inferior lobe –

Esophagus

Right crus
of lumbar part
of diaphragm

Right lobe of liver

Azygos vein

Costodiaphragmatic
recess

Abdominal aorta

Inferior vena cava

Descending part
of duodenum

Right colic flexure

Thoracic duct

Trachea

Superior lobe
of left lung

Arch of aorta

Carina of trachea

Left pulmonary
artery

Left main bronchus

Oblique fissure
of left lung

Left atrium of heart
with openings
of pulmonary veins

Pericardial cavity,
Parietal layer
of serous pericardium
(internal aspect)

Inferior lobe
of left lung

Fundus of stomach

Spleen

Pancreas

Left colic flexure

Duodenojejunal
flexure

Jejunum

155 Upper part of the trunk (40%)
Coronal section through the trunk in the plane
of the tracheal bifurcation and the esophageal hiatus,
drawing of an anatomical section, ventral aspect

a

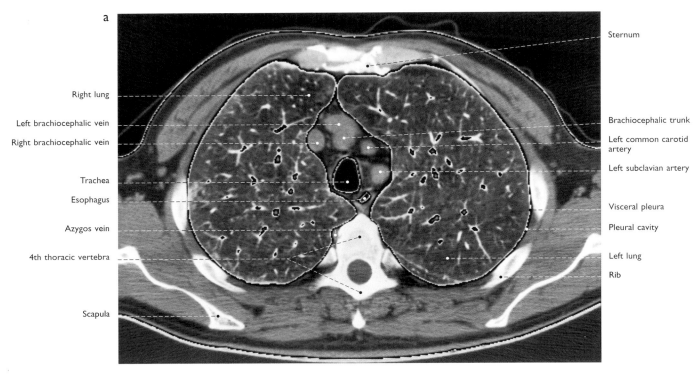

Sternum

Right lung

Left brachiocephalic vein

Right brachiocephalic vein

Brachiocephalic trunk

Left common carotid artery

Left subclavian artery

Trachea

Esophagus

Visceral pleura

Azygos vein

Pleural cavity

4th thoracic vertebra

Left lung

Rib

Scapula

b

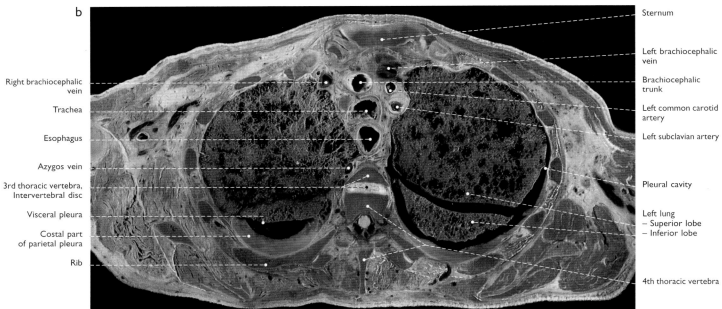

Sternum

Right brachiocephalic vein

Left brachiocephalic vein

Trachea

Brachiocephalic trunk

Esophagus

Left common carotid artery

Left subclavian artery

Azygos vein

3rd thoracic vertebra, Intervertebral disc

Pleural cavity

Visceral pleura

Left lung
– Superior lobe
– Inferior lobe

Costal part of parietal pleura

Rib

4th thoracic vertebra

156 Thorax (50%)

Transverse sections through the lungs and the upper mediastinum
at the level of the fourth (Th IV, a) and the third/fourth (Th III/IV, b)
thoracic vertebral bodies, respectively, inferior aspect

a Computed tomogram (CT) after injection of contrast medium
(combined mediastinal and lung window settings)

b Anatomical section

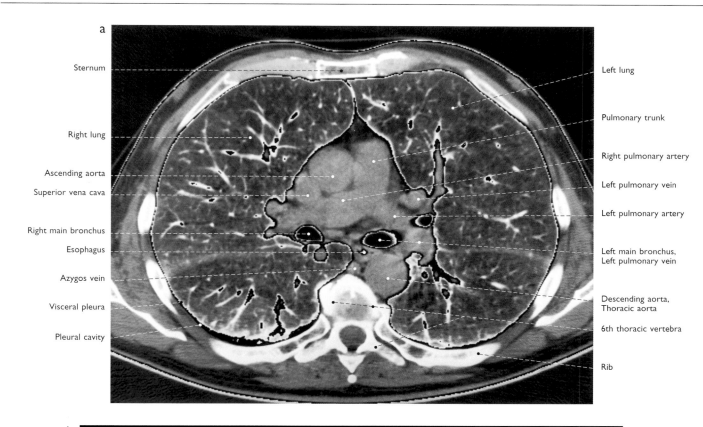

a

Sternum — Left lung

Right lung — Pulmonary trunk

Ascending aorta — Right pulmonary artery
Superior vena cava — Left pulmonary vein

Left pulmonary artery

Right main bronchus — Left main bronchus,
Esophagus — Left pulmonary vein

Azygos vein

Visceral pleura — Descending aorta,
Thoracic aorta

Pleural cavity — 6th thoracic vertebra

Rib

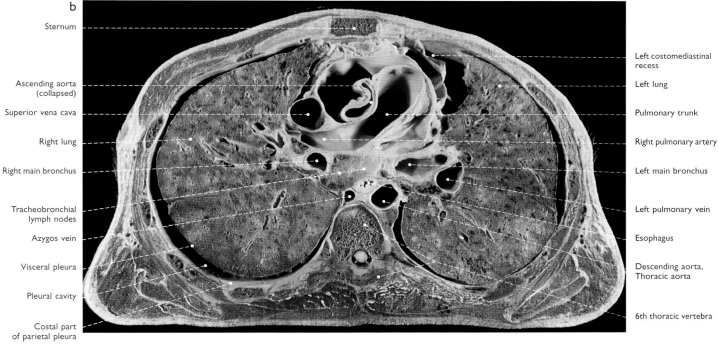

b

Sternum — Left costomediastinal
recess

Ascending aorta — Left lung
(collapsed)

Superior vena cava — Pulmonary trunk

Right lung — Right pulmonary artery

Right main bronchus — Left main bronchus

Tracheobronchial — Left pulmonary vein
lymph nodes

Azygos vein — Esophagus

Visceral pleura — Descending aorta,
Thoracic aorta

Pleural cavity — 6th thoracic vertebra

Costal part
of parietal pleura

157   Thorax (50%)

Transverse sections through the lungs and the mediastinum
at the level of the sixth thoracic vertebral body (Th VI),
inferior aspect

a   Computed tomogram (CT) after injection of contrast medium
(combined mediastinal and lung window settings)

b   Anatomical section

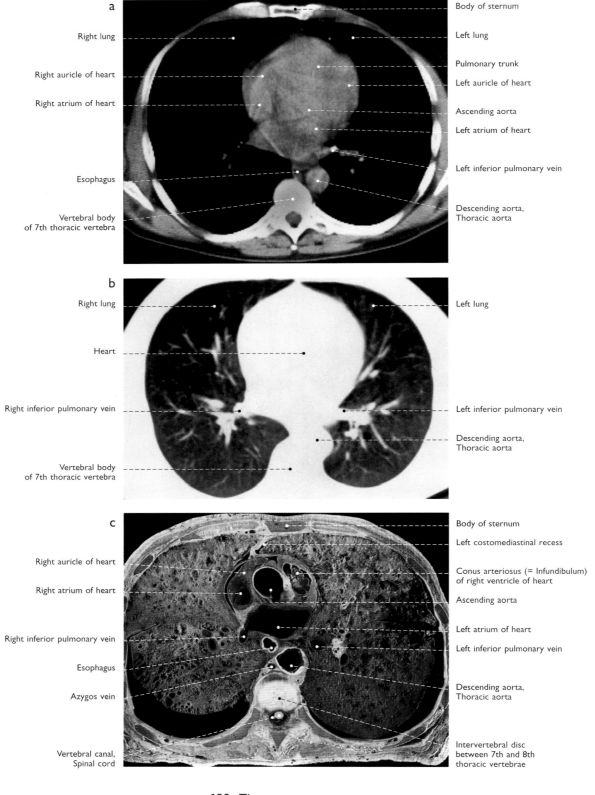

a
Right lung
Right auricle of heart
Right atrium of heart
Esophagus
Vertebral body
of 7th thoracic vertebra

Body of sternum
Left lung
Pulmonary trunk
Left auricle of heart
Ascending aorta
Left atrium of heart
Left inferior pulmonary vein
Descending aorta,
Thoracic aorta

b
Right lung
Heart
Right inferior pulmonary vein
Vertebral body
of 7th thoracic vertebra

Left lung
Left inferior pulmonary vein
Descending aorta,
Thoracic aorta

c
Right auricle of heart
Right atrium of heart
Right inferior pulmonary vein
Esophagus
Azygos vein
Vertebral canal,
Spinal cord

Body of sternum
Left costomediastinal recess
Conus arteriosus (= Infundibulum)
of right ventricle of heart
Ascending aorta
Left atrium of heart
Left inferior pulmonary vein
Descending aorta,
Thoracic aorta
Intervertebral disc
between 7th and 8th
thoracic vertebrae

158 Thorax (35%)

Transverse sections at the level of the seventh
thoracic vertebral body (Th VII), inferior aspect
a, b   Computed tomograms (CT)
   a   Mediastinal window setting
   b   Lung window setting
   c   Anatomical section

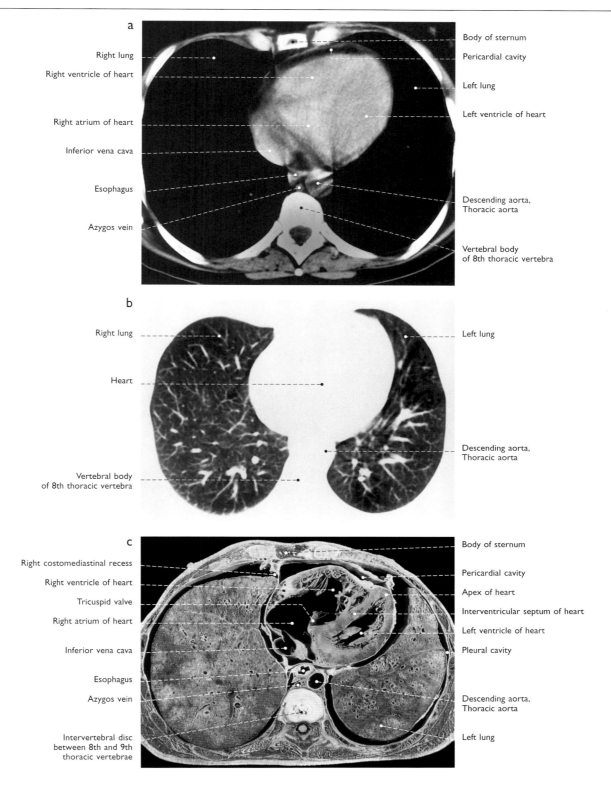

a

Right lung

Right ventricle of heart

Right atrium of heart

Inferior vena cava

Esophagus

Azygos vein

Body of sternum

Pericardial cavity

Left lung

Left ventricle of heart

Descending aorta,
Thoracic aorta

Vertebral body
of 8th thoracic vertebra

b

Right lung

Heart

Vertebral body
of 8th thoracic vertebra

Left lung

Descending aorta,
Thoracic aorta

c

Right costomediastinal recess

Right ventricle of heart

Tricuspid valve

Right atrium of heart

Inferior vena cava

Esophagus

Azygos vein

Intervertebral disc
between 8th and 9th
thoracic vertebrae

Body of sternum

Pericardial cavity

Apex of heart

Interventricular septum of heart

Left ventricle of heart

Pleural cavity

Descending aorta,
Thoracic aorta

Left lung

159　Thorax (35%)

Transverse sections at the level of the eighth
thoracic vertebral body (Th VIII), inferior aspect

a, b　Computed tomograms (CT)

　　a　Mediastinal window setting

　　b　Lung window setting

　　c　Anatomical section

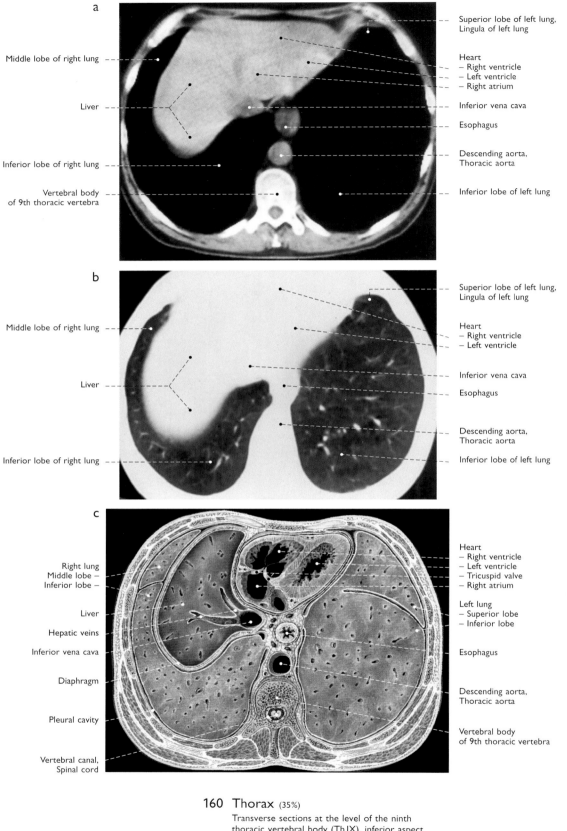

a

Middle lobe of right lung

Liver

Inferior lobe of right lung

Vertebral body
of 9th thoracic vertebra

Superior lobe of left lung,
Lingula of left lung

Heart
– Right ventricle
– Left ventricle
– Right atrium

Inferior vena cava

Esophagus

Descending aorta,
Thoracic aorta

Inferior lobe of left lung

b

Middle lobe of right lung

Liver

Inferior lobe of right lung

Superior lobe of left lung,
Lingula of left lung

Heart
– Right ventricle
– Left ventricle

Inferior vena cava

Esophagus

Descending aorta,
Thoracic aorta

Inferior lobe of left lung

c

Right lung
Middle lobe –
Inferior lobe –

Liver

Hepatic veins

Inferior vena cava

Diaphragm

Pleural cavity

Vertebral canal,
Spinal cord

Heart
– Right ventricle
– Left ventricle
– Tricuspid valve
– Right atrium

Left lung
– Superior lobe
– Inferior lobe

Esophagus

Descending aorta,
Thoracic aorta

Vertebral body
of 9th thoracic vertebra

160 Thorax (35%)

Transverse sections at the level of the ninth
thoracic vertebral body (Th IX), inferior aspect
a, b   Computed tomograms (CT)
   a   Mediastinal window setting
   b   Lung window setting
   c   Anatomical section (painted)

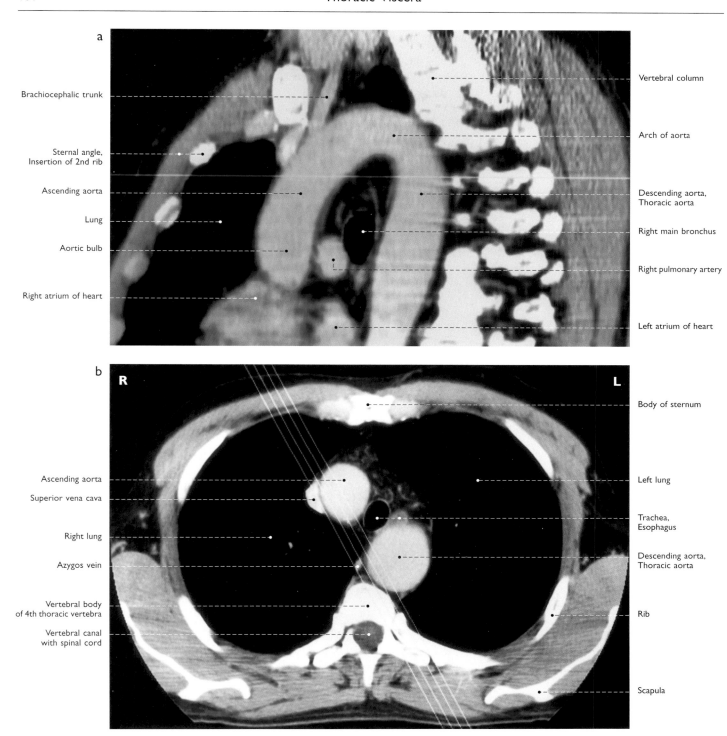

a

Brachiocephalic trunk

Sternal angle,
Insertion of 2nd rib

Ascending aorta

Lung

Aortic bulb

Right atrium of heart

Vertebral column

Arch of aorta

Descending aorta,
Thoracic aorta

Right main bronchus

Right pulmonary artery

Left atrium of heart

b

R   L

Ascending aorta

Superior vena cava

Right lung

Azygos vein

Vertebral body
of 4th thoracic vertebra

Vertebral canal
with spinal cord

Body of sternum

Left lung

Trachea,
Esophagus

Descending aorta,
Thoracic aorta

Rib

Scapula

161 Thorax (50%)

Computed tomograms (CT) showing the aorta

a Oblique section through the arch of aorta from right anterior
to left posterior as indicated in fig. b (oblique sagittal reconstruction)

b Transverse section at the level of the sternal angle and the body
of the fourth thoracic vertebra (Th IV) in the plane as indicated in fig. a

a

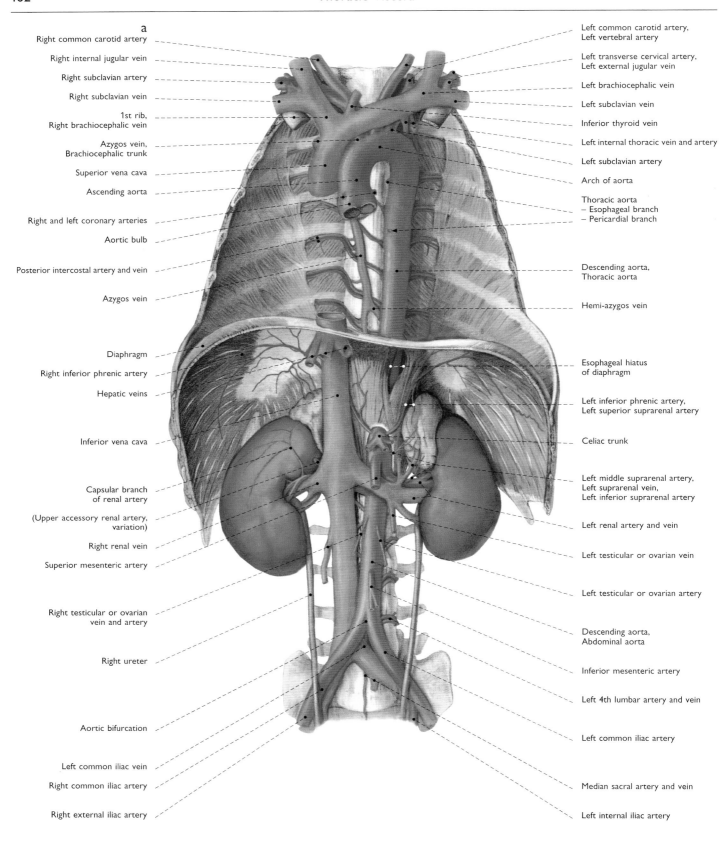

Right common carotid artery

Right internal jugular vein

Right subclavian artery

Right subclavian vein

1st rib,
Right brachiocephalic vein

Azygos vein,
Brachiocephalic trunk

Superior vena cava

Ascending aorta

Right and left coronary arteries

Aortic bulb

Posterior intercostal artery and vein

Azygos vein

Diaphragm

Right inferior phrenic artery

Hepatic veins

Inferior vena cava

Capsular branch
of renal artery

(Upper accessory renal artery,
variation)

Right renal vein

Superior mesenteric artery

Right testicular or ovarian
vein and artery

Right ureter

Aortic bifurcation

Left common iliac vein

Right common iliac artery

Right external iliac artery

Left common carotid artery,
Left vertebral artery

Left transverse cervical artery,
Left external jugular vein

Left brachiocephalic vein

Left subclavian vein

Inferior thyroid vein

Left internal thoracic vein and artery

Left subclavian artery

Arch of aorta

Thoracic aorta
– Esophageal branch
– Pericardial branch

Descending aorta,
Thoracic aorta

Hemi-azygos vein

Esophageal hiatus
of diaphragm

Left inferior phrenic artery,
Left superior suprarenal artery

Celiac trunk

Left middle suprarenal artery,
Left suprarenal vein,
Left inferior suprarenal artery

Left renal artery and vein

Left testicular or ovarian vein

Left testicular or ovarian artery

Descending aorta,
Abdominal aorta

Inferior mesenteric artery

Left 4th lumbar artery and vein

Left common iliac artery

Median sacral artery and vein

Left internal iliac artery

**162   Blood vessels on the anterior side
of the dorsal body wall**
Ventral aspect (40%)

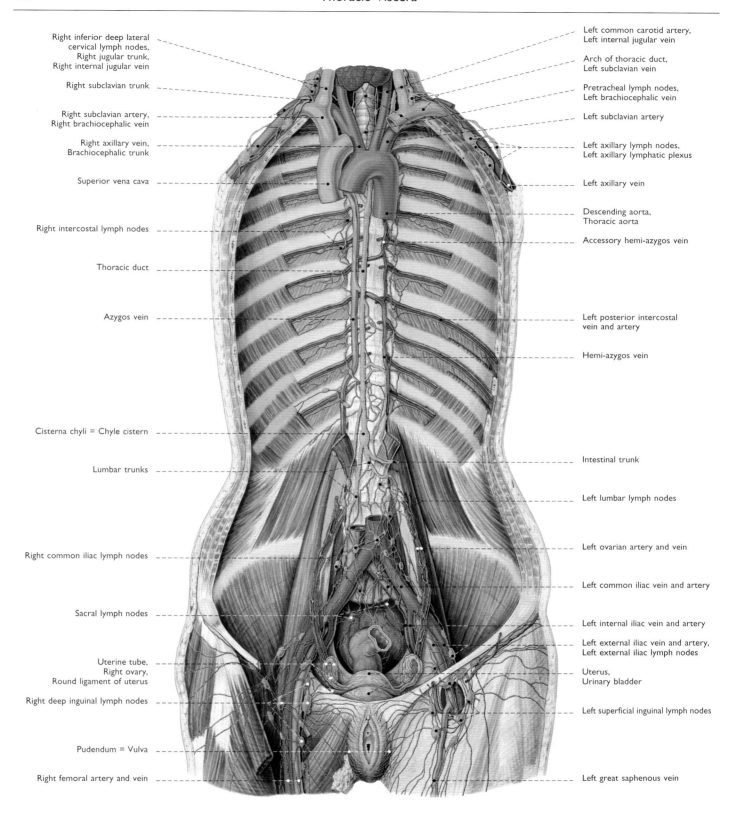

Right inferior deep lateral cervical lymph nodes, Right jugular trunk, Right internal jugular vein

Right subclavian trunk

Right subclavian artery, Right brachiocephalic vein

Right axillary vein, Brachiocephalic trunk

Superior vena cava

Right intercostal lymph nodes

Thoracic duct

Azygos vein

Cisterna chyli = Chyle cistern

Lumbar trunks

Right common iliac lymph nodes

Sacral lymph nodes

Uterine tube, Right ovary, Round ligament of uterus

Right deep inguinal lymph nodes

Pudendum = Vulva

Right femoral artery and vein

Left common carotid artery, Left internal jugular vein

Arch of thoracic duct, Left subclavian vein

Pretracheal lymph nodes, Left brachiocephalic vein

Left subclavian artery

Left axillary lymph nodes, Left axillary lymphatic plexus

Left axillary vein

Descending aorta, Thoracic aorta

Accessory hemi-azygos vein

Left posterior intercostal vein and artery

Hemi-azygos vein

Intestinal trunk

Left lumbar lymph nodes

Left ovarian artery and vein

Left common iliac vein and artery

Left internal iliac vein and artery

Left external iliac vein and artery, Left external iliac lymph nodes

Uterus, Urinary bladder

Left superficial inguinal lymph nodes

Left great saphenous vein

163 Lymphatic vessels and lymph nodes of the thorax, abdomen, and pelvis of a female (30%)
Lymphatic vessels and lymph nodes on the anterior surface of the dorsal body wall, pelvis, and inguinal region, ventral aspect

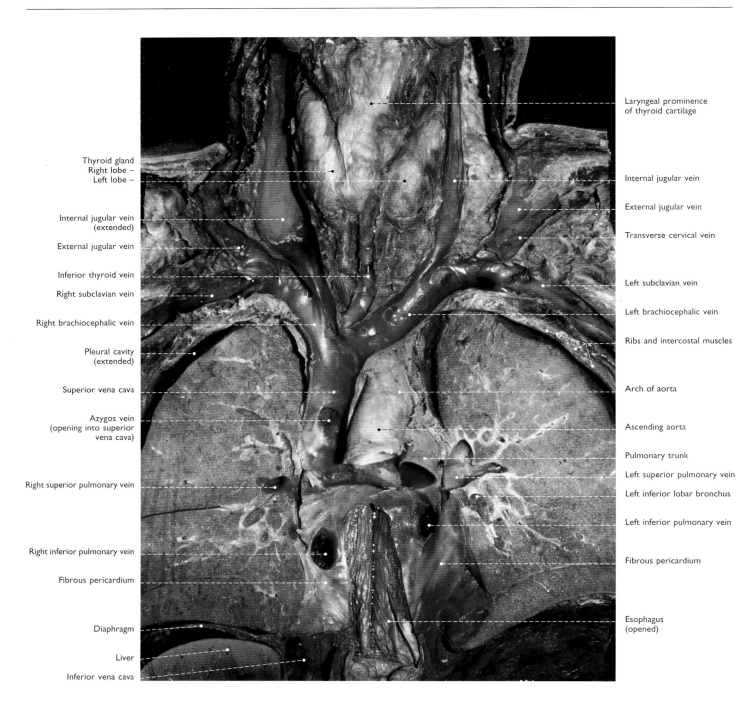

Laryngeal prominence
of thyroid cartilage

Thyroid gland
Right lobe –
Left lobe –

Internal jugular vein

External jugular vein

Transverse cervical vein

Internal jugular vein
(extended)

External jugular vein

Inferior thyroid vein

Right subclavian vein

Left subclavian vein

Left brachiocephalic vein

Right brachiocephalic vein

Ribs and intercostal muscles

Pleural cavity
(extended)

Superior vena cava

Arch of aorta

Azygos vein
(opening into superior
vena cava)

Ascending aorta

Pulmonary trunk

Left superior pulmonary vein

Right superior pulmonary vein

Left inferior lobar bronchus

Left inferior pulmonary vein

Right inferior pulmonary vein

Fibrous pericardium

Fibrous pericardium

Diaphragm

Esophagus
(opened)

Liver

Inferior vena cava

164 Mediastinum and large vein trunks (55%)
Coronal section through the thorax and the lower neck
in the plane of the superior vena cava and the two internal
jugular veins, anatomical section, ventral aspect

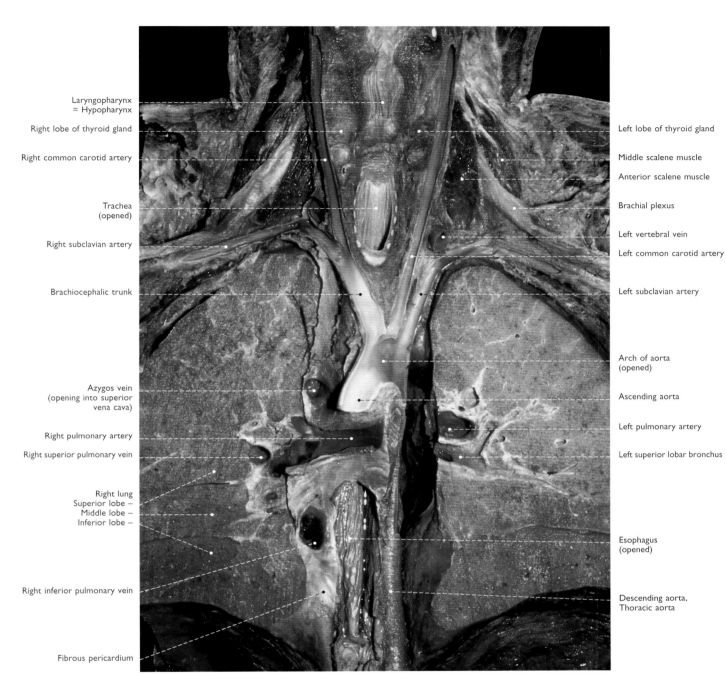

Laryngopharynx = Hypopharynx

Right lobe of thyroid gland

Right common carotid artery

Trachea (opened)

Right subclavian artery

Brachiocephalic trunk

Azygos vein (opening into superior vena cava)

Right pulmonary artery

Right superior pulmonary vein

Right lung
Superior lobe –
Middle lobe –
Inferior lobe –

Right inferior pulmonary vein

Fibrous pericardium

Left lobe of thyroid gland

Middle scalene muscle

Anterior scalene muscle

Brachial plexus

Left vertebral vein

Left common carotid artery

Left subclavian artery

Arch of aorta (opened)

Ascending aorta

Left pulmonary artery

Left superior lobar bronchus

Esophagus (opened)

Descending aorta, Thoracic aorta

165 Mediastinum and large artery trunks (55%)
Coronal section through the thorax and the lower neck
in the plane of the arch of aorta and the two common carotid arteries,
anatomical section, ventral aspect

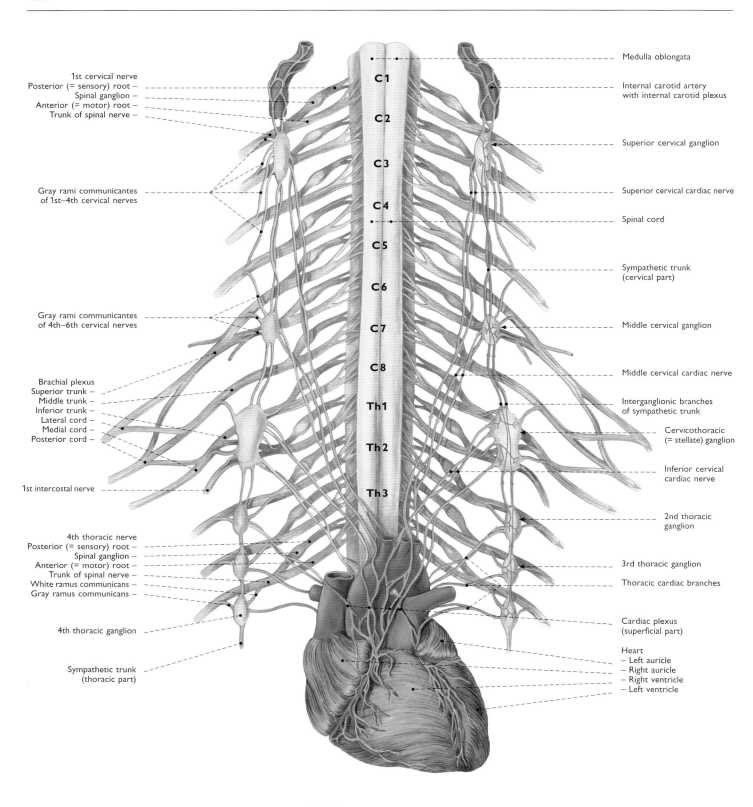

1st cervical nerve
Posterior (= sensory) root –
Spinal ganglion –
Anterior (= motor) root –
Trunk of spinal nerve –

Gray rami communicantes
of 1st–4th cervical nerves

Gray rami communicantes
of 4th–6th cervical nerves

Brachial plexus
Superior trunk –
Middle trunk –
Inferior trunk –
Lateral cord –
Medial cord –
Posterior cord –

1st intercostal nerve

4th thoracic nerve
Posterior (= sensory) root –
Spinal ganglion –
Anterior (= motor) root –
Trunk of spinal nerve –
White ramus communicans –
Gray ramus communicans –

4th thoracic ganglion

Sympathetic trunk
(thoracic part)

C1
C2
C3
C4
C5
C6
C7
C8
Th1
Th2
Th3

Medulla oblongata

Internal carotid artery
with internal carotid plexus

Superior cervical ganglion

Superior cervical cardiac nerve

Spinal cord

Sympathetic trunk
(cervical part)

Middle cervical ganglion

Middle cervical cardiac nerve

Interganglionic branches
of sympathetic trunk

Cervicothoracic
(= stellate) ganglion

Inferior cervical
cardiac nerve

2nd thoracic
ganglion

3rd thoracic ganglion

Thoracic cardiac branches

Cardiac plexus
(superficial part)

Heart
– Left auricle
– Right auricle
– Right ventricle
– Left ventricle

**166 Sympathetic part of the autonomic division
of peripheral nervous system
in the neck and the upper thorax**
Schematic representation, ventral aspect
On the right side of the picture, the preganglionic neurons
of the sympathetic efferent nervous system are indicated
by blue lines, the postganglionic neurons by green ones.

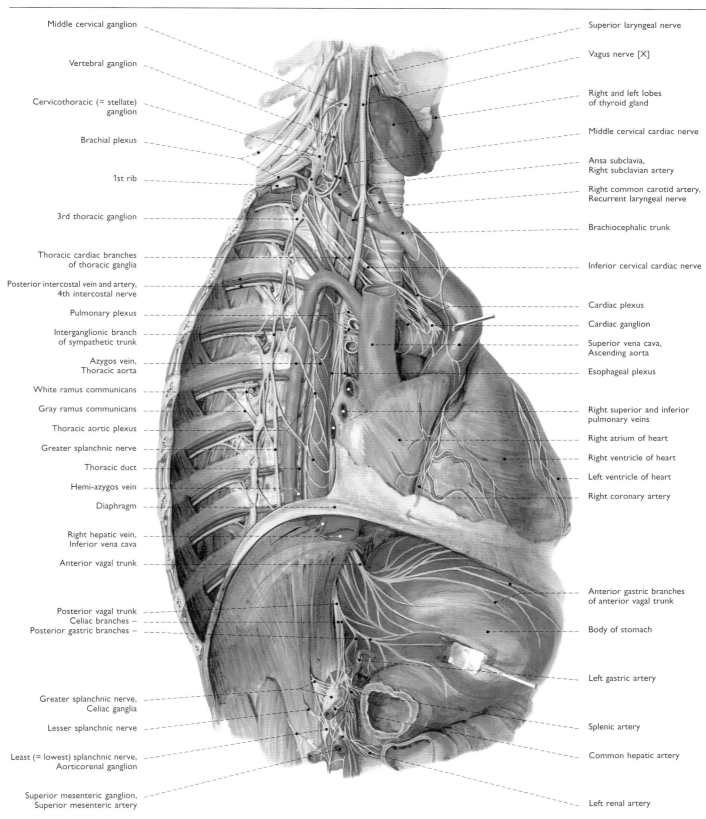

Middle cervical ganglion

Vertebral ganglion

Cervicothoracic (= stellate) ganglion

Brachial plexus

1st rib

3rd thoracic ganglion

Thoracic cardiac branches of thoracic ganglia

Posterior intercostal vein and artery, 4th intercostal nerve

Pulmonary plexus

Interganglionic branch of sympathetic trunk

Azygos vein, Thoracic aorta

White ramus communicans

Gray ramus communicans

Thoracic aortic plexus

Greater splanchnic nerve

Thoracic duct

Hemi-azygos vein

Diaphragm

Right hepatic vein, Inferior vena cava

Anterior vagal trunk

Posterior vagal trunk
Celiac branches –
Posterior gastric branches –

Greater splanchnic nerve, Celiac ganglia

Lesser splanchnic nerve

Least (= lowest) splanchnic nerve, Aorticorenal ganglion

Superior mesenteric ganglion, Superior mesenteric artery

Superior laryngeal nerve

Vagus nerve [X]

Right and left lobes of thyroid gland

Middle cervical cardiac nerve

Ansa subclavia, Right subclavian artery

Right common carotid artery, Recurrent laryngeal nerve

Brachiocephalic trunk

Inferior cervical cardiac nerve

Cardiac plexus

Cardiac ganglion

Superior vena cava, Ascending aorta

Esophageal plexus

Right superior and inferior pulmonary veins

Right atrium of heart

Right ventricle of heart

Left ventricle of heart

Right coronary artery

Anterior gastric branches of anterior vagal trunk

Body of stomach

Left gastric artery

Splenic artery

Common hepatic artery

Left renal artery

167 Autonomic division of the peripheral nervous system in the thorax and the upper abdomen (50%)
Anterolateral aspect

Abdominal and Pelvic Viscera

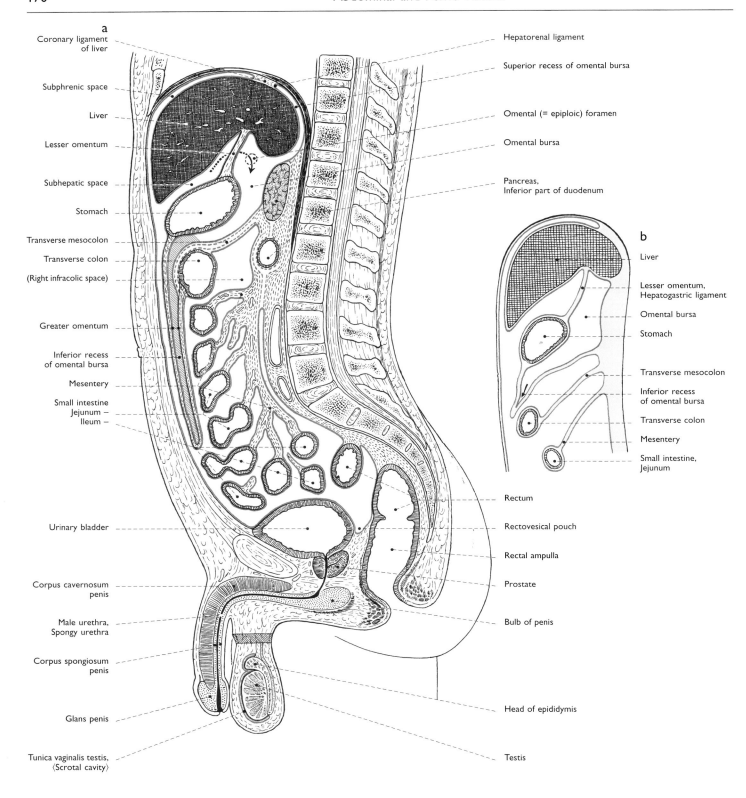

a

Coronary ligament of liver

Subphrenic space

Liver

Lesser omentum

Subhepatic space

Stomach

Transverse mesocolon

Transverse colon

(Right infracolic space)

Greater omentum

Inferior recess of omental bursa

Mesentery

Small intestine
Jejunum —
Ileum —

Urinary bladder

Corpus cavernosum penis

Male urethra, Spongy urethra

Corpus spongiosum penis

Glans penis

Tunica vaginalis testis, ⟨Scrotal cavity⟩

Hepatorenal ligament

Superior recess of omental bursa

Omental (= epiploic) foramen

Omental bursa

Pancreas, Inferior part of duodenum

b

Liver

Lesser omentum, Hepatogastric ligament

Omental bursa

Stomach

Transverse mesocolon

Inferior recess of omental bursa

Transverse colon

Mesentery

Small intestine, Jejunum

Rectum

Rectovesical pouch

Rectal ampulla

Prostate

Bulb of penis

Head of epididymis

Testis

170 Peritoneal cavity

Schematized median sections
a Adult stage of a male. Step-cut in the scrotum in order to expose the right cavity of the tunica vaginalis
b Fetal stage

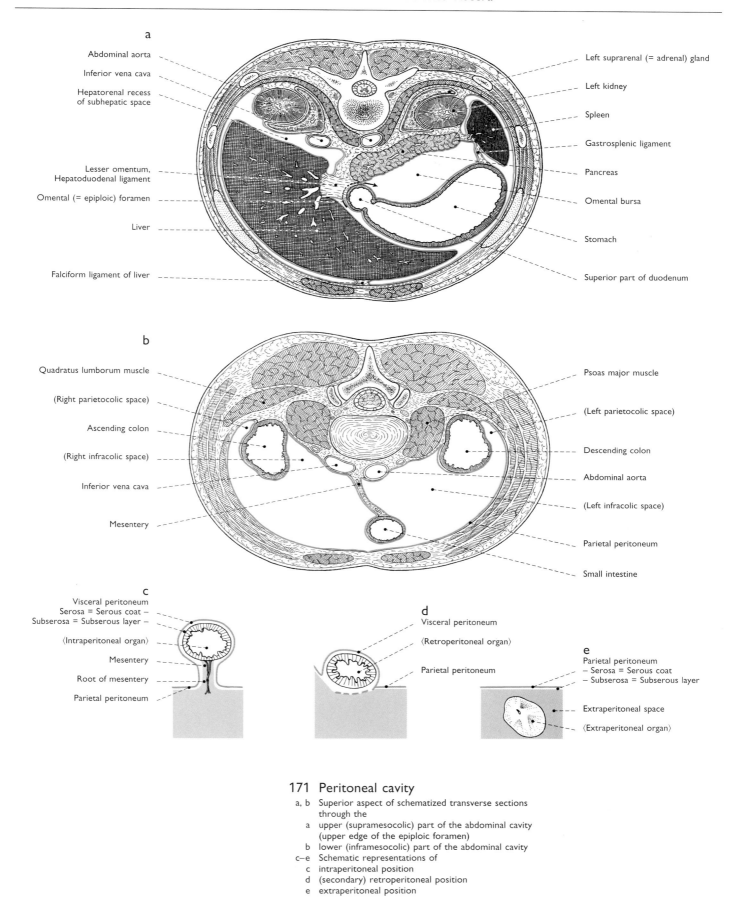

a

Abdominal aorta

Inferior vena cava

Hepatorenal recess of subhepatic space

Lesser omentum, Hepatoduodenal ligament

Omental (= epiploic) foramen

Liver

Falciform ligament of liver

Left suprarenal (= adrenal) gland

Left kidney

Spleen

Gastrosplenic ligament

Pancreas

Omental bursa

Stomach

Superior part of duodenum

b

Quadratus lumborum muscle

(Right parietocolic space)

Ascending colon

(Right infracolic space)

Inferior vena cava

Mesentery

Psoas major muscle

(Left parietocolic space)

Descending colon

Abdominal aorta

(Left infracolic space)

Parietal peritoneum

Small intestine

c

Visceral peritoneum
Serosa = Serous coat –
Subserosa = Subserous layer –

⟨Intraperitoneal organ⟩

Mesentery

Root of mesentery

Parietal peritoneum

d

Visceral peritoneum

⟨Retroperitoneal organ⟩

Parietal peritoneum

e

Parietal peritoneum
– Serosa = Serous coat
– Subserosa = Subserous layer

Extraperitoneal space

⟨Extraperitoneal organ⟩

171 Peritoneal cavity

a, b   Superior aspect of schematized transverse sections through the

a   upper (supramesocolic) part of the abdominal cavity (upper edge of the epiploic foramen)

b   lower (inframesocolic) part of the abdominal cavity

c–e   Schematic representations of

c   intraperitoneal position

d   (secondary) retroperitoneal position

e   extraperitoneal position

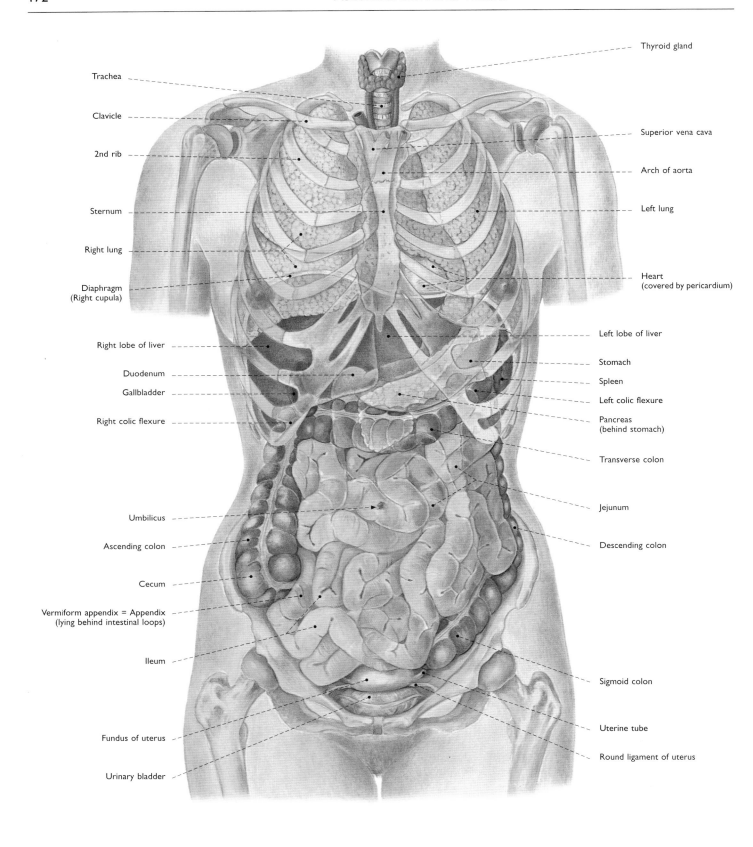

Thyroid gland

Trachea

Clavicle

2nd rib

Sternum

Right lung

Diaphragm
(Right cupula)

Superior vena cava

Arch of aorta

Left lung

Heart
(covered by pericardium)

Right lobe of liver

Duodenum

Gallbladder

Right colic flexure

Left lobe of liver

Stomach

Spleen

Left colic flexure

Pancreas
(behind stomach)

Transverse colon

Umbilicus

Ascending colon

Cecum

Vermiform appendix = Appendix
(lying behind intestinal loops)

Ileum

Jejunum

Descending colon

Fundus of uterus

Urinary bladder

Sigmoid colon

Uterine tube

Round ligament of uterus

172   Thoracic and abdominal viscera (30%)
Surface projections onto the chest and
anterior abdominal walls, ventral aspect

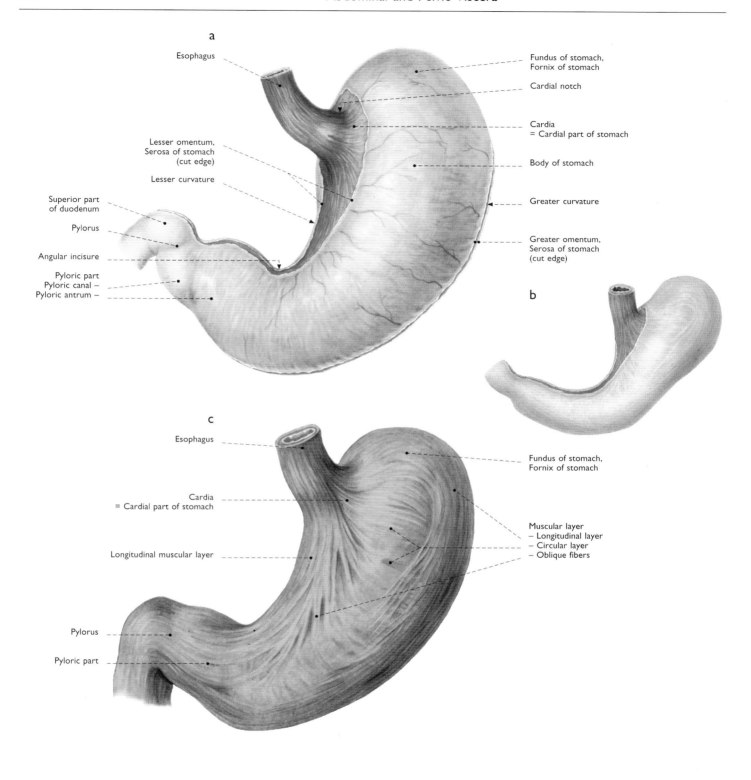

a

Esophagus

Fundus of stomach,
Fornix of stomach

Cardial notch

Cardia
= Cardial part of stomach

Lesser omentum,
Serosa of stomach
(cut edge)

Body of stomach

Lesser curvature

Greater curvature

Superior part
of duodenum

Pylorus

Greater omentum,
Serosa of stomach
(cut edge)

Angular incisure

Pyloric part
Pyloric canal —
Pyloric antrum —

b

c

Esophagus

Fundus of stomach,
Fornix of stomach

Cardia
= Cardial part of stomach

Muscular layer
– Longitudinal layer
– Circular layer
– Oblique fibers

Longitudinal muscular layer

Pylorus

Pyloric part

173 Stomach (55%)

Ventral aspect
a External aspect of a completely filled stomach with distended walls
b Empty stomach with extremely contracted walls
c Muscle tracts in the anterior wall of the stomach after removal
of the serosa and subserosa

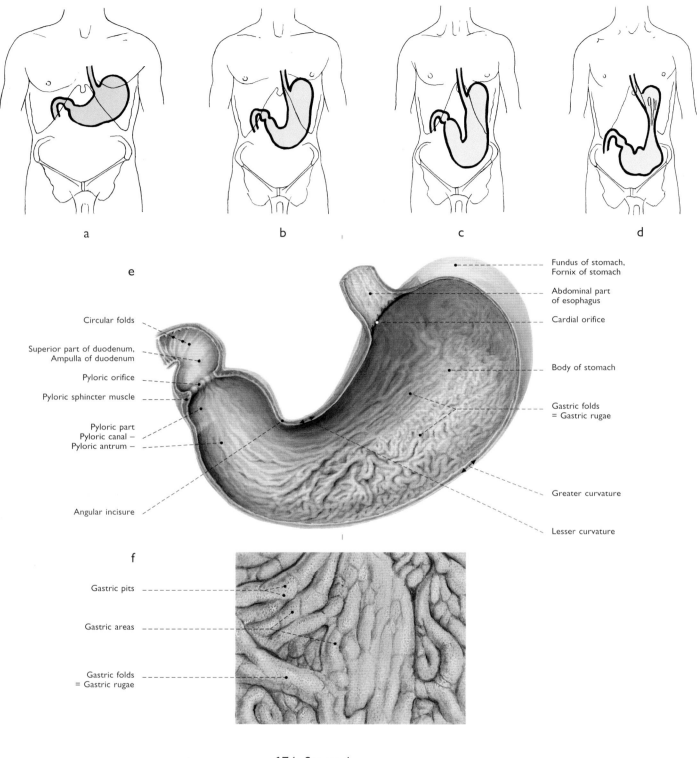

a

b

c

d

e

Circular folds

Superior part of duodenum,
Ampulla of duodenum

Pyloric orifice

Pyloric sphincter muscle

Pyloric part
Pyloric canal —
Pyloric antrum —

Angular incisure

Fundus of stomach,
Fornix of stomach

Abdominal part
of esophagus

Cardial orifice

Body of stomach

Gastric folds
= Gastric rugae

Greater curvature

Lesser curvature

f

Gastric pits

Gastric areas

Gastric folds
= Gastric rugae

174 Stomach

a–d Schematic representations of some important functional forms
of the stomach
a Hypertonic stomach
b Orthotonic stomach
c Hypotonic stomach
d Atonic stomach
e, f Internal aspect of the stomach
e Internal aspect of the posterior wall after removal
of the anterior wall (50%)
f Mucosa of the body of stomach (300%)

a

Cardial notch

Abdominal part
of esophagus

Lesser curvature

Angular incisure

Superior part of duodenum,
Ampulla of duodenum
= Duodenal cap

Pyloric orifice

Inferior (= horizontal) part
of duodenum

Fundus of stomach,
Fornix of stomach

Body of stomach

Greater curvature

Jejunum

Pyloric part

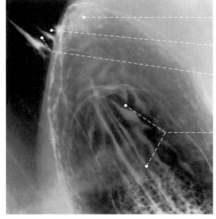

b

Fundus of stomach,
Fornix of stomach

Cardial notch

Abdominal part
of esophagus

Gastric folds

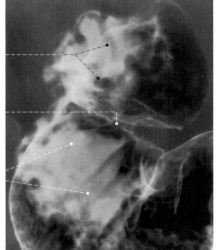

c

Superior part of duodenum,
Ampulla of duodenum
= Duodenal cap

Pyloric orifice

Pyloric part
Pyloric canal –
Pyloric antrum –

175 Stomach (50%)

Double-contrast radiographs after barium meal
and distension by air
a   Postero-anterior radiograph of the stomach
    and the ampulla of duodenum
b   Spot film radiograph of the fundus of stomach
c   Oblique radiograph of the pyloric part of stomach and
    the ampulla of duodenum from right anterior (RAO projection)

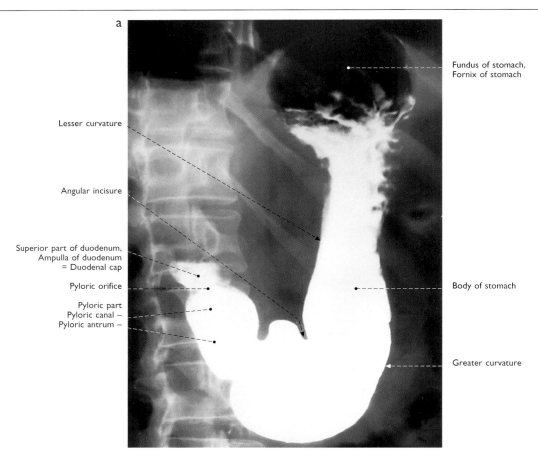

a

Fundus of stomach,
Fornix of stomach

Lesser curvature

Angular incisure

Superior part of duodenum,
Ampulla of duodenum
= Duodenal cap

Pyloric orifice

Pyloric part
Pyloric canal –
Pyloric antrum –

Body of stomach

Greater curvature

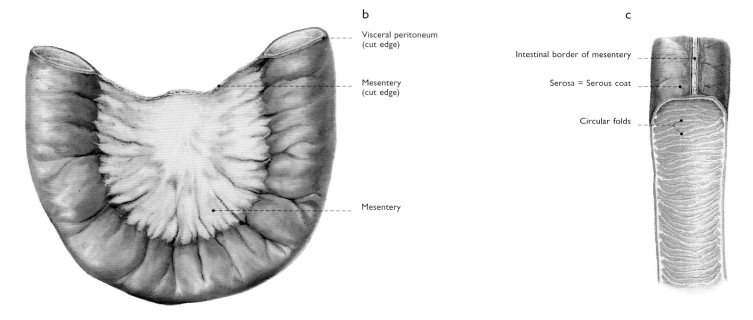

b

Visceral peritoneum
(cut edge)

Mesentery
(cut edge)

Mesentery

c

Intestinal border of mesentery

Serosa = Serous coat

Circular folds

176 Stomach and small intestine (50%)

a Postero-anterior radiograph of the stomach
and the ampulla of duodenum after barium meal
b Jejunal loop with its mesentery, external aspect
c Jejunum partially opened

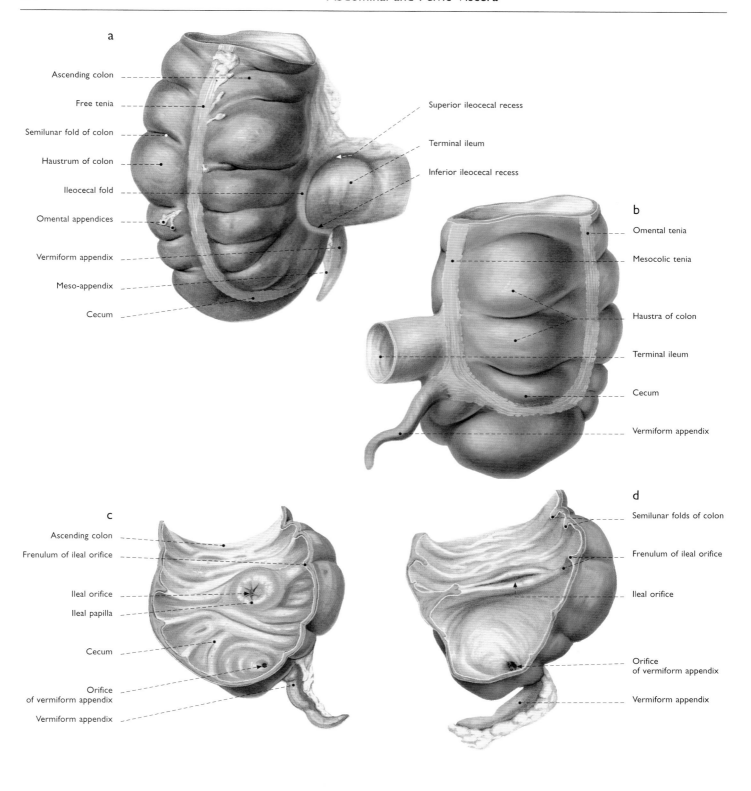

a

Ascending colon

Free tenia

Semilunar fold of colon

Haustrum of colon

Ileocecal fold

Omental appendices

Vermiform appendix

Meso-appendix

Cecum

Superior ileocecal recess

Terminal ileum

Inferior ileocecal recess

b

Omental tenia

Mesocolic tenia

Haustra of colon

Terminal ileum

Cecum

Vermiform appendix

c

Ascending colon

Frenulum of ileal orifice

Ileal orifice

Ileal papilla

Cecum

Orifice
of vermiform appendix

Vermiform appendix

d

Semilunar folds of colon

Frenulum of ileal orifice

Ileal orifice

Orifice
of vermiform appendix

Vermiform appendix

177 Cecum and vermiform appendix (70%)

a   Ventral aspect
b   Dorsal aspect
c, d   Ileal orifice and orifice of vermiform appendix after removal
     of the ventrolateral wall of the cecum and the ascending colon
c   View during life
d   View of the relaxed intestine after death

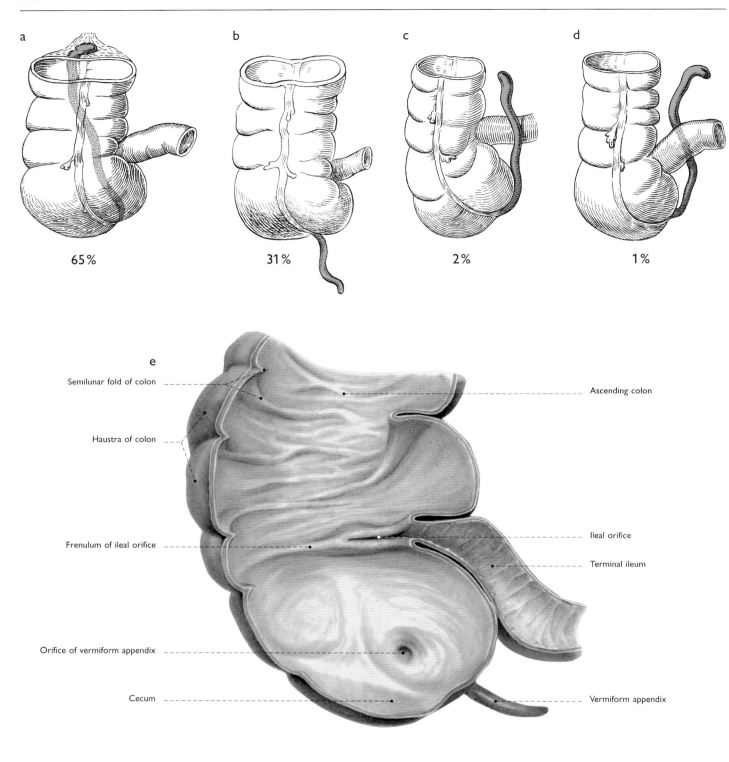

a   b   c   d

65%   31%   2%   1%

e

Semilunar fold of colon

Haustra of colon

Frenulum of ileal orifice

Orifice of vermiform appendix

Cecum

Ascending colon

Ileal orifice

Terminal ileum

Vermiform appendix

178 Cecum and vermiform appendix

a–d   Four possible positions of the vermiform appendix.
The percentile numbers beneath the pictures indicate
the approximate frequency.
a   Retrocecal and retrocolic position
b   Pendulous position into the lesser pelvis
c   Pre-ileal position
d   Retro-ileal position
e   Internal aspect of the dorsal wall of the cecum
after removal of the ventral intestinal wall (80%)

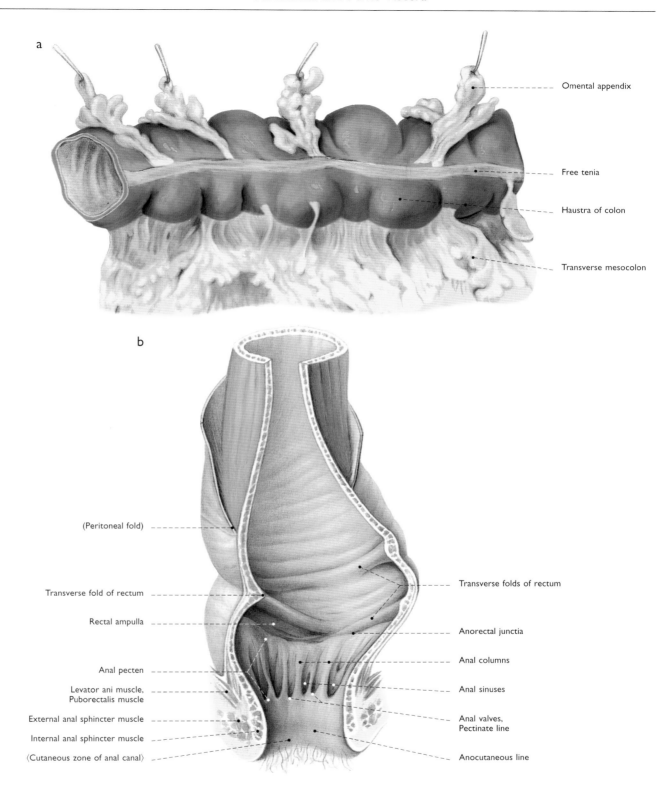

Omental appendix

Free tenia

Haustra of colon

Transverse mesocolon

(Peritoneal fold)

Transverse fold of rectum

Rectal ampulla

Anal pecten

Levator ani muscle,
Puborectalis muscle

External anal sphincter muscle

Internal anal sphincter muscle

(Cutaneous zone of anal canal)

Transverse folds of rectum

Anorectal junctia

Anal columns

Anal sinuses

Anal valves,
Pectinate line

Anocutaneous line

179 Transverse colon and rectum (70%)
a   Dorsal aspect of the middle part of the transverse colon
b   Interior of the rectum revealed by incising along the midventral line

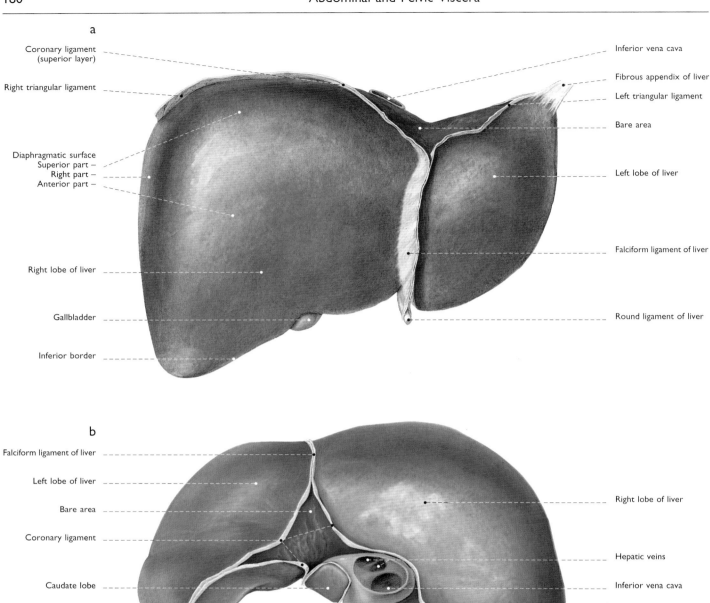

a

Coronary ligament
(superior layer)

Right triangular ligament

Diaphragmatic surface
Superior part –
Right part –
Anterior part –

Right lobe of liver

Gallbladder

Inferior border

Inferior vena cava

Fibrous appendix of liver

Left triangular ligament

Bare area

Left lobe of liver

Falciform ligament of liver

Round ligament of liver

b

Falciform ligament of liver

Left lobe of liver

Bare area

Coronary ligament

Caudate lobe

Fibrous appendix of liver

Right lobe of liver

Hepatic veins

Inferior vena cava

Coronary ligament
(superior layer)

Bare area

Right triangular ligament

Coronary ligament
(inferior layer)

180 Liver (45%)
Diaphragmatic surface
a   Ventral aspect
b   Superior aspect

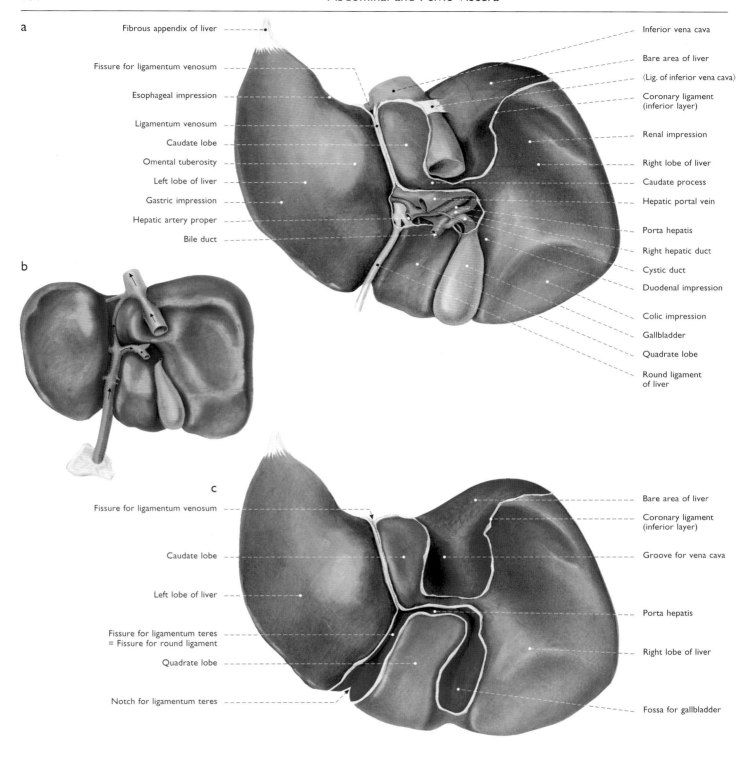

a

Fibrous appendix of liver

Fissure for ligamentum venosum

Esophageal impression

Ligamentum venosum

Caudate lobe

Omental tuberosity

Left lobe of liver

Gastric impression

Hepatic artery proper

Bile duct

Inferior vena cava

Bare area of liver

⟨Lig. of inferior vena cava⟩

Coronary ligament
(inferior layer)

Renal impression

Right lobe of liver

Caudate process

Hepatic portal vein

Porta hepatis

Right hepatic duct

Cystic duct

Duodenal impression

Colic impression

Gallbladder

Quadrate lobe

Round ligament
of liver

b

c

Fissure for ligamentum venosum

Caudate lobe

Left lobe of liver

Fissure for ligamentum teres
= Fissure for round ligament

Quadrate lobe

Notch for ligamentum teres

Bare area of liver

Coronary ligament
(inferior layer)

Groove for vena cava

Porta hepatis

Right lobe of liver

Fossa for gallbladder

181 Liver (45%)
Visceral surface, dorsal aspect
a Liver of an adult
b Liver of a newborn child
c Liver of an adult after removal of the gallbladder,
   the inferior vena cava, the hepatic portal vein,
   and the remnants of embryonal vessels

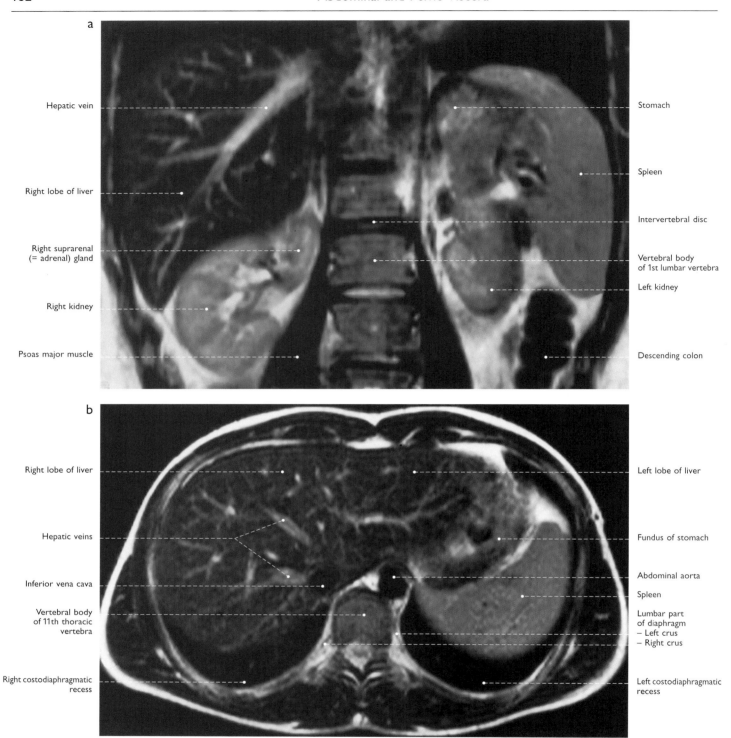

a
Hepatic vein
Right lobe of liver
Right suprarenal (= adrenal) gland
Right kidney
Psoas major muscle

Stomach
Spleen
Intervertebral disc
Vertebral body of 1st lumbar vertebra
Left kidney
Descending colon

b
Right lobe of liver
Hepatic veins
Inferior vena cava
Vertebral body of 11th thoracic vertebra
Right costodiaphragmatic recess

Left lobe of liver
Fundus of stomach
Abdominal aorta
Spleen
Lumbar part of diaphragm – Left crus – Right crus
Left costodiaphragmatic recess

182 Liver and adjacent organs (50%)

Magnetic resonance images (MRI, T$_2$-weighted)
a Coronal section through the abdomen in the plane of lumbar vertebral bodies, ventral aspect
b Transverse section through the epigastric region at the level of the eleventh thoracic vertebral body (Th XI), inferior aspect

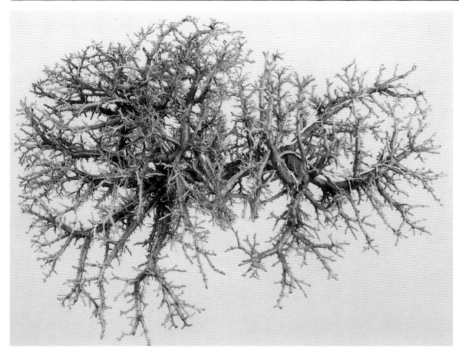

a

Blue: Hepatic portal vein with ramifications
Red: Hepatic artery proper with branches
Yellow: Intrahepatic bile ducts,
              Right and left hepatic ducts

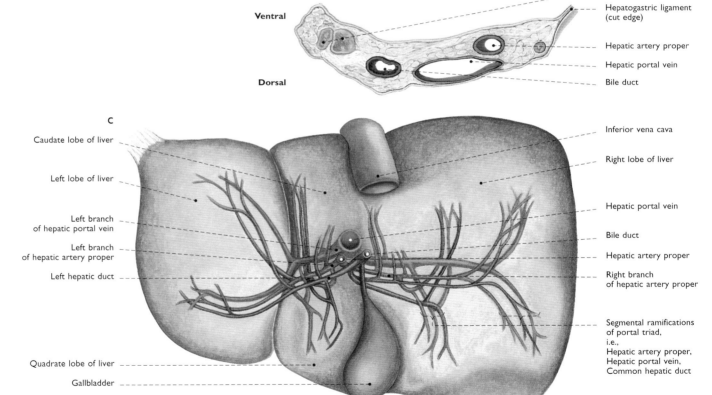

b

Ventral

Dorsal

— Hepatic lymph nodes

— Hepatogastric ligament
   (cut edge)

— Hepatic artery proper

— Hepatic portal vein

— Bile duct

c

Caudate lobe of liver

Left lobe of liver

Left branch
of hepatic portal vein

Left branch
of hepatic artery proper

Left hepatic duct

Quadrate lobe of liver

Gallbladder

Inferior vena cava

Right lobe of liver

Hepatic portal vein

Bile duct

Hepatic artery proper

Right branch
of hepatic artery proper

Segmental ramifications
of portal triad,
i.e.,
Hepatic artery proper,
Hepatic portal vein,
Common hepatic duct

**183 Hepatic blood vessels and
        intrahepatic bile duct system**

a Corrosion cast (50%), ventral aspect
b Hepatoduodenal ligament (150%), transverse section,
   inferior aspect
c Distribution pattern of the blood vessels and bile ducts
   in the liver (50%), schematic representation,
   dorsal aspect

a

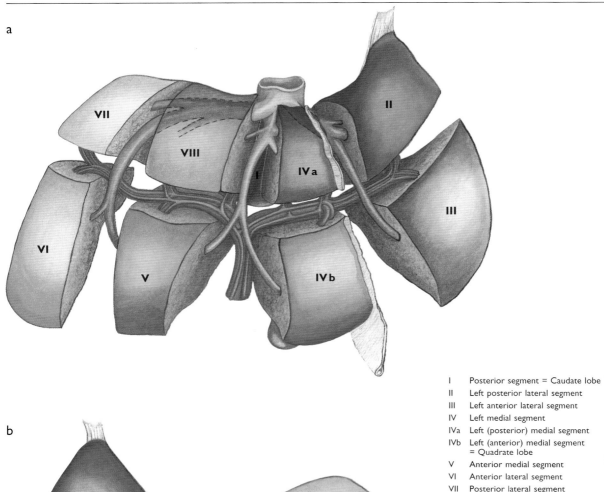

I	Posterior segment = Caudate lobe
II	Left posterior lateral segment
III	Left anterior lateral segment
IV	Left medial segment
IVa	Left (posterior) medial segment
IVb	Left (anterior) medial segment = Quadrate lobe
V	Anterior medial segment
VI	Anterior lateral segment
VII	Posterior lateral segment
VIII	Posterior medial segment

Left branch of hepatic artery proper

Right branch of hepatic artery proper

b

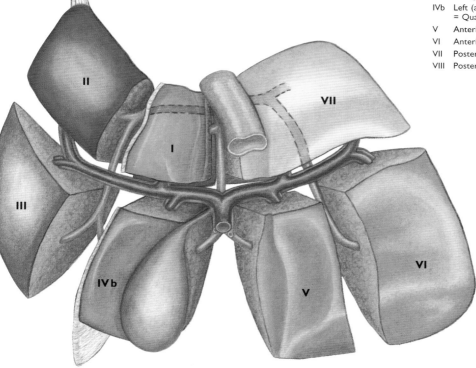

184 Segmentation of liver (50%)

Schematic representations
(according to Heberer, Köle, and Tscherne, 1986)
a Diaphragmatic surface of the liver, ventral aspect
b Visceral surface of the liver, dorsal aspect

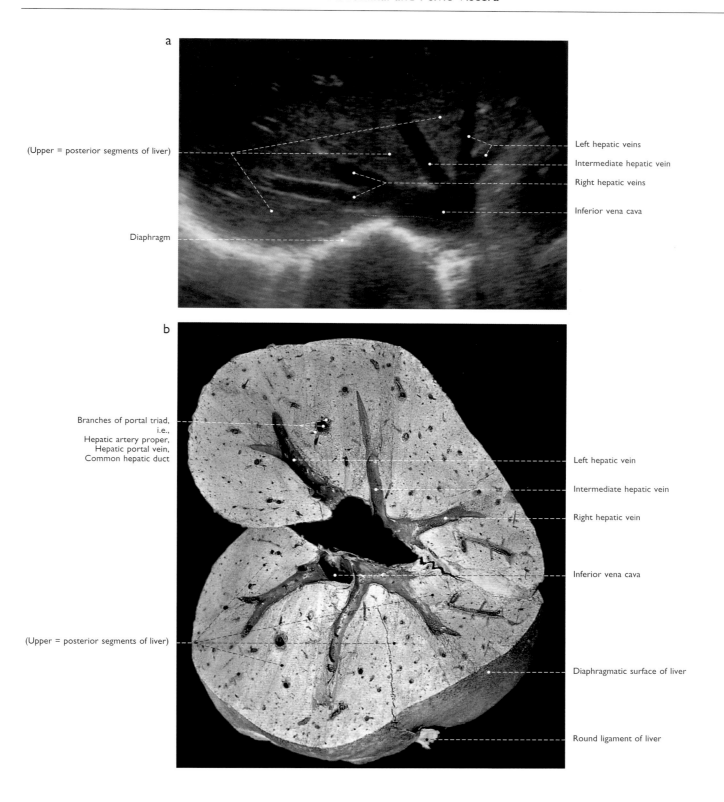

a

(Upper = posterior segments of liver) ····· Left hepatic veins

Intermediate hepatic vein

Right hepatic veins

Inferior vena cava

Diaphragm

b

Branches of portal triad,
i.e.,
Hepatic artery proper,
Hepatic portal vein,
Common hepatic duct

Left hepatic vein

Intermediate hepatic vein

Right hepatic vein

Inferior vena cava

(Upper = posterior segments of liver)

Diaphragmatic surface of liver

Round ligament of liver

185 Liver

a Ultrasound image showing the hepatic veins (40%),
   subcostal oblique section
b Section through the upper part of a human liver,
   opening the four cranial liver segments.
   The ventral part of the liver is turned upwards (30%).
   Ventral aspect

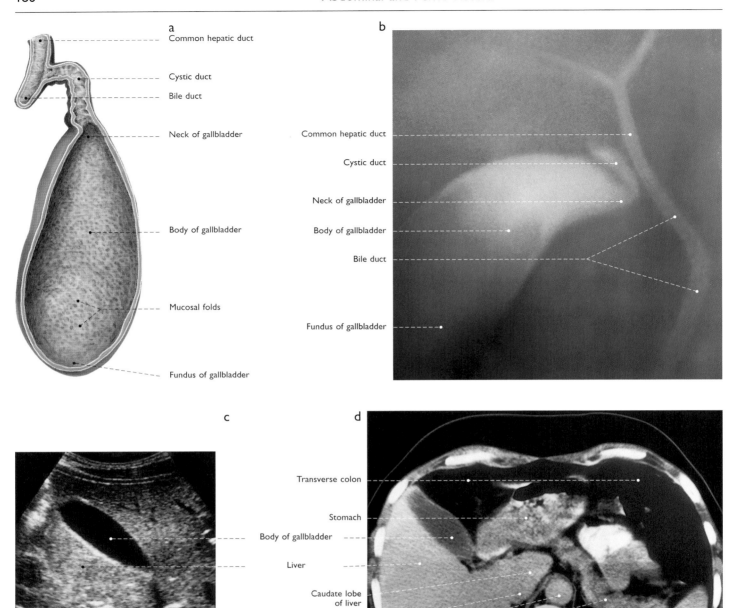

a

Common hepatic duct

Cystic duct

Bile duct

Neck of gallbladder

Body of gallbladder

Mucosal folds

Fundus of gallbladder

b

Common hepatic duct

Cystic duct

Neck of gallbladder

Body of gallbladder

Bile duct

Fundus of gallbladder

c

Body of gallbladder

Liver

d

Transverse colon

Stomach

Body of gallbladder

Liver

Caudate lobe of liver

Inferior vena cava

Abdominal aorta

Body of pancreas

Left kidney

Spleen

186 Gallbladder and extrahepatic bile duct system
a Gallbladder and bile ducts after removal of their dorsal walls (90%), dorsal aspect
b Cholecystocholangiography after intravenous injection of contrast medium (100%), postero-anterior radiograph
c Ultrasound image of the gallbladder (50%), subcostal oblique section
d Transverse computed tomogram (CT) at the level of the twelfth thoracic vertebral body (Th XII) (35%), inferior aspect

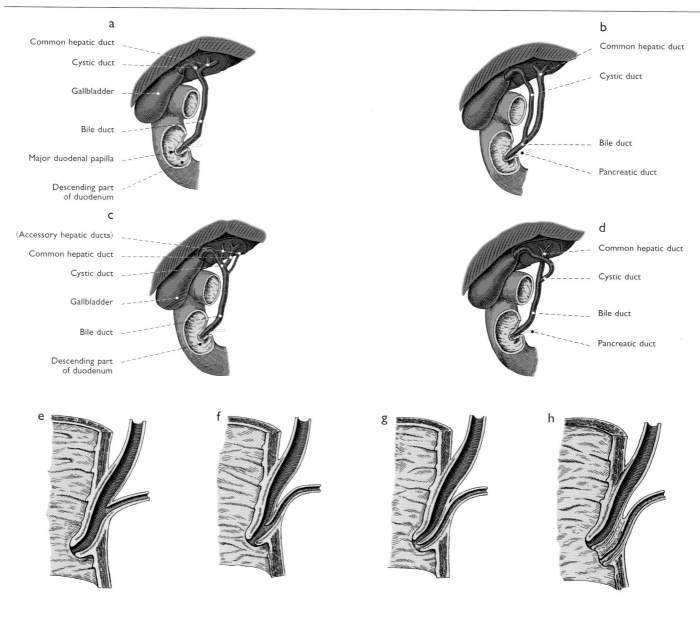

a

Common hepatic duct
Cystic duct
Gallbladder
Bile duct
Major duodenal papilla
Descending part of duodenum

b

Common hepatic duct
Cystic duct
Bile duct
Pancreatic duct

c

⟨Accessory hepatic ducts⟩
Common hepatic duct
Cystic duct
Gallbladder
Bile duct
Descending part of duodenum

d

Common hepatic duct
Cystic duct
Bile duct
Pancreatic duct

e   f   g   h

187   Extrahepatic bile duct system

a–d   Variations of the hepatic and cystic ducts, schematic representations
  a   The hepatic and cystic ducts joining at a high level close to the liver
  b   The hepatic and cystic ducts joining at a low level distant from the liver
  c   Accessory hepatic ducts joining the main ducts at a high level
  d   The cystic duct winding ventrodorsally around the common hepatic duct prior to their junction
e–h   Variations of the orifices of the bile and pancreatic ducts, schematic representations
  e   The pancreatic duct merging with the bile duct before they penetrate the duodenal wall
  f   Common opening of the bile duct and the pancreatic duct joining within the duodenal wall
  g   The two independent ducts ending in one common opening at the major duodenal papilla
  h   The two independent ducts open separately into the duodenum creating a bipartite papilla

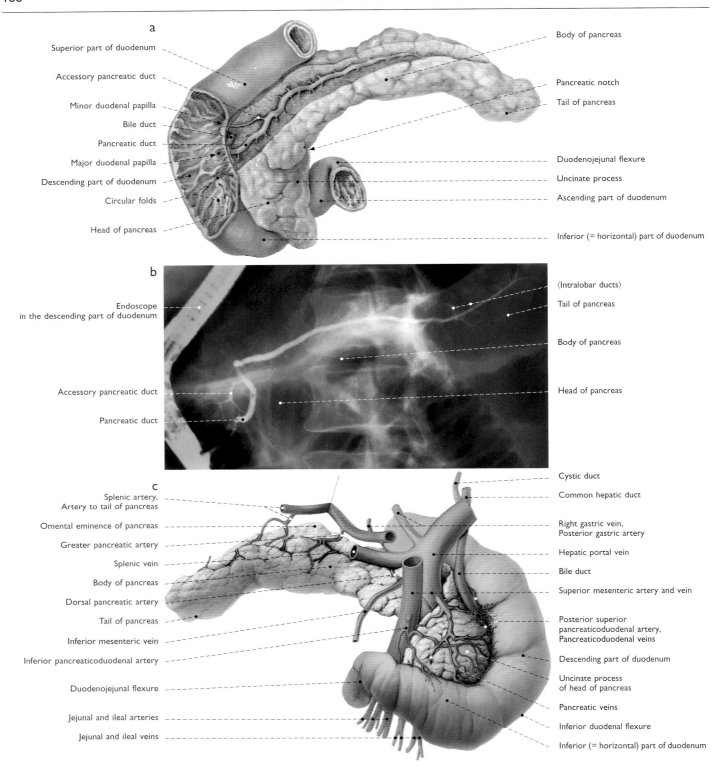

a

Superior part of duodenum
Accessory pancreatic duct
Minor duodenal papilla
Bile duct
Pancreatic duct
Major duodenal papilla
Descending part of duodenum
Circular folds
Head of pancreas

Body of pancreas
Pancreatic notch
Tail of pancreas
Duodenojejunal flexure
Uncinate process
Ascending part of duodenum
Inferior (= horizontal) part of duodenum

b

Endoscope
in the descending part of duodenum
Accessory pancreatic duct
Pancreatic duct

⟨Intralobar ducts⟩
Tail of pancreas
Body of pancreas
Head of pancreas

c

Splenic artery,
Artery to tail of pancreas
Omental eminence of pancreas
Greater pancreatic artery
Splenic vein
Body of pancreas
Dorsal pancreatic artery
Tail of pancreas
Inferior mesenteric vein
Inferior pancreaticoduodenal artery
Duodenojejunal flexure
Jejunal and ileal arteries
Jejunal and ileal veins

Cystic duct
Common hepatic duct
Right gastric vein,
Posterior gastric artery
Hepatic portal vein
Bile duct
Superior mesenteric artery and vein
Posterior superior
pancreaticoduodenal artery,
Pancreaticoduodenal veins
Descending part of duodenum
Uncinate process
of head of pancreas
Pancreatic veins
Inferior duodenal flexure
Inferior (= horizontal) part of duodenum

188 Pancreas and duodenum (60%)

a The anterior wall of the descending part of the duodenum
   was removed. The pancreatic duct and the accessory pancreatic duct
   are exposed. Ventral aspect
b Endoscopic retrograde cholangiopancreatography (ERCP)
   imaging the pancreatic and accessory pancreatic ducts,
   postero-anterior radiograph
c Pancreas, duodenum, bile duct, and adjacent blood vessels,
   dorsal aspect

a

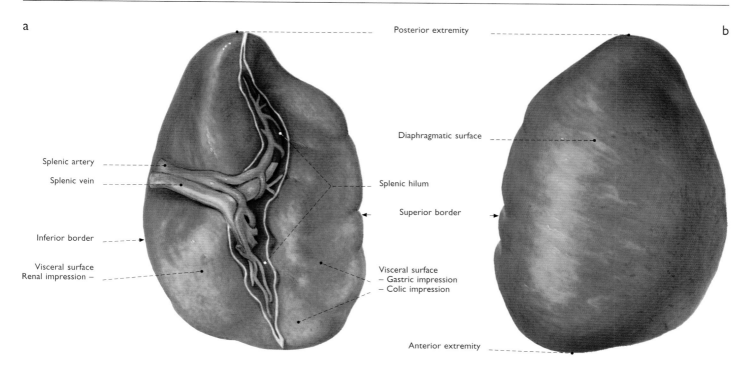

Posterior extremity

b

Splenic artery

Splenic vein

Diaphragmatic surface

Splenic hilum

Superior border

Inferior border

Visceral surface
Renal impression –

Visceral surface
– Gastric impression
– Colic impression

Anterior extremity

c

d

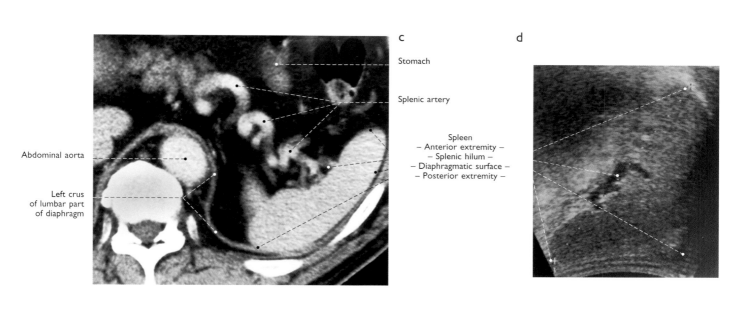

Stomach

Splenic artery

Abdominal aorta

Left crus
of lumbar part
of diaphragm

Spleen
– Anterior extremity –
– Splenic hilum –
– Diaphragmatic surface –
– Posterior extremity –

189 Spleen
  a   Visceral surface
  b   Diaphragmatic surface
  c   Transverse computed tomogram (CT) after injection
     of contrast medium (50%), inferior aspect
  d   Ultrasound image of the spleen (60%), subcostal oblique section

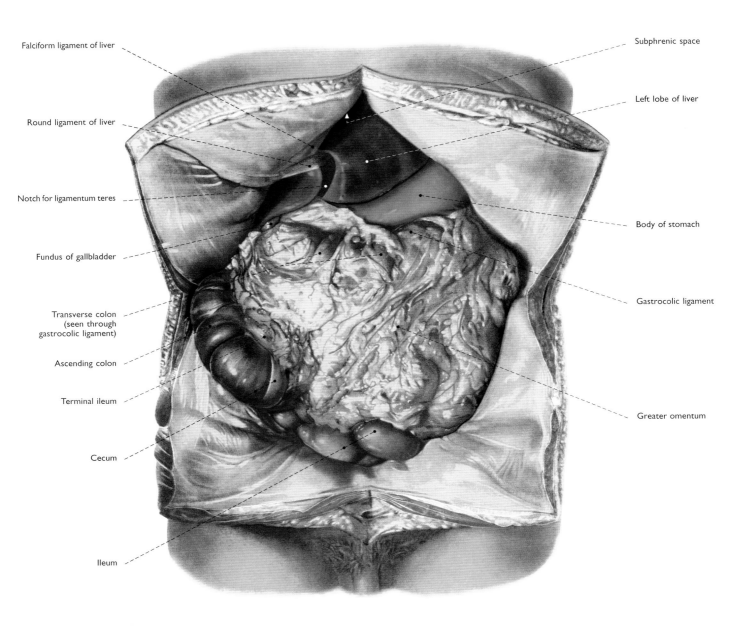

Falciform ligament of liver

Round ligament of liver

Notch for ligamentum teres

Fundus of gallbladder

Transverse colon
(seen through
gastrocolic ligament)

Ascending colon

Terminal ileum

Cecum

Ileum

Subphrenic space

Left lobe of liver

Body of stomach

Gastrocolic ligament

Greater omentum

190 Superficial abdominal viscera (30%)
The abdominal wall was opened by a cruciate incision
and retracted. Ventral aspect

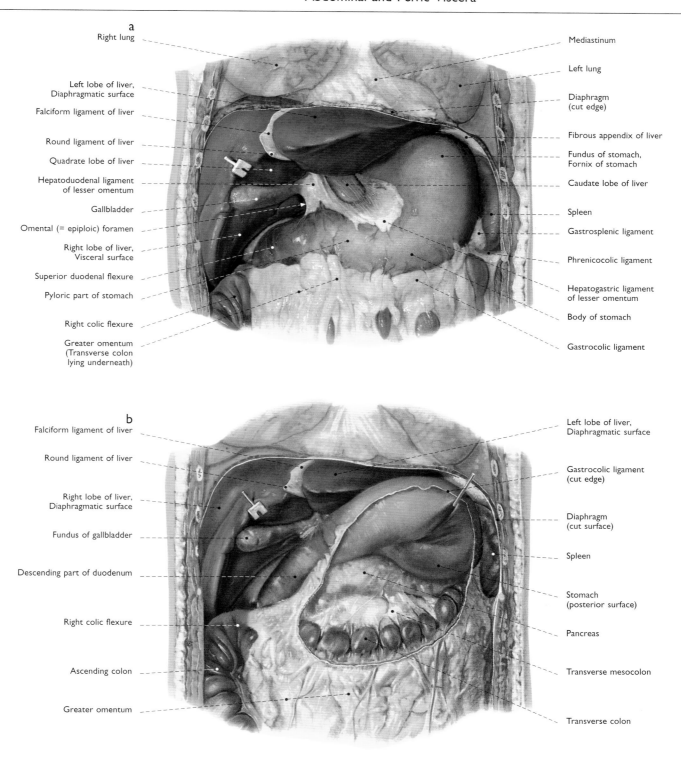

a

Right lung — Mediastinum

Left lobe of liver, Diaphragmatic surface — Left lung

Falciform ligament of liver — Diaphragm (cut edge)

Round ligament of liver — Fibrous appendix of liver

Quadrate lobe of liver — Fundus of stomach, Fornix of stomach

Hepatoduodenal ligament of lesser omentum — Caudate lobe of liver

Gallbladder — Spleen

Omental (= epiploic) foramen — Gastrosplenic ligament

Right lobe of liver, Visceral surface — Phrenicocolic ligament

Superior duodenal flexure — Hepatogastric ligament of lesser omentum

Pyloric part of stomach — Body of stomach

Right colic flexure — Gastrocolic ligament

Greater omentum (Transverse colon lying underneath)

b

Falciform ligament of liver — Left lobe of liver, Diaphragmatic surface

Round ligament of liver — Gastrocolic ligament (cut edge)

Right lobe of liver, Diaphragmatic surface — Diaphragm (cut surface)

Fundus of gallbladder — Spleen

Descending part of duodenum — Stomach (posterior surface)

Right colic flexure — Pancreas

Ascending colon — Transverse mesocolon

Greater omentum — Transverse colon

191 Viscera of the upper abdomen (35%)
The ventral body wall was removed, the liver is raised by hooks.
a Ventral aspect
b The gastrocolic ligament was additionally cut transversely
and the stomach retracted cranially. By this, the dorsal wall
of the omental bursa is exposed. Ventral aspect

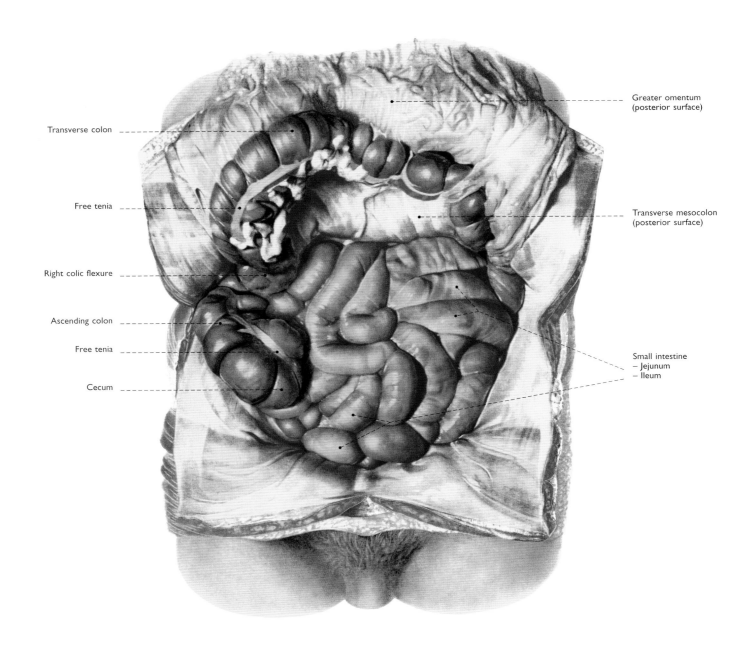

Transverse colon

Free tenia

Right colic flexure

Ascending colon

Free tenia

Cecum

Greater omentum
(posterior surface)

Transverse mesocolon
(posterior surface)

Small intestine
– Jejunum
– Ileum

192   Intraperitoneal viscera of the lower abdomen (30%)
The greater omentum and the transverse colon
are retracted upwards. Ventral aspect

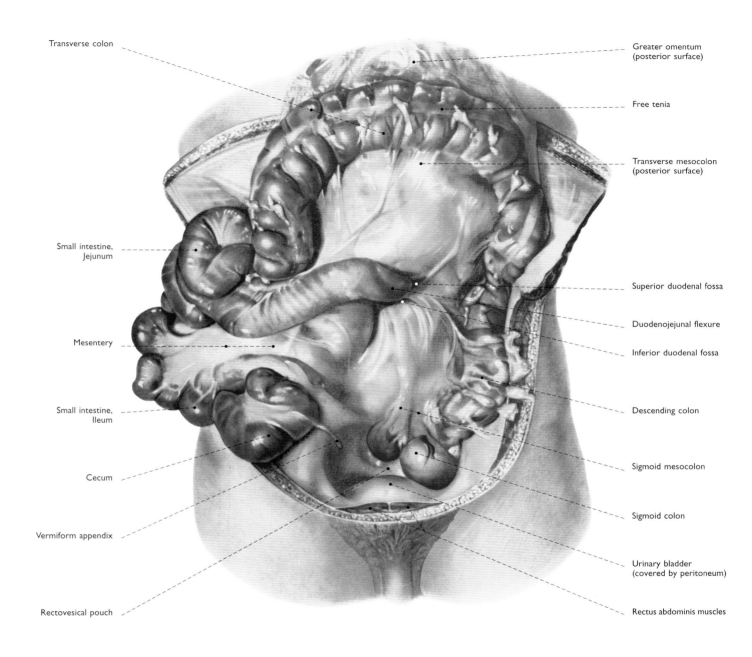

Transverse colon

Small intestine, Jejunum

Mesentery

Small intestine, Ileum

Cecum

Vermiform appendix

Rectovesical pouch

Greater omentum (posterior surface)

Free tenia

Transverse mesocolon (posterior surface)

Superior duodenal fossa

Duodenojejunal flexure

Inferior duodenal fossa

Descending colon

Sigmoid mesocolon

Sigmoid colon

Urinary bladder (covered by peritoneum)

Rectus abdominis muscles

193 Intraperitoneal viscera of the lower abdomen (30%)
The transverse colon and the greater omentum are turned upwards,
the ileum and jejunum drawn to the right. Ventral aspect

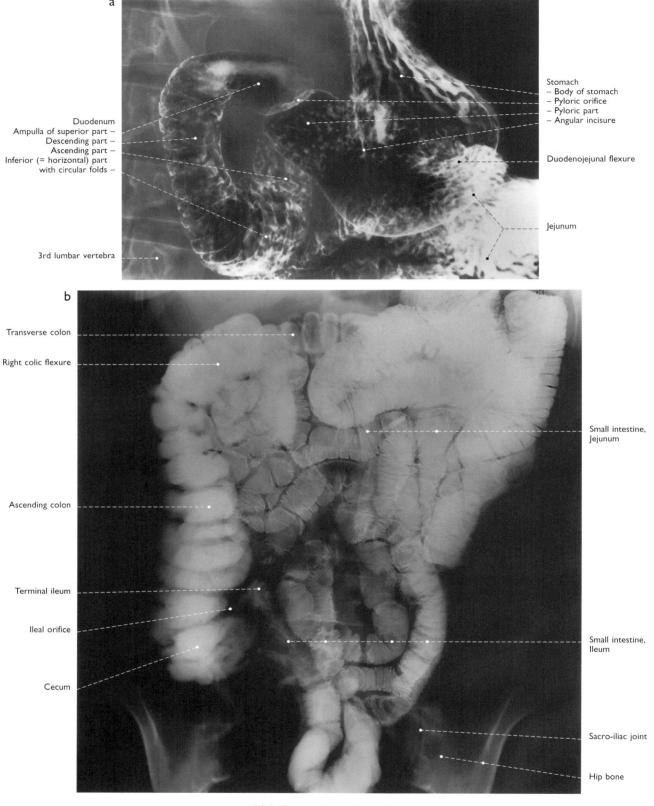

a

Duodenum
Ampulla of superior part –
Descending part –
Ascending part –
Inferior (= horizontal) part
with circular folds –

3rd lumbar vertebra

Stomach
– Body of stomach
– Pyloric orifice
– Pyloric part
– Angular incisure

Duodenojejunal flexure

Jejunum

b

Transverse colon

Right colic flexure

Ascending colon

Terminal ileum

Ileal orifice

Cecum

Small intestine,
Jejunum

Small intestine,
Ileum

Sacro-iliac joint

Hip bone

194 Stomach and small intestine (50%)

a   Double-contrast radiograph of the stomach and the duodenum
    after barium meal and distension by air,
    right anterior oblique (RAO) projection
b   Postero-anterior radiograph of the small intestine
    and the ascending colon after barium meal

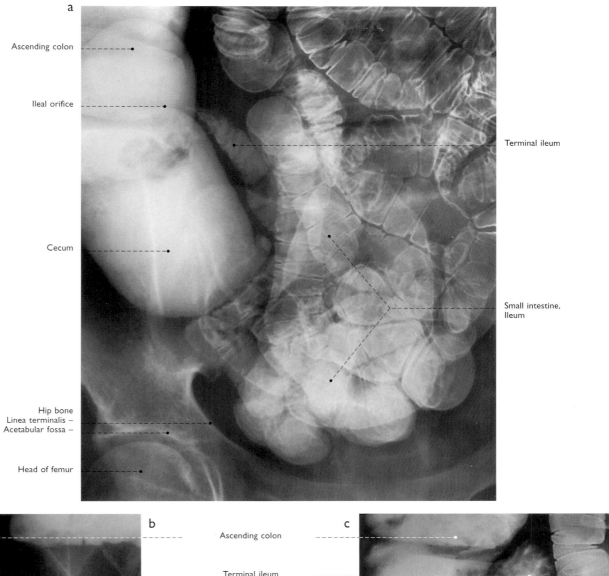

a

Ascending colon

Ileal orifice

Terminal ileum

Cecum

Small intestine,
Ileum

Hip bone
Linea terminalis –
Acetabular fossa –

Head of femur

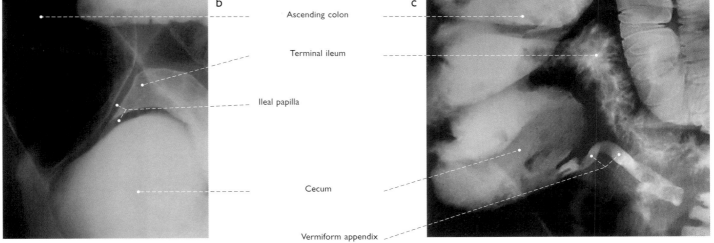

b

Ascending colon

Terminal ileum

Ileal papilla

c

Cecum

Vermiform appendix

195 Ileum and cecum (50%)

Postero-anterior radiographs of the small intestine and
the ascending colon after barium meal and distension by air
(double-contrast radiography)

a Ileum, cecum, and ascending colon
b Ileal papilla
c Terminal ileum, cecum, and vermiform appendix

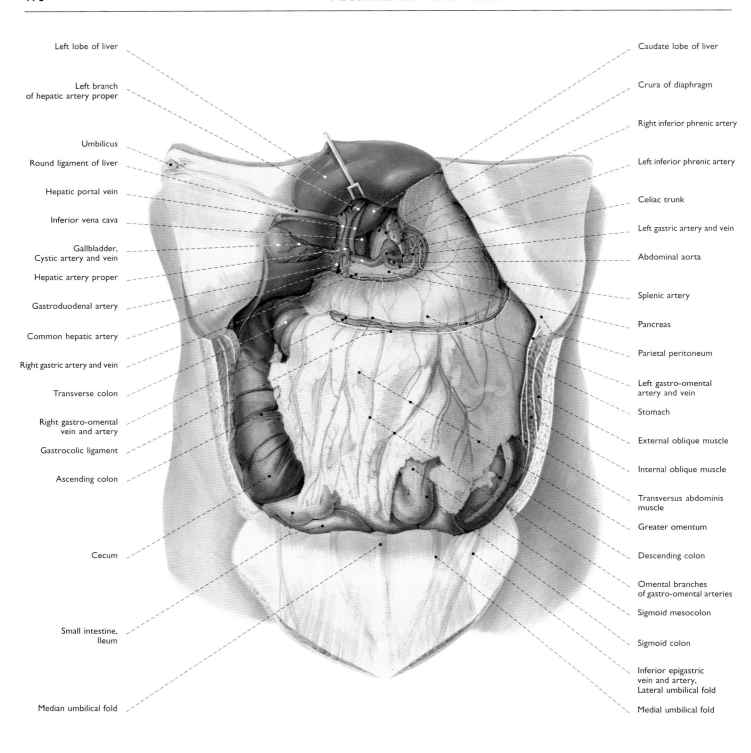

Left lobe of liver

Left branch
of hepatic artery proper

Umbilicus
Round ligament of liver

Hepatic portal vein

Inferior vena cava

Gallbladder,
Cystic artery and vein

Hepatic artery proper

Gastroduodenal artery

Common hepatic artery

Right gastric artery and vein

Transverse colon

Right gastro-omental
vein and artery

Gastrocolic ligament

Ascending colon

Cecum

Small intestine,
Ileum

Median umbilical fold

Caudate lobe of liver

Crura of diaphragm

Right inferior phrenic artery

Left inferior phrenic artery

Celiac trunk

Left gastric artery and vein

Abdominal aorta

Splenic artery

Pancreas

Parietal peritoneum

Left gastro-omental
artery and vein

Stomach

External oblique muscle

Internal oblique muscle

Transversus abdominis
muscle

Greater omentum

Descending colon

Omental branches
of gastro-omental arteries

Sigmoid mesocolon

Sigmoid colon

Inferior epigastric
vein and artery,
Lateral umbilical fold

Medial umbilical fold

196 Celiac trunk and its branches (30%)
The lesser omentum was removed,
the liver is retracted upwards. Ventral aspect

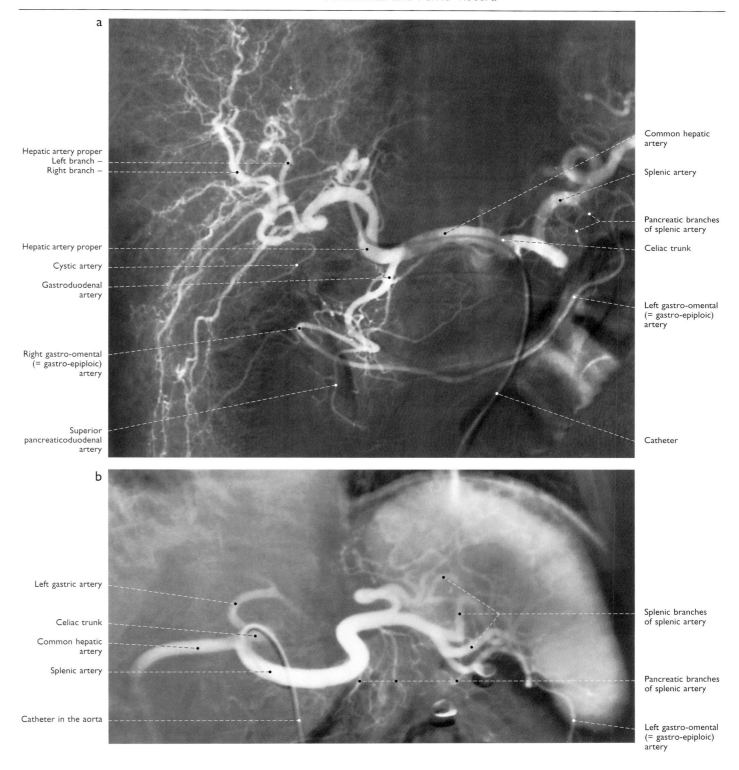

a

Hepatic artery proper
Left branch –
Right branch –

Common hepatic
artery

Splenic artery

Pancreatic branches
of splenic artery

Celiac trunk

Hepatic artery proper

Cystic artery

Gastroduodenal
artery

Left gastro-omental
(= gastro-epiploic)
artery

Right gastro-omental
(= gastro-epiploic)
artery

Superior
pancreaticoduodenal
artery

Catheter

b

Left gastric artery

Splenic branches
of splenic artery

Celiac trunk

Common hepatic
artery

Splenic artery

Pancreatic branches
of splenic artery

Catheter in the aorta

Left gastro-omental
(= gastro-epiploic)
artery

197 Celiac trunk and its branches

Anteroposterior radiographs
a   Celiacography, selective arteriogram of the celiac trunk (70%)
b   Splenography, selective arteriogram of the splenic artery (90%)

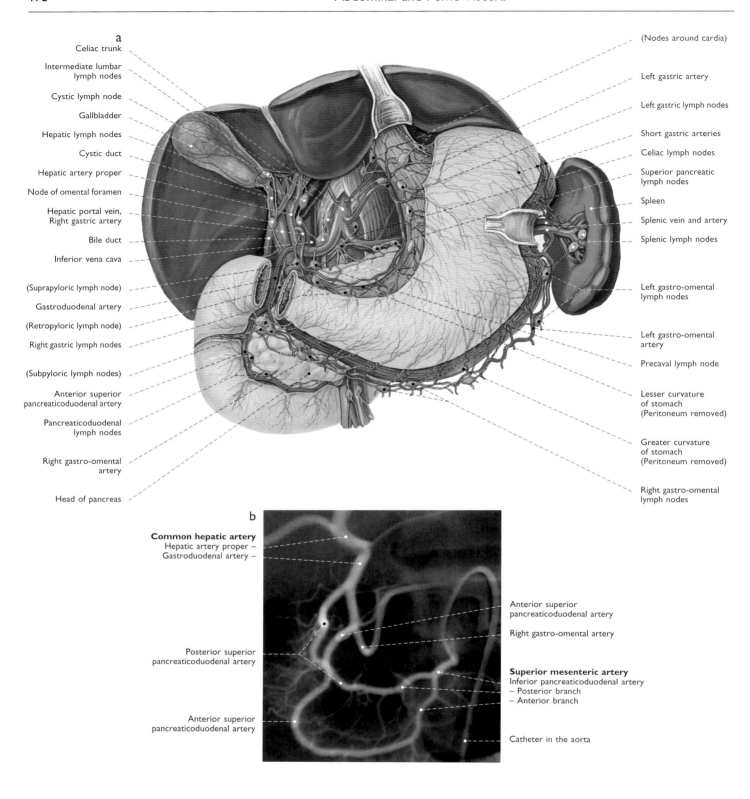

a

Celiac trunk

Intermediate lumbar
lymph nodes

Cystic lymph node

Gallbladder

Hepatic lymph nodes

Cystic duct

Hepatic artery proper

Node of omental foramen

Hepatic portal vein,
Right gastric artery

Bile duct

Inferior vena cava

(Suprapyloric lymph node)

Gastroduodenal artery

(Retropyloric lymph node)

Right gastric lymph nodes

(Subpyloric lymph nodes)

Anterior superior
pancreaticoduodenal artery

Pancreaticoduodenal
lymph nodes

Right gastro-omental
artery

Head of pancreas

(Nodes around cardia)

Left gastric artery

Left gastric lymph nodes

Short gastric arteries

Celiac lymph nodes

Superior pancreatic
lymph nodes

Spleen

Splenic vein and artery

Splenic lymph nodes

Left gastro-omental
lymph nodes

Left gastro-omental
artery

Precaval lymph node

Lesser curvature
of stomach
(Peritoneum removed)

Greater curvature
of stomach
(Peritoneum removed)

Right gastro-omental
lymph nodes

b

Common hepatic artery
Hepatic artery proper –
Gastroduodenal artery –

Posterior superior
pancreaticoduodenal artery

Anterior superior
pancreaticoduodenal artery

Anterior superior
pancreaticoduodenal artery

Right gastro-omental artery

Superior mesenteric artery
Inferior pancreaticoduodenal artery
– Posterior branch
– Anterior branch

Catheter in the aorta

198 Arteries, lymphatic vessels, and lymph nodes
     in the upper abdomen (40%)
   a Ventral aspect
   b Arteriogram of the common hepatic artery and
      the superior mesenteric artery in order to show
      the arterial supply of the head of pancreas

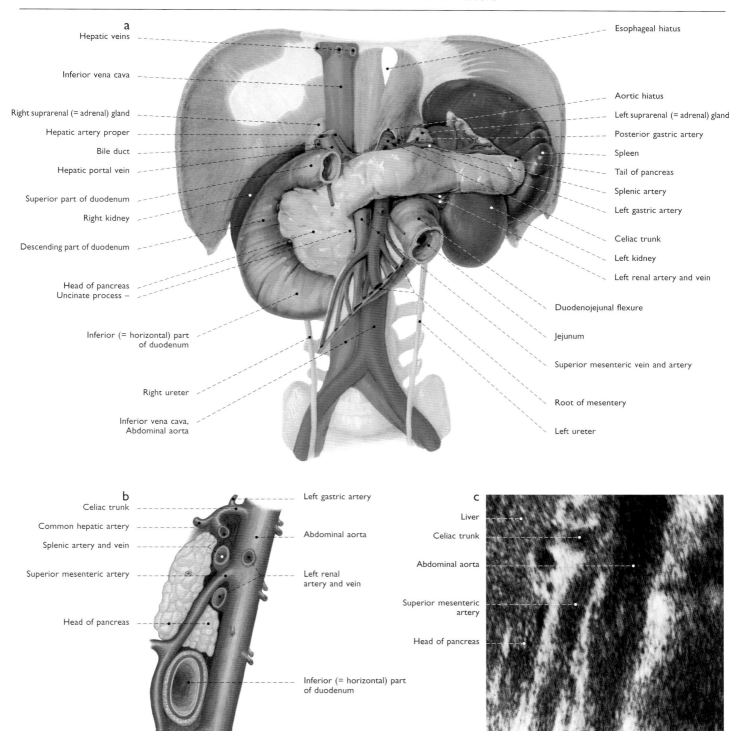

a

Hepatic veins
Inferior vena cava
Right suprarenal (= adrenal) gland
Hepatic artery proper
Bile duct
Hepatic portal vein
Superior part of duodenum
Right kidney
Descending part of duodenum
Head of pancreas
Uncinate process
Inferior (= horizontal) part of duodenum
Right ureter
Inferior vena cava, Abdominal aorta

Esophageal hiatus
Aortic hiatus
Left suprarenal (= adrenal) gland
Posterior gastric artery
Spleen
Tail of pancreas
Splenic artery
Left gastric artery
Celiac trunk
Left kidney
Left renal artery and vein
Duodenojejunal flexure
Jejunum
Superior mesenteric vein and artery
Root of mesentery
Left ureter

b

Celiac trunk
Common hepatic artery
Splenic artery and vein
Superior mesenteric artery
Head of pancreas
Inferior mesenteric artery

Left gastric artery
Abdominal aorta
Left renal artery and vein
Inferior (= horizontal) part of duodenum

c

Liver
Celiac trunk
Abdominal aorta
Superior mesenteric artery
Head of pancreas

199 Retroperitoneal organs of the upper abdomen and spleen

a Ventral aspect (60%)
b Scissor-like arrangement of the abdominal aorta and the superior mesenteric artery around the duodenum (70%), medial aspect of the right half
c Ultrasound image of the abdominal aorta and the superior mesenteric artery (70%), midsagittal longitudinal section

Left lobe of liver

Right gastro-omental
vein and artery

Round ligament of liver

Quadrate lobe of liver

Common hepatic artery

Gallbladder

Cystic vein and artery

Pyloric part of stomach

Gastroduodenal artery

Splenic artery

Anterior superior
pancreaticoduodenal artery

Transverse colon

Middle colic vein and artery

Inferior pancreatico-
duodenal artery

Head of pancreas

Parietal peritoneum
(cut edge)

Descending part
of duodenum

Superior mesenteric vein

Ascending colon

Right colic artery

Ileocolic artery

Terminal ileum

Inferior epigastric
veins and artery,
Lateral umbilical fold

Body of stomach

Left gastric artery and vein

Left crus of diaphragm

Celiac trunk

Inferior phrenic artery

Splenic artery

Splenic vein

Left colic flexure

Tail of pancreas

Superior mesenteric artery

Root
of transverse mesocolon

Inferior mesenteric vein

Jejunal and ileal
veins and arteries

Small intestine

Jejunal and ileal
arteries and veins

Median umbilical fold

Medial umbilical fold

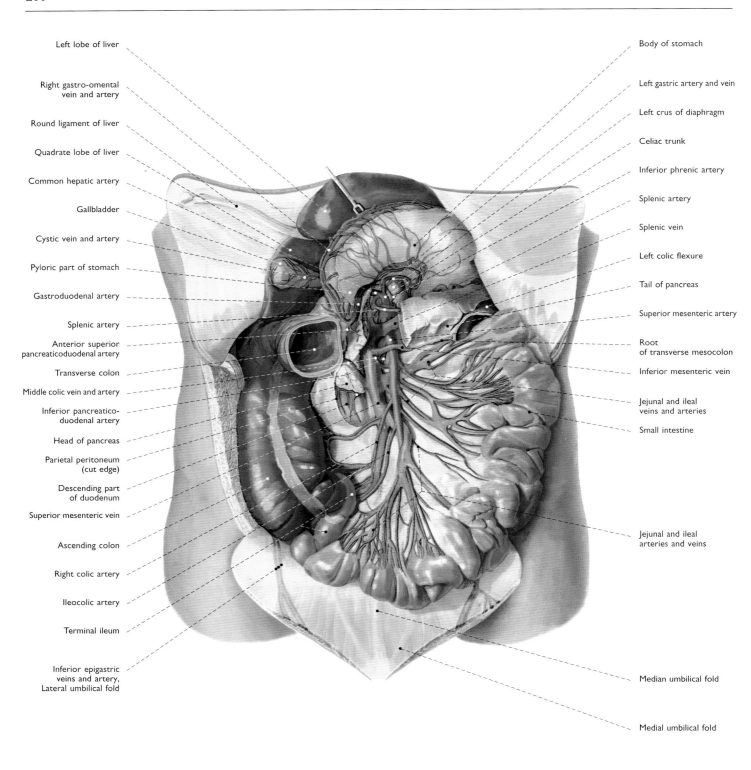

200 Celiac trunk and superior mesenteric vessels
with their branches (30%)
The greater omentum and the transverse colon were removed,
the stomach is retracted upwards and the small intestine
drawn to the left. Ventral aspect

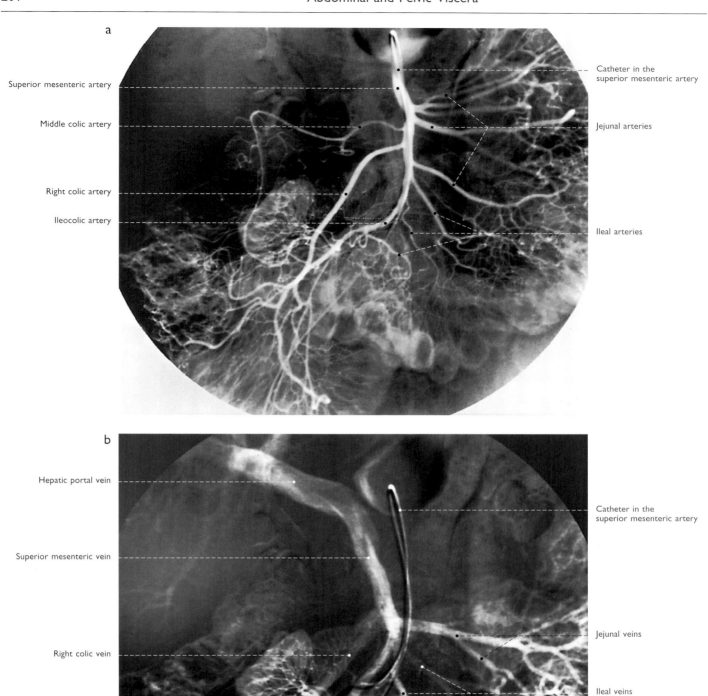

a

Superior mesenteric artery

Middle colic artery

Right colic artery

Ileocolic artery

Catheter in the
superior mesenteric artery

Jejunal arteries

Ileal arteries

b

Hepatic portal vein

Superior mesenteric vein

Right colic vein

Ileocolic vein

Catheter in the
superior mesenteric artery

Jejunal veins

Ileal veins

**201 Superior mesenteric vessels and
hepatic portal vein** (60%)

Postero-anterior radiographs
a   Selective arteriogram of the superior mesenteric artery
b   Venous phase of the superior mesenteric arteriogram
     showing the superior mesenteric and hepatic portal veins

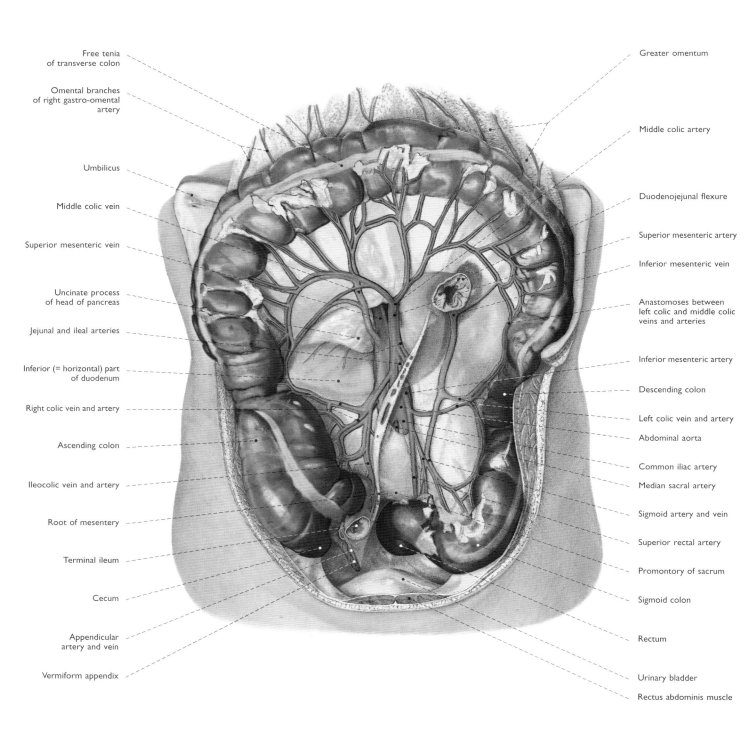

Free tenia
of transverse colon

Omental branches
of right gastro-omental
artery

Umbilicus

Middle colic vein

Superior mesenteric vein

Uncinate process
of head of pancreas

Jejunal and ileal arteries

Inferior (= horizontal) part
of duodenum

Right colic vein and artery

Ascending colon

Ileocolic vein and artery

Root of mesentery

Terminal ileum

Cecum

Appendicular
artery and vein

Vermiform appendix

Greater omentum

Middle colic artery

Duodenojejunal flexure

Superior mesenteric artery

Inferior mesenteric vein

Anastomoses between
left colic and middle colic
veins and arteries

Inferior mesenteric artery

Descending colon

Left colic vein and artery

Abdominal aorta

Common iliac artery

Median sacral artery

Sigmoid artery and vein

Superior rectal artery

Promontory of sacrum

Sigmoid colon

Rectum

Urinary bladder

Rectus abdominis muscle

202 Vascular supply of the large intestine (30%)
The greater omentum and the transverse colon are retracted upwards.
The small intestine was transected both at the duodenojejunal flexure
and the ileocecal transition, and removed along with its mesentery
which was severed at the root of mesentery. Ventral aspect

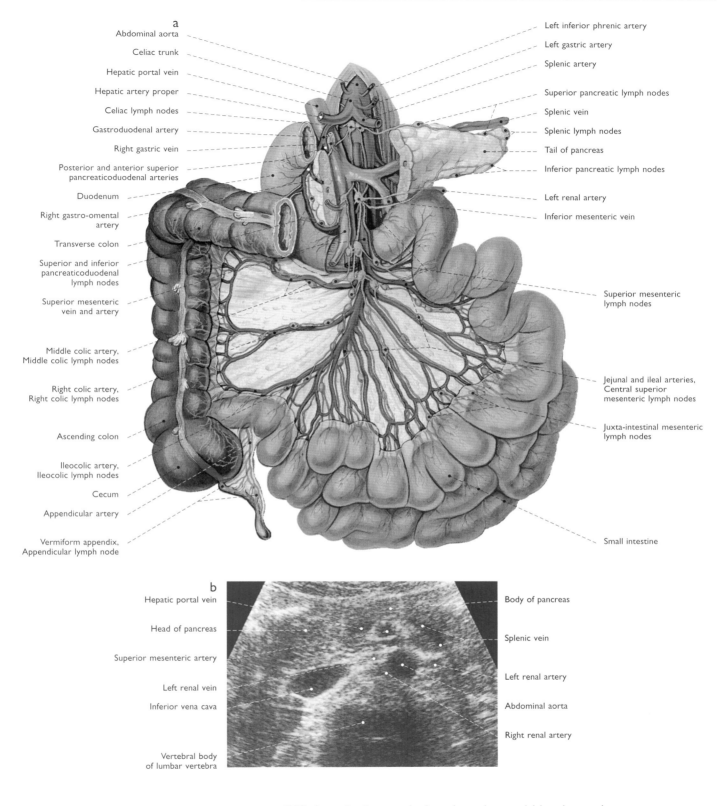

a

Abdominal aorta

Celiac trunk

Hepatic portal vein

Hepatic artery proper

Celiac lymph nodes

Gastroduodenal artery

Right gastric vein

Posterior and anterior superior pancreaticoduodenal arteries

Duodenum

Right gastro-omental artery

Transverse colon

Superior and inferior pancreaticoduodenal lymph nodes

Superior mesenteric vein and artery

Middle colic artery, Middle colic lymph nodes

Right colic artery, Right colic lymph nodes

Ascending colon

Ileocolic artery, Ileocolic lymph nodes

Cecum

Appendicular artery

Vermiform appendix, Appendicular lymph node

Left inferior phrenic artery

Left gastric artery

Splenic artery

Superior pancreatic lymph nodes

Splenic vein

Splenic lymph nodes

Tail of pancreas

Inferior pancreatic lymph nodes

Left renal artery

Inferior mesenteric vein

Superior mesenteric lymph nodes

Jejunal and ileal arteries, Central superior mesenteric lymph nodes

Juxta-intestinal mesenteric lymph nodes

Small intestine

b

Hepatic portal vein

Head of pancreas

Superior mesenteric artery

Left renal vein

Inferior vena cava

Vertebral body of lumbar vertebra

Body of pancreas

Splenic vein

Left renal artery

Abdominal aorta

Right renal artery

203 Lymphatic vessels, lymph nodes, and blood vessels of the mesentery and the retroperitoneal organs of the upper abdomen

a Ventral aspect (40%)
b Ultrasound image (60%), transverse section through the upper abdomen

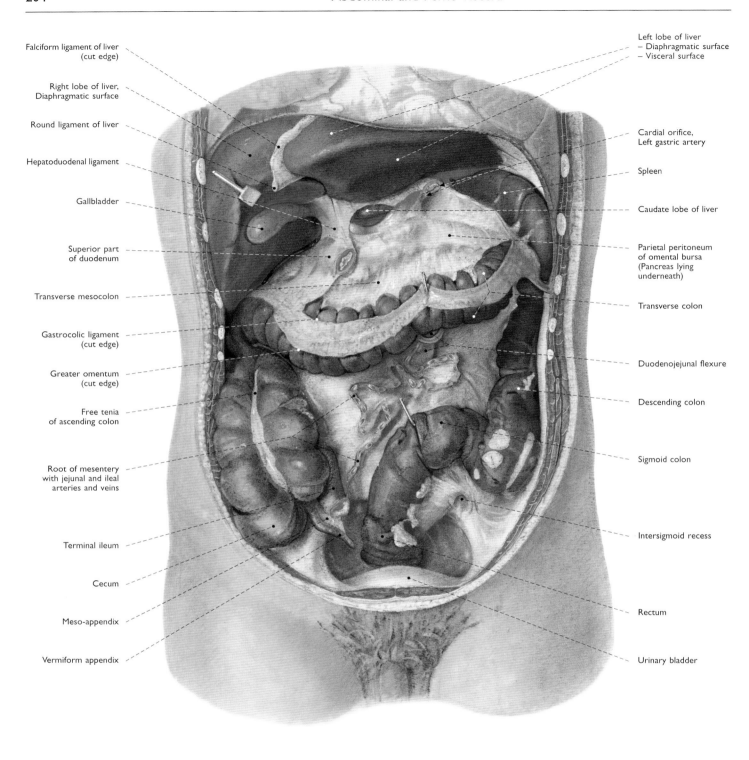

Falciform ligament of liver (cut edge)

Right lobe of liver, Diaphragmatic surface

Round ligament of liver

Hepatoduodenal ligament

Gallbladder

Superior part of duodenum

Transverse mesocolon

Gastrocolic ligament (cut edge)

Greater omentum (cut edge)

Free tenia of ascending colon

Root of mesentery with jejunal and ileal arteries and veins

Terminal ileum

Cecum

Meso-appendix

Vermiform appendix

Left lobe of liver
– Diaphragmatic surface
– Visceral surface

Cardial orifice, Left gastric artery

Spleen

Caudate lobe of liver

Parietal peritoneum of omental bursa (Pancreas lying underneath)

Transverse colon

Duodenojejunal flexure

Descending colon

Sigmoid colon

Intersigmoid recess

Rectum

Urinary bladder

204   Large intestine and mesenteries (30%)

The anterior body wall was removed. The stomach was taken away
by severing the hepatogastric, gastrosplenic, and gastrocolic ligaments.
The greater omentum, the jejunum, and the ileum with their mesenteries,
excepting the terminal ileum, were also removed. Ventral aspect

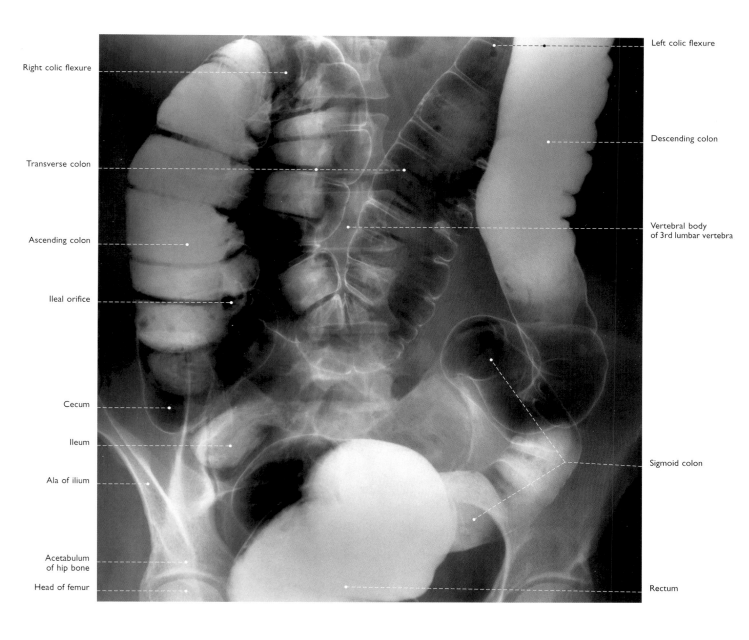

Right colic flexure

Transverse colon

Ascending colon

Ileal orifice

Cecum

Ileum

Ala of ilium

Acetabulum
of hip bone

Head of femur

Left colic flexure

Descending colon

Vertebral body
of 3rd lumbar vertebra

Sigmoid colon

Rectum

205 Large intestine (50%)
Double-contrast barium enema of the large bowel (colon)
with a V-shaped, pendulous transverse colon,
postero-anterior radiograph

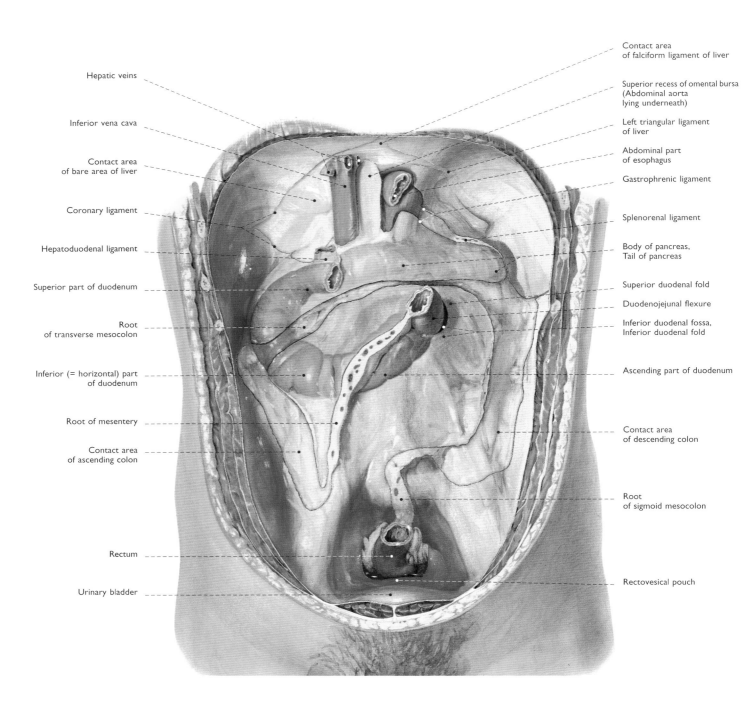

Hepatic veins

Inferior vena cava

Contact area
of bare area of liver

Coronary ligament

Hepatoduodenal ligament

Superior part of duodenum

Root
of transverse mesocolon

Inferior (= horizontal) part
of duodenum

Root of mesentery

Contact area
of ascending colon

Rectum

Urinary bladder

Contact area
of falciform ligament of liver

Superior recess of omental bursa
(Abdominal aorta
lying underneath)

Left triangular ligament
of liver

Abdominal part
of esophagus

Gastrophrenic ligament

Splenorenal ligament

Body of pancreas,
Tail of pancreas

Superior duodenal fold

Duodenojejunal flexure

Inferior duodenal fossa,
Inferior duodenal fold

Ascending part of duodenum

Contact area
of descending colon

Root
of sigmoid mesocolon

Rectovesical pouch

206　Posterior abdominal wall (30%)
Duodenum and pancreas remaining in situ.
The contact areas of the retroperitoneal parts of colon
and the liver as well as the roots of mesenteries are shown.
Ventral aspect

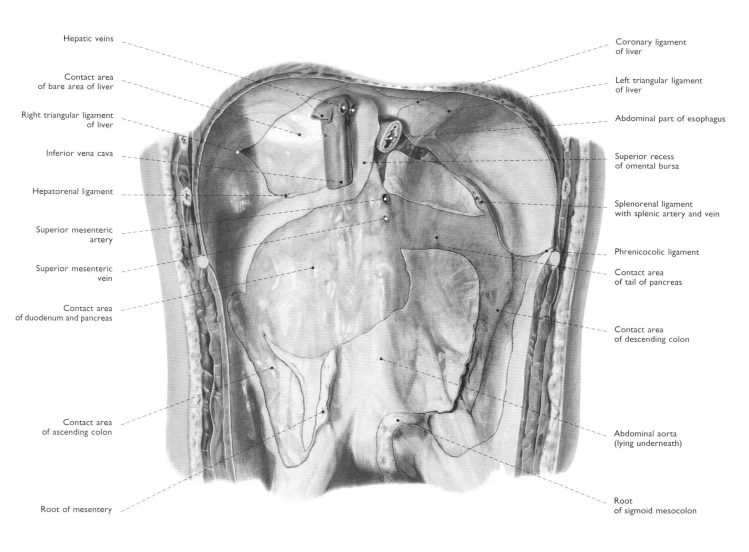

Hepatic veins

Contact area
of bare area of liver

Right triangular ligament
of liver

Inferior vena cava

Hepatorenal ligament

Superior mesenteric
artery

Superior mesenteric
vein

Contact area
of duodenum and pancreas

Contact area
of ascending colon

Root of mesentery

Coronary ligament
of liver

Left triangular ligament
of liver

Abdominal part of esophagus

Superior recess
of omental bursa

Splenorenal ligament
with splenic artery and vein

Phrenicocolic ligament

Contact area
of tail of pancreas

Contact area
of descending colon

Abdominal aorta
(lying underneath)

Root
of sigmoid mesocolon

207 Posterior abdominal wall (30%)
Lines of peritoneal reflexion after removal of the intraperitoneal
organs and contact areas of the retroperitoneal organs.
Duodenum and pancreas were removed. Ventral aspect

a

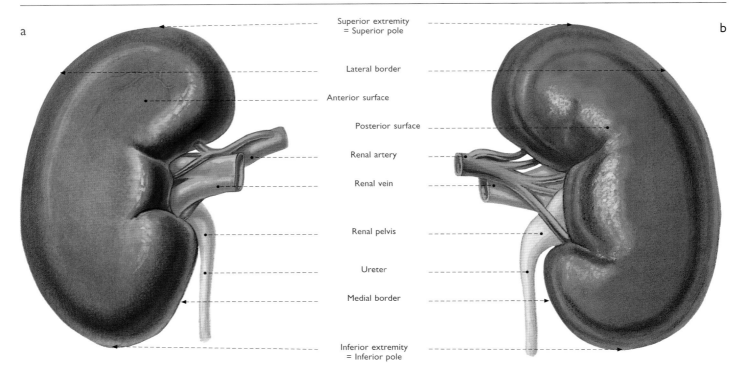

Superior extremity
= Superior pole

Lateral border

Anterior surface

Posterior surface

Renal artery

Renal vein

Renal pelvis

Ureter

Medial border

Inferior extremity
= Inferior pole

b

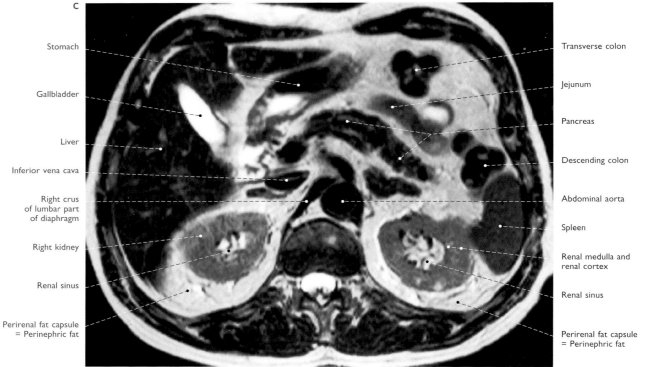

c

Stomach

Gallbladder

Liver

Inferior vena cava

Right crus
of lumbar part
of diaphragm

Right kidney

Renal sinus

Perirenal fat capsule
= Perinephric fat

Transverse colon

Jejunum

Pancreas

Descending colon

Abdominal aorta

Spleen

Renal medulla and
renal cortex

Renal sinus

Perirenal fat capsule
= Perinephric fat

208 Kidney of an adult

a, b The main hilar structures of the right kidney were separated
       from each other (90%).
   a Ventral aspect
   b Dorsal aspect
   c Transverse magnetic resonance image (MRI, T$_2$-weighted)
       through the upper abdomen at the level of the first lumbar
       vertebral body (LI) to show both kidneys and the perinephric fat (40%),
       inferior aspect

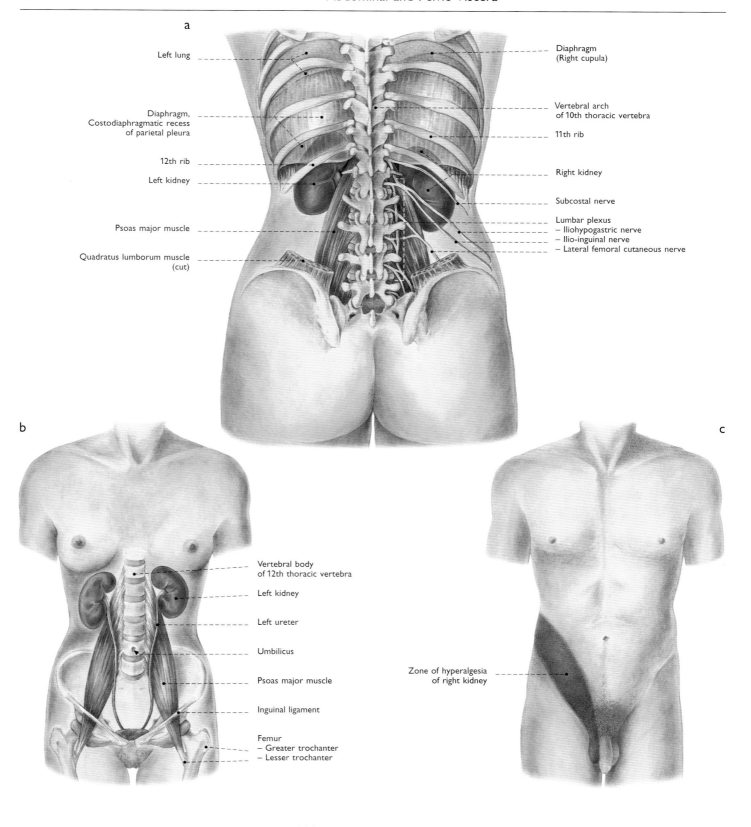

a

Left lung

Diaphragm,
Costodiaphragmatic recess
of parietal pleura

12th rib

Left kidney

Psoas major muscle

Quadratus lumborum muscle
(cut)

Diaphragm
(Right cupula)

Vertebral arch
of 10th thoracic vertebra

11th rib

Right kidney

Subcostal nerve

Lumbar plexus
– Iliohypogastric nerve
– Ilio-inguinal nerve
– Lateral femoral cutaneous nerve

b

Vertebral body
of 12th thoracic vertebra

Left kidney

Left ureter

Umbilicus

Psoas major muscle

Inguinal ligament

Femur
– Greater trochanter
– Lesser trochanter

c

Zone of hyperalgesia
of right kidney

209 Kidneys

a Kidneys and adjacent structures projected to
   the posterior abdominal wall (25%), dorsal aspect
b Projection of the kidneys and both psoas major muscles
   onto the anterior abdominal wall (15%), ventral aspect
c Zone of hyperalgesia of the right kidney (15%), ventral aspect

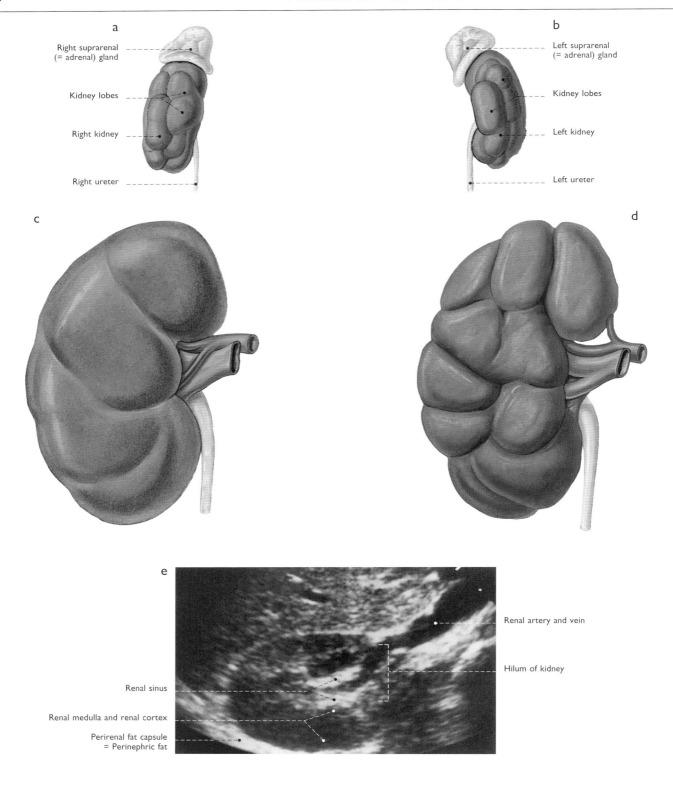

a
Right suprarenal (= adrenal) gland
Kidney lobes
Right kidney
Right ureter

b
Left suprarenal (= adrenal) gland
Kidney lobes
Left kidney
Left ureter

c

d

e
Renal artery and vein
Hilum of kidney
Renal sinus
Renal medulla and renal cortex
Perirenal fat capsule = Perinephric fat

210 Fetal and lobulated kidneys

a, b Kidneys and suprarenal (= adrenal) glands of a human fetus,
　　seventh month of pregnancy (100%), ventral aspect
c, d Right kidney, ventral aspect (80%)
　c Faintly persisting fetal lobulation of the renal surface of an adult
　d Markedly persisting fetal lobulation of the renal surface of an adult
　e Ultrasound image of the right kidney (80%), transverse section

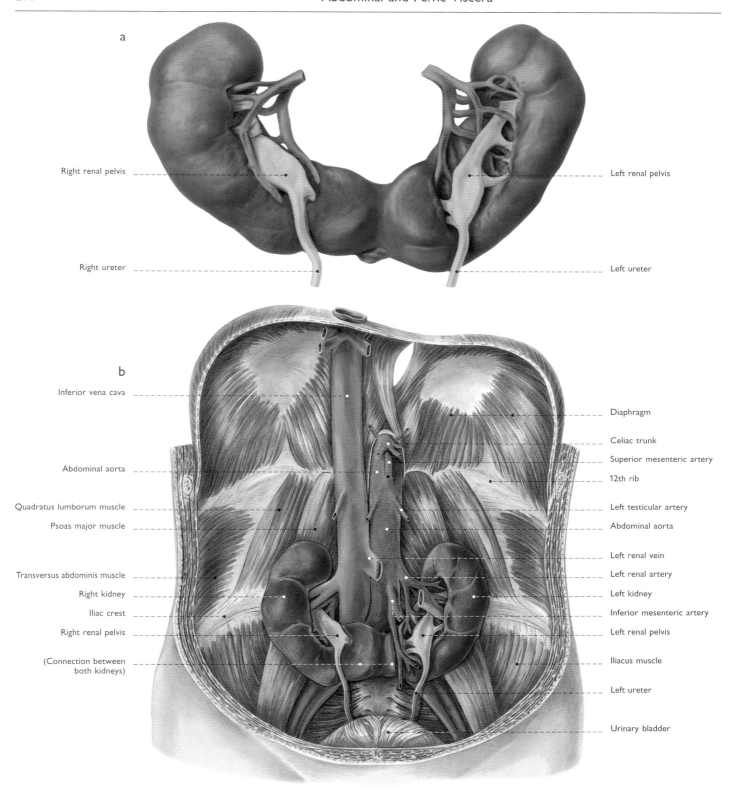

a

Right renal pelvis

Right ureter

Left renal pelvis

Left ureter

b

Inferior vena cava

Abdominal aorta

Quadratus lumborum muscle

Psoas major muscle

Transversus abdominis muscle

Right kidney

Iliac crest

Right renal pelvis

(Connection between both kidneys)

Diaphragm

Celiac trunk

Superior mesenteric artery

12th rib

Left testicular artery

Abdominal aorta

Left renal vein

Left renal artery

Left kidney

Inferior mesenteric artery

Left renal pelvis

Iliacus muscle

Left ureter

Urinary bladder

211 Horseshoe kidney

a   Isolated horseshoe kidney (60%), ventral aspect
b   Horseshoe kidney in situ (30%), ventral aspect

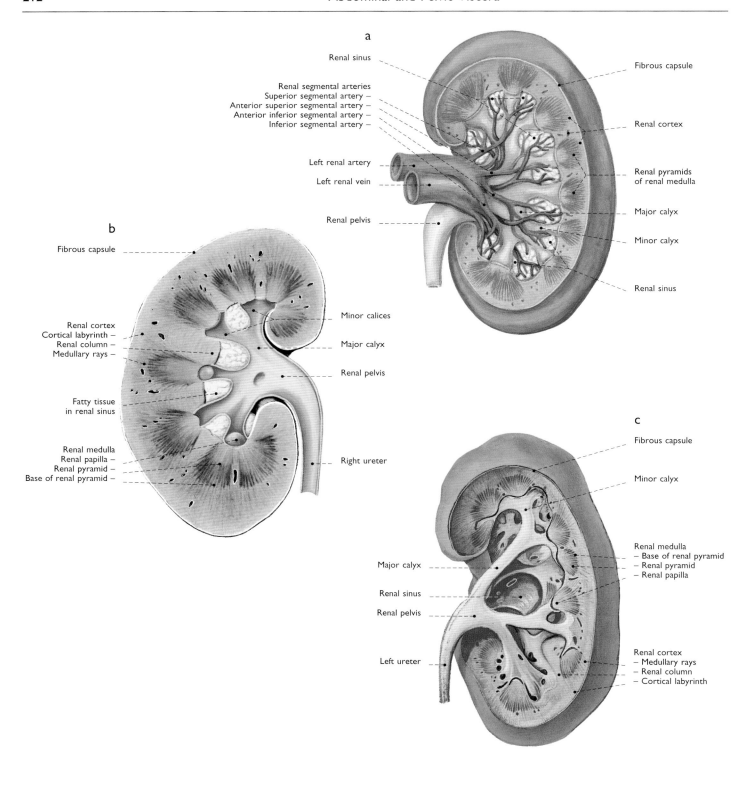

a

Renal sinus

Renal segmental arteries
Superior segmental artery –
Anterior superior segmental artery –
Anterior inferior segmental artery –
Inferior segmental artery –

Left renal artery

Left renal vein

Renal pelvis

Fibrous capsule

Renal cortex

Renal pyramids
of renal medulla

Major calyx

Minor calyx

Renal sinus

b

Fibrous capsule

Renal cortex
Cortical labyrinth –
Renal column –
Medullary rays –

Fatty tissue
in renal sinus

Renal medulla
Renal papilla –
Renal pyramid –
Base of renal pyramid –

Minor calices

Major calyx

Renal pelvis

Right ureter

c

Fibrous capsule

Minor calyx

Renal medulla
– Base of renal pyramid
– Renal pyramid
– Renal papilla

Major calyx

Renal sinus

Renal pelvis

Left ureter

Renal cortex
– Medullary rays
– Renal column
– Cortical labyrinth

212 Kidney (80%)
Ventral aspect
a Left renal sinus with renal pelvis and renal blood vessels.
   The renal parenchyma of the anterior part of kidney was removed.
b Longitudinal section through the right kidney, cut surface
   of the posterior part
c Left renal sinus with the renal pelvis and its division into calices.
   The fatty tissue and blood vessels in the renal sinus were removed.

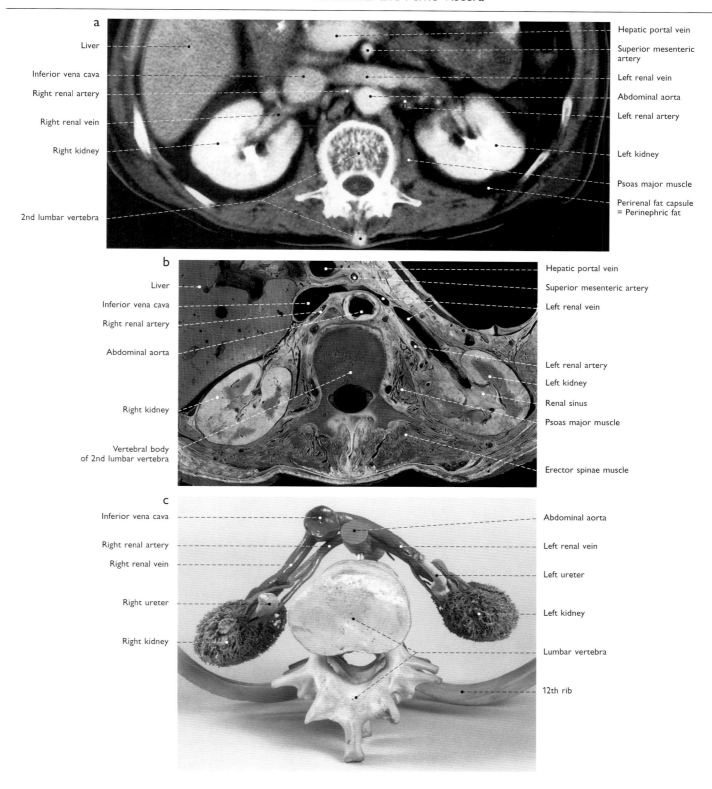

a

Liver

Inferior vena cava

Right renal artery

Right renal vein

Right kidney

2nd lumbar vertebra

Hepatic portal vein

Superior mesenteric artery

Left renal vein

Abdominal aorta

Left renal artery

Left kidney

Psoas major muscle

Perirenal fat capsule = Perinephric fat

b

Liver

Inferior vena cava

Right renal artery

Abdominal aorta

Right kidney

Vertebral body of 2nd lumbar vertebra

Hepatic portal vein

Superior mesenteric artery

Left renal vein

Left renal artery

Left kidney

Renal sinus

Psoas major muscle

Erector spinae muscle

c

Inferior vena cava

Right renal artery

Right renal vein

Right ureter

Right kidney

Abdominal aorta

Left renal vein

Left ureter

Left kidney

Lumbar vertebra

12th rib

213   Kidneys and renal blood vessels (40%)

Inferior aspect

a   Transverse computed tomogram (CT) at the level of the second lumbar vertebral body (L II)

b   Transverse anatomical section at the same level as in fig. a

c   Corrosion cast of the renal blood vessels and the ureters of both kidneys of a 15-year-old girl (Anatomical Collection, Basel)

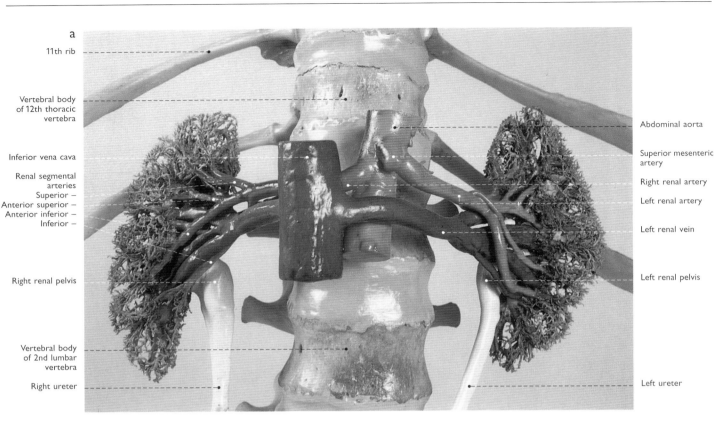

a
- 11th rib
- Vertebral body of 12th thoracic vertebra
- Inferior vena cava
- Renal segmental arteries
  Superior –
  Anterior superior –
  Anterior inferior –
  Inferior –
- Right renal pelvis
- Vertebral body of 2nd lumbar vertebra
- Right ureter
- Abdominal aorta
- Superior mesenteric artery
- Right renal artery
- Left renal artery
- Left renal vein
- Left renal pelvis
- Left ureter

b   60%

c   8%

d   6%

e   5%

214 Kidneys and renal blood vessels

Ventral aspect
a Corrosion cast of the renal blood vessels and the ureters of both kidneys of a 15-year-old girl (60%) (Anatomical Collection, Basel)
b–e Variations of the renal artery. The percentile numbers beneath the pictures indicate the approximate frequency.
b 'Normal pattern' with only one renal artery from the aorta on the left side of the body
c Additional upper accessory renal artery from the aorta
d Additional lower accessory renal artery from the aorta
c Multiple (more than two) renal arteries from the aorta

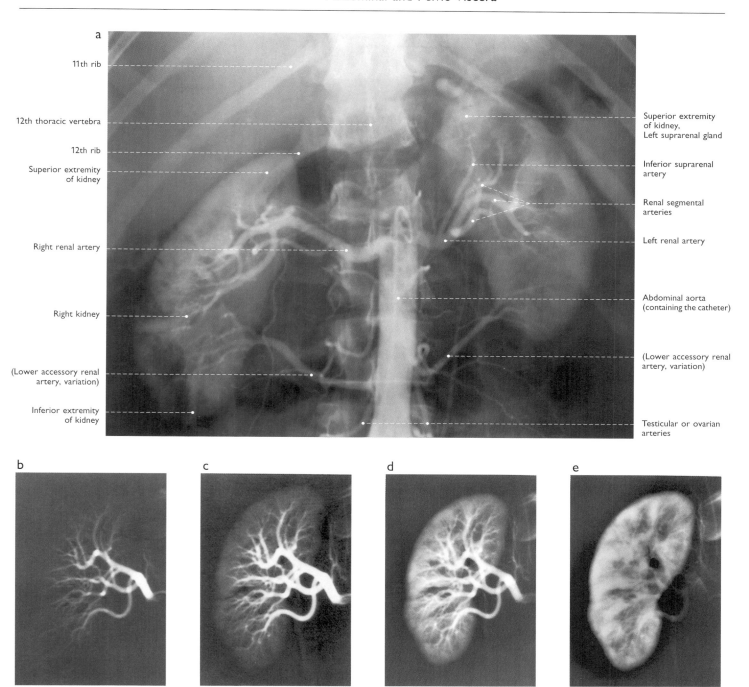

a

11th rib

12th thoracic vertebra

12th rib

Superior extremity
of kidney

Right renal artery

Right kidney

(Lower accessory renal
artery, variation)

Inferior extremity
of kidney

Superior extremity
of kidney,
Left suprarenal gland

Inferior suprarenal
artery

Renal segmental
arteries

Left renal artery

Abdominal aorta
(containing the catheter)

(Lower accessory renal
artery, variation)

Testicular or ovarian
arteries

b

c

d

e

215 Kidneys and renal blood vessels
      Ventral aspect
  a Renal arteriogram of the renal arteries,
      at both sides lower polar arteries from the aorta (60%),
      postero-anterior radiograph
  b–e Selective arteriogram of the right renal artery,
      stages of increasing enrichment of contrast medium
      in the renal parenchyma (30%)

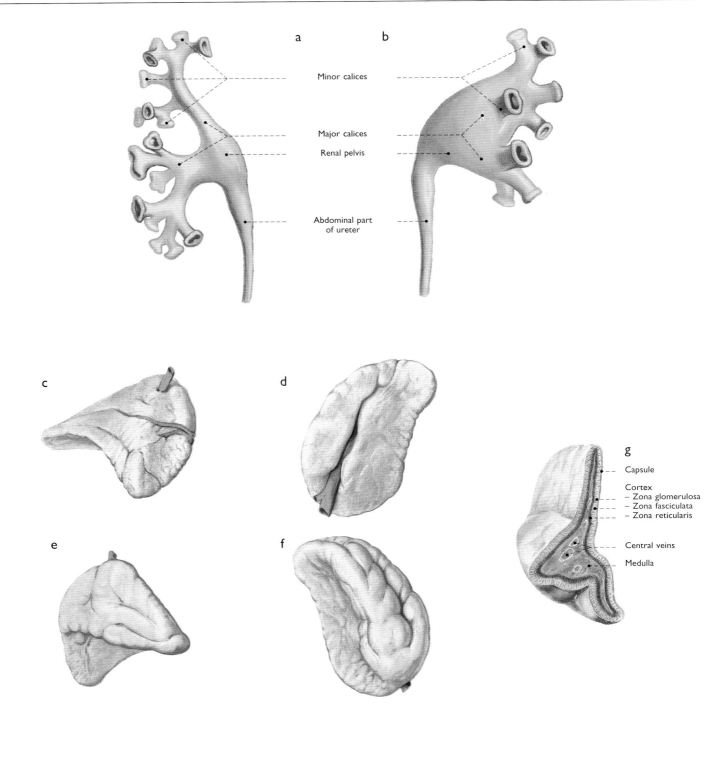

a

b

Minor calices

Major calices

Renal pelvis

Abdominal part
of ureter

c

d

e

f

g

Capsule

Cortex
– Zona glomerulosa
– Zona fasciculata
– Zona reticularis

Central veins

Medulla

216   Renal pelvis and suprarenal (= adrenal) gland

a, b   Renal pelves (100%), ventral aspect
   a   Right renal pelvis, dendritic type
   b   Left renal pelvis, ampullary type
c–g   Suprarenal (= adrenal) glands
c, e   Right suprarenal gland (80%)
d, f   Left suprarenal gland (80%)
c, d   Anterior surface
e, f   Posterior surface
   g   Longitudinal section through a suprarenal gland (200%)

a

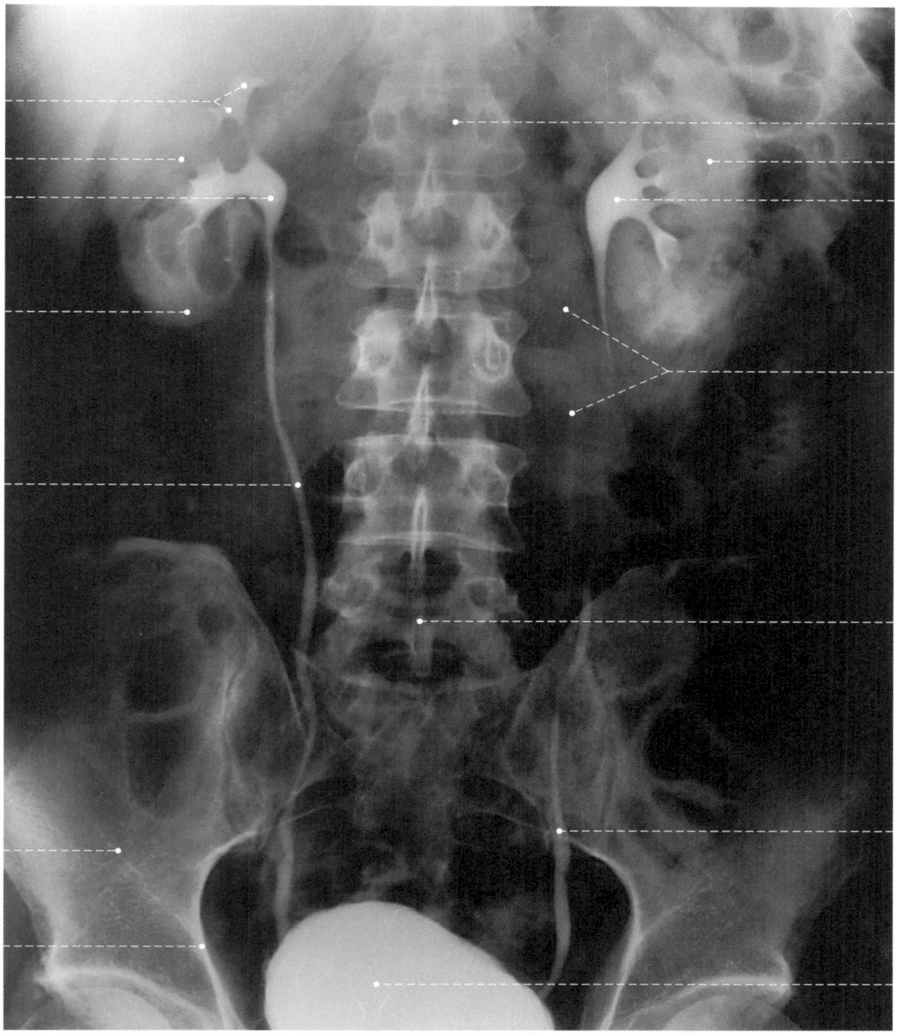

Renal calices

Right kidney

Right renal pelvis

Inferior extremity
of kidney

Right ureter

Hip bone

Linea terminalis
of pelvis

1st lumbar vertebra

Left kidney

Left renal pelvis

Psoas major muscle

5th lumbar vertebra

Left ureter

Urinary bladder

b

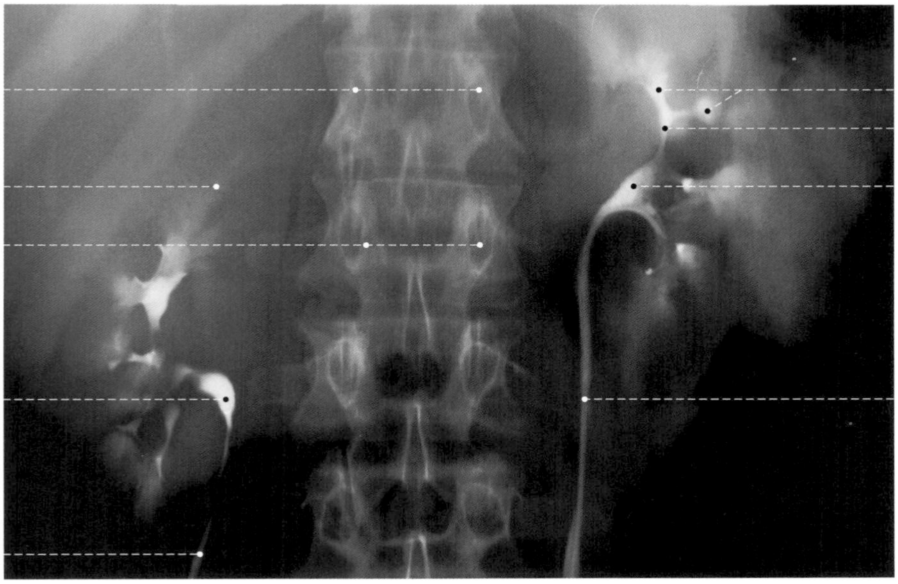

12th thoracic vertebra

12th rib

1st lumbar vertebra

Right renal pelvis

Right ureter

Minor calices

Major calyx

Left renal pelvis

Left ureter

217   Renal pelvis and ureter

Intravenous excretion urograms
a   Anteroposterior radiograph (30%)
b   Anteroposterior tomogram of renal pelves and calices (40%)

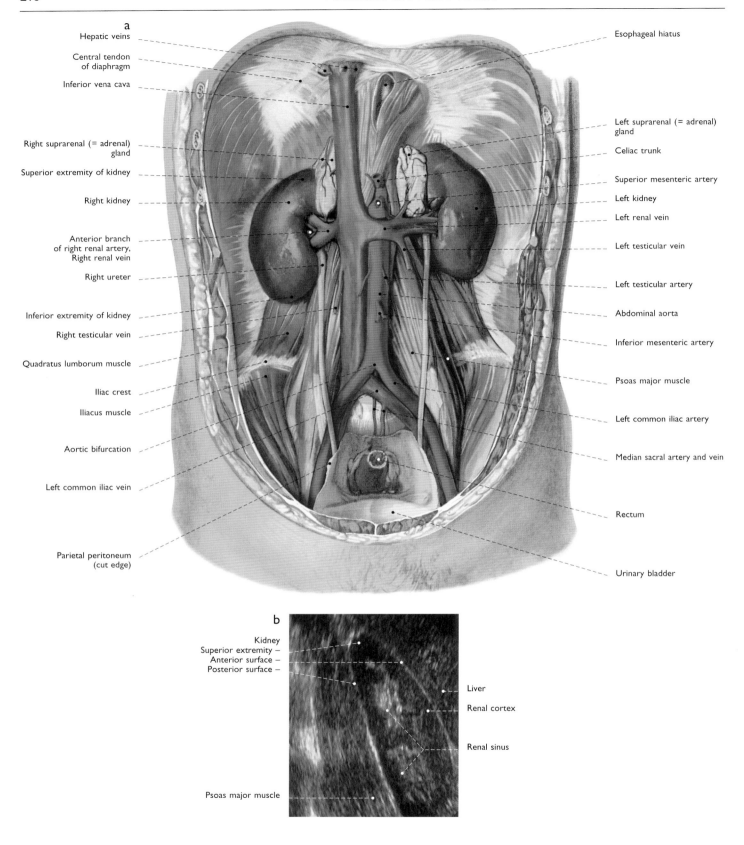

a

Hepatic veins

Central tendon of diaphragm

Inferior vena cava

Right suprarenal (= adrenal) gland

Superior extremity of kidney

Right kidney

Anterior branch of right renal artery, Right renal vein

Right ureter

Inferior extremity of kidney

Right testicular vein

Quadratus lumborum muscle

Iliac crest

Iliacus muscle

Aortic bifurcation

Left common iliac vein

Parietal peritoneum (cut edge)

Esophageal hiatus

Left suprarenal (= adrenal) gland

Celiac trunk

Superior mesenteric artery

Left kidney

Left renal vein

Left testicular vein

Left testicular artery

Abdominal aorta

Inferior mesenteric artery

Psoas major muscle

Left common iliac artery

Median sacral artery and vein

Rectum

Urinary bladder

b

Kidney
Superior extremity –
Anterior surface –
Posterior surface –

Psoas major muscle

Liver

Renal cortex

Renal sinus

218   Urinary system and great abdominal blood vessels

a   Ventral aspect (30%)
b   Ultrasound image (50%), subcostal longitudinal section

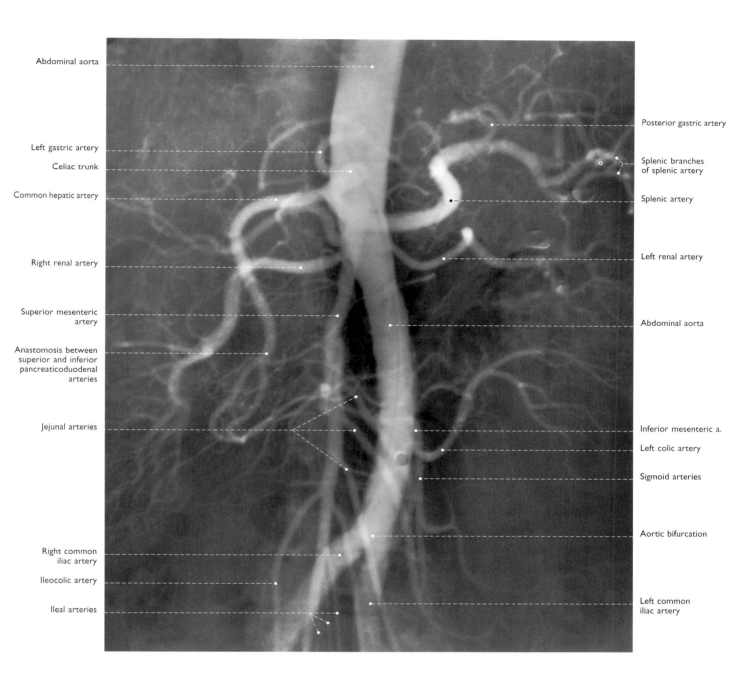

Abdominal aorta

Left gastric artery

Celiac trunk

Common hepatic artery

Right renal artery

Superior mesenteric
artery

Anastomosis between
superior and inferior
pancreaticoduodenal
arteries

Jejunal arteries

Right common
iliac artery

Ileocolic artery

Ileal arteries

Posterior gastric artery

Splenic branches
of splenic artery

Splenic artery

Left renal artery

Abdominal aorta

Inferior mesenteric a.

Left colic artery

Sigmoid arteries

Aortic bifurcation

Left common
iliac artery

219 Abdominal arteries (80%)
Abdominal aortogram, postero-anterior radiograph.
The abdominal aorta is slightly displaced to the left.

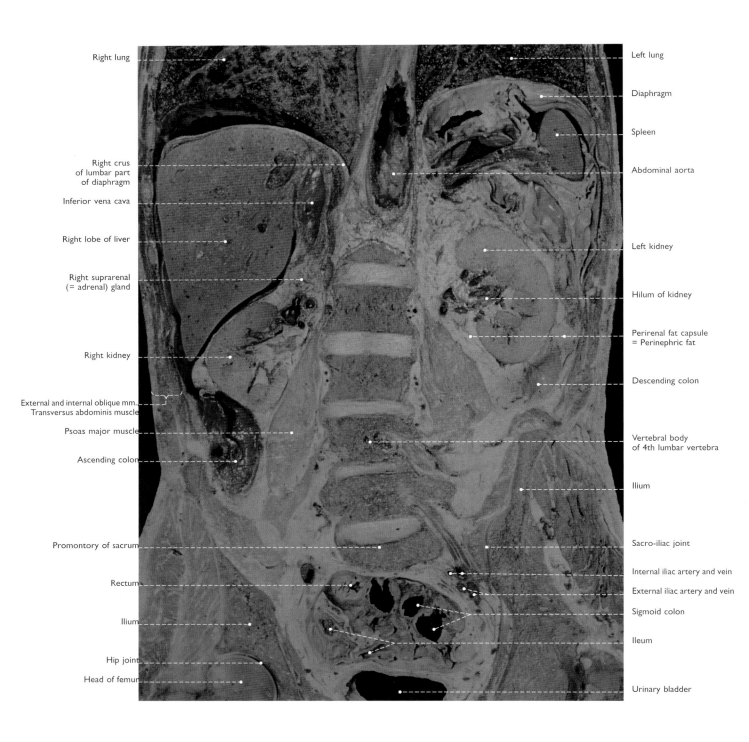

Right lung

Right crus
of lumbar part
of diaphragm

Inferior vena cava

Right lobe of liver

Right suprarenal
(= adrenal) gland

Right kidney

External and internal oblique mm.
Transversus abdominis muscle

Psoas major muscle

Ascending colon

Promontory of sacrum

Rectum

Ilium

Hip joint

Head of femur

Left lung

Diaphragm

Spleen

Abdominal aorta

Left kidney

Hilum of kidney

Perirenal fat capsule
= Perinephric fat

Descending colon

Vertebral body
of 4th lumbar vertebra

Ilium

Sacro-iliac joint

Internal iliac artery and vein

External iliac artery and vein

Sigmoid colon

Ileum

Urinary bladder

220 Abdomen (30%)
Coronal anatomical section through the abdomen
in the plane of lumbar vertebral bodies, ventral aspect

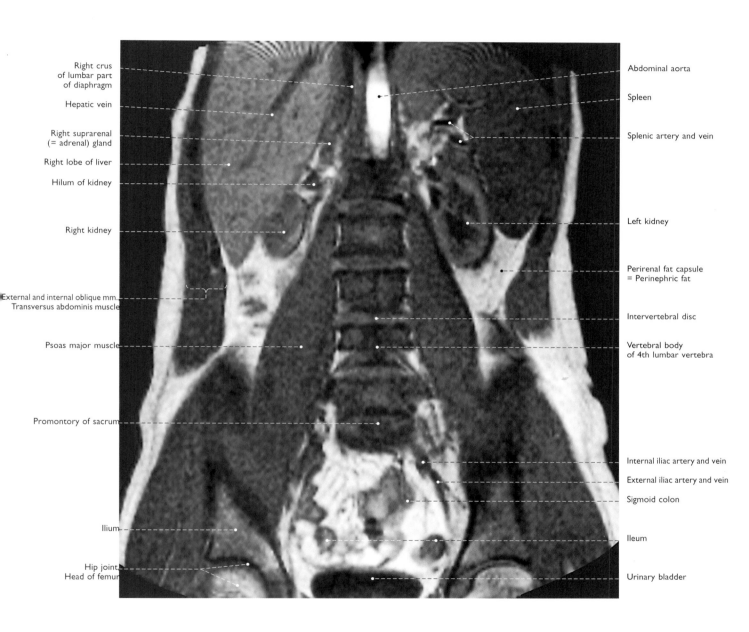

Right crus of lumbar part of diaphragm

Hepatic vein

Right suprarenal (= adrenal) gland

Right lobe of liver

Hilum of kidney

Right kidney

External and internal oblique mm. Transversus abdominis muscle

Psoas major muscle

Promontory of sacrum

Ilium

Hip joint
Head of femur

Abdominal aorta

Spleen

Splenic artery and vein

Left kidney

Perirenal fat capsule = Perinephric fat

Intervertebral disc

Vertebral body of 4th lumbar vertebra

Internal iliac artery and vein

External iliac artery and vein

Sigmoid colon

Ileum

Urinary bladder

221 Abdomen (30%)
Coronal magnetic resonance image (MRI, T$_1$-weighted)
through the abdomen in the plane of lumbar vertebral bodies
and the heads of femur, ventral aspect

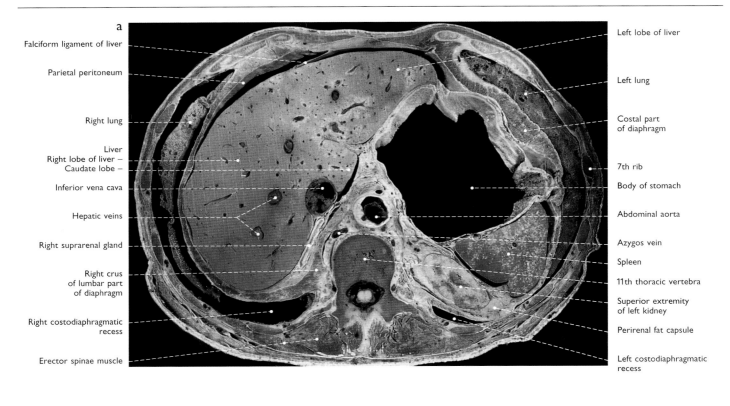

a

Falciform ligament of liver

Parietal peritoneum

Right lung

Liver
Right lobe of liver –
Caudate lobe –

Inferior vena cava

Hepatic veins

Right suprarenal gland

Right crus
of lumbar part
of diaphragm

Right costodiaphragmatic
recess

Erector spinae muscle

Left lobe of liver

Left lung

Costal part
of diaphragm

7th rib

Body of stomach

Abdominal aorta

Azygos vein

Spleen

11th thoracic vertebra

Superior extremity
of left kidney

Perirenal fat capsule

Left costodiaphragmatic
recess

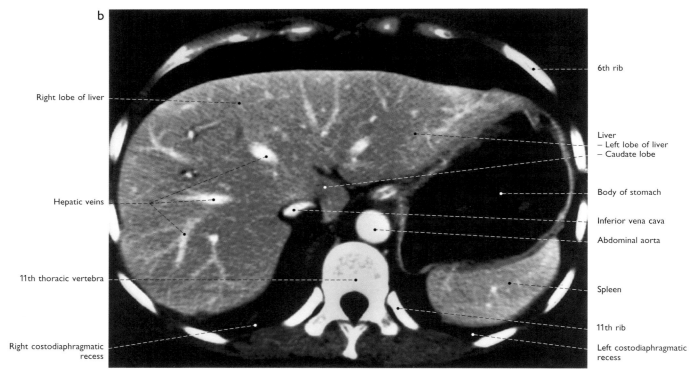

b

Right lobe of liver

Hepatic veins

11th thoracic vertebra

Right costodiaphragmatic
recess

6th rib

Liver
– Left lobe of liver
– Caudate lobe

Body of stomach

Inferior vena cava

Abdominal aorta

Spleen

11th rib

Left costodiaphragmatic
recess

222   Abdomen (40%)

Transverse sections through the upper abdomen at the level
of the eleventh thoracic vertebral body (Th XI), inferior aspect
a   Anatomical section
b   Computed tomogram (CT) after injection of contrast medium

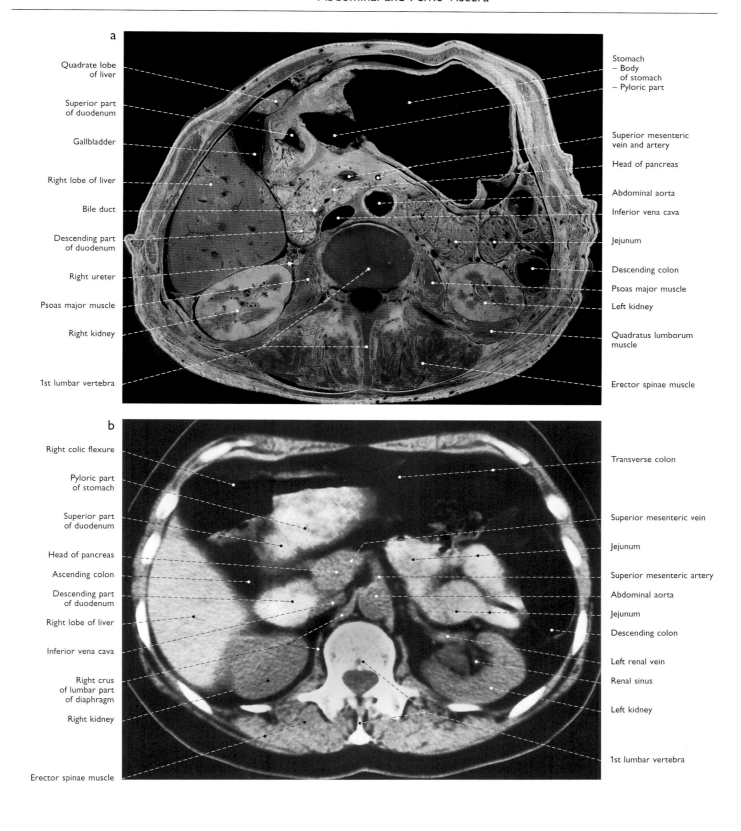

a

Quadrate lobe of liver

Superior part of duodenum

Gallbladder

Right lobe of liver

Bile duct

Descending part of duodenum

Right ureter

Psoas major muscle

Right kidney

1st lumbar vertebra

Stomach
- Body of stomach
- Pyloric part

Superior mesenteric vein and artery

Head of pancreas

Abdominal aorta

Inferior vena cava

Jejunum

Descending colon

Psoas major muscle

Left kidney

Quadratus lumborum muscle

Erector spinae muscle

b

Right colic flexure

Pyloric part of stomach

Superior part of duodenum

Head of pancreas

Ascending colon

Descending part of duodenum

Right lobe of liver

Inferior vena cava

Right crus of lumbar part of diaphragm

Right kidney

Erector spinae muscle

Transverse colon

Superior mesenteric vein

Jejunum

Superior mesenteric artery

Abdominal aorta

Jejunum

Descending colon

Left renal vein

Renal sinus

Left kidney

1st lumbar vertebra

223 Abdomen (40%)
Transverse sections through the upper abdomen at the level of the first lumbar vertebral body (LI), inferior aspect
a Anatomical section
b Computed tomogram (CT)

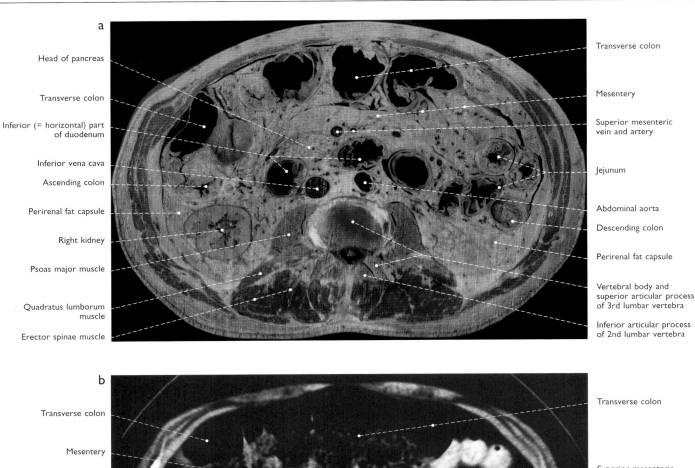

a

Head of pancreas

Transverse colon

Inferior (= horizontal) part of duodenum

Inferior vena cava

Ascending colon

Perirenal fat capsule

Right kidney

Psoas major muscle

Quadratus lumborum muscle

Erector spinae muscle

Transverse colon

Mesentery

Superior mesenteric vein and artery

Jejunum

Abdominal aorta

Descending colon

Perirenal fat capsule

Vertebral body and superior articular process of 3rd lumbar vertebra

Inferior articular process of 2nd lumbar vertebra

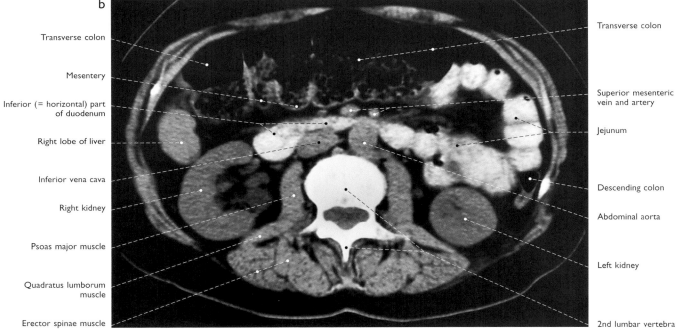

b

Transverse colon

Mesentery

Inferior (= horizontal) part of duodenum

Right lobe of liver

Inferior vena cava

Right kidney

Psoas major muscle

Quadratus lumborum muscle

Erector spinae muscle

Transverse colon

Superior mesenteric vein and artery

Jejunum

Descending colon

Abdominal aorta

Left kidney

2nd lumbar vertebra

224   Abdomen (40%)
Transverse sections through the abdomen at the level
of the second (LII, b) and third (LIII, a) lumbar vertebral body,
respectively, inferior aspect
a   Anatomical section
b   Computed tomogram (CT)

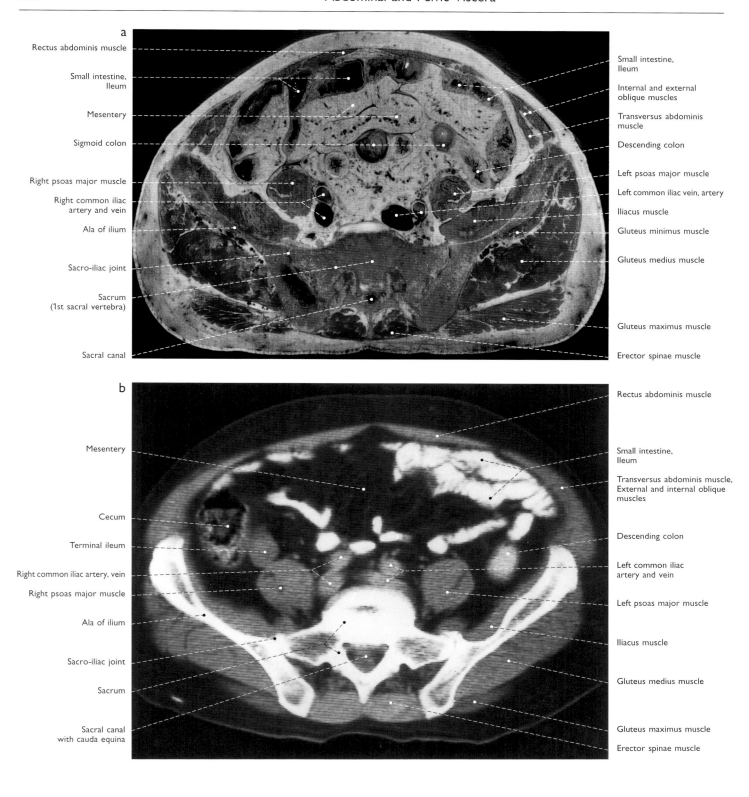

a

Rectus abdominis muscle

Small intestine, Ileum

Mesentery

Sigmoid colon

Right psoas major muscle

Right common iliac artery and vein

Ala of ilium

Sacro-iliac joint

Sacrum (1st sacral vertebra)

Sacral canal

Small intestine, Ileum

Internal and external oblique muscles

Transversus abdominis muscle

Descending colon

Left psoas major muscle

Left common iliac vein, artery

Iliacus muscle

Gluteus minimus muscle

Gluteus medius muscle

Gluteus maximus muscle

Erector spinae muscle

b

Mesentery

Cecum

Terminal ileum

Right common iliac artery, vein

Right psoas major muscle

Ala of ilium

Sacro-iliac joint

Sacrum

Sacral canal with cauda equina

Rectus abdominis muscle

Small intestine, Ileum

Transversus abdominis muscle, External and internal oblique muscles

Descending colon

Left common iliac artery and vein

Left psoas major muscle

Iliacus muscle

Gluteus medius muscle

Gluteus maximus muscle

Erector spinae muscle

225 Abdomen (40%)
Transverse sections through the lower abdomen at the level
of the first sacral vertebra (S1) and the sacro-iliac joints,
inferior aspect
a Anatomical section
b Computed tomogram (CT)

a

12th rib

Subcostal nerve

Anterior (= ventral) ramus
of 1st lumbar nerve

Iliohypogastric nerve

Ilio-inguinal nerve

Lateral femoral cutaneous nerve

Femoral nerve

Genitofemoral nerve

Th XII

L I

L II

L III

L IV

LV

Lumbosacral trunk

Obturator nerve

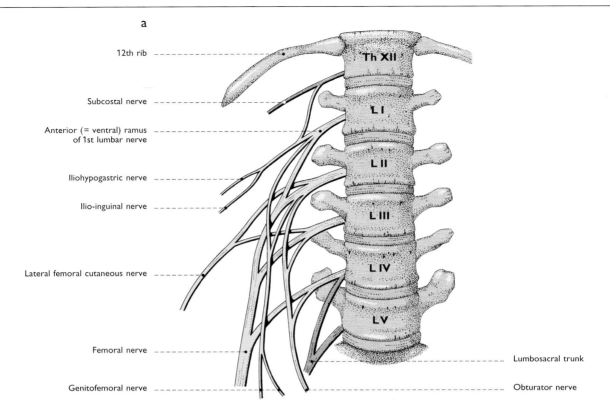

b

Anterior (= ventral) ramus
of 4th lumbar nerve

Lumbosacral trunk

Superior gluteal nerve

Inferior gluteal nerve

Sciatic nerve

Posterior femoral cutaneous nerve

LV

Pelvic splanchnic nerves
(= Parasympathetic root of pelvic ganglia)

Pudendal nerve

Coccygeal nerve

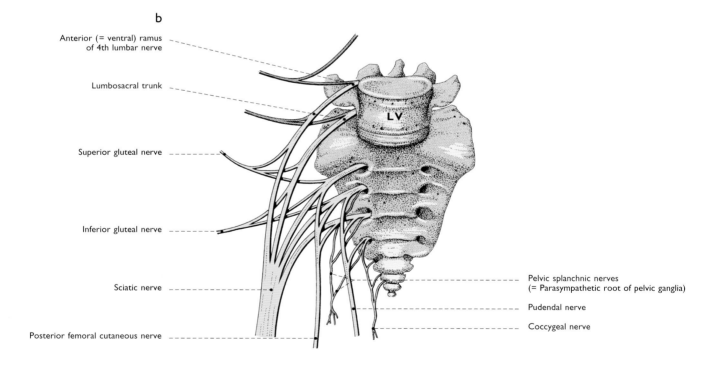

226 Lumbar and sacral plexuses
Schematic representations, ventral aspect
a   Lumbar plexus
b   Sacral plexus

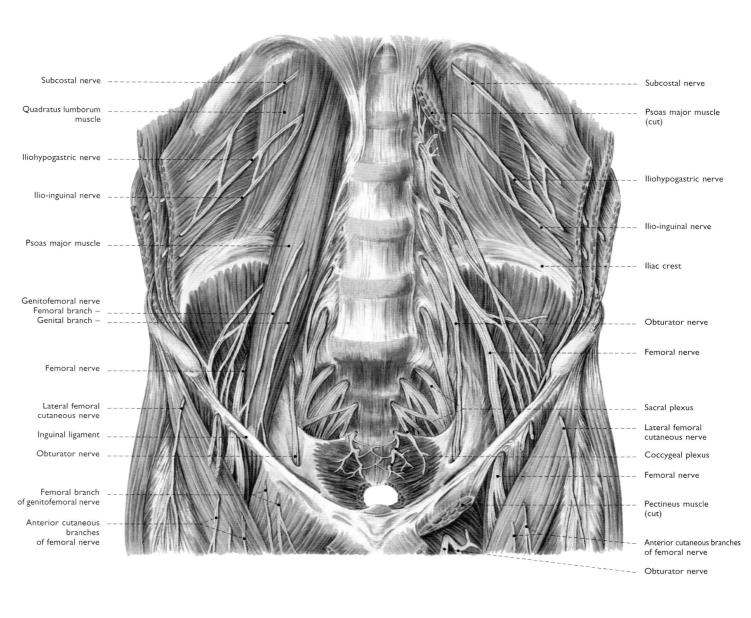

Subcostal nerve

Quadratus lumborum
muscle

Iliohypogastric nerve

Ilio-inguinal nerve

Psoas major muscle

Genitofemoral nerve
Femoral branch —
Genital branch —

Femoral nerve

Lateral femoral
cutaneous nerve

Inguinal ligament

Obturator nerve

Femoral branch
of genitofemoral nerve

Anterior cutaneous
branches
of femoral nerve

Subcostal nerve

Psoas major muscle
(cut)

Iliohypogastric nerve

Ilio-inguinal nerve

Iliac crest

Obturator nerve

Femoral nerve

Sacral plexus

Lateral femoral
cutaneous nerve

Coccygeal plexus

Femoral nerve

Pectineus muscle
(cut)

Anterior cutaneous branches
of femoral nerve

Obturator nerve

227 Lumbosacral plexus (40%)
On the left side of the body, the psoas major muscle was removed
and the pectineus muscle cut near to its origin. Ventral aspect

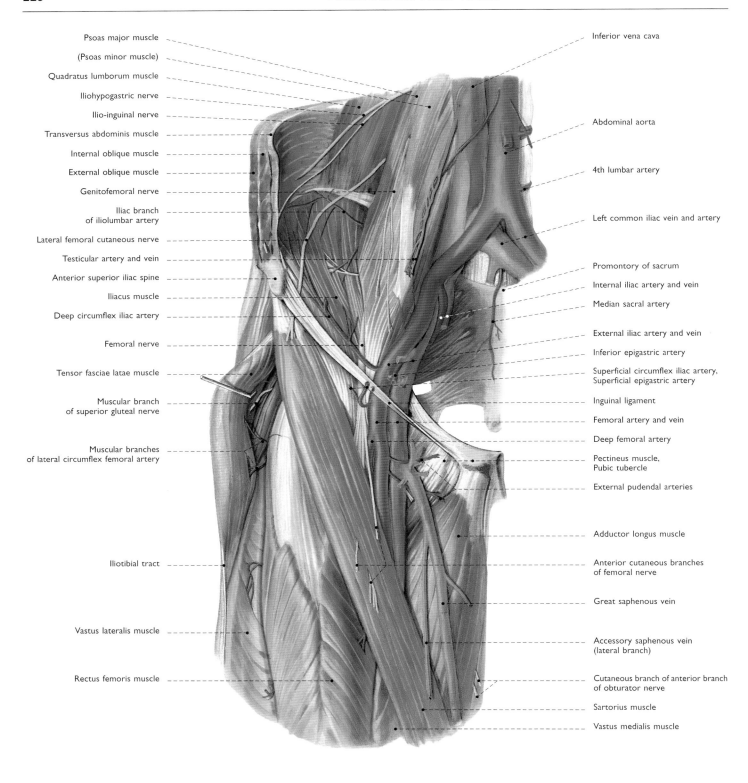

Psoas major muscle

(Psoas minor muscle)

Quadratus lumborum muscle

Iliohypogastric nerve

Ilio-inguinal nerve

Transversus abdominis muscle

Internal oblique muscle

External oblique muscle

Genitofemoral nerve

Iliac branch
of iliolumbar artery

Lateral femoral cutaneous nerve

Testicular artery and vein

Anterior superior iliac spine

Iliacus muscle

Deep circumflex iliac artery

Femoral nerve

Tensor fasciae latae muscle

Muscular branch
of superior gluteal nerve

Muscular branches
of lateral circumflex femoral artery

Iliotibial tract

Vastus lateralis muscle

Rectus femoris muscle

Inferior vena cava

Abdominal aorta

4th lumbar artery

Left common iliac vein and artery

Promontory of sacrum

Internal iliac artery and vein

Median sacral artery

External iliac artery and vein

Inferior epigastric artery

Superficial circumflex iliac artery,
Superficial epigastric artery

Inguinal ligament

Femoral artery and vein

Deep femoral artery

Pectineus muscle,
Pubic tubercle

External pudendal arteries

Adductor longus muscle

Anterior cutaneous branches
of femoral nerve

Great saphenous vein

Accessory saphenous vein
(lateral branch)

Cutaneous branch of anterior branch
of obturator nerve

Sartorius muscle

Vastus medialis muscle

228 Blood vessels and nerves
of the posterior abdominal wall
and the thigh of a male (50%)
Ventral aspect

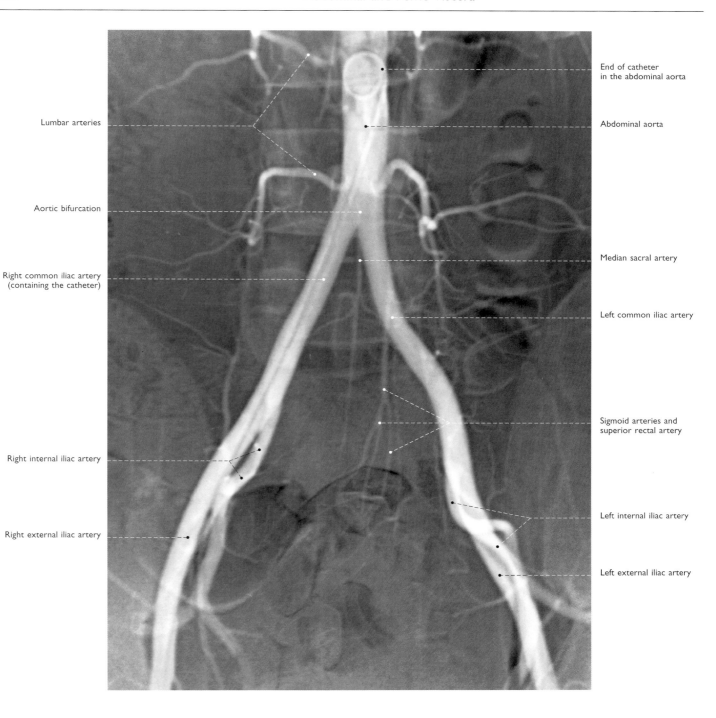

Lumbar arteries

Aortic bifurcation

Right common iliac artery
(containing the catheter)

Right internal iliac artery

Right external iliac artery

End of catheter
in the abdominal aorta

Abdominal aorta

Median sacral artery

Left common iliac artery

Sigmoid arteries and
superior rectal artery

Left internal iliac artery

Left external iliac artery

229 Abdominal arteries (80%)
Arteriogram of the caudal abdominal aorta,
the aortic bifurcation and the iliac arteries,
postero-anterior radiograph

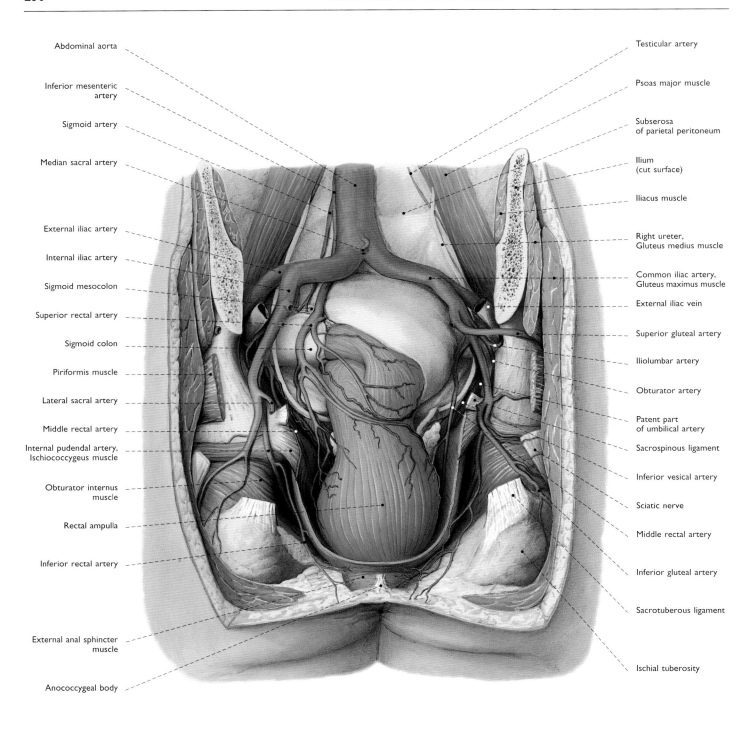

Abdominal aorta

Inferior mesenteric artery

Sigmoid artery

Median sacral artery

External iliac artery

Internal iliac artery

Sigmoid mesocolon

Superior rectal artery

Sigmoid colon

Piriformis muscle

Lateral sacral artery

Middle rectal artery

Internal pudendal artery, Ischiococcygeus muscle

Obturator internus muscle

Rectal ampulla

Inferior rectal artery

External anal sphincter muscle

Anococcygeal body

Testicular artery

Psoas major muscle

Subserosa of parietal peritoneum

Ilium (cut surface)

Iliacus muscle

Right ureter, Gluteus medius muscle

Common iliac artery, Gluteus maximus muscle

External iliac vein

Superior gluteal artery

Iliolumbar artery

Obturator artery

Patent part of umbilical artery

Sacrospinous ligament

Inferior vesical artery

Sciatic nerve

Middle rectal artery

Inferior gluteal artery

Sacrotuberous ligament

Ischial tuberosity

230　Arterial supply of the rectum of a male (60%)
The sacrum was removed, the coccygeus muscle,
the muscles of the gluteal region, the sacrospinous and
sacrotuberous ligaments were cut off and partially excised.
Dorsal aspect

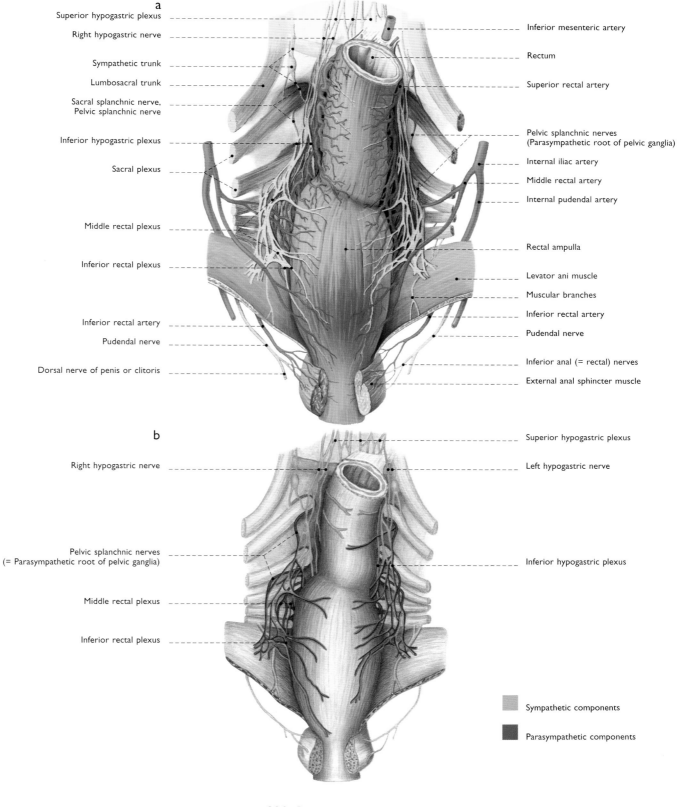

a

Superior hypogastric plexus

Right hypogastric nerve

Sympathetic trunk

Lumbosacral trunk

Sacral splanchnic nerve, Pelvic splanchnic nerve

Inferior hypogastric plexus

Sacral plexus

Middle rectal plexus

Inferior rectal plexus

Inferior rectal artery

Pudendal nerve

Dorsal nerve of penis or clitoris

Inferior mesenteric artery

Rectum

Superior rectal artery

Pelvic splanchnic nerves (Parasympathetic root of pelvic ganglia)

Internal iliac artery

Middle rectal artery

Internal pudendal artery

Rectal ampulla

Levator ani muscle

Muscular branches

Inferior rectal artery

Pudendal nerve

Inferior anal (= rectal) nerves

External anal sphincter muscle

b

Right hypogastric nerve

Pelvic splanchnic nerves (= Parasympathetic root of pelvic ganglia)

Middle rectal plexus

Inferior rectal plexus

Superior hypogastric plexus

Left hypogastric nerve

Inferior hypogastric plexus

Sympathetic components

Parasympathetic components

231   Rectum (45%)

Ventral aspect
a   Arteries and nerves of the rectum
b   Explanatory drawing as to fig. a.
    Sympathetic fibers are shown by **orange**,
    parasympathetic ones by **brown** color.

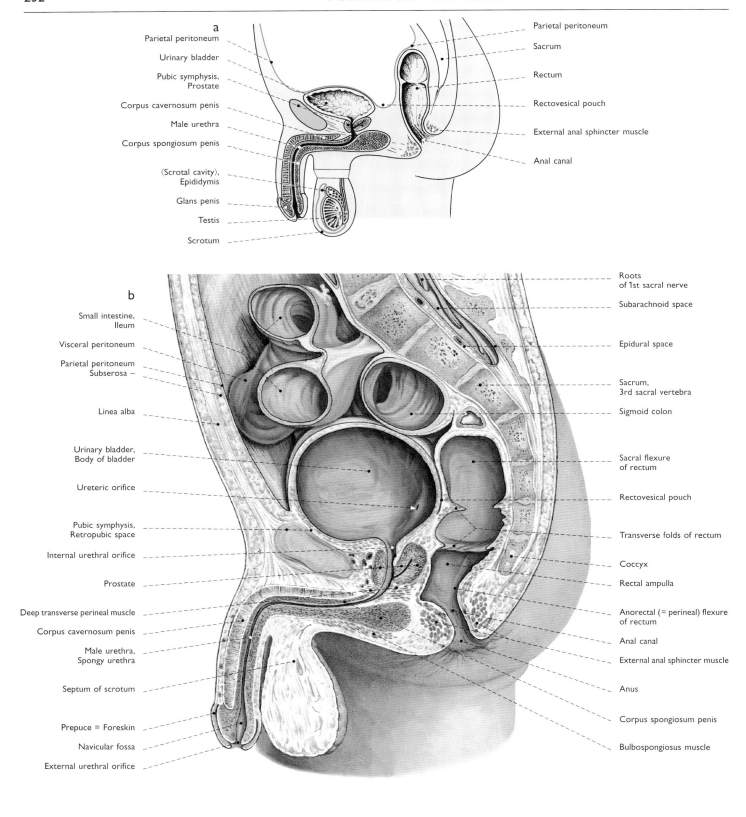

a

Parietal peritoneum

Urinary bladder

Pubic symphysis,
Prostate

Corpus cavernosum penis

Male urethra

Corpus spongiosum penis

⟨Scrotal cavity⟩,
Epididymis

Glans penis

Testis

Scrotum

Parietal peritoneum

Sacrum

Rectum

Rectovesical pouch

External anal sphincter muscle

Anal canal

b

Small intestine,
Ileum

Visceral peritoneum

Parietal peritoneum
Subserosa —

Linea alba

Urinary bladder,
Body of bladder

Ureteric orifice

Pubic symphysis,
Retropubic space

Internal urethral orifice

Prostate

Deep transverse perineal muscle

Corpus cavernosum penis

Male urethra,
Spongy urethra

Septum of scrotum

Prepuce = Foreskin

Navicular fossa

External urethral orifice

Roots
of 1st sacral nerve

Subarachnoid space

Epidural space

Sacrum,
3rd sacral vertebra

Sigmoid colon

Sacral flexure
of rectum

Rectovesical pouch

Transverse folds of rectum

Coccyx

Rectal ampulla

Anorectal (= perineal) flexure
of rectum

Anal canal

External anal sphincter muscle

Anus

Corpus spongiosum penis

Bulbospongiosus muscle

232   Male pelvis and urogenital system

a   Male pelvis, schematized median section, medial aspect
b   Pelvic viscera of an 18-year-old male,
median section (55%), medial aspect of the right half
(Anatomical Collection, Basel)

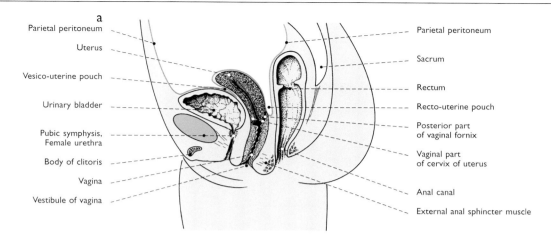

a

Parietal peritoneum

Uterus

Vesico-uterine pouch

Urinary bladder

Pubic symphysis,
Female urethra

Body of clitoris

Vagina

Vestibule of vagina

Parietal peritoneum

Sacrum

Rectum

Recto-uterine pouch

Posterior part
of vaginal fornix

Vaginal part
of cervix of uterus

Anal canal

External anal sphincter muscle

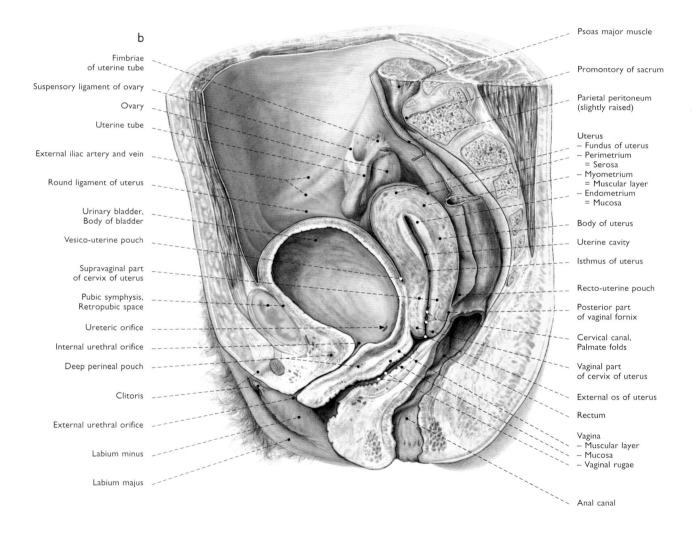

b

Fimbriae
of uterine tube

Suspensory ligament of ovary

Ovary

Uterine tube

External iliac artery and vein

Round ligament of uterus

Urinary bladder,
Body of bladder

Vesico-uterine pouch

Supravaginal part
of cervix of uterus

Pubic symphysis,
Retropubic space

Ureteric orifice

Internal urethral orifice

Deep perineal pouch

Clitoris

External urethral orifice

Labium minus

Labium majus

Psoas major muscle

Promontory of sacrum

Parietal peritoneum
(slightly raised)

Uterus
– Fundus of uterus
– Perimetrium
  = Serosa
– Myometrium
  = Muscular layer
– Endometrium
  = Mucosa

Body of uterus

Uterine cavity

Isthmus of uterus

Recto-uterine pouch

Posterior part
of vaginal fornix

Cervical canal,
Palmate folds

Vaginal part
of cervix of uterus

External os of uterus

Rectum

Vagina
– Muscular layer
– Mucosa
– Vaginal rugae

Anal canal

233   Female pelvis and urogenital apparatus

   a   Female pelvis, schematized median section, medial aspect
   b   Pelvic viscera of a 23-year-old female, median section (55%),
       medial aspect of the right half (Anatomical Collection, Basel)

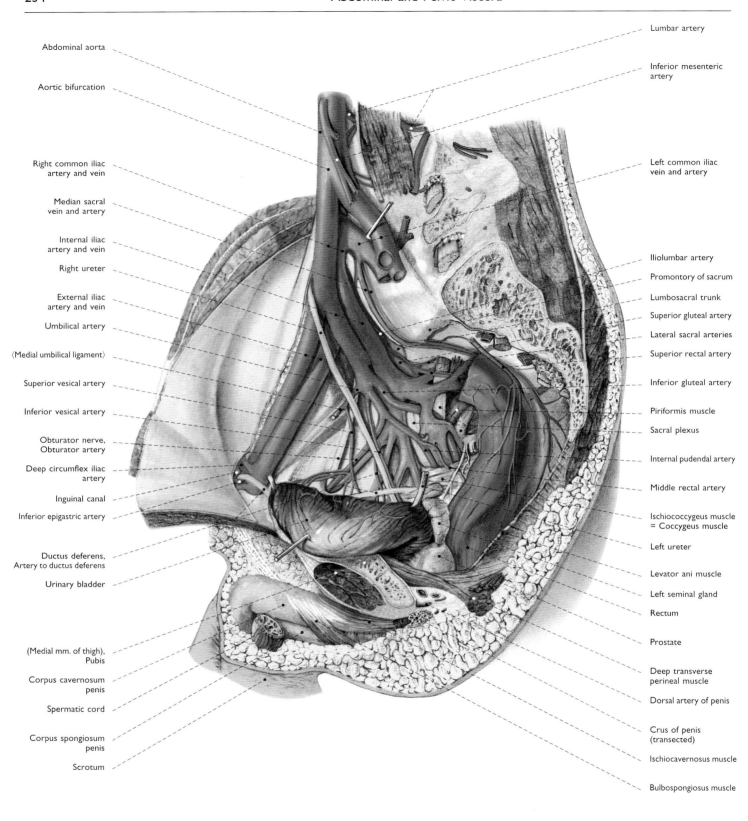

Abdominal aorta

Aortic bifurcation

Right common iliac
artery and vein

Median sacral
vein and artery

Internal iliac
artery and vein

Right ureter

External iliac
artery and vein

Umbilical artery

⟨Medial umbilical ligament⟩

Superior vesical artery

Inferior vesical artery

Obturator nerve,
Obturator artery

Deep circumflex iliac
artery

Inguinal canal

Inferior epigastric artery

Ductus deferens,
Artery to ductus deferens

Urinary bladder

(Medial mm. of thigh),
Pubis

Corpus cavernosum
penis

Spermatic cord

Corpus spongiosum
penis

Scrotum

Lumbar artery

Inferior mesenteric
artery

Left common iliac
vein and artery

Iliolumbar artery

Promontory of sacrum

Lumbosacral trunk

Superior gluteal artery

Lateral sacral arteries

Superior rectal artery

Inferior gluteal artery

Piriformis muscle

Sacral plexus

Internal pudendal artery

Middle rectal artery

Ischiococcygeus muscle
= Coccygeus muscle

Left ureter

Levator ani muscle

Left seminal gland

Rectum

Prostate

Deep transverse
perineal muscle

Dorsal artery of penis

Crus of penis
(transected)

Ischiocavernosus muscle

Bulbospongiosus muscle

234 Blood vessels and nerves of the male pelvis (70%)
Sagittal section to the left of the median plane,
medial aspect of the right part

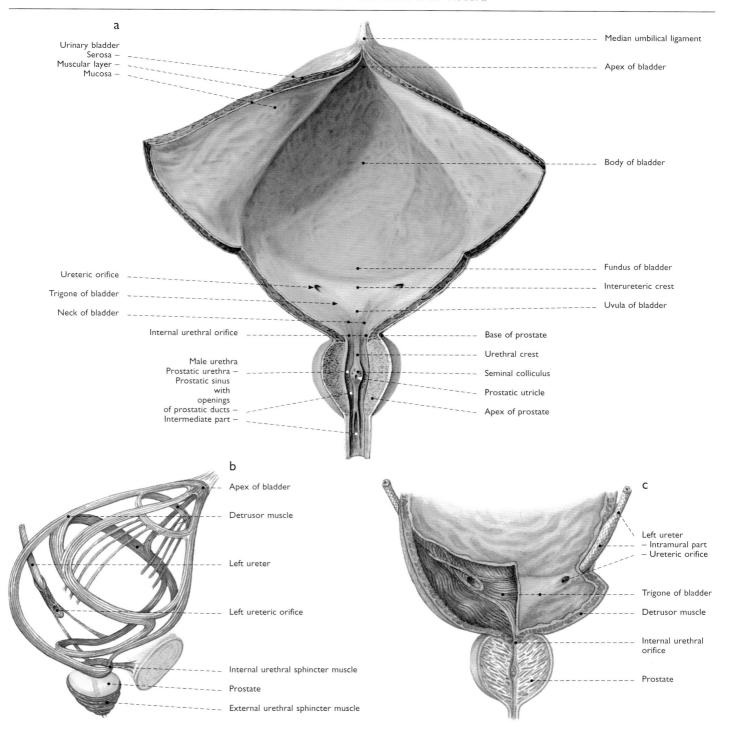

a

Urinary bladder
Serosa —
Muscular layer —
Mucosa —

Median umbilical ligament

Apex of bladder

Body of bladder

Ureteric orifice

Trigone of bladder

Neck of bladder

Internal urethral orifice

Male urethra
Prostatic urethra —
Prostatic sinus
with
openings
of prostatic ducts —
Intermediate part —

Fundus of bladder

Interureteric crest

Uvula of bladder

Base of prostate

Urethral crest

Seminal colliculus

Prostatic utricle

Apex of prostate

b

Apex of bladder

Detrusor muscle

Left ureter

Left ureteric orifice

Internal urethral sphincter muscle

Prostate

External urethral sphincter muscle

c

Left ureter
– Intramural part
– Ureteric orifice

Trigone of bladder

Detrusor muscle

Internal urethral
orifice

Prostate

235   Urinary bladder

a   Urinary bladder and urethra of a male. The bladder and prostate
    were incised along the midsagittal plane and opened (80%). Ventral aspect
b   Arrangement of the muscles in the bladder wall (according to Ferner,
    1975) (60%), schematic representation, right lateral aspect
c   Ureteric orifices and trigone of bladder (according to Ferner, 1975,
    and Leonhardt, 1987). In the left half of the bladder, a step-cut
    in the bladder wall for showing the intramural part of ureter.
    On the right side of the bladder, the mucosa was removed
    in order to demonstrate the muscle arrangement in the trigone (80%),
    ventral aspect

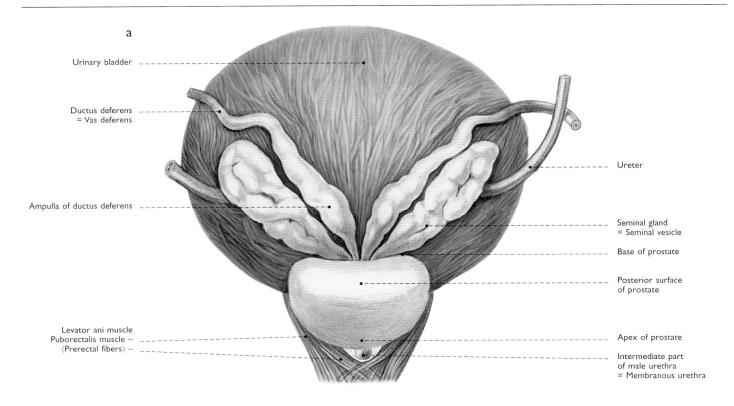

a

Urinary bladder

Ductus deferens
= Vas deferens

Ampulla of ductus deferens

Levator ani muscle
Puborectalis muscle –
⟨Prerectal fibers⟩ –

Ureter

Seminal gland
= Seminal vesicle

Base of prostate

Posterior surface
of prostate

Apex of prostate

Intermediate part
of male urethra
= Membranous urethra

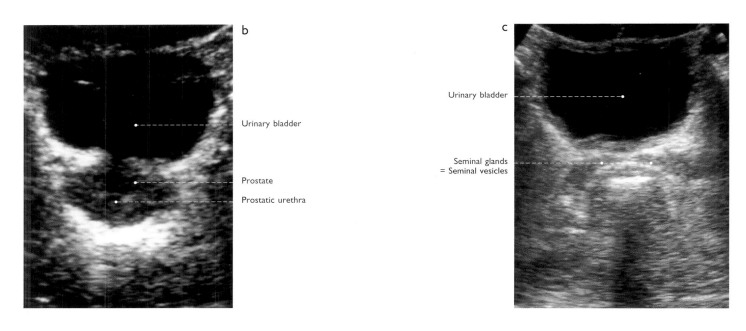

b

Urinary bladder

Prostate

Prostatic urethra

c

Urinary bladder

Seminal glands
= Seminal vesicles

236 Urinary bladder, deferent duct, seminal gland, and prostate

a Dorsal aspect (100%)
b, c Ultrasound images (80%), transverse sections above the symphysis through
b the filled urinary bladder and the prostate
c the filled urinary bladder and the seminal glands

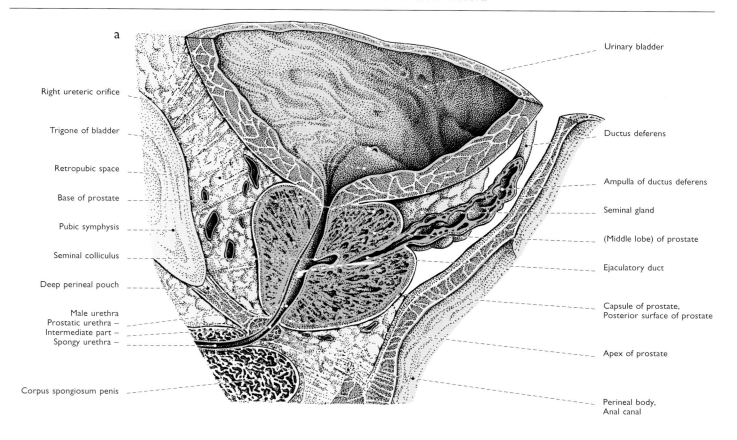

a

Right ureteric orifice

Trigone of bladder

Retropubic space

Base of prostate

Pubic symphysis

Seminal colliculus

Deep perineal pouch

Male urethra
Prostatic urethra –
Intermediate part –
Spongy urethra –

Corpus spongiosum penis

Urinary bladder

Ductus deferens

Ampulla of ductus deferens

Seminal gland

(Middle lobe) of prostate

Ejaculatory duct

Capsule of prostate,
Posterior surface of prostate

Apex of prostate

Perineal body,
Anal canal

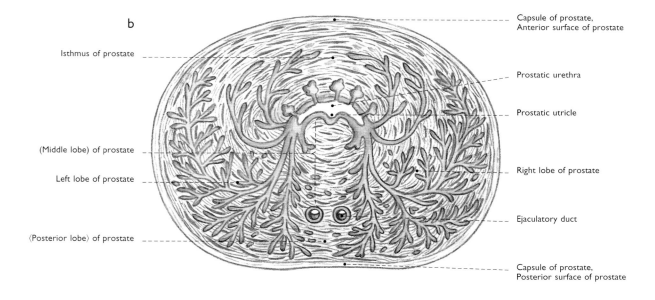

b

Isthmus of prostate

(Middle lobe) of prostate

Left lobe of prostate

(Posterior lobe) of prostate

Capsule of prostate,
Anterior surface of prostate

Prostatic urethra

Prostatic utricle

Right lobe of prostate

Ejaculatory duct

Capsule of prostate,
Posterior surface of prostate

237 Urinary bladder, deferent duct,
     seminal gland, and prostate
  a Median section, medial aspect of the right half (120%)
  b Transverse section through the prostate (250%),
     schematic representation, superior aspect

a

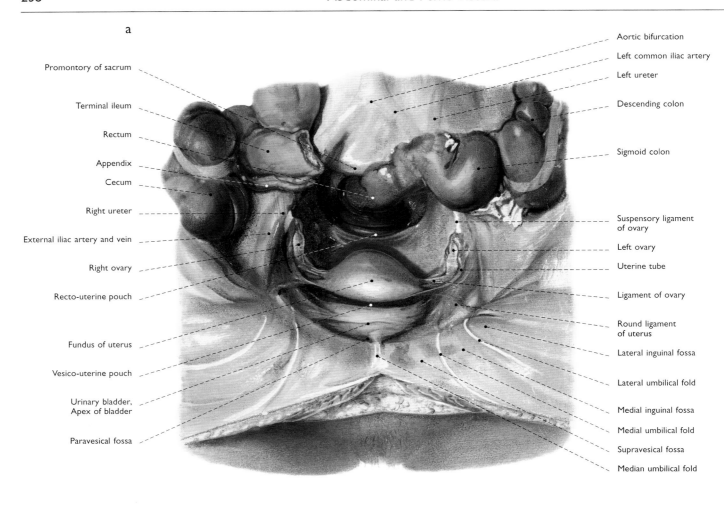

Promontory of sacrum

Terminal ileum

Rectum

Appendix

Cecum

Right ureter

External iliac artery and vein

Right ovary

Recto-uterine pouch

Fundus of uterus

Vesico-uterine pouch

Urinary bladder,
Apex of bladder

Paravesical fossa

Aortic bifurcation

Left common iliac artery

Left ureter

Descending colon

Sigmoid colon

Suspensory ligament
of ovary

Left ovary

Uterine tube

Ligament of ovary

Round ligament
of uterus

Lateral inguinal fossa

Lateral umbilical fold

Medial inguinal fossa

Medial umbilical fold

Supravesical fossa

Median umbilical fold

b

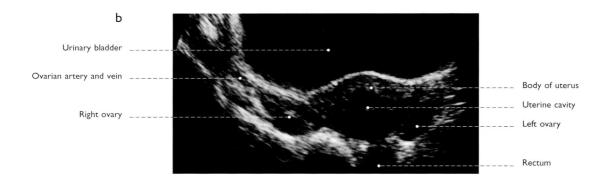

Urinary bladder

Ovarian artery and vein

Right ovary

Body of uterus

Uterine cavity

Left ovary

Rectum

238   Pelvic viscera and anterior abdominal wall

a   Pelvic viscera of a female in situ. The ventral abdominal wall
was opened by a median incision and the small intestine
nearly completely removed (45%). Cranioventral aspect

b   Ultrasound image of uterus and ovaries (60%),
transverse section above the symphysis

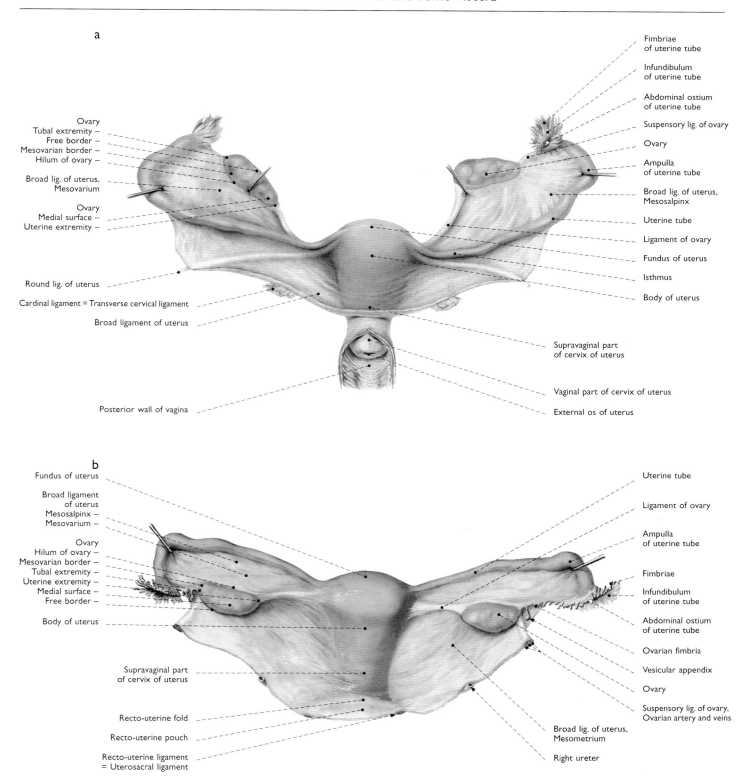

a

Ovary
Tubal extremity —
Free border —
Mesovarian border —
Hilum of ovary —

Broad lig. of uterus,
Mesovarium

Ovary
Medial surface —
Uterine extremity —

Round lig. of uterus

Cardinal ligament = Transverse cervical ligament

Broad ligament of uterus

Posterior wall of vagina

Fimbriae
of uterine tube

Infundibulum
of uterine tube

Abdominal ostium
of uterine tube

Suspensory lig. of ovary

Ovary

Ampulla
of uterine tube

Broad lig. of uterus,
Mesosalpinx

Uterine tube

Ligament of ovary

Fundus of uterus

Isthmus

Body of uterus

Supravaginal part
of cervix of uterus

Vaginal part of cervix of uterus

External os of uterus

b

Fundus of uterus

Broad ligament
of uterus
Mesosalpinx —
Mesovarium —

Ovary
Hilum of ovary —
Mesovarian border —
Tubal extremity —
Uterine extremity —
Medial surface —
Free border —

Body of uterus

Supravaginal part
of cervix of uterus

Recto-uterine fold

Recto-uterine pouch

Recto-uterine ligament
= Uterosacral ligament

Uterine tube

Ligament of ovary

Ampulla
of uterine tube

Fimbriae

Infundibulum
of uterine tube

Abdominal ostium
of uterine tube

Ovarian fimbria

Vesicular appendix

Ovary

Suspensory lig. of ovary,
Ovarian artery and veins

Broad lig. of uterus,
Mesometrium

Right ureter

239 Internal genitalia of a young woman (60%)
The ovaries and uterine tubes are drawn apart.
The broad ligament of uterus was cut off from its parietal
attachment. In fig. a the anterior vaginal wall was opened in front.
a Ventral aspect
b Dorsal aspect

a

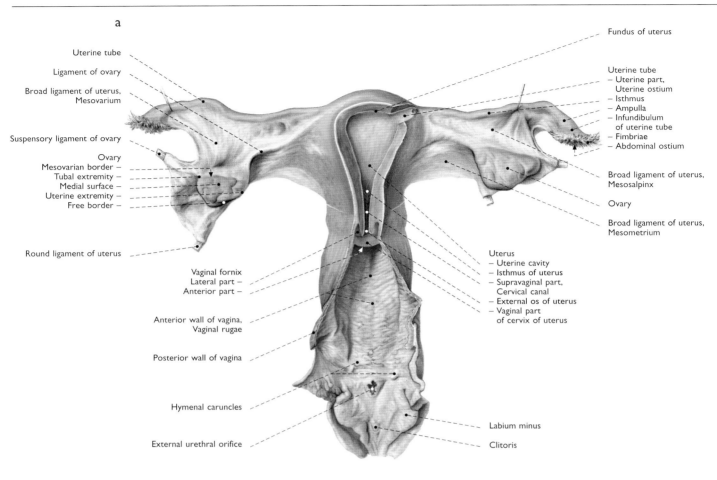

Uterine tube

Ligament of ovary

Broad ligament of uterus,
Mesovarium

Suspensory ligament of ovary

Ovary
Mesovarian border –
Tubal extremity –
Medial surface –
Uterine extremity –
Free border –

Round ligament of uterus

Vaginal fornix
Lateral part –
Anterior part –

Anterior wall of vagina,
Vaginal rugae

Posterior wall of vagina

Hymenal caruncles

External urethral orifice

Fundus of uterus

Uterine tube
– Uterine part,
Uterine ostium
– Isthmus
– Ampulla
– Infundibulum
of uterine tube
– Fimbriae
– Abdominal ostium

Broad ligament of uterus,
Mesosalpinx

Ovary

Broad ligament of uterus,
Mesometrium

Uterus
– Uterine cavity
– Isthmus of uterus
– Supravaginal part,
Cervical canal
– External os of uterus
– Vaginal part
of cervix of uterus

Labium minus

Clitoris

b

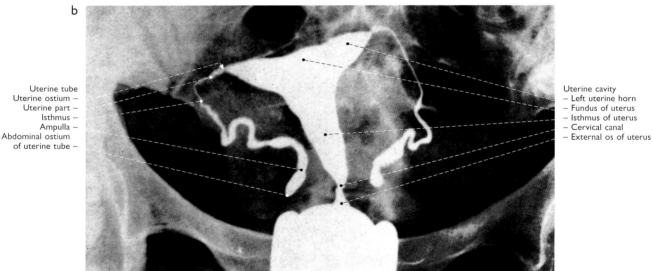

Uterine tube
Uterine ostium –
Uterine part –
Isthmus –
Ampulla –
Abdominal ostium
of uterine tube –

Uterine cavity
– Left uterine horn
– Fundus of uterus
– Isthmus of uterus
– Cervical canal
– External os of uterus

240 Female internal genitalia

a   A triangular window was cut in the dorsal wall of uterus.
The dorsal vaginal wall was opened by a median incision (60%).
Dorsal aspect

b   Radiograph of the uterus and uterine tubes filled with
contrast medium (hysterosalpingography). Slight displacement
of the female internal genitalia to the right (70%)

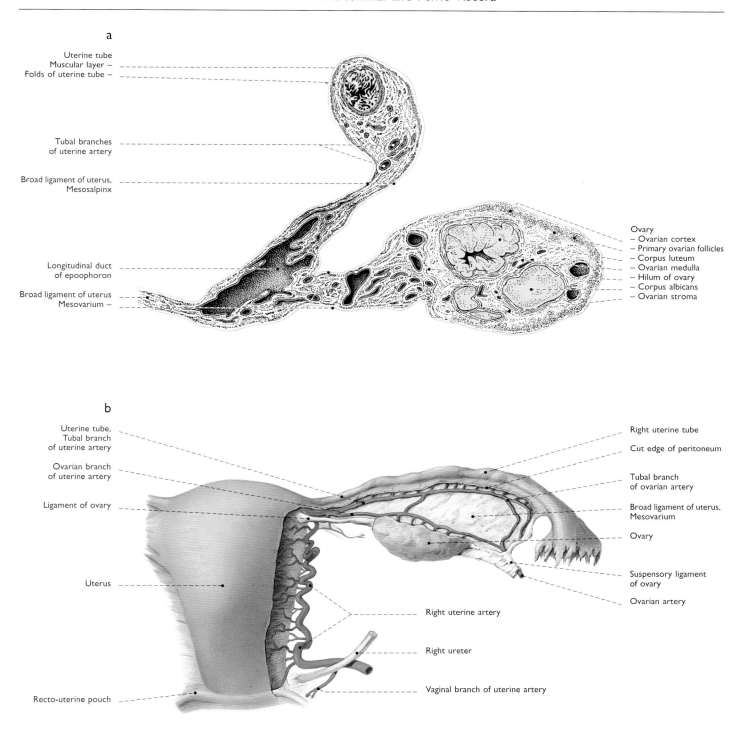

a

Uterine tube
Muscular layer –
Folds of uterine tube –

Tubal branches
of uterine artery

Broad ligament of uterus,
Mesosalpinx

Longitudinal duct
of epoophoron

Broad ligament of uterus
Mesovarium –

Ovary
– Ovarian cortex
– Primary ovarian follicles
– Corpus luteum
– Ovarian medulla
– Hilum of ovary
– Corpus albicans
– Ovarian stroma

b

Uterine tube,
Tubal branch
of uterine artery

Ovarian branch
of uterine artery

Ligament of ovary

Uterus

Recto-uterine pouch

Right uterine tube

Cut edge of peritoneum

Tubal branch
of ovarian artery

Broad ligament of uterus,
Mesovarium

Ovary

Suspensory ligament
of ovary

Ovarian artery

Right uterine artery

Right ureter

Vaginal branch of uterine artery

241 Female internal genitalia
a   Sagittal section through the ovary and the uterine tube (230%)
b   Blood supply of the uterus, the uterine tubes, and the ovary (70%),
    dorsal aspect

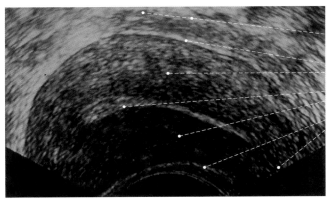

a

Intestinal loops

Uterus
– Intestinal surface
– Body of uterus,
  Myometrium
– Uterine cavity and endometrium
– Body of uterus,
  Myometrium
– Vesical surface
– Cervix of uterus

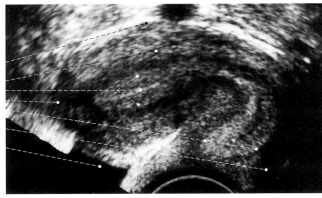

b

Uterus
Intestinal surface –
Body of uterus,
Myometrium –
Uterine cavity and endometrium –
Fundus of uterus –
Cervix of uterus –

Recto-uterine pouch

Urinary bladder

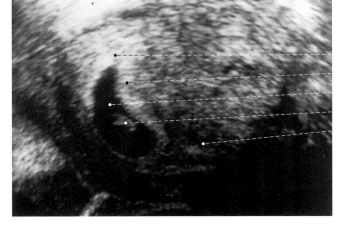

c

Fundus of uterus

Chorionic villi

Amniotic cavity

Embryo

Body of uterus,
Myometrium

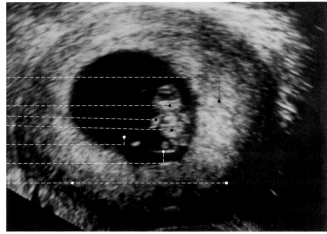

d

Chorionic villi

Embryo
Head –
Upper limb –
Trunk –

Amniotic cavity

Umbilical cord

Body of uterus,
Myometrium

242 Female internal genitalia
Ultrasound images of the uterus
a Longitudinal section through the body of uterus
  during early proliferative stage (100%)
b Longitudinal section through the body and cervix of uterus
  during secretory stage (70%)
c, d Sections through the uterus during early pregnancy (100%)
c in the seventh week of pregnancy (fifth week after conception)
d in the ninth week of pregnancy (seventh week after conception)

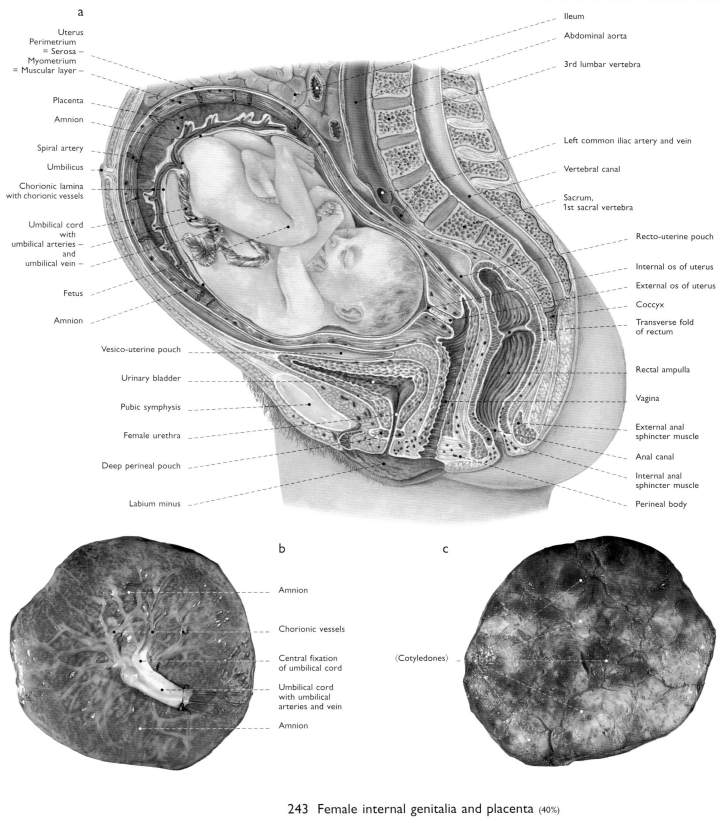

a

Uterus
Perimetrium
= Serosa
Myometrium
= Muscular layer

Placenta

Amnion

Spiral artery

Umbilicus

Chorionic lamina
with chorionic vessels

Umbilical cord
with
umbilical arteries
and
umbilical vein

Fetus

Amnion

Vesico-uterine pouch

Urinary bladder

Pubic symphysis

Female urethra

Deep perineal pouch

Labium minus

Ileum

Abdominal aorta

3rd lumbar vertebra

Left common iliac artery and vein

Vertebral canal

Sacrum,
1st sacral vertebra

Recto-uterine pouch

Internal os of uterus

External os of uterus

Coccyx

Transverse fold
of rectum

Rectal ampulla

Vagina

External anal
sphincter muscle

Anal canal

Internal anal
sphincter muscle

Perineal body

b

Amnion

Chorionic vessels

Central fixation
of umbilical cord

Umbilical cord
with umbilical
arteries and vein

Amnion

c

⟨Cotyledones⟩

243 Female internal genitalia and placenta (40%)

a Female pelvis with an uterus advanced in pregnancy, medial aspect of a median section (fetus and umbilical cord were left intact)

b, c Recently delivered placenta

b Fetal surface with umbilical cord

c Maternal surface

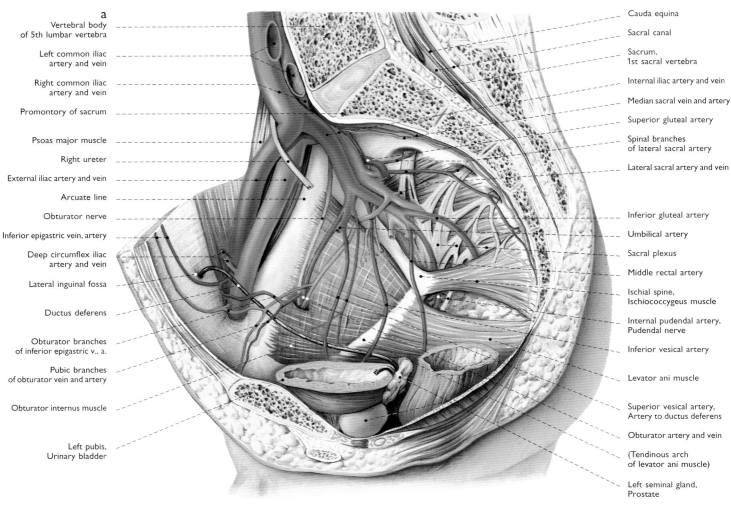

a
Vertebral body
of 5th lumbar vertebra
Left common iliac
artery and vein
Right common iliac
artery and vein
Promontory of sacrum

Psoas major muscle
Right ureter
External iliac artery and vein
Arcuate line
Obturator nerve
Inferior epigastric vein, artery
Deep circumflex iliac
artery and vein
Lateral inguinal fossa
Ductus deferens
Obturator branches
of inferior epigastric v., a.
Pubic branches
of obturator vein and artery
Obturator internus muscle

Left pubis,
Urinary bladder

Cauda equina
Sacral canal
Sacrum,
1st sacral vertebra
Internal iliac artery and vein
Median sacral vein and artery
Superior gluteal artery
Spinal branches
of lateral sacral artery
Lateral sacral artery and vein

Inferior gluteal artery
Umbilical artery
Sacral plexus
Middle rectal artery
Ischial spine,
Ischiococcygeus muscle
Internal pudendal artery,
Pudendal nerve
Inferior vesical artery
Levator ani muscle
Superior vesical artery,
Artery to ductus deferens
Obturator artery and vein
(Tendinous arch
of levator ani muscle)
Left seminal gland,
Prostate

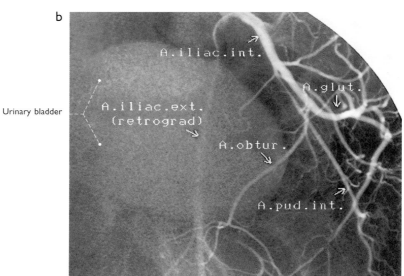

b

Urinary bladder

A.iliac.int.

A.glut.

A.iliac.ext.
(retrograd)

A.obtur.

A.pud.int.

244 Arteries, nerves, and viscera
of the male pelvis (70%)
   a Sagittal section slightly to the left of the median plane
      through a male pelvis, medial aspect of the right part
   b Arteriogram of the right internal iliac artery
      and its branches in a male, medial aspect

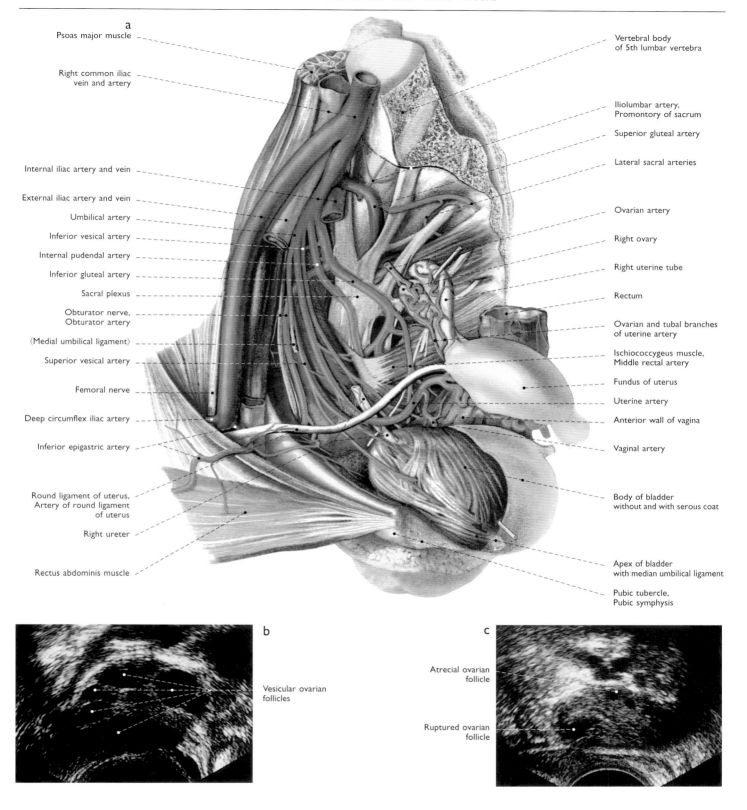

a

Psoas major muscle

Right common iliac vein and artery

Internal iliac artery and vein

External iliac artery and vein

Umbilical artery

Inferior vesical artery

Internal pudendal artery

Inferior gluteal artery

Sacral plexus

Obturator nerve, Obturator artery

(Medial umbilical ligament)

Superior vesical artery

Femoral nerve

Deep circumflex iliac artery

Inferior epigastric artery

Round ligament of uterus, Artery of round ligament of uterus

Right ureter

Rectus abdominis muscle

Vertebral body of 5th lumbar vertebra

Iliolumbar artery, Promontory of sacrum

Superior gluteal artery

Lateral sacral arteries

Ovarian artery

Right ovary

Right uterine tube

Rectum

Ovarian and tubal branches of uterine artery

Ischiococcygeus muscle, Middle rectal artery

Fundus of uterus

Uterine artery

Anterior wall of vagina

Vaginal artery

Body of bladder without and with serous coat

Apex of bladder with median umbilical ligament

Pubic tubercle, Pubic symphysis

b

Vesicular ovarian follicles

c

Atrecial ovarian follicle

Ruptured ovarian follicle

245 Arteries, nerves, and viscera of the female pelvis

a   Median section. The unpaired viscera were left intact (70%). Oblique aspect from the left, above and anterior

b, c   Ultrasound images of the ovaries of a female in the phase of sexual maturity (100%)

a

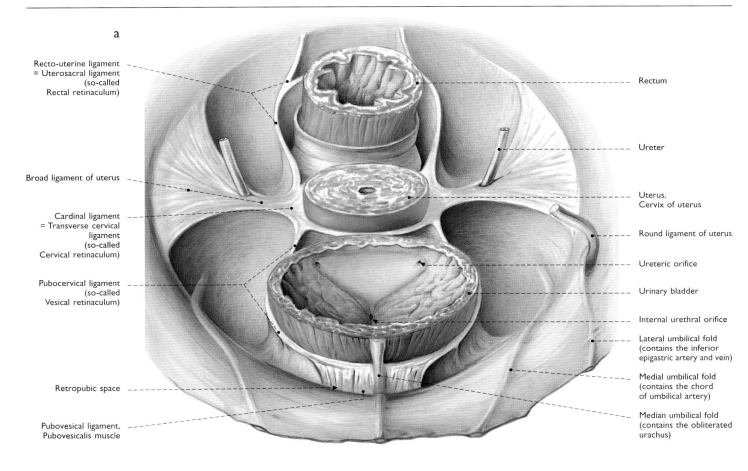

Recto-uterine ligament
= Uterosacral ligament
(so-called
Rectal retinaculum)

Broad ligament of uterus

Cardinal ligament
= Transverse cervical
ligament
(so-called
Cervical retinaculum)

Pubocervical ligament
(so-called
Vesical retinaculum)

Retropubic space

Pubovesical ligament,
Pubovesicalis muscle

Rectum

Ureter

Uterus,
Cervix of uterus

Round ligament of uterus

Ureteric orifice

Urinary bladder

Internal urethral orifice

Lateral umbilical fold
(contains the inferior
epigastric artery and vein)

Medial umbilical fold
(contains the chord
of umbilical artery)

Median umbilical fold
(contains the obliterated
urachus)

b   c

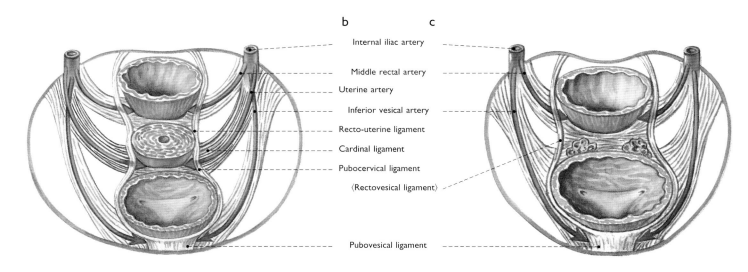

Internal iliac artery

Middle rectal artery

Uterine artery

Inferior vesical artery

Recto-uterine ligament

Cardinal ligament

Pubocervical ligament

⟨Rectovesical ligament⟩

Pubovesical ligament

246   Viscera and connective tissue of the lesser pelvis
       Schematic representations, cranioventral aspect
a   Connective tissue in the lesser pelvis of a female (70%)
b, c   Sagittal and frontal connective tissue strands
       (according to Lierse, 1984) (40%)
b   in the lesser pelvis of a female
c   in the lesser pelvis of a male
       The arrows indicate the course
       of the main supplying vessels and nerves.

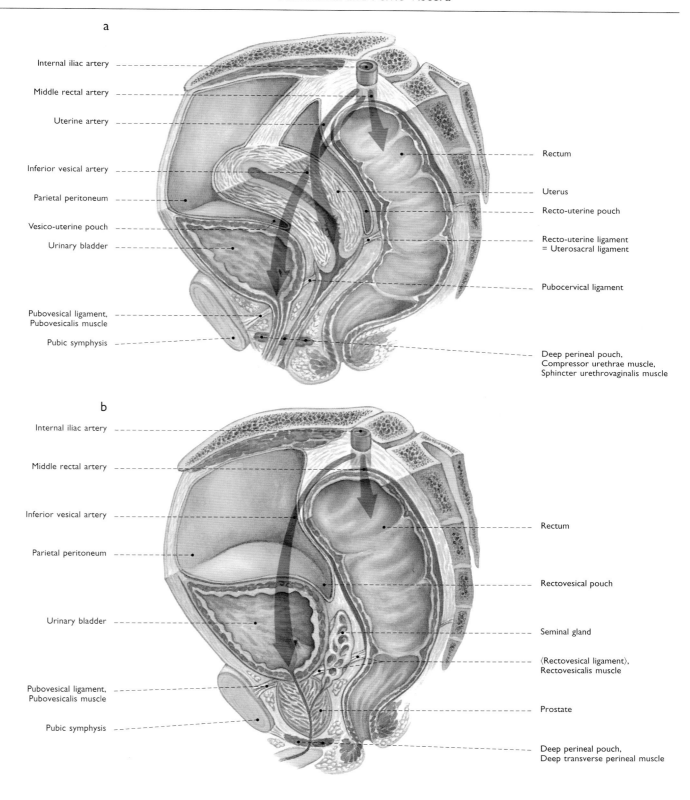

a

Internal iliac artery

Middle rectal artery

Uterine artery

Inferior vesical artery

Parietal peritoneum

Vesico-uterine pouch

Urinary bladder

Pubovesical ligament,
Pubovesicalis muscle

Pubic symphysis

Rectum

Uterus

Recto-uterine pouch

Recto-uterine ligament
= Uterosacral ligament

Pubocervical ligament

Deep perineal pouch,
Compressor urethrae muscle,
Sphincter urethrovaginalis muscle

b

Internal iliac artery

Middle rectal artery

Inferior vesical artery

Parietal peritoneum

Urinary bladder

Pubovesical ligament,
Pubovesicalis muscle

Pubic symphysis

Rectum

Rectovesical pouch

Seminal gland

⟨Rectovesical ligament⟩,
Rectovesicalis muscle

Prostate

Deep perineal pouch,
Deep transverse perineal muscle

**247 Viscera and connective tissue
of the lesser pelvis** (50%)
Schematic representations (according to Lierse, 1984),
midsagittal sections, medial aspect of the right halfs
a Female lesser pelvis
b Male lesser pelvis
The arrows indicate the course
of the main supplying vessels and nerves.

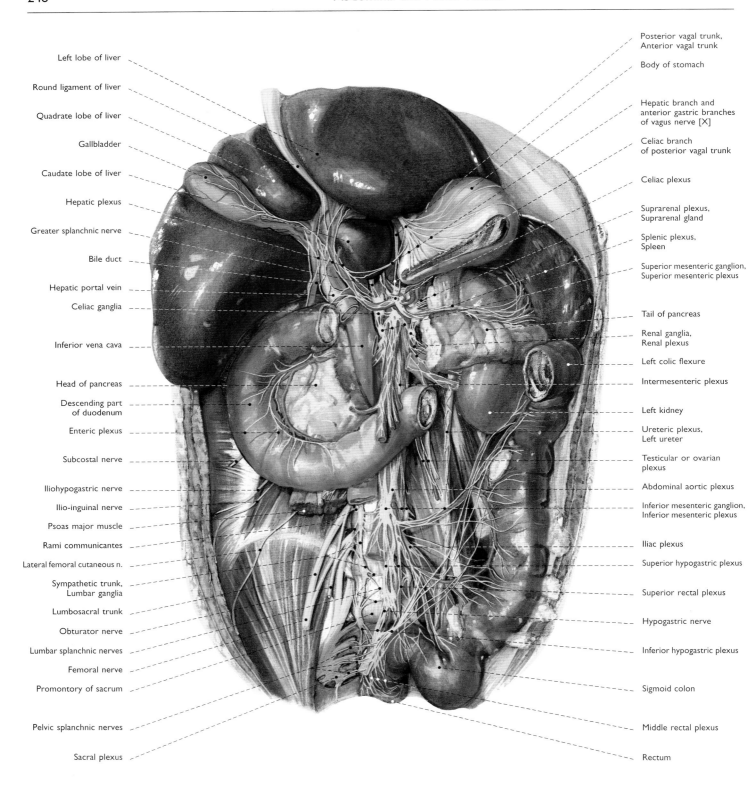

Left lobe of liver

Round ligament of liver

Quadrate lobe of liver

Gallbladder

Caudate lobe of liver

Hepatic plexus

Greater splanchnic nerve

Bile duct

Hepatic portal vein

Celiac ganglia

Inferior vena cava

Head of pancreas

Descending part of duodenum

Enteric plexus

Subcostal nerve

Iliohypogastric nerve

Ilio-inguinal nerve

Psoas major muscle

Rami communicantes

Lateral femoral cutaneous n.

Sympathetic trunk, Lumbar ganglia

Lumbosacral trunk

Obturator nerve

Lumbar splanchnic nerves

Femoral nerve

Promontory of sacrum

Pelvic splanchnic nerves

Sacral plexus

Posterior vagal trunk, Anterior vagal trunk

Body of stomach

Hepatic branch and anterior gastric branches of vagus nerve [X]

Celiac branch of posterior vagal trunk

Celiac plexus

Suprarenal plexus, Suprarenal gland

Splenic plexus, Spleen

Superior mesenteric ganglion, Superior mesenteric plexus

Tail of pancreas

Renal ganglia, Renal plexus

Left colic flexure

Intermesenteric plexus

Left kidney

Ureteric plexus, Left ureter

Testicular or ovarian plexus

Abdominal aortic plexus

Inferior mesenteric ganglion, Inferior mesenteric plexus

Iliac plexus

Superior hypogastric plexus

Superior rectal plexus

Hypogastric nerve

Inferior hypogastric plexus

Sigmoid colon

Middle rectal plexus

Rectum

248 Autonomic division of peripheral nervous system in the retroperitoneal space (40%)
Ventral aspect

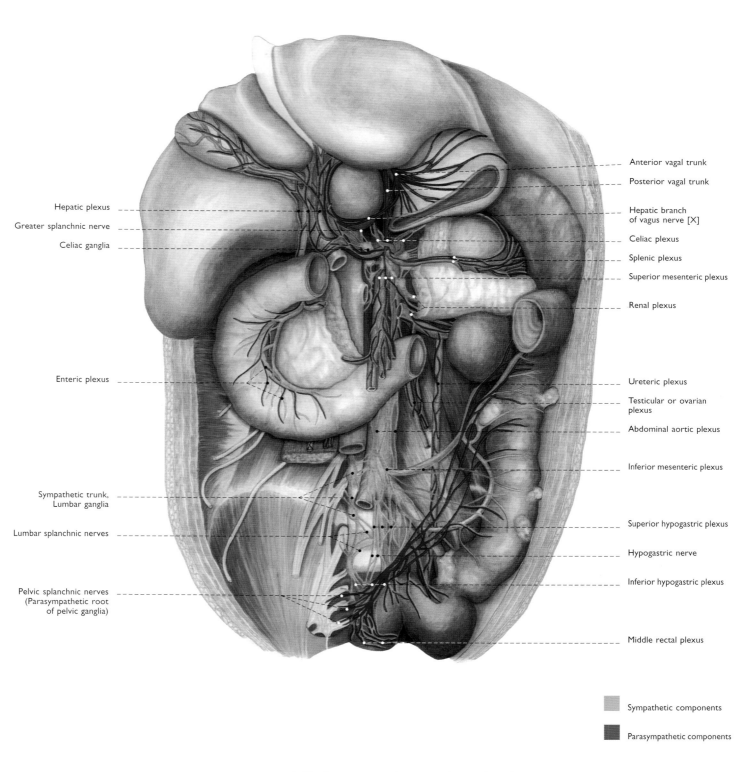

Hepatic plexus

Greater splanchnic nerve

Celiac ganglia

Enteric plexus

Sympathetic trunk,
Lumbar ganglia

Lumbar splanchnic nerves

Pelvic splanchnic nerves
(Parasympathetic root
of pelvic ganglia)

Anterior vagal trunk

Posterior vagal trunk

Hepatic branch
of vagus nerve [X]

Celiac plexus

Splenic plexus

Superior mesenteric plexus

Renal plexus

Ureteric plexus

Testicular or ovarian
plexus

Abdominal aortic plexus

Inferior mesenteric plexus

Superior hypogastric plexus

Hypogastric nerve

Inferior hypogastric plexus

Middle rectal plexus

Sympathetic components

Parasympathetic components

249   **Autonomic division of peripheral nervous system
in the retroperitoneal space** (40%)
Explanatory drawing as to fig. 248.
Sympathetic fibers are shown by **orange**,
parasympathetic ones by **brown** color.
Ventral aspect

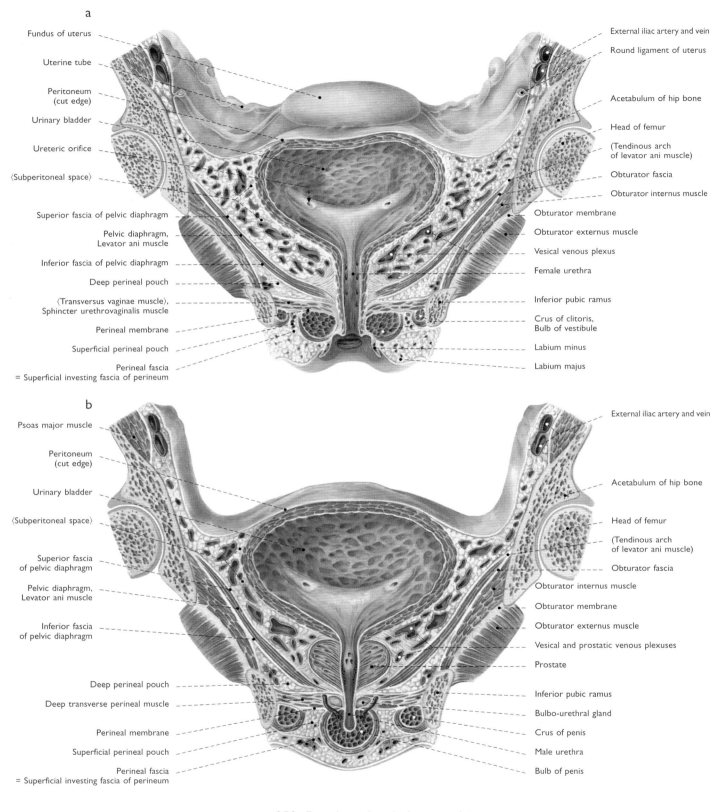

a

Fundus of uterus

Uterine tube

Peritoneum
(cut edge)

Urinary bladder

Ureteric orifice

⟨Subperitoneal space⟩

Superior fascia of pelvic diaphragm

Pelvic diaphragm,
Levator ani muscle

Inferior fascia of pelvic diaphragm

Deep perineal pouch

⟨Transversus vaginae muscle⟩,
Sphincter urethrovaginalis muscle

Perineal membrane

Superficial perineal pouch

Perineal fascia
= Superficial investing fascia of perineum

External iliac artery and vein

Round ligament of uterus

Acetabulum of hip bone

Head of femur

(Tendinous arch
of levator ani muscle)

Obturator fascia

Obturator internus muscle

Obturator membrane

Obturator externus muscle

Vesical venous plexus

Female urethra

Inferior pubic ramus

Crus of clitoris,
Bulb of vestibule

Labium minus

Labium majus

b

Psoas major muscle

Peritoneum
(cut edge)

Urinary bladder

⟨Subperitoneal space⟩

Superior fascia
of pelvic diaphragm

Pelvic diaphragm,
Levator ani muscle

Inferior fascia
of pelvic diaphragm

Deep perineal pouch

Deep transverse perineal muscle

Perineal membrane

Superficial perineal pouch

Perineal fascia
= Superficial investing fascia of perineum

External iliac artery and vein

Acetabulum of hip bone

Head of femur

(Tendinous arch
of levator ani muscle)

Obturator fascia

Obturator internus muscle

Obturator membrane

Obturator externus muscle

Vesical and prostatic venous plexuses

Prostate

Inferior pubic ramus

Bulbo-urethral gland

Crus of penis

Male urethra

Bulb of penis

250   Female and male lesser pelvis (60%)
Ventral aspect
Coronal sections through the lesser pelvis
in the plane of the urethra and urinary bladder
a   of a female
b   of a male

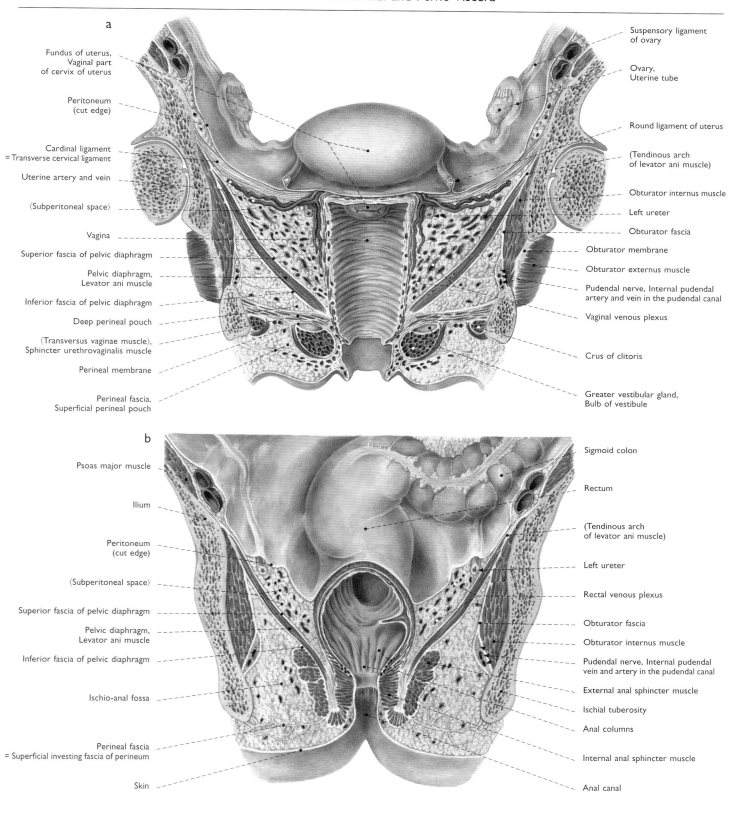

a

Fundus of uterus,
Vaginal part
of cervix of uterus

Peritoneum
(cut edge)

Cardinal ligament
= Transverse cervical ligament

Uterine artery and vein

⟨Subperitoneal space⟩

Vagina

Superior fascia of pelvic diaphragm

Pelvic diaphragm,
Levator ani muscle

Inferior fascia of pelvic diaphragm

Deep perineal pouch

⟨Transversus vaginae muscle⟩,
Sphincter urethrovaginalis muscle

Perineal membrane

Perineal fascia,
Superficial perineal pouch

Suspensory ligament
of ovary

Ovary,
Uterine tube

Round ligament of uterus

(Tendinous arch
of levator ani muscle)

Obturator internus muscle

Left ureter

Obturator fascia

Obturator membrane

Obturator externus muscle

Pudendal nerve, Internal pudendal
artery and vein in the pudendal canal

Vaginal venous plexus

Crus of clitoris

Greater vestibular gland,
Bulb of vestibule

b

Psoas major muscle

Ilium

Peritoneum
(cut edge)

⟨Subperitoneal space⟩

Superior fascia of pelvic diaphragm

Pelvic diaphragm,
Levator ani muscle

Inferior fascia of pelvic diaphragm

Ischio-anal fossa

Perineal fascia
= Superficial investing fascia of perineum

Skin

Sigmoid colon

Rectum

(Tendinous arch
of levator ani muscle)

Left ureter

Rectal venous plexus

Obturator fascia

Obturator internus muscle

Pudendal nerve, Internal pudendal
vein and artery in the pudendal canal

External anal sphincter muscle

Ischial tuberosity

Anal columns

Internal anal sphincter muscle

Anal canal

251   Female and male lesser pelvis
      Ventral aspect
      Coronal sections through the lesser pelvis
   a in the plane of the vagina of a female (60%)
   b in the plane of the rectum and anal canal
      of a male or female (50%)

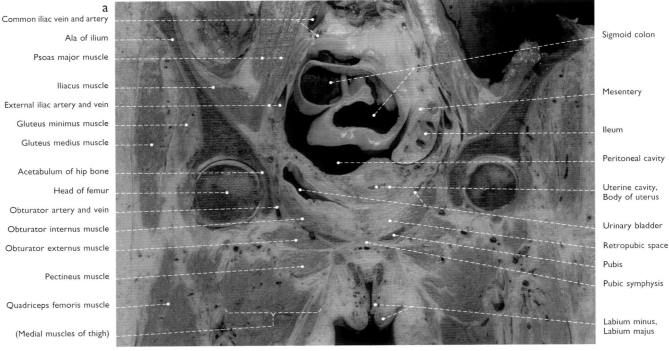

a

Common iliac vein and artery
Ala of ilium
Psoas major muscle
Iliacus muscle
External iliac artery and vein
Gluteus minimus muscle
Gluteus medius muscle
Acetabulum of hip bone
Head of femur
Obturator artery and vein
Obturator internus muscle
Obturator externus muscle
Pectineus muscle
Quadriceps femoris muscle
(Medial muscles of thigh)

Sigmoid colon
Mesentery
Ileum
Peritoneal cavity
Uterine cavity, Body of uterus
Urinary bladder
Retropubic space
Pubis
Pubic symphysis
Labium minus, Labium majus

b

Common iliac vein and artery
Gluteus minimus m.
Gluteus medius m.
External iliac artery, vein
Uterine cavity
Body of uterus
Obturator internus m.
Obturator externus m.
Pubis
Quadriceps femoris m.
(Medial muscles of thigh)

Sigmoid colon
Ileum
Ovary, Uterine tube
Urinary bladder
Retropubic space
Clitoris
Labium majus

252 Lesser pelvis of a female (40%)

Coronal sections through ventral parts of the lesser pelvis
of a female just behind the symphysis, ventral aspect
a   Anatomical section
b   Magnetic resonance image (MRI, T$_2$-weighted)

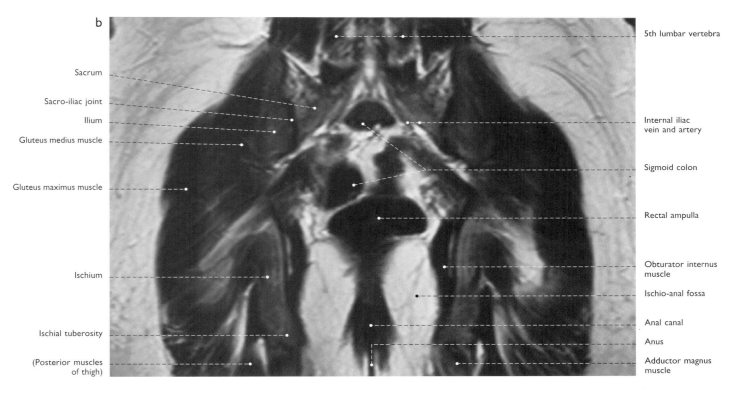

a

Ilium
Sacro-iliac joint
Sacrum

Gluteus minimus muscle

Gluteus medius muscle

Gemellus superior muscle,
Obturator internus m. (tendon),
Gemellus inferior muscle

Greater trochanter
of femur

Quadratus femoris muscle,
Obturator internus muscle

Ischio-anal fossa

Ischial tuberosity

Levator ani muscle

Vertebral canal

Sciatic nerve

Sigmoid colon

Peritoneal cavity

Ischium

Rectal ampulla

Anal canal

Anus

b

Sacrum

Sacro-iliac joint

Ilium

Gluteus medius muscle

Gluteus maximus muscle

Ischium

Ischial tuberosity

(Posterior muscles
of thigh)

5th lumbar vertebra

Internal iliac
vein and artery

Sigmoid colon

Rectal ampulla

Obturator internus
muscle

Ischio-anal fossa

Anal canal

Anus

Adductor magnus
muscle

253 Lesser pelvis of a female (40%)
Coronal sections through dorsal parts of the lesser pelvis
of a female in the plane of the anal canal, ventral aspect
a Anatomical section
b Magnetic resonance image (MRI, T₂-weighted)

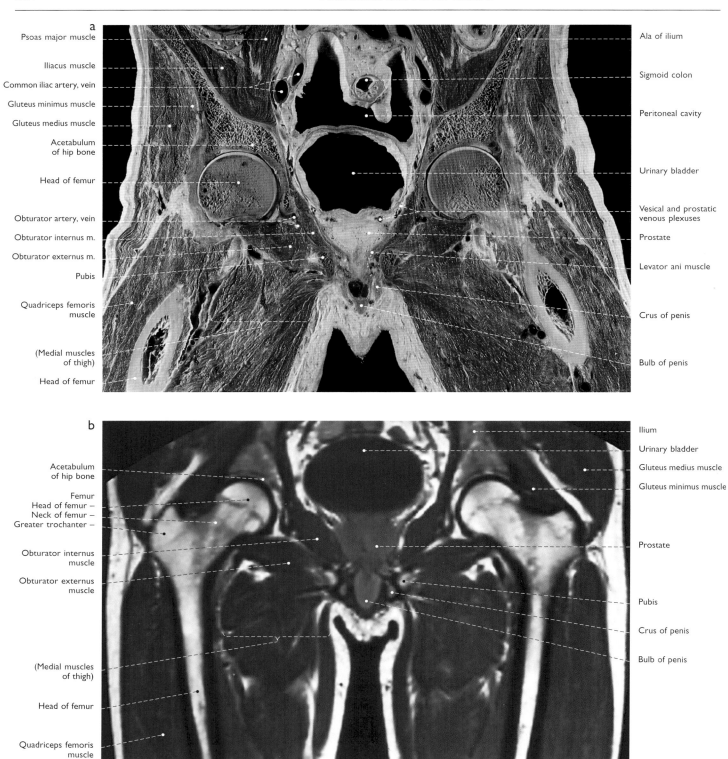

a

Psoas major muscle

Iliacus muscle

Common iliac artery, vein

Gluteus minimus muscle

Gluteus medius muscle

Acetabulum
of hip bone

Head of femur

Obturator artery, vein

Obturator internus m.

Obturator externus m.

Pubis

Quadriceps femoris
muscle

(Medial muscles
of thigh)

Head of femur

Ala of ilium

Sigmoid colon

Peritoneal cavity

Urinary bladder

Vesical and prostatic
venous plexuses

Prostate

Levator ani muscle

Crus of penis

Bulb of penis

b

Acetabulum
of hip bone

Femur
Head of femur –
Neck of femur –
Greater trochanter –

Obturator internus
muscle

Obturator externus
muscle

(Medial muscles
of thigh)

Head of femur

Quadriceps femoris
muscle

Ilium

Urinary bladder

Gluteus medius muscle

Gluteus minimus muscle

Prostate

Pubis

Crus of penis

Bulb of penis

254 Lesser pelvis of a male (40%)

Coronal sections through ventral parts of the lesser pelvis
of a male just behind the symphysis, ventral aspect
a   Anatomical section
b   Magnetic resonance image (MRI, T$_1$-weighted)

a

Sacrum
Sacro-iliac joint
Ilium
Internal iliac artery, vein
Gluteus medius muscle
Gluteus minimus muscle
Obturator internus muscle
(Tendinous arch of levator ani muscle)
Levator ani muscle
Internal pudendal artery and vein in the pudendal canal
Quadratus femoris m., Ischial tuberosity
Ischio-anal fossa
Quadriceps femoris m.
Adductor magnus m.
(Posterior muscles of thigh)

Median sacral vein and artery
Sigmoid colon
Peritoneal cavity
Ductus deferens
Seminal gland
Femur
Rectal ampulla
Levator ani muscle
Anal canal
Anus

b

Gluteus maximus muscle
Levator ani muscle
Ilium
Obturator internus muscle
Ischium
Ischial tuberosity
Quadriceps femoris muscle
(Posterior muscles of thigh)
Adductor magnus muscle

Median sacral vein, artery
Sigmoid colon
Internal iliac artery, vein
Ductus deferens
Seminal gland
Rectal ampulla
Femur
Internal pudendal artery and vein in the pudendal canal
Ischio-anal fossa
Anal canal
Anus

255 Lesser pelvis of a male (40%)
Coronal sections through dorsal parts of the lesser pelvis of a male in the plane of the anal canal, ventral aspect
a Anatomical section
b Magnetic resonance image (MRI, T$_1$-weighted)

a

Rectus abdominis muscle

External iliac artery and vein

Uterus
Uterine cavity –
Body of uterus –
Isthmus of uterus –
Cervix of uterus –

Vaginal fornix

Recto-uterine pouch

Gluteus maximus muscle

Coccyx

Sartorius muscle

Ileum

Iliopsoas muscle

Ilium

Gluteus minimus muscle,
Gluteus medius muscle

Cardinal ligament
= Transverse cervical ligament

Rectum

b

Femoral nerve

Femoral artery and vein

Iliopsoas muscle

Obturator nerve,
Obturator artery and vein

Hip joint

Levator ani muscle

Obturator internus muscle

Pudendal nerve,
Internal pudendal artery and vein

Coccyx

Rectus abdominis muscle

Sartorius muscle

Urinary bladder

Vagina

Ligament of head of femur,
Head of femur

Rectum

Sciatic nerve

Ischio-anal fossa

Gluteus maximus muscle

c

Pubic symphysis

Pubis

External urethral sphincter muscle,
Female urethra

Vagina

Quadratus femoris muscle

Sciatic nerve

Rectum

Intergluteal cleft

Great saphenous vein

Femoral vein, artery, and nerve

Tensor fasciae latae muscle

Iliopsoas muscle,
Lesser trochanter of femur

Obturator membrane

Obturator internus muscle,
Obturator externus muscle

Levator ani muscle

Ischio-anal fossa

Ischial tuberosity

Gluteus maximus muscle

256   Lesser pelvis of a female (40%)

Inferior aspect
Transverse anatomical sections (painted) through
a   cranial
b   middle
c   caudal
horizontal planes of the lesser pelvis of a female.
Slight displacement of the uterus to the right in fig. a

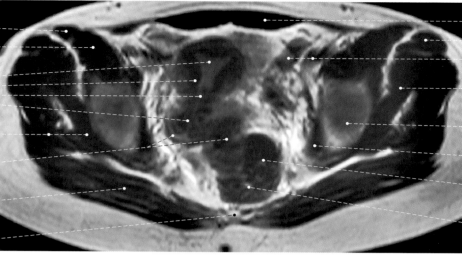

a

Sartorius muscle
Iliopsoas muscle
Uterus
Uterine cavity –
Body of uterus –
Isthmus of uterus –
Cervix of uterus –
Gluteus medius muscle,
Gluteus minimus muscle
Vaginal fornix,
Recto-uterine pouch
Gluteus maximus muscle
Coccyx

Rectus abdominis muscle
Tensor fasciae latae muscle
Ileum
Rectus femoris muscle
Ilium
Obturator internus muscle
Sigmoid colon
Rectum

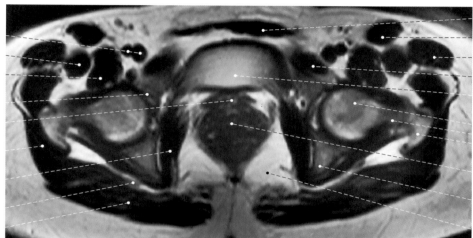

b

Femoral artery and vein
Rectus femoris muscle
Iliopsoas muscle
Acetabular fossa
Vagina
Gluteus medius muscle
Obturator internus muscle
Sciatic nerve
Gluteus maximus muscle

Rectus abdominis muscle
Sartorius muscle
Tensor fasciae latae muscle
Pectineus muscle
Urinary bladder
Femur
– Head of femur
– Neck of femur
– Greater trochanter
Rectum
Ischium
Ischio-anal fossa

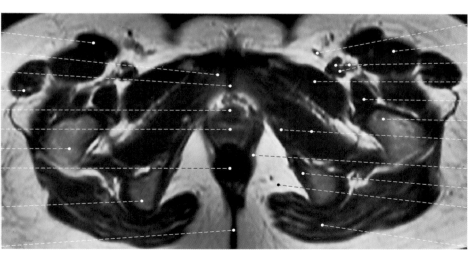

c

Sartorius muscle
Pubis
Pubic symphysis
Tensor fasciae latae muscle
Female urethra
Vagina
Femur
Rectum
Ischial tuberosity
Intergluteal cleft

Great saphenous vein
Rectus femoris muscle
Femoral vein, nerve, and artery
Pectineus muscle
Iliopsoas muscle
Lesser trochanter of femur
Obturator membrane,
Obturator externus muscle
Levator ani muscle
Obturator internus muscle
Ischio-anal fossa
Gluteus maximus muscle

257 Lesser pelvis of a female (40%)

Inferior aspect
Transverse magnetic resonance images (MRI, T_2-weighted) through
a cranial
b middle
c caudal
   horizontal planes of the lesser pelvis of a female.
   Slight displacement of the uterus to the right in fig. a

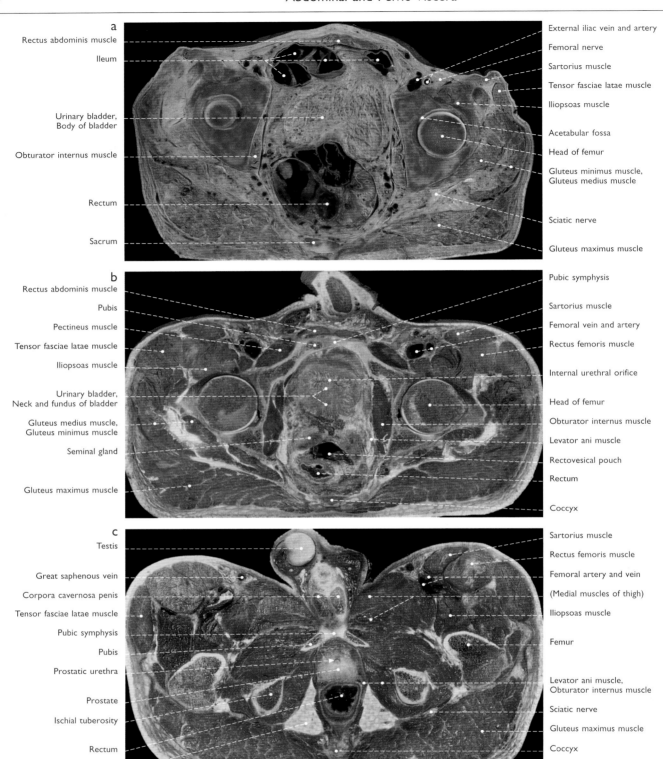

a
- Rectus abdominis muscle
- Ileum
- Urinary bladder, Body of bladder
- Obturator internus muscle
- Rectum
- Sacrum

- External iliac vein and artery
- Femoral nerve
- Sartorius muscle
- Tensor fasciae latae muscle
- Iliopsoas muscle
- Acetabular fossa
- Head of femur
- Gluteus minimus muscle, Gluteus medius muscle
- Sciatic nerve
- Gluteus maximus muscle

b
- Rectus abdominis muscle
- Pubis
- Pectineus muscle
- Tensor fasciae latae muscle
- Iliopsoas muscle
- Urinary bladder, Neck and fundus of bladder
- Gluteus medius muscle, Gluteus minimus muscle
- Seminal gland
- Gluteus maximus muscle

- Pubic symphysis
- Sartorius muscle
- Femoral vein and artery
- Rectus femoris muscle
- Internal urethral orifice
- Head of femur
- Obturator internus muscle
- Levator ani muscle
- Rectovesical pouch
- Rectum
- Coccyx

c
- Testis
- Great saphenous vein
- Corpora cavernosa penis
- Tensor fasciae latae muscle
- Pubic symphysis
- Pubis
- Prostatic urethra
- Prostate
- Ischial tuberosity
- Rectum
- Ischio-anal fossa

- Sartorius muscle
- Rectus femoris muscle
- Femoral artery and vein
- (Medial muscles of thigh)
- Iliopsoas muscle
- Femur
- Levator ani muscle, Obturator internus muscle
- Sciatic nerve
- Gluteus maximus muscle
- Coccyx
- Intergluteal cleft

258 Lesser pelvis of a male (40%)

Transverse anatomical sections through
a   cranial
b   middle
c   caudal
horizontal planes of the lesser pelvis of a male
a, c   Inferior aspect
b   Superior aspect

a

Rectus abdominis muscle

Tensor fasciae latae muscle

Ileum

Urinary bladder,
Body of bladder

Acetabular fossa

Gluteus maximus muscle

Sacrum

Sartorius muscle

Iliopsoas muscle

External iliac artery and vein

Head of femur

Gluteus minimus muscle

Gluteus medius muscle

Obturator internus muscle

Rectum

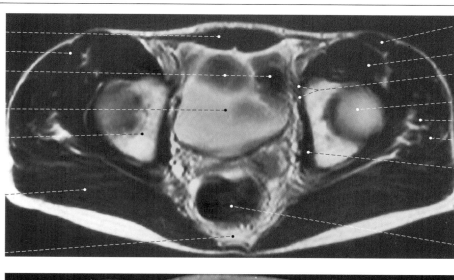

b

Rectus abdominis muscle

Tensor fasciae latae muscle

Urinary bladder

Gluteus medius muscle,
Gluteus minimus muscle

Seminal gland

Gluteus maximus muscle

Coccyx

Sartorius muscle

Femoral artery and vein

Iliopsoas muscle

Rectus femoris muscle

Acetabular fossa,
Head of femur

Obturator internus muscle

Rectum

Intergluteal cleft

c

Corpora cavernosa penis

Great saphenous vein

Pubis,
Pubic symphysis

Tensor fasciae latae muscle

Pectineus muscle

Femur
Neck of femur —
Greater trochanter —

Prostate
with male urethra

Obturator internus muscle

Ischial tuberosity

Ischio-anal fossa

Penis

Sartorius muscle

Femoral vein and artery

Rectus femoris muscle

Iliopsoas muscle

Obturator externus muscle

Levator ani muscle

Rectum

Sciatic nerve

Gluteus maximus muscle

Intergluteal cleft

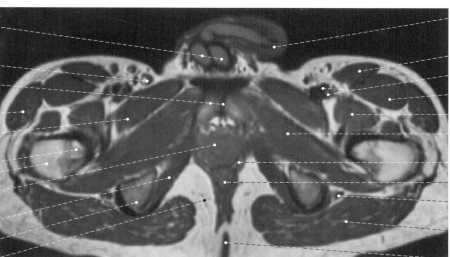

259 Lesser pelvis of a male (40%)

Inferior aspect
Transverse magnetic resonance images (MRI, T$_2$- or T$_1$-weighted,
respectively) through
a   cranial
b   middle
c   caudal
     horizontal planes of the lesser pelvis of a male

a

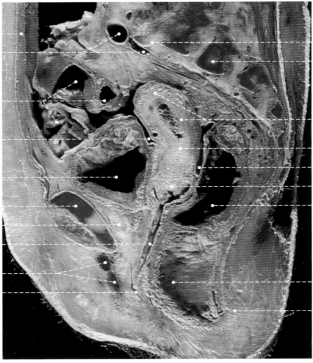

Rectus abdominis muscle

Left common iliac artery and vein

Ileum

Vesico-uterine pouch

Urinary bladder

Pubis

Retropubic space

Vagina

Crus and body of clitoris

Female urethra

Promontory of sacrum

Sacrum,
2nd sacral vertebra

Fundus and body of uterus

Isthmus of uterus

Recto-uterine pouch

Cervix of uterus

Rectum

Rectal ampulla

External anal sphincter muscle

b

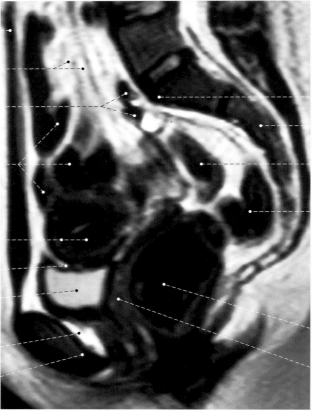

Rectus abdominis muscle

Mesentery

Left common iliac artery and vein

Ileum

Fundus and body of uterus

Vesico-uterine pouch

Urinary bladder

Retropubic space

Pubis,
Pubic symphysis

Promontory of sacrum

Sacrum,
2nd sacral vertebra

Sigmoid colon

Rectum

Rectal ampulla

Vagina

260 **Pelvis of a female** (45%)
Midsagittal sections
a Anatomical section, medial aspect of the right half of the body
b Magnetic resonance image (MRI, T$_2$-weighted)

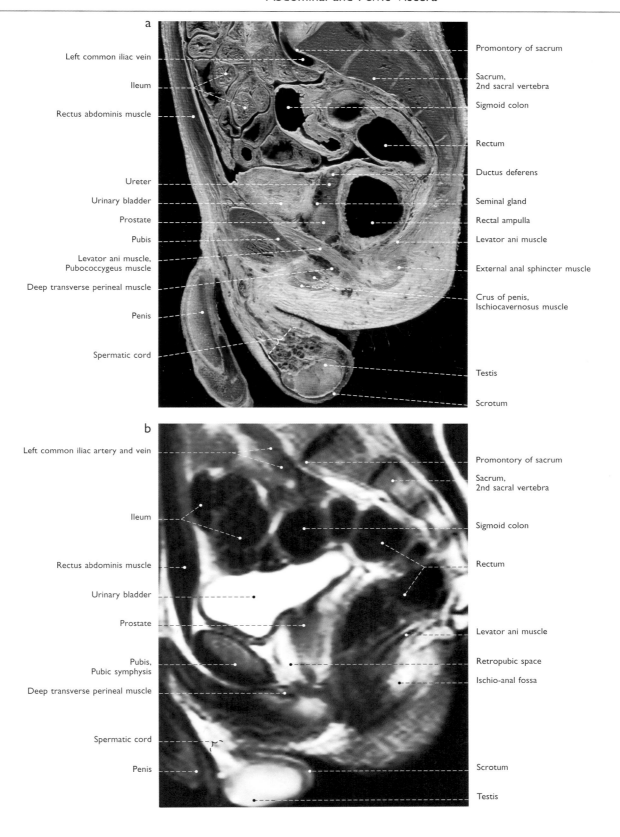

a

Left common iliac vein

Ileum

Rectus abdominis muscle

Ureter

Urinary bladder

Prostate

Pubis

Levator ani muscle,
Pubococcygeus muscle

Deep transverse perineal muscle

Penis

Spermatic cord

Promontory of sacrum

Sacrum,
2nd sacral vertebra

Sigmoid colon

Rectum

Ductus deferens

Seminal gland

Rectal ampulla

Levator ani muscle

External anal sphincter muscle

Crus of penis,
Ischiocavernosus muscle

Testis

Scrotum

b

Left common iliac artery and vein

Ileum

Rectus abdominis muscle

Urinary bladder

Prostate

Pubis,
Pubic symphysis

Deep transverse perineal muscle

Spermatic cord

Penis

Promontory of sacrum

Sacrum,
2nd sacral vertebra

Sigmoid colon

Rectum

Levator ani muscle

Retropubic space

Ischio-anal fossa

Scrotum

Testis

261 Pelvis of a male (45%)

Midsagittal sections
a Anatomical section, medial aspect of the right half of the body
b Magnetic resonance image (MRI, T$_2$-weighted)

Pelvic Diaphragm and External Genitalia

a

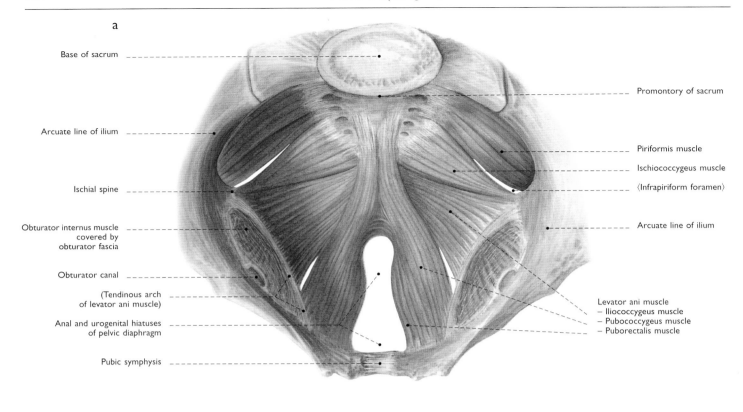

Base of sacrum

Promontory of sacrum

Arcuate line of ilium

Piriformis muscle

Ischiococcygeus muscle

⟨Infrapiriform foramen⟩

Ischial spine

Arcuate line of ilium

Obturator internus muscle
covered by
obturator fascia

Obturator canal

(Tendinous arch
of levator ani muscle)

Levator ani muscle
– Iliococcygeus muscle
– Pubococcygeus muscle
– Puborectalis muscle

Anal and urogenital hiatuses
of pelvic diaphragm

Pubic symphysis

b

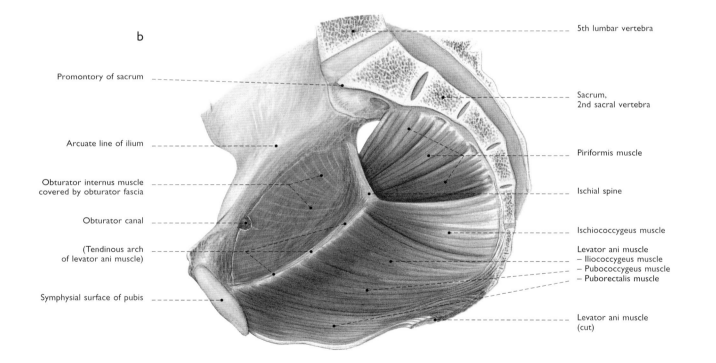

5th lumbar vertebra

Promontory of sacrum

Sacrum,
2nd sacral vertebra

Arcuate line of ilium

Piriformis muscle

Obturator internus muscle
covered by obturator fascia

Ischial spine

Obturator canal

Ischiococcygeus muscle

(Tendinous arch
of levator ani muscle)

Levator ani muscle
– Iliococcygeus muscle
– Pubococcygeus muscle
– Puborectalis muscle

Symphysial surface of pubis

Levator ani muscle
(cut)

264 Pelvic diaphragm (60%)

Muscles of the pelvic diaphragm (= pelvic floor)
a Superior aspect
b Medial aspect of the right half of the pelvis

a

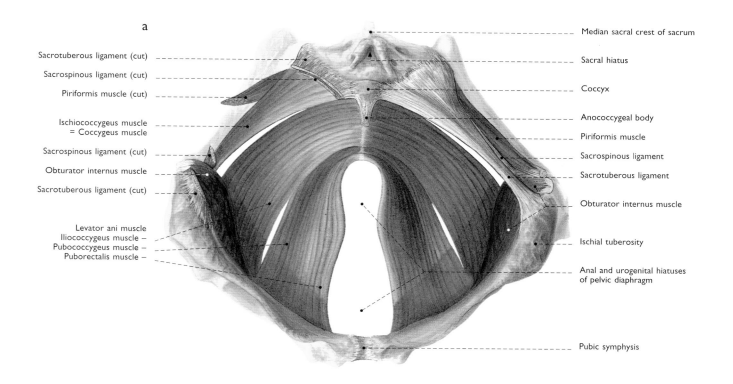

Sacrotuberous ligament (cut)

Sacrospinous ligament (cut)

Piriformis muscle (cut)

Ischiococcygeus muscle
= Coccygeus muscle

Sacrospinous ligament (cut)

Obturator internus muscle

Sacrotuberous ligament (cut)

Levator ani muscle
Iliococcygeus muscle –
Pubococcygeus muscle –
Puborectalis muscle –

Median sacral crest of sacrum

Sacral hiatus

Coccyx

Anococcygeal body

Piriformis muscle

Sacrospinous ligament

Sacrotuberous ligament

Obturator internus muscle

Ischial tuberosity

Anal and urogenital hiatuses
of pelvic diaphragm

Pubic symphysis

b

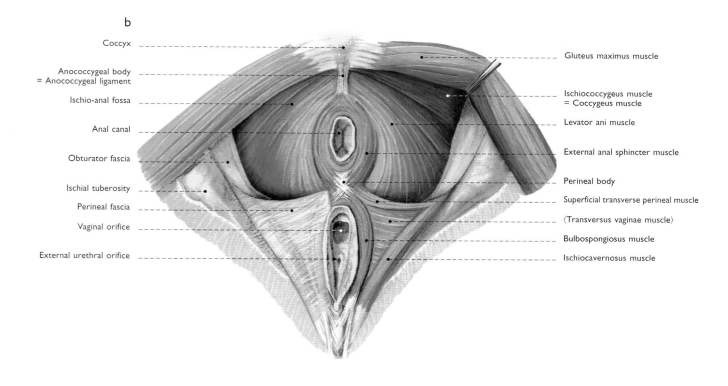

Coccyx

Anococcygeal body
= Anococcygeal ligament

Ischio-anal fossa

Anal canal

Obturator fascia

Ischial tuberosity

Perineal fascia

Vaginal orifice

External urethral orifice

Gluteus maximus muscle

Ischiococcygeus muscle
= Coccygeus muscle

Levator ani muscle

External anal sphincter muscle

Perineal body

Superficial transverse perineal muscle

⟨Transversus vaginae muscle⟩

Bulbospongiosus muscle

Ischiocavernosus muscle

265 Pelvic diaphragm and perineum of a female (60%)
Inferior aspect
a Muscles of the pelvic diaphragm (= pelvic floor)
b Muscles of the pelvic diaphragm and perineal muscles

a

Coccyx

Anococcygeal body
= Anococcygeal ligament

Ischial tuberosity

Anal canal

External anal sphincter muscle

Perineal body

⟨Urethral hiatus⟩

Intermediate part of urethra
= Membranous urethra
(cut margin)

Spongy urethra
(cut margin)

Corpus spongiosum penis

Ischiococcygeus muscle
= Coccygeus muscle

Levator ani muscle
– Iliococcygeus muscle
– Pubococcygeus muscle
– Puborectalis muscle
– ⟨Prerectal fibers⟩

Ischiocavernosus muscle

Prostate

Transverse perineal ligament

b

Gluteus maximus muscle

Ischio-anal fossa

Obturator fascia

External anal sphincter muscle

Anal canal

Perineal fascia
= Superficial investing fascia
of perineum

Coccyx

Anococcygeal body
= Anococcygeal ligament

Levator ani muscle

Obturator internus muscle
(fascia removed)

Ischial tuberosity

Superficial transverse perineal muscle

Deep transverse perineal muscle

Ischiocavernosus muscle

Bulbospongiosus muscle

Corpus spongiosum penis

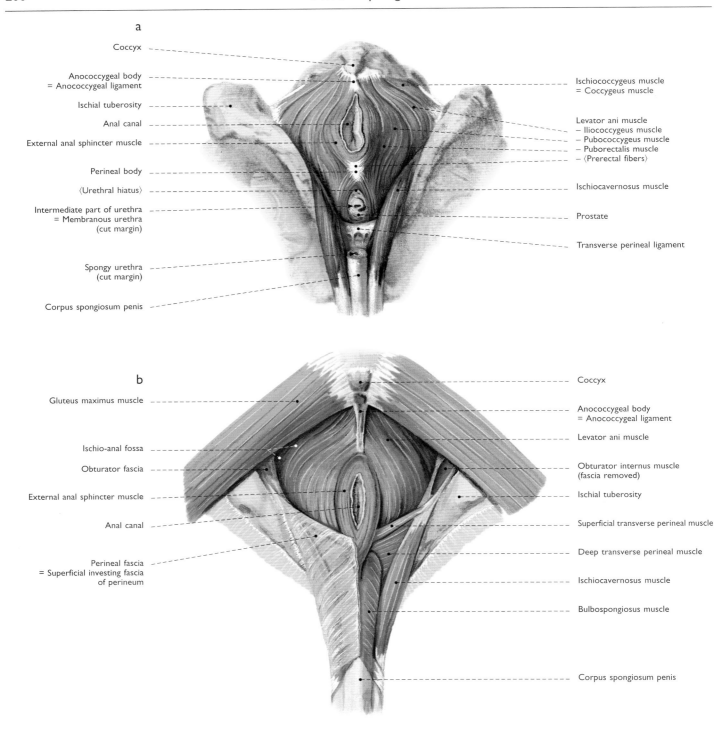

266 Pelvic diaphragm and perineum of a male (60%)
Inferior aspect
a Muscles of the pelvic diaphragm (= pelvic floor)
b Muscles of the pelvic diaphragm and perineal muscles

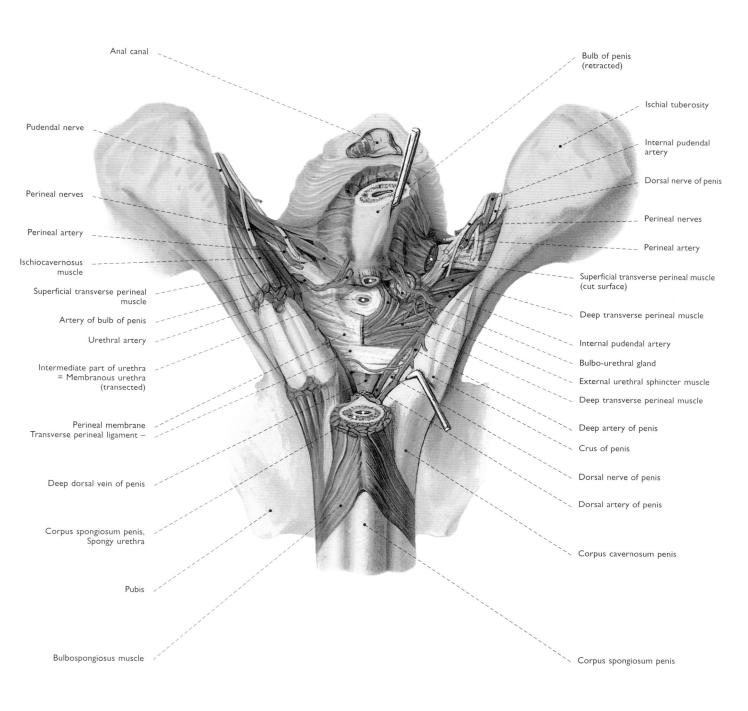

Anal canal

Pudendal nerve

Perineal nerves

Perineal artery

Ischiocavernosus muscle

Superficial transverse perineal muscle

Artery of bulb of penis

Urethral artery

Intermediate part of urethra = Membranous urethra (transected)

Perineal membrane
Transverse perineal ligament

Deep dorsal vein of penis

Corpus spongiosum penis, Spongy urethra

Pubis

Bulbospongiosus muscle

Bulb of penis (retracted)

Ischial tuberosity

Internal pudendal artery

Dorsal nerve of penis

Perineal nerves

Perineal artery

Superficial transverse perineal muscle (cut surface)

Deep transverse perineal muscle

Internal pudendal artery

Bulbo-urethral gland

External urethral sphincter muscle

Deep transverse perineal muscle

Deep artery of penis

Crus of penis

Dorsal nerve of penis

Dorsal artery of penis

Corpus cavernosum penis

Corpus spongiosum penis

267 Penis and deep perineal space (90%)
Inferior aspect
The corpus spongiosum penis was transected
and the bulb of penis retracted.

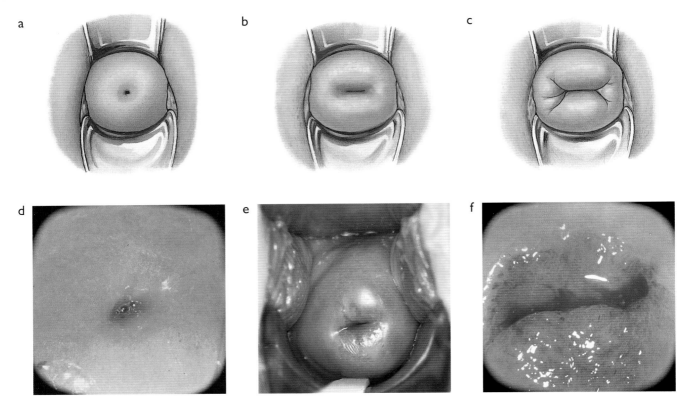

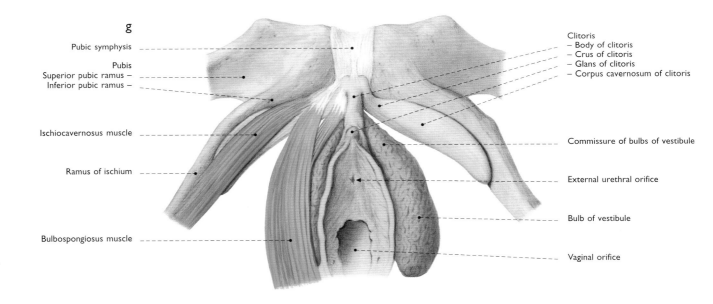

Pubic symphysis

Pubis
Superior pubic ramus –
Inferior pubic ramus –

Ischiocavernosus muscle

Ramus of ischium

Bulbospongiosus muscle

Clitoris
– Body of clitoris
– Crus of clitoris
– Glans of clitoris
– Corpus cavernosum of clitoris

Commissure of bulbs of vestibule

External urethral orifice

Bulb of vestibule

Vaginal orifice

268 Vaginal part of the cervix of uterus and clitoris

a–f Vaginal aspect of the external os of uterus
a, b, d, e of a nulliparous woman (a, b, e, 100%; d, 200%)
c, f of a multiparous woman (c, 100%; f, 200%)
d–f Original photographs
g Erectile bodies of the clitoris (100%), inferior aspect

a

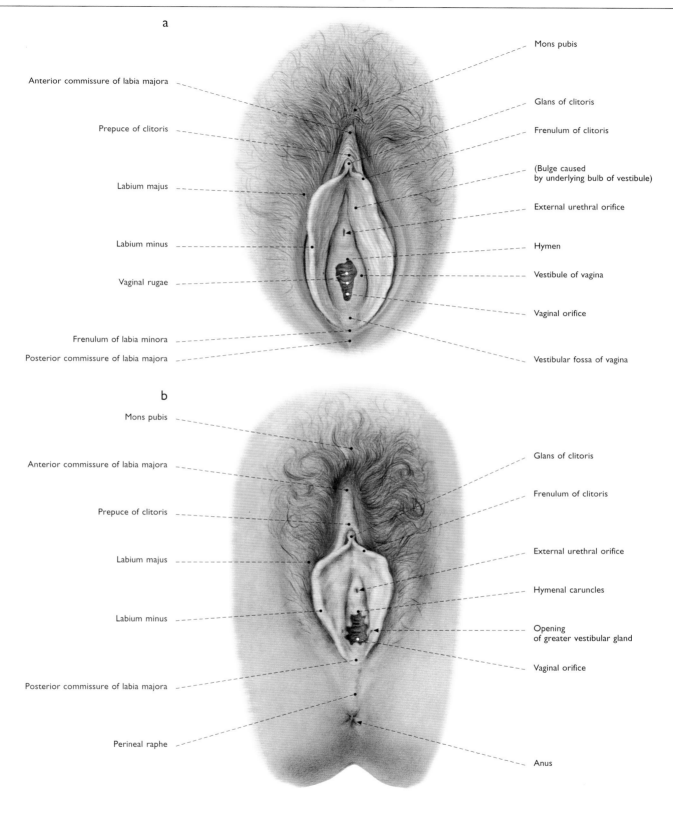

Anterior commissure of labia majora

Prepuce of clitoris

Labium majus

Labium minus

Vaginal rugae

Frenulum of labia minora

Posterior commissure of labia majora

Mons pubis

Glans of clitoris

Frenulum of clitoris

(Bulge caused
by underlying bulb of vestibule)

External urethral orifice

Hymen

Vestibule of vagina

Vaginal orifice

Vestibular fossa of vagina

b

Mons pubis

Anterior commissure of labia majora

Prepuce of clitoris

Labium majus

Labium minus

Posterior commissure of labia majora

Perineal raphe

Glans of clitoris

Frenulum of clitoris

External urethral orifice

Hymenal caruncles

Opening
of greater vestibular gland

Vaginal orifice

Anus

269 Female external genitalia (80%)
Inferior aspect
a Female genitals of a virgin
b Female genitals after defloration

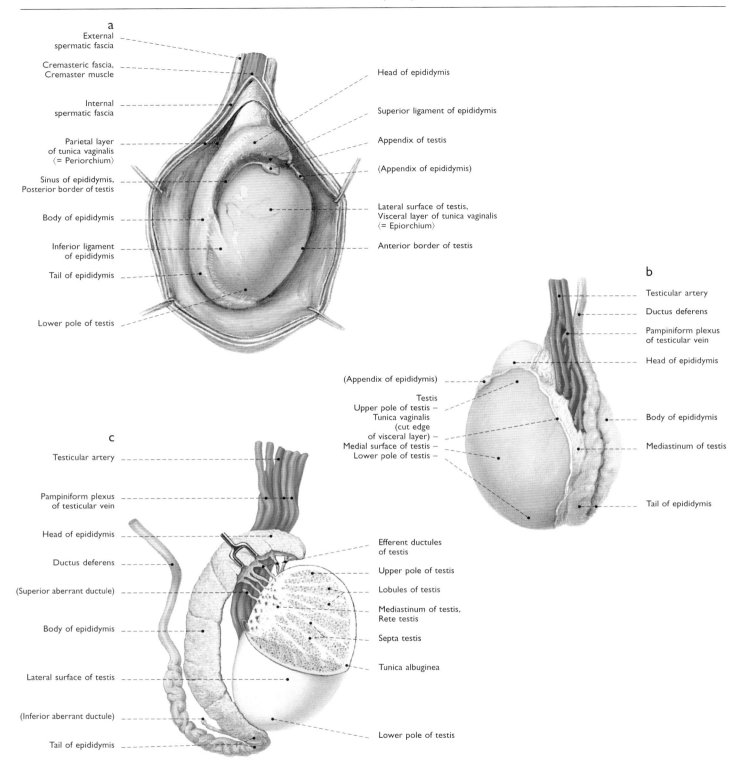

a

External spermatic fascia

Cremasteric fascia, Cremaster muscle

Internal spermatic fascia

Parietal layer of tunica vaginalis ⟨= Periorchium⟩

Sinus of epididymis, Posterior border of testis

Body of epididymis

Inferior ligament of epididymis

Tail of epididymis

Lower pole of testis

Head of epididymis

Superior ligament of epididymis

Appendix of testis

(Appendix of epididymis)

Lateral surface of testis, Visceral layer of tunica vaginalis ⟨= Epiorchium⟩

Anterior border of testis

b

Testicular artery

Ductus deferens

Pampiniform plexus of testicular vein

Head of epididymis

Body of epididymis

Mediastinum of testis

Tail of epididymis

(Appendix of epididymis)

Testis
Upper pole of testis –
Tunica vaginalis (cut edge of visceral layer) –
Medial surface of testis –
Lower pole of testis –

c

Testicular artery

Pampiniform plexus of testicular vein

Head of epididymis

Ductus deferens

(Superior aberrant ductule)

Body of epididymis

Lateral surface of testis

(Inferior aberrant ductule)

Tail of epididymis

Efferent ductules of testis

Upper pole of testis

Lobules of testis

Mediastinum of testis, Rete testis

Septa testis

Tunica albuginea

Lower pole of testis

270 Testis and epididymis (100%)

a, b   The coverings of the right testis were opened (a) and removed (b).
a   Right lateral aspect
b   Medial aspect
c   The lateral superior quadrant of the right testis was excised by a rectangular incision. Right lateral aspect

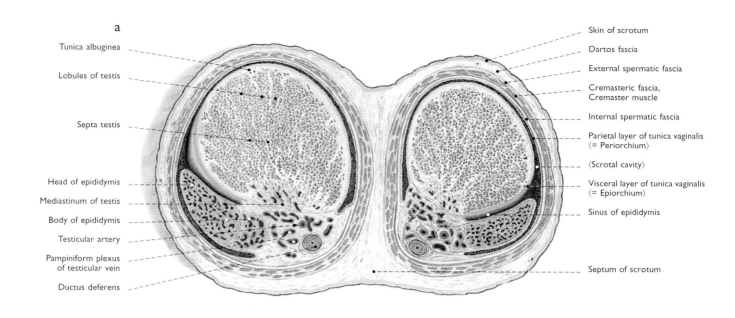

a

Tunica albuginea

Lobules of testis

Septa testis

Head of epididymis

Mediastinum of testis

Body of epididymis

Testicular artery

Pampiniform plexus
of testicular vein

Ductus deferens

Skin of scrotum

Dartos fascia

External spermatic fascia

Cremasteric fascia,
Cremaster muscle

Internal spermatic fascia

Parietal layer of tunica vaginalis
⟨= Periorchium⟩

⟨Scrotal cavity⟩

Visceral layer of tunica vaginalis
⟨= Epiorchium⟩

Sinus of epididymis

Septum of scrotum

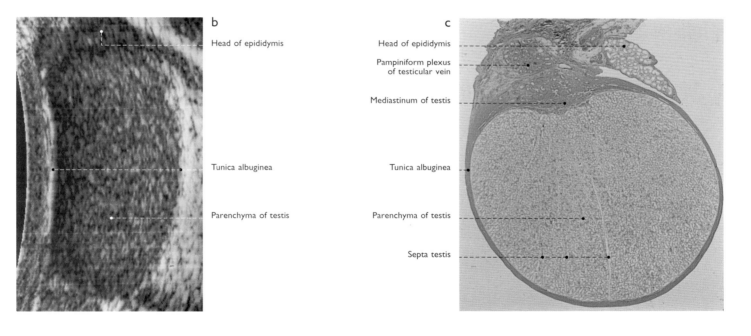

b

Head of epididymis

Tunica albuginea

Parenchyma of testis

c

Head of epididymis

Pampiniform plexus
of testicular vein

Mediastinum of testis

Tunica albuginea

Parenchyma of testis

Septa testis

271 Scrotum and testis

a   Transverse section through the scrotum and its contents (150%)
b   Longitudinal ultrasound image of the testis (150%)
c   Histological picture of the testis and the head
    of epididymis sectioned in a transverse plane (260%)

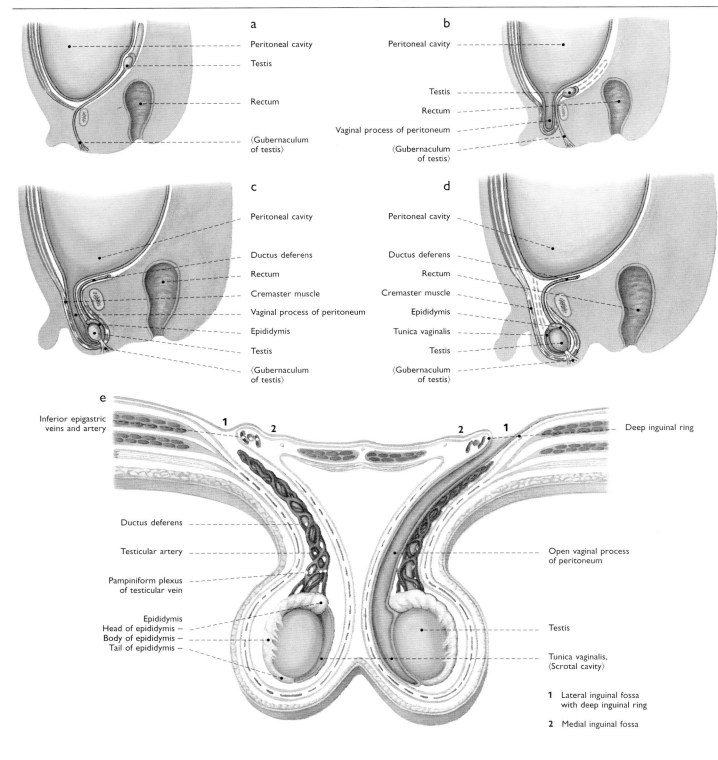

a

Peritoneal cavity

Testis

Rectum

⟨Gubernaculum of testis⟩

b

Peritoneal cavity

Testis

Rectum

Vaginal process of peritoneum

⟨Gubernaculum of testis⟩

c

Peritoneal cavity

Ductus deferens

Rectum

Cremaster muscle

Vaginal process of peritoneum

Epididymis

Testis

⟨Gubernaculum of testis⟩

d

Peritoneal cavity

Ductus deferens

Rectum

Cremaster muscle

Epididymis

Tunica vaginalis

Testis

⟨Gubernaculum of testis⟩

e

Inferior epigastric veins and artery

Ductus deferens

Testicular artery

Pampiniform plexus of testicular vein

Epididymis
Head of epididymis –
Body of epididymis –
Tail of epididymis –

Deep inguinal ring

Open vaginal process of peritoneum

Testis

Tunica vaginalis, ⟨Scrotal cavity⟩

1 Lateral inguinal fossa with deep inguinal ring

2 Medial inguinal fossa

272 Prenatal descent of the testis and inguinal region after birth

a–d   Diverse stages of the prenatal descent of the testis. Medial aspect of the right halfs of paramedian sagittal sections

e   Inguinal region of a male. On the right side of the body, normal situation. On the left side of the body, persistent vaginal process of peritoneum. Schematized section through the anterior abdominal wall on the level of the inguinal canal and through the scrotum (according to Benninghoff, 1985), ventral aspect

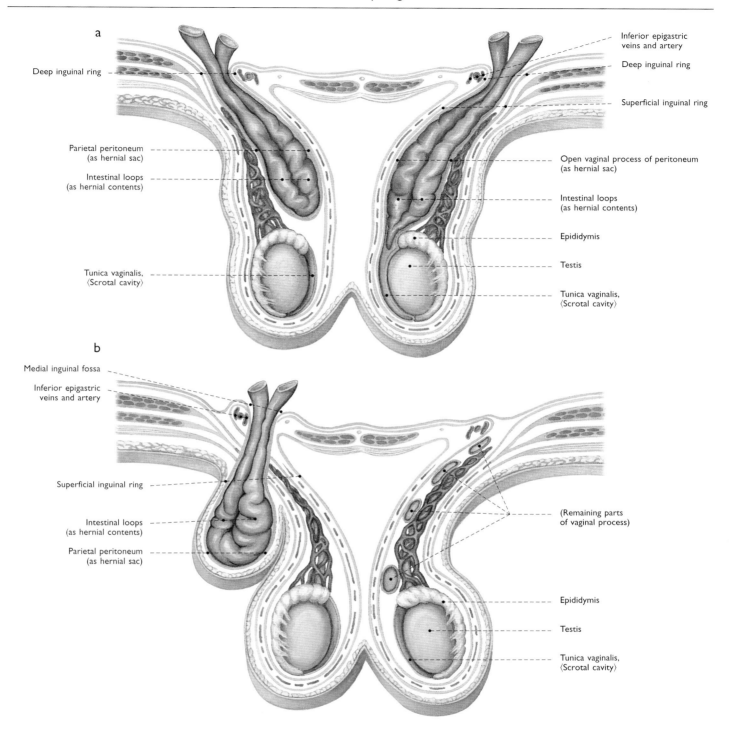

a

Deep inguinal ring

Inferior epigastric
veins and artery

Deep inguinal ring

Superficial inguinal ring

Parietal peritoneum
(as hernial sac)

Open vaginal process of peritoneum
(as hernial sac)

Intestinal loops
(as hernial contents)

Intestinal loops
(as hernial contents)

Epididymis

Testis

Tunica vaginalis,
⟨Scrotal cavity⟩

Tunica vaginalis,
⟨Scrotal cavity⟩

b

Medial inguinal fossa

Inferior epigastric
veins and artery

Superficial inguinal ring

(Remaining parts
of vaginal process)

Intestinal loops
(as hernial contents)

Parietal peritoneum
(as hernial sac)

Epididymis

Testis

Tunica vaginalis,
⟨Scrotal cavity⟩

273   Inguinal region of a male

Schematized sections through the anterior abdominal wall
on the level of the inguinal canal and through the scrotum
(according to Benninghoff, 1985), ventral aspect

a   On both sides, lateral indirect inguinal herniae descending along
the inguinal canal, the inner hernial ring being the deep inguinal ring.
On the left side of the body, persistent vaginal process of peritoneum
and complete congenital hernia.

b   On the right side of the body, medial direct inguinal hernia.
The inner hernial ring is the medial inguinal fossa. On the left side
of the body, persistent cysts in the spermatic cord as remainders
of the vaginal process of peritoneum.

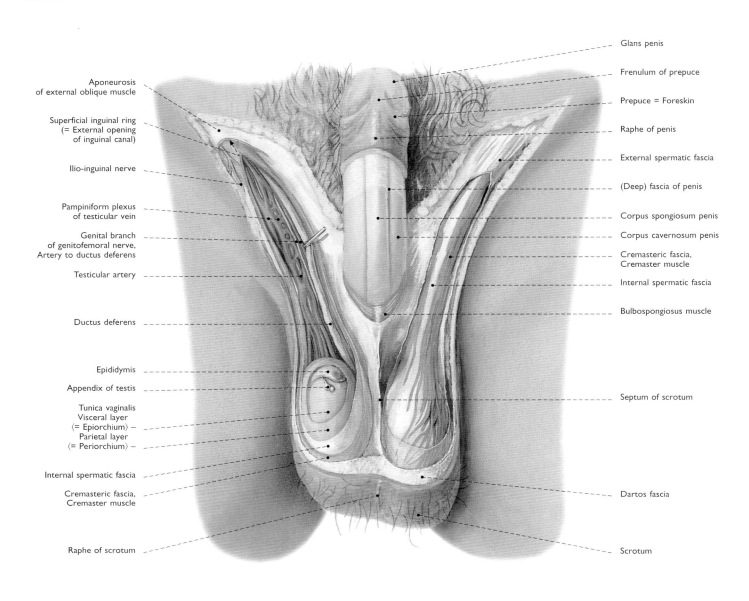

Aponeurosis
of external oblique muscle

Superficial inguinal ring
(= External opening
of inguinal canal)

Ilio-inguinal nerve

Pampiniform plexus
of testicular vein

Genital branch
of genitofemoral nerve,
Artery to ductus deferens

Testicular artery

Ductus deferens

Epididymis

Appendix of testis

Tunica vaginalis
Visceral layer
⟨= Epiorchium⟩ –
Parietal layer
⟨= Periorchium⟩ –

Internal spermatic fascia

Cremasteric fascia,
Cremaster muscle

Raphe of scrotum

Glans penis

Frenulum of prepuce

Prepuce = Foreskin

Raphe of penis

External spermatic fascia

(Deep) fascia of penis

Corpus spongiosum penis

Corpus cavernosum penis

Cremasteric fascia,
Cremaster muscle

Internal spermatic fascia

Bulbospongiosus muscle

Septum of scrotum

Dartos fascia

Scrotum

274   Male external genitalia (70%)

The penis was turned upwards, the skin and the deep fascia of penis
were largely removed from the body of penis. The skin of the scrotum
was excised in the region of both spermatic cords. On the right side
of the body, the structures of the spermatic cord are exposed by
opening the external and internal spermatic fasciae, the interposed
cremasteric fascia, and the cremaster muscle. On the left side of the body,
the cremaster muscle is shown after having removed the external spermatic
and the cremasteric fasciae. Ventral aspect

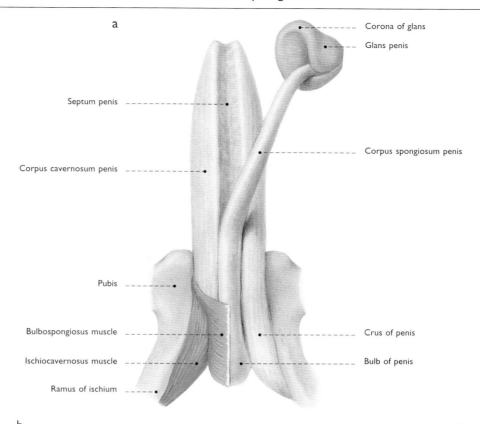

a

Corona of glans

Glans penis

Septum penis

Corpus spongiosum penis

Corpus cavernosum penis

Pubis

Bulbospongiosus muscle

Crus of penis

Ischiocavernosus muscle

Bulb of penis

Ramus of ischium

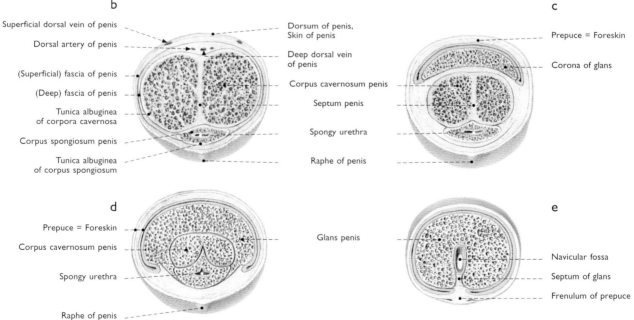

b

Superficial dorsal vein of penis

Dorsal artery of penis

(Superficial) fascia of penis

(Deep) fascia of penis

Tunica albuginea of corpora cavernosa

Corpus spongiosum penis

Tunica albuginea of corpus spongiosum

Dorsum of penis, Skin of penis

Deep dorsal vein of penis

Corpus cavernosum penis

Septum penis

Spongy urethra

Raphe of penis

c

Prepuce = Foreskin

Corona of glans

d

Prepuce = Foreskin

Corpus cavernosum penis

Spongy urethra

Raphe of penis

Glans penis

e

Navicular fossa

Septum of glans

Frenulum of prepuce

275 Penis (80%)

a Erectile bodies of the penis. The glans penis and the distal part of the corpus spongiosum penis were detached from the corpora cavernosa penis and displaced to the left. Inferior aspect

b–e Distal aspect of transverse sections
  b through the body of penis
  c at the level of the neck of glans penis
  d through the posterior part of the glans penis
  e through the anterior part of the glans penis

a

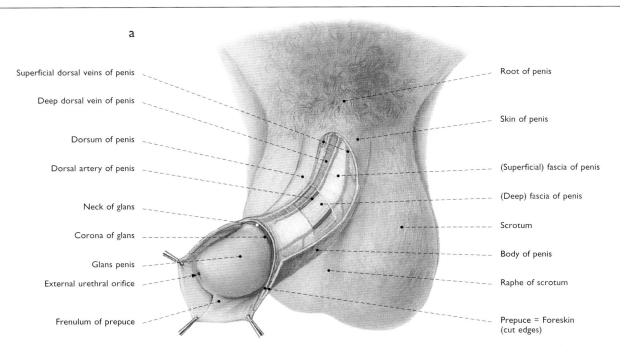

Superficial dorsal veins of penis

Deep dorsal vein of penis

Dorsum of penis

Dorsal artery of penis

Neck of glans

Corona of glans

Glans penis

External urethral orifice

Frenulum of prepuce

Root of penis

Skin of penis

(Superficial) fascia of penis

(Deep) fascia of penis

Scrotum

Body of penis

Raphe of scrotum

Prepuce = Foreskin
(cut edges)

b

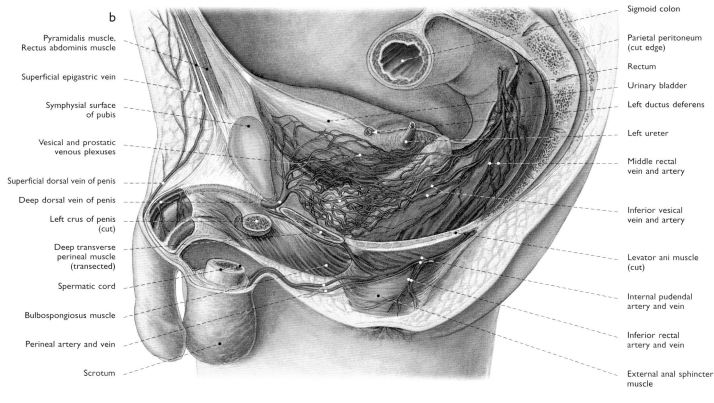

Pyramidalis muscle,
Rectus abdominis muscle

Superficial epigastric vein

Symphysial surface
of pubis

Vesical and prostatic
venous plexuses

Superficial dorsal vein of penis

Deep dorsal vein of penis

Left crus of penis
(cut)

Deep transverse
perineal muscle
(transected)

Spermatic cord

Bulbospongiosus muscle

Perineal artery and vein

Scrotum

Sigmoid colon

Parietal peritoneum
(cut edge)

Rectum

Urinary bladder

Left ductus deferens

Left ureter

Middle rectal
vein and artery

Inferior vesical
vein and artery

Levator ani muscle
(cut)

Internal pudendal
artery and vein

Inferior rectal
artery and vein

External anal sphincter
muscle

276   Male external genitalia

a   The preputial sac was opened and a longitudinal strip of skin removed from the left side of the prepuce and the body of penis. A small rectangular window was cut into the (superficial) fascia of penis (80%). Ventral aspect

b   Drainage of superficial and deep dorsal veins of penis (60%). Left paramedian section through the lesser pelvis, medial aspect of the right part

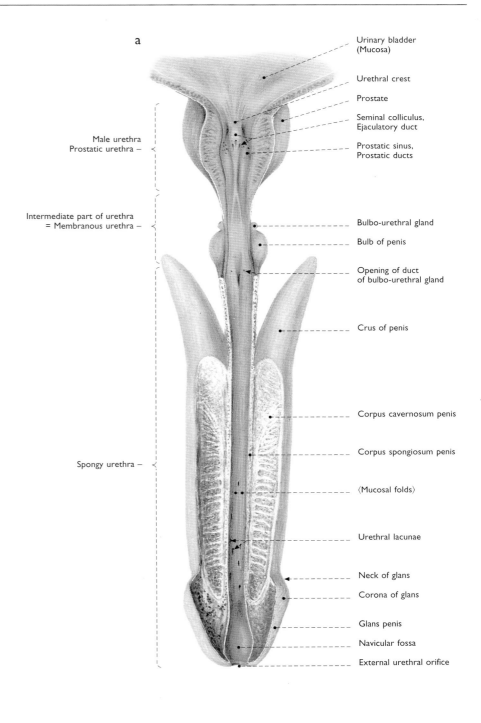

a

Urinary bladder
(Mucosa)

Urethral crest

Prostate

Seminal colliculus,
Ejaculatory duct

Male urethra
Prostatic urethra —

Prostatic sinus,
Prostatic ducts

Intermediate part of urethra
= Membranous urethra —

Bulbo-urethral gland

Bulb of penis

Opening of duct
of bulbo-urethral gland

Crus of penis

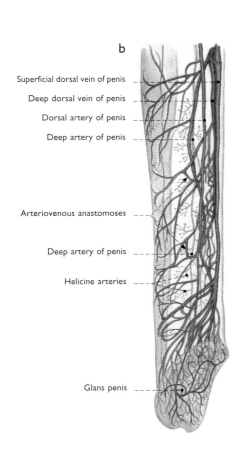

b

Superficial dorsal vein of penis

Deep dorsal vein of penis

Dorsal artery of penis

Deep artery of penis

Corpus cavernosum penis

Corpus spongiosum penis

⟨Mucosal folds⟩

Spongy urethra —

Arteriovenous anastomoses

Urethral lacunae

Deep artery of penis

Helicine arteries

Neck of glans

Corona of glans

Glans penis

Navicular fossa

Glans penis

External urethral orifice

277 Male urethra and arteries of the penis (80%)

a The urethra was opened by a median section
   from the internal to the external urethral orifices.
   The cut surfaces were turned outwards. Ventral aspect
b Arteries of the penis including the helicine arteries
   (according to Ferner, 1975, and Lierse, 1984),
   schematic representation, right lateral aspect

a

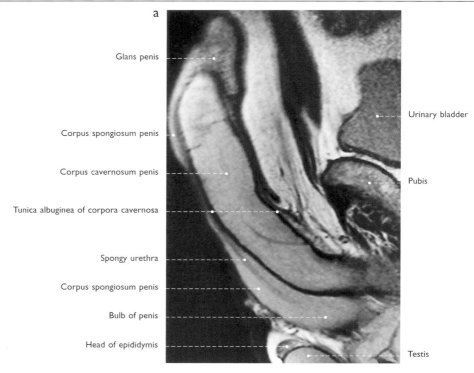

Glans penis

Corpus spongiosum penis

Corpus cavernosum penis

Tunica albuginea of corpora cavernosa

Spongy urethra

Corpus spongiosum penis

Bulb of penis

Head of epididymis

Urinary bladder

Pubis

Testis

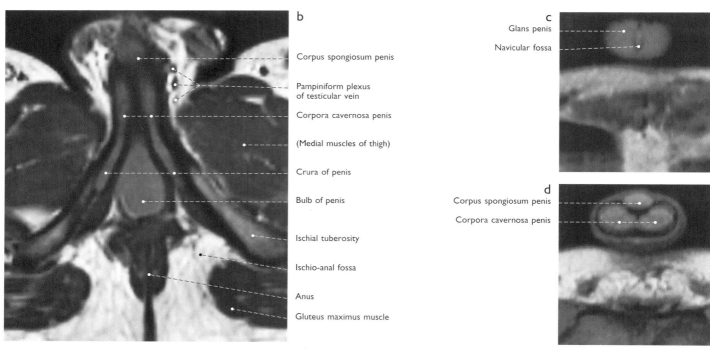

b

Corpus spongiosum penis

Pampiniform plexus of testicular vein

Corpora cavernosa penis

(Medial muscles of thigh)

Crura of penis

Bulb of penis

Ischial tuberosity

Ischio-anal fossa

Anus

Gluteus maximus muscle

c

Glans penis

Navicular fossa

d

Corpus spongiosum penis

Corpora cavernosa penis

278 Penis and male urethra

a   Sagittal magnetic resonance image (MRI, T_2-weighted)
    of an erected penis lying on the anterior abdominal wall (80%),
    medial aspect of the right half

b–d Transverse magnetic resonance images (MRI, T_1-weighted),
     inferior aspect,

b   through the root of penis, the anus,
    and the ischiopubic rami (50%)

c, d through the penis put on the anterior abdominal wall (90%)

c   distally through the glans penis

d   proximally through the body of penis

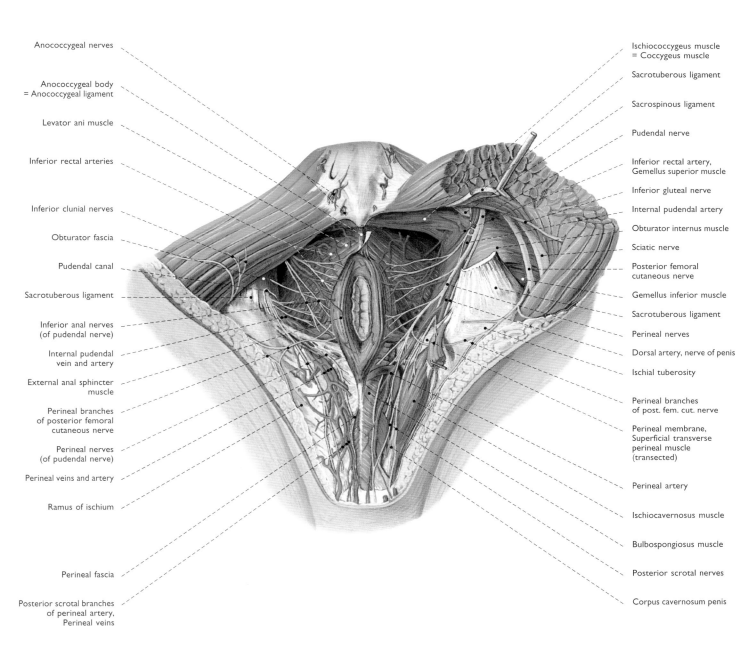

Anococcygeal nerves

Anococcygeal body
= Anococcygeal ligament

Levator ani muscle

Inferior rectal arteries

Inferior clunial nerves

Obturator fascia

Pudendal canal

Sacrotuberous ligament

Inferior anal nerves
(of pudendal nerve)

Internal pudendal
vein and artery

External anal sphincter
muscle

Perineal branches
of posterior femoral
cutaneous nerve

Perineal nerves
(of pudendal nerve)

Perineal veins and artery

Ramus of ischium

Perineal fascia

Posterior scrotal branches
of perineal artery,
Perineal veins

Ischiococcygeus muscle
= Coccygeus muscle

Sacrotuberous ligament

Sacrospinous ligament

Pudendal nerve

Inferior rectal artery,
Gemellus superior muscle

Inferior gluteal nerve

Internal pudendal artery

Obturator internus muscle

Sciatic nerve

Posterior femoral
cutaneous nerve

Gemellus inferior muscle

Sacrotuberous ligament

Perineal nerves

Dorsal artery, nerve of penis

Ischial tuberosity

Perineal branches
of post. fem. cut. nerve

Perineal membrane,
Superficial transverse
perineal muscle
(transected)

Perineal artery

Ischiocavernosus muscle

Bulbospongiosus muscle

Posterior scrotal nerves

Corpus cavernosum penis

279 Blood vessels and nerves
of the perineal region of a male (70%)
Inferior aspect

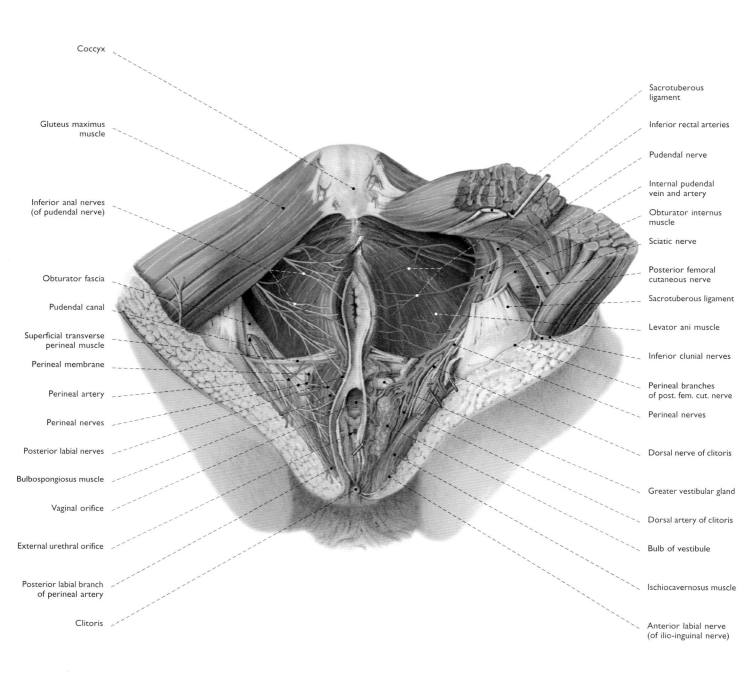

Coccyx

Gluteus maximus
muscle

Inferior anal nerves
(of pudendal nerve)

Obturator fascia

Pudendal canal

Superficial transverse
perineal muscle

Perineal membrane

Perineal artery

Perineal nerves

Posterior labial nerves

Bulbospongiosus muscle

Vaginal orifice

External urethral orifice

Posterior labial branch
of perineal artery

Clitoris

Sacrotuberous
ligament

Inferior rectal arteries

Pudendal nerve

Internal pudendal
vein and artery

Obturator internus
muscle

Sciatic nerve

Posterior femoral
cutaneous nerve

Sacrotuberous ligament

Levator ani muscle

Inferior clunial nerves

Perineal branches
of post. fem. cut. nerve

Perineal nerves

Dorsal nerve of clitoris

Greater vestibular gland

Dorsal artery of clitoris

Bulb of vestibule

Ischiocavernosus muscle

Anterior labial nerve
(of ilio-inguinal nerve)

280   Blood vessels and nerves
of the perineal region of a female (70%)
Inferior aspect

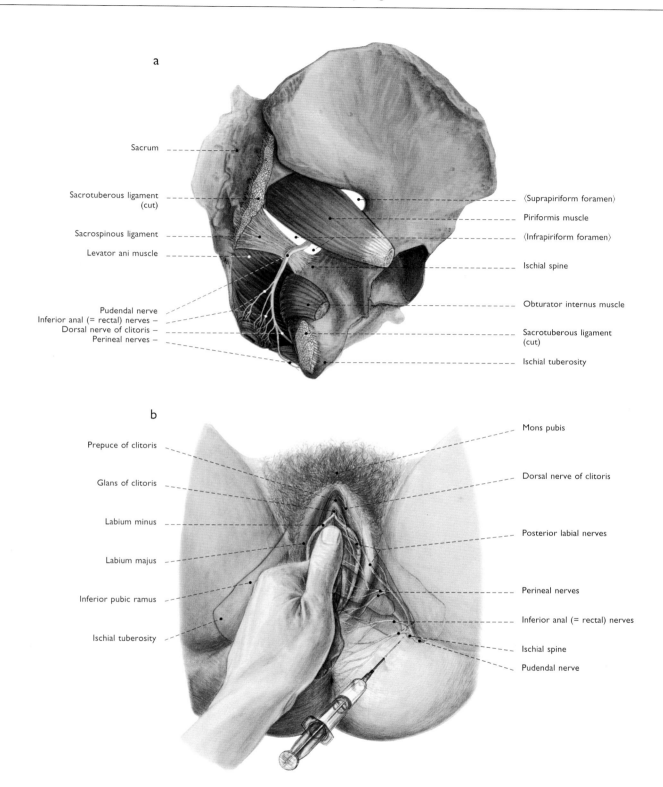

a

Sacrum

Sacrotuberous ligament (cut)

Sacrospinous ligament

Levator ani muscle

Pudendal nerve
Inferior anal (= rectal) nerves –
Dorsal nerve of clitoris –
Perineal nerves –

⟨Suprapiriform foramen⟩

Piriformis muscle

⟨Infrapiriform foramen⟩

Ischial spine

Obturator internus muscle

Sacrotuberous ligament (cut)

Ischial tuberosity

b

Prepuce of clitoris

Glans of clitoris

Labium minus

Labium majus

Inferior pubic ramus

Ischial tuberosity

Mons pubis

Dorsal nerve of clitoris

Posterior labial nerves

Perineal nerves

Inferior anal (= rectal) nerves

Ischial spine

Pudendal nerve

281 Nerves of the perineal region of a female (40%)
    a Course of the right pudendal nerve, right dorsolateral aspect
    b Anesthesia of the pudendal nerve on the left side of the body,
       schematic representation, inferior aspect

Central Nervous System

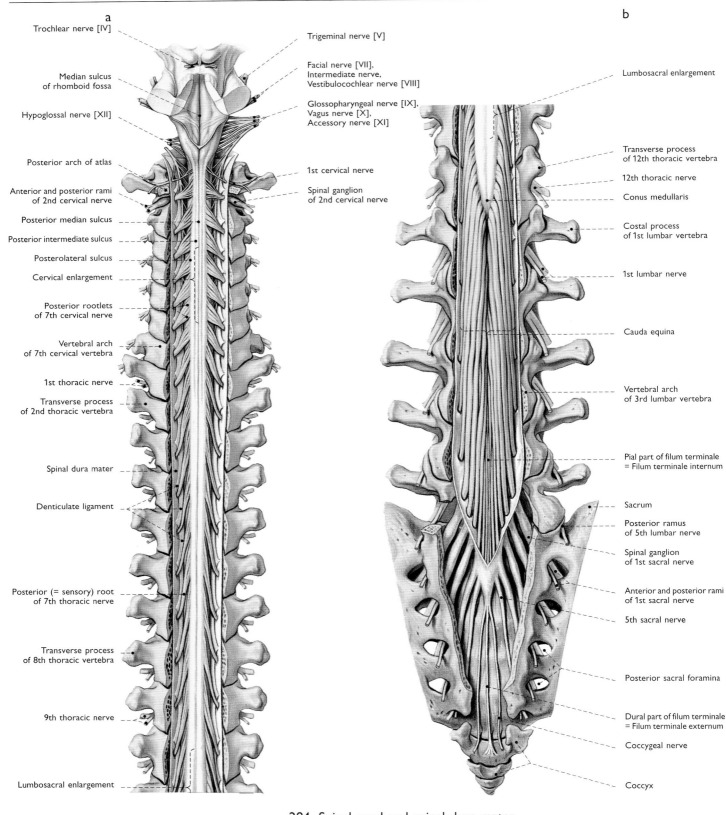

a

Trochlear nerve [IV]

Median sulcus
of rhomboid fossa

Hypoglossal nerve [XII]

Posterior arch of atlas

Anterior and posterior rami
of 2nd cervical nerve

Posterior median sulcus

Posterior intermediate sulcus

Posterolateral sulcus

Cervical enlargement

Posterior rootlets
of 7th cervical nerve

Vertebral arch
of 7th cervical vertebra

1st thoracic nerve

Transverse process
of 2nd thoracic vertebra

Spinal dura mater

Denticulate ligament

Posterior (= sensory) root
of 7th thoracic nerve

Transverse process
of 8th thoracic vertebra

9th thoracic nerve

Lumbosacral enlargement

Trigeminal nerve [V]

Facial nerve [VII],
Intermediate nerve,
Vestibulocochlear nerve [VIII]

Glossopharyngeal nerve [IX],
Vagus nerve [X],
Accessory nerve [XI]

1st cervical nerve

Spinal ganglion
of 2nd cervical nerve

b

Lumbosacral enlargement

Transverse process
of 12th thoracic vertebra

12th thoracic nerve

Conus medullaris

Costal process
of 1st lumbar vertebra

1st lumbar nerve

Cauda equina

Vertebral arch
of 3rd lumbar vertebra

Pial part of filum terminale
= Filum terminale internum

Sacrum

Posterior ramus
of 5th lumbar nerve

Spinal ganglion
of 1st sacral nerve

Anterior and posterior rami
of 1st sacral nerve

5th sacral nerve

Posterior sacral foramina

Dural part of filum terminale
= Filum terminale externum

Coccygeal nerve

Coccyx

284 Spinal cord and spinal dura mater
     in the vertebral canal (50%)
     The vertebral canal was opened dorsally.
     Dorsal aspect
   a Spinal cord
   b Cauda equina

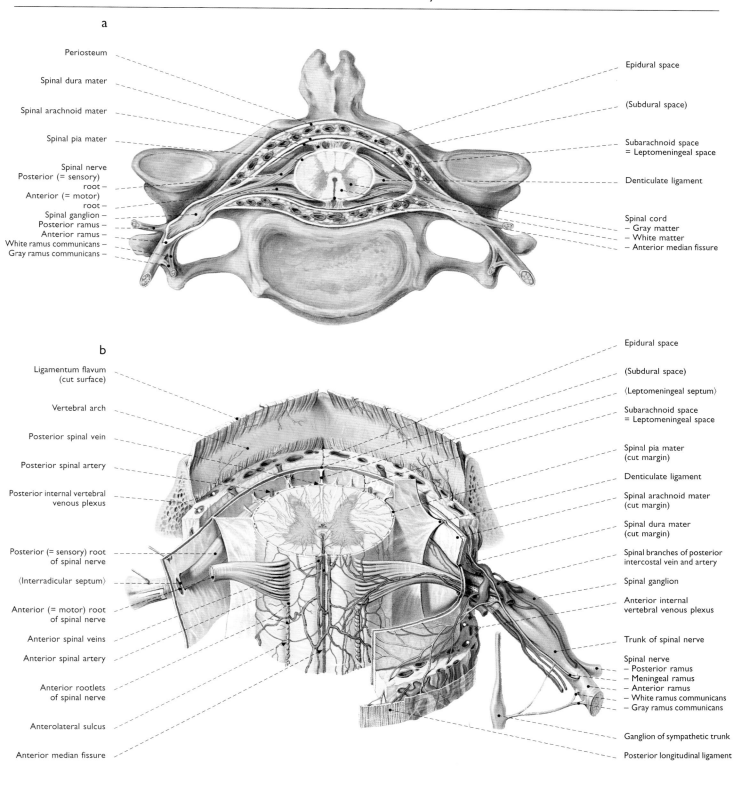

a

Periosteum
Spinal dura mater
Spinal arachnoid mater
Spinal pia mater
Spinal nerve
Posterior (= sensory) root
Anterior (= motor) root
Spinal ganglion
Posterior ramus
Anterior ramus
White ramus communicans
Gray ramus communicans

Epidural space
(Subdural space)
Subarachnoid space
= Leptomeningeal space
Denticulate ligament
Spinal cord
– Gray matter
– White matter
– Anterior median fissure

b

Ligamentum flavum (cut surface)
Vertebral arch
Posterior spinal vein
Posterior spinal artery
Posterior internal vertebral venous plexus
Posterior (= sensory) root of spinal nerve
⟨Interradicular septum⟩
Anterior (= motor) root of spinal nerve
Anterior spinal veins
Anterior spinal artery
Anterior rootlets of spinal nerve
Anterolateral sulcus
Anterior median fissure

Epidural space
(Subdural space)
⟨Leptomeningeal septum⟩
Subarachnoid space = Leptomeningeal space
Spinal pia mater (cut margin)
Denticulate ligament
Spinal arachnoid mater (cut margin)
Spinal dura mater (cut margin)
Spinal branches of posterior intercostal vein and artery
Spinal ganglion
Anterior internal vertebral venous plexus
Trunk of spinal nerve
Spinal nerve
– Posterior ramus
– Meningeal ramus
– Anterior ramus
– White ramus communicans
– Gray ramus communicans
Ganglion of sympathetic trunk
Posterior longitudinal ligament

285 Spinal cord, meninges, and roots of spinal nerve
Transverse sections of the spinal cord and the roots of spinal nerve
a Section through the vertebral canal of cervical spine (230%), superior aspect
b Schematized three-dimensional representation after removal of vertebral bodies and transverse processes of vertebrae (400%), ventrocranial aspect

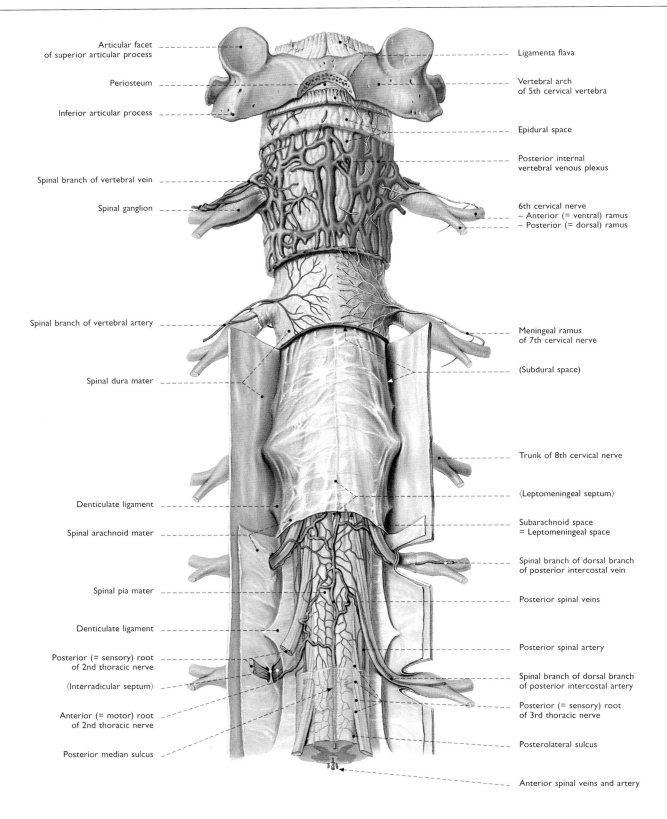

Articular facet
of superior articular process

Periosteum

Inferior articular process

Spinal branch of vertebral vein

Spinal ganglion

Spinal branch of vertebral artery

Spinal dura mater

Denticulate ligament

Spinal arachnoid mater

Spinal pia mater

Denticulate ligament

Posterior (= sensory) root
of 2nd thoracic nerve

⟨Interradicular septum⟩

Anterior (= motor) root
of 2nd thoracic nerve

Posterior median sulcus

Ligamenta flava

Vertebral arch
of 5th cervical vertebra

Epidural space

Posterior internal
vertebral venous plexus

6th cervical nerve
– Anterior (= ventral) ramus
– Posterior (= dorsal) ramus

Meningeal ramus
of 7th cervical nerve

(Subdural space)

Trunk of 8th cervical nerve

⟨Leptomeningeal septum⟩

Subarachnoid space
= Leptomeningeal space

Spinal branch of dorsal branch
of posterior intercostal vein

Posterior spinal veins

Posterior spinal artery

Spinal branch of dorsal branch
of posterior intercostal artery

Posterior (= sensory) root
of 3rd thoracic nerve

Posterolateral sulcus

Anterior spinal veins and artery

286 Spinal cord, meninges, and spinal nerves
The investing structures of the spinal cord and
the blood vessels are demonstrated in layers (150%).
Dorsal aspect

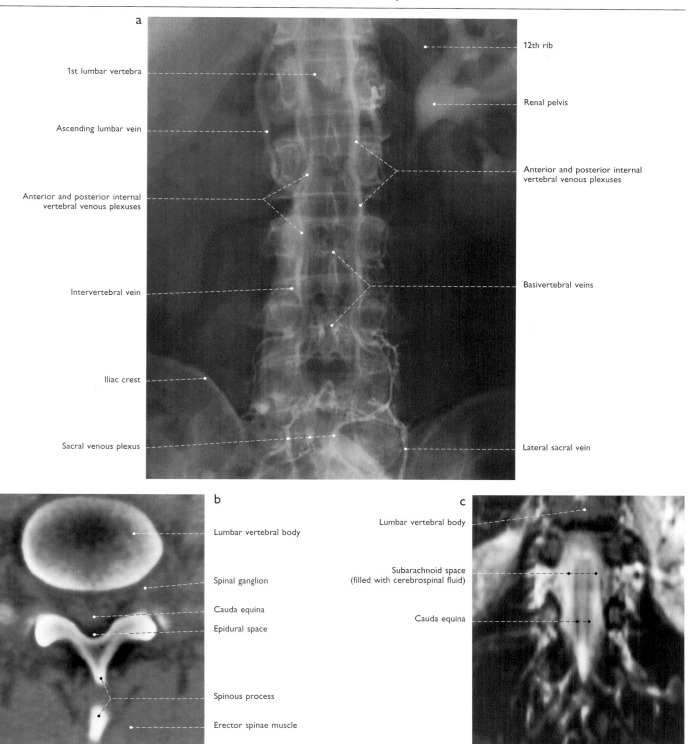

a

12th rib

1st lumbar vertebra

Renal pelvis

Ascending lumbar vein

Anterior and posterior internal
vertebral venous plexuses

Anterior and posterior internal
vertebral venous plexuses

Basivertebral veins

Intervertebral vein

Iliac crest

Sacral venous plexus

Lateral sacral vein

b

Lumbar vertebral body

Spinal ganglion

Cauda equina

Epidural space

Spinous process

Erector spinae muscle

c

Lumbar vertebral body

Subarachnoid space
(filled with cerebrospinal fluid)

Cauda equina

287   Veins of the vertebral column and cauda equina

a   Lumbar venogram and filling of the internal vertebral venous plexuses,
     postero-anterior radiograph (60%)
b   Transverse computed tomogram (CT) through
     the fifth lumbar vertebra and the cauda equina (80%),
     inferior aspect
c   Coronal magnetic resonance image (MRI, T$_2$-weighted)
     of the lumbar spine (60%)

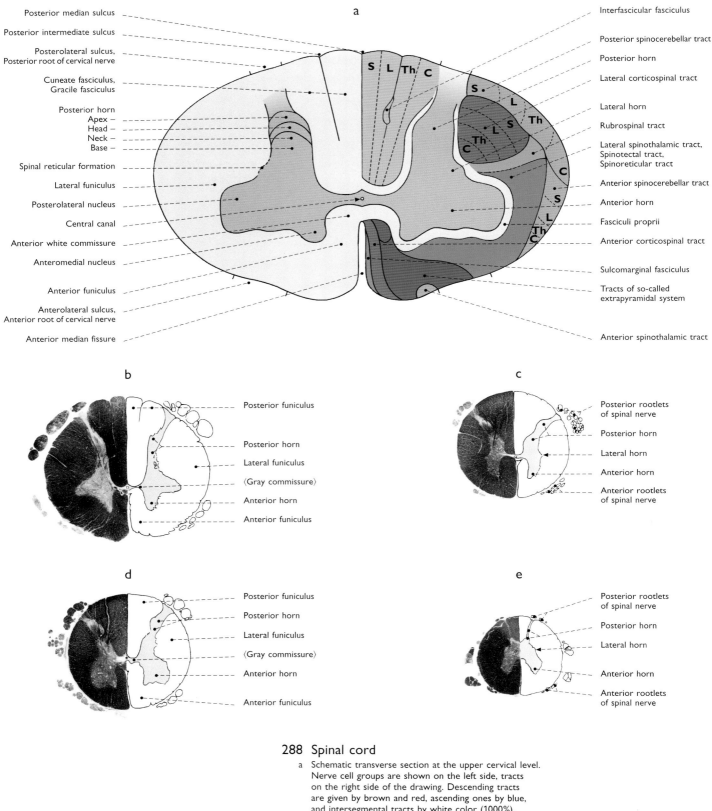

a

Posterior median sulcus

Posterior intermediate sulcus

Posterolateral sulcus,
Posterior root of cervical nerve

Cuneate fasciculus,
Gracile fasciculus

Posterior horn
Apex —
Head —
Neck —
Base —

Spinal reticular formation

Lateral funiculus

Posterolateral nucleus

Central canal

Anterior white commissure

Anteromedial nucleus

Anterior funiculus

Anterolateral sulcus,
Anterior root of cervical nerve

Anterior median fissure

Interfascicular fasciculus

Posterior spinocerebellar tract

Posterior horn

Lateral corticospinal tract

Lateral horn

Rubrospinal tract

Lateral spinothalamic tract,
Spinotectal tract,
Spinoreticular tract

Anterior spinocerebellar tract

Anterior horn

Fasciculi proprii

Anterior corticospinal tract

Sulcomarginal fasciculus

Tracts of so-called
extrapyramidal system

Anterior spinothalamic tract

b

Posterior funiculus

Posterior horn

Lateral funiculus

⟨Gray commissure⟩

Anterior horn

Anterior funiculus

c

Posterior rootlets
of spinal nerve

Posterior horn

Lateral horn

Anterior horn

Anterior rootlets
of spinal nerve

d

Posterior funiculus

Posterior horn

Lateral funiculus

⟨Gray commissure⟩

Anterior horn

Anterior funiculus

e

Posterior rootlets
of spinal nerve

Posterior horn

Lateral horn

Anterior horn

Anterior rootlets
of spinal nerve

288 Spinal cord

a Schematic transverse section at the upper cervical level.
   Nerve cell groups are shown on the left side, tracts
   on the right side of the drawing. Descending tracts
   are given by brown and red, ascending ones by blue,
   and intersegmental tracts by white color (1000%).
b–e Transverse sections of the spinal cord (400%)
   at the levels of the
b cervical part
c thoracic part
d lumbar part
e sacral part

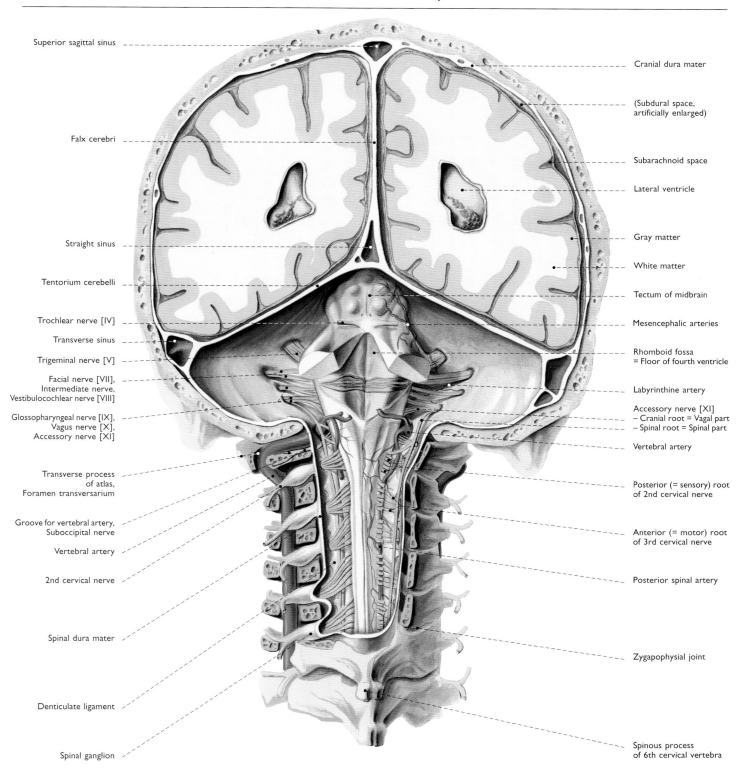

Superior sagittal sinus

Falx cerebri

Straight sinus

Tentorium cerebelli

Trochlear nerve [IV]

Transverse sinus

Trigeminal nerve [V]

Facial nerve [VII],
Intermediate nerve,
Vestibulocochlear nerve [VIII]

Glossopharyngeal nerve [IX],
Vagus nerve [X],
Accessory nerve [XI]

Transverse process
of atlas,
Foramen transversarium

Groove for vertebral artery,
Suboccipital nerve

Vertebral artery

2nd cervical nerve

Spinal dura mater

Denticulate ligament

Spinal ganglion

Cranial dura mater

(Subdural space,
artificially enlarged)

Subarachnoid space

Lateral ventricle

Gray matter

White matter

Tectum of midbrain

Mesencephalic arteries

Rhomboid fossa
= Floor of fourth ventricle

Labyrinthine artery

Accessory nerve [XI]
– Cranial root = Vagal part
– Spinal root = Spinal part

Vertebral artery

Posterior (= sensory) root
of 2nd cervical nerve

Anterior (= motor) root
of 3rd cervical nerve

Posterior spinal artery

Zygapophysial joint

Spinous process
of 6th cervical vertebra

289 Brainstem and dura mater (75%)
Coronal section through the head and neck.
The vertebral arches were removed. Dorsal aspect

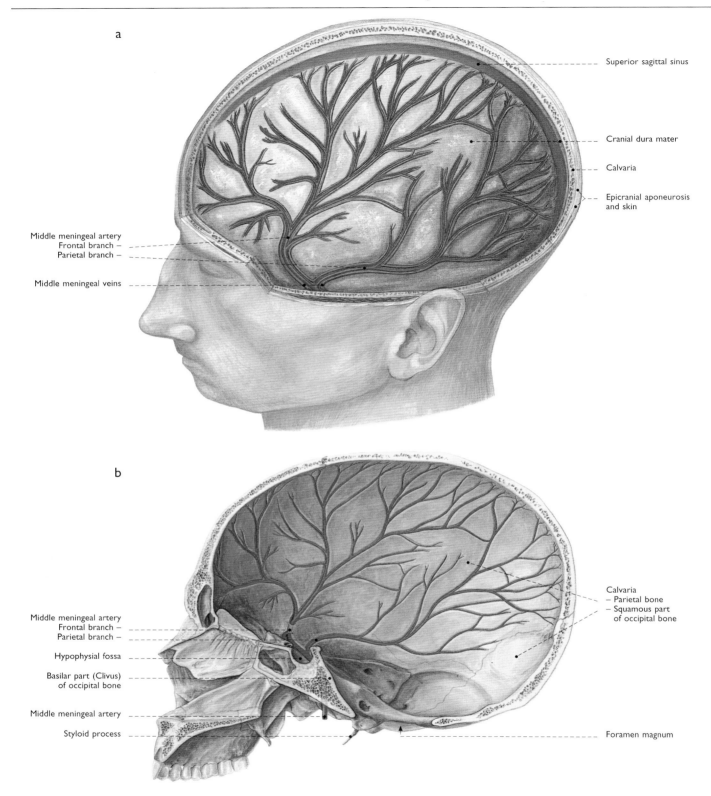

a

Superior sagittal sinus

Cranial dura mater

Calvaria

Epicranial aponeurosis
and skin

Middle meningeal artery
Frontal branch −
Parietal branch −

Middle meningeal veins

b

Middle meningeal artery
Frontal branch −
Parietal branch −

Hypophysial fossa

Basilar part (Clivus)
of occipital bone

Middle meningeal artery

Styloid process

Calvaria
− Parietal bone
− Squamous part
of occipital bone

Foramen magnum

290 Meningeal arteries (50%)

  a   Meningeal arteries and veins apposed externally
      to the cranial dura mater. The lateral bones of cranium
      were removed. Left parietolateral aspect
  b   Meningeal arteries lying in osseous grooves of the lateral bones
      of cranium, medial aspect of the right half of cranium

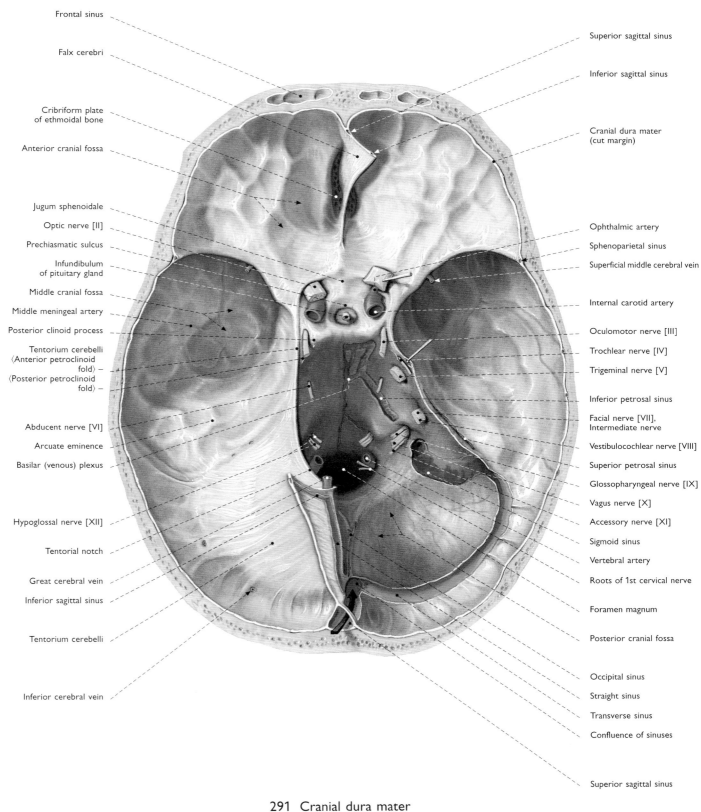

Frontal sinus

Falx cerebri

Cribriform plate
of ethmoidal bone

Anterior cranial fossa

Jugum sphenoidale

Optic nerve [II]

Prechiasmatic sulcus

Infundibulum
of pituitary gland

Middle cranial fossa

Middle meningeal artery

Posterior clinoid process

Tentorium cerebelli
⟨Anterior petroclinoid
fold⟩ —
⟨Posterior petroclinoid
fold⟩ —

Abducent nerve [VI]

Arcuate eminence

Basilar (venous) plexus

Hypoglossal nerve [XII]

Tentorial notch

Great cerebral vein

Inferior sagittal sinus

Tentorium cerebelli

Inferior cerebral vein

Superior sagittal sinus

Inferior sagittal sinus

Cranial dura mater
(cut margin)

Ophthalmic artery

Sphenoparietal sinus

Superficial middle cerebral vein

Internal carotid artery

Oculomotor nerve [III]

Trochlear nerve [IV]

Trigeminal nerve [V]

Inferior petrosal sinus

Facial nerve [VII],
Intermediate nerve

Vestibulocochlear nerve [VIII]

Superior petrosal sinus

Glossopharyngeal nerve [IX]

Vagus nerve [X]

Accessory nerve [XI]

Sigmoid sinus

Vertebral artery

Roots of 1st cervical nerve

Foramen magnum

Posterior cranial fossa

Occipital sinus

Straight sinus

Transverse sinus

Confluence of sinuses

Superior sagittal sinus

**291   Cranial dura mater
and dural venous sinuses** (80%)

The right half of the tentorium cerebelli was removed,
as well as the falx cerebri except for its anterior and
posterior attachments. Some of the dural venous sinuses
were opened. Superior aspect

a

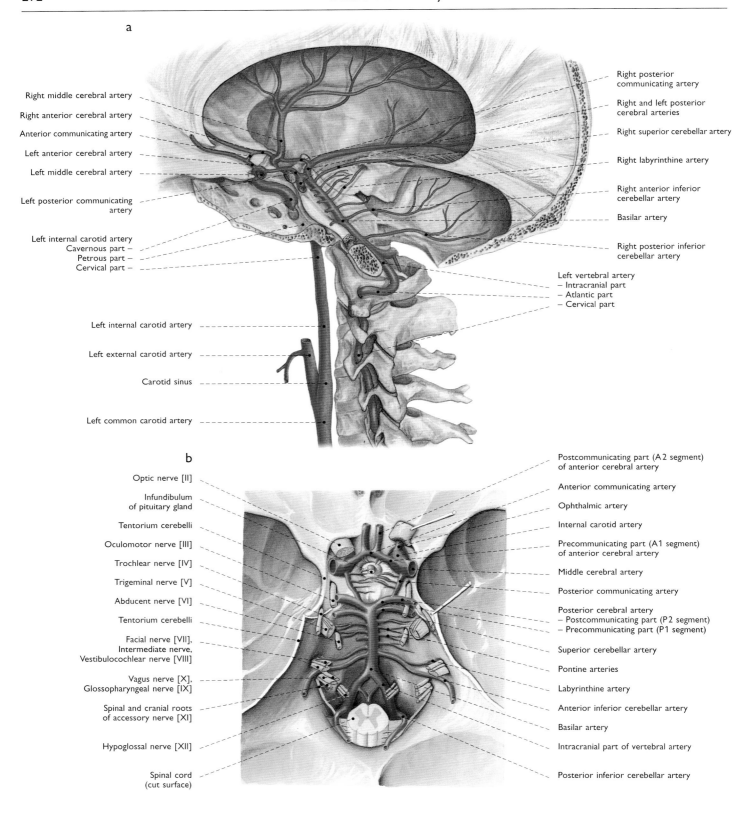

Right middle cerebral artery

Right anterior cerebral artery

Anterior communicating artery

Left anterior cerebral artery

Left middle cerebral artery

Left posterior communicating
artery

Left internal carotid artery
Cavernous part –
Petrous part –
Cervical part –

Left internal carotid artery

Left external carotid artery

Carotid sinus

Left common carotid artery

Right posterior
communicating artery

Right and left posterior
cerebral arteries

Right superior cerebellar artery

Right labyrinthine artery

Right anterior inferior
cerebellar artery

Basilar artery

Right posterior inferior
cerebellar artery

Left vertebral artery
– Intracranial part
– Atlantic part
– Cervical part

b

Optic nerve [II]

Infundibulum
of pituitary gland

Tentorium cerebelli

Oculomotor nerve [III]

Trochlear nerve [IV]

Trigeminal nerve [V]

Abducent nerve [VI]

Tentorium cerebelli

Facial nerve [VII],
Intermediate nerve,
Vestibulocochlear nerve [VIII]

Vagus nerve [X],
Glossopharyngeal nerve [IX]

Spinal and cranial roots
of accessory nerve [XI]

Hypoglossal nerve [XII]

Spinal cord
(cut surface)

Postcommunicating part (A2 segment)
of anterior cerebral artery

Anterior communicating artery

Ophthalmic artery

Internal carotid artery

Precommunicating part (A1 segment)
of anterior cerebral artery

Middle cerebral artery

Posterior communicating artery

Posterior cerebral artery
– Postcommunicating part (P2 segment)
– Precommunicating part (P1 segment)

Superior cerebellar artery

Pontine arteries

Labyrinthine artery

Anterior inferior cerebellar artery

Basilar artery

Intracranial part of vertebral artery

Posterior inferior cerebellar artery

292 Cranial dura mater and cerebral arterial circle
    a Internal carotid and vertebral arteries, cerebral arterial circle (60%),
       sagittal section to the left of the median plane,
       parietomedial aspect of the right half
    b Cerebral arterial circle (90%), superior aspect

a

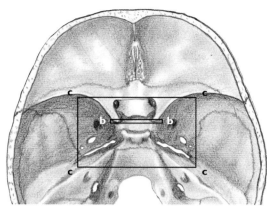

b

Infundibular recess,
Infundibulum of pituitary gland

Diaphragma sellae

Neurohypophysis

Adenohypophysis

Intercavernous sinus

Cavernous sinus

Sphenoidal sinuses

Septum
of sphenoidal sinuses

Anterior clinoid process

Cavernous sinus

Cavernous part
of internal carotid artery

Oculomotor nerve [III]

Trochlear nerve [IV]

Abducent nerve [VI]

Ophthalmic nerve [V₁]

Maxillary nerve [V₂]

c

Optic nerve [II]

Optic chiasm

Internal carotid artery

Ophthalmic nerve [V₁]

Infundibulum of pituitary gland,
Diaphragma sellae

Maxillary nerve [V₂]

Optic tract

Mandibular nerve [V₃]

Trigeminal ganglion

Trigeminal nerve [V]

Basilar (venous) plexus

Clivus

Anterior clinoid process
(transected)

Ophthalmic artery

Trochlear nerve [IV]

Ophthalmic nerve [V₁]

Tentorial nerve
(of ophthalmic nerve)

Oculomotor nerve [III]

Tentorium cerebelli,
⟨Anterior petroclinoid fold⟩

Dorsum sellae

⟨Posterior petroclinoid fold⟩

Trochlear nerve [IV]

Trigeminal nerve [V]

Abducent nerve [VI]

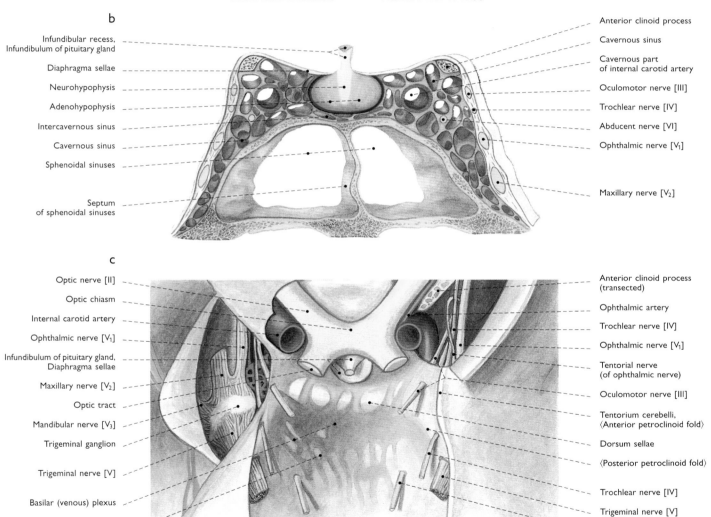

293   Cavernous sinus

a   Internal surface of the cranial base. The section planes
of figs. b and c are indicated.

b   Coronal section through the cavernous sinuses, the pituitary gland,
and the sphenoidal sinuses (300%)

c   View of central areas of the cranial base. On the left side,
the cranial dura mater is turned upwards, the cavernous sinus opened,
and the trigeminal ganglion exposed (200%). Superior aspect

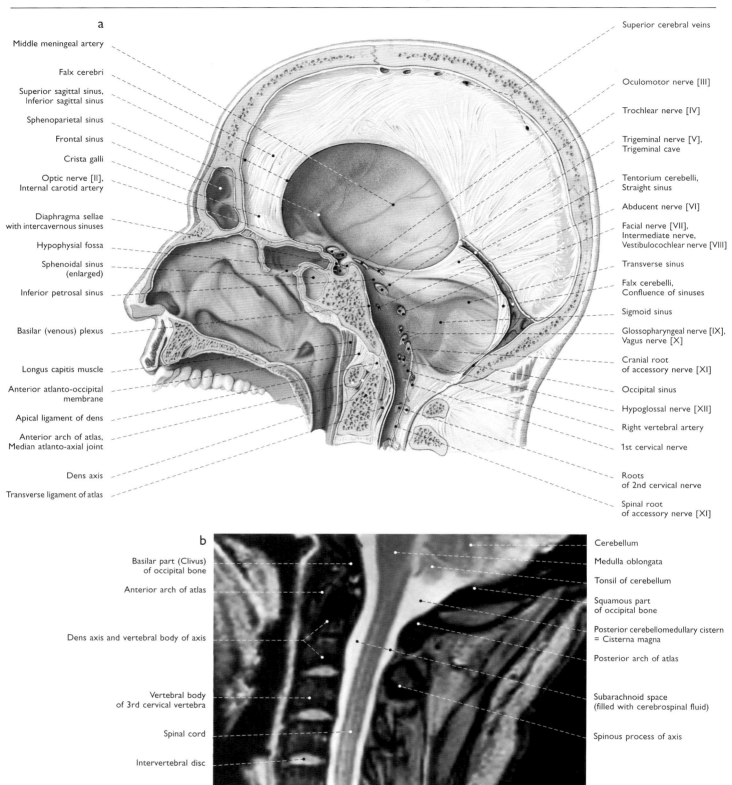

a

Middle meningeal artery

Falx cerebri

Superior sagittal sinus,
Inferior sagittal sinus

Sphenoparietal sinus

Frontal sinus

Crista galli

Optic nerve [II],
Internal carotid artery

Diaphragma sellae
with intercavernous sinuses

Hypophysial fossa

Sphenoidal sinus
(enlarged)

Inferior petrosal sinus

Basilar (venous) plexus

Longus capitis muscle

Anterior atlanto-occipital
membrane

Apical ligament of dens

Anterior arch of atlas,
Median atlanto-axial joint

Dens axis

Transverse ligament of atlas

Superior cerebral veins

Oculomotor nerve [III]

Trochlear nerve [IV]

Trigeminal nerve [V],
Trigeminal cave

Tentorium cerebelli,
Straight sinus

Abducent nerve [VI]

Facial nerve [VII],
Intermediate nerve,
Vestibulocochlear nerve [VIII]

Transverse sinus

Falx cerebelli,
Confluence of sinuses

Sigmoid sinus

Glossopharyngeal nerve [IX],
Vagus nerve [X]

Cranial root
of accessory nerve [XI]

Occipital sinus

Hypoglossal nerve [XII]

Right vertebral artery

1st cervical nerve

Roots
of 2nd cervical nerve

Spinal root
of accessory nerve [XI]

b

Basilar part (Clivus)
of occipital bone

Anterior arch of atlas

Dens axis and vertebral body of axis

Vertebral body
of 3rd cervical vertebra

Spinal cord

Intervertebral disc

Cerebellum

Medulla oblongata

Tonsil of cerebellum

Squamous part
of occipital bone

Posterior cerebellomedullary cistern
= Cisterna magna

Posterior arch of atlas

Subarachnoid space
(filled with cerebrospinal fluid)

Spinous process of axis

294 Cranial cavity and meninges

a Cranial cavity sectioned slightly to the left
of the median plane. The nasal septum was removed (50%).
Medial aspect of the right half

b Sagittal magnetic resonance image (MRI, T$_2$-weighted)
of the brainstem, the posterior cerebellomedullary cistern,
and adjacent structures (70%)

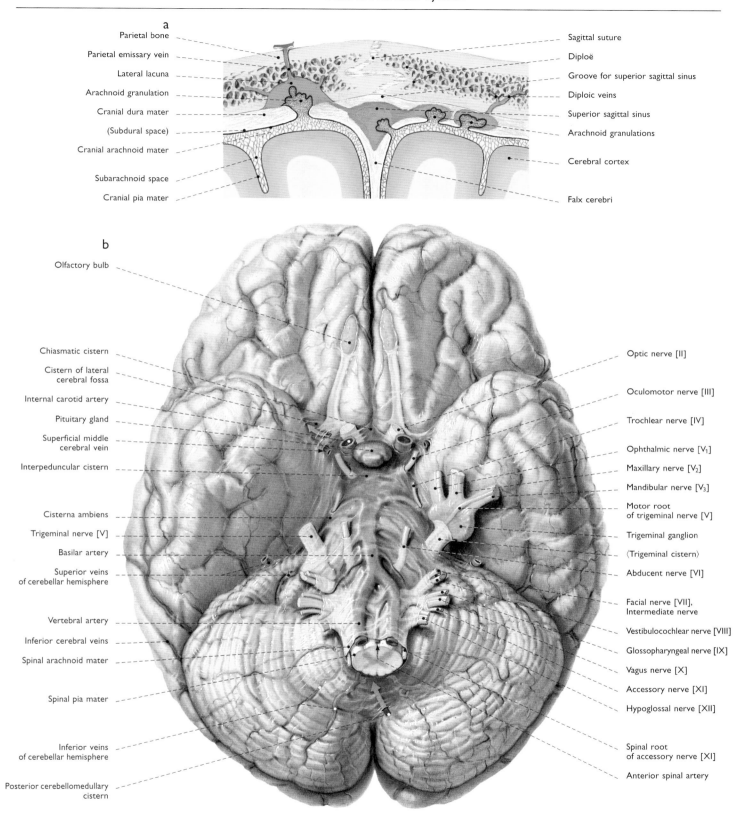

a

Parietal bone

Parietal emissary vein

Lateral lacuna

Arachnoid granulation

Cranial dura mater

(Subdural space)

Cranial arachnoid mater

Subarachnoid space

Cranial pia mater

Sagittal suture

Diploë

Groove for superior sagittal sinus

Diploic veins

Superior sagittal sinus

Arachnoid granulations

Cerebral cortex

Falx cerebri

b

Olfactory bulb

Chiasmatic cistern

Cistern of lateral cerebral fossa

Internal carotid artery

Pituitary gland

Superficial middle cerebral vein

Interpeduncular cistern

Cisterna ambiens

Trigeminal nerve [V]

Basilar artery

Superior veins of cerebellar hemisphere

Vertebral artery

Inferior cerebral veins

Spinal arachnoid mater

Spinal pia mater

Inferior veins of cerebellar hemisphere

Posterior cerebellomedullary cistern

Optic nerve [II]

Oculomotor nerve [III]

Trochlear nerve [IV]

Ophthalmic nerve [V₁]

Maxillary nerve [V₂]

Mandibular nerve [V₃]

Motor root of trigeminal nerve [V]

Trigeminal ganglion

⟨Trigeminal cistern⟩

Abducent nerve [VI]

Facial nerve [VII], Intermediate nerve

Vestibulocochlear nerve [VIII]

Glossopharyngeal nerve [IX]

Vagus nerve [X]

Accessory nerve [XI]

Hypoglossal nerve [XII]

Spinal root of accessory nerve [XI]

Anterior spinal artery

295 Brain and meninges (100%)

a   Meninges on the cerebral vault, schematic coronal section
b   Brain with leptomeninx (100%), inferior aspect

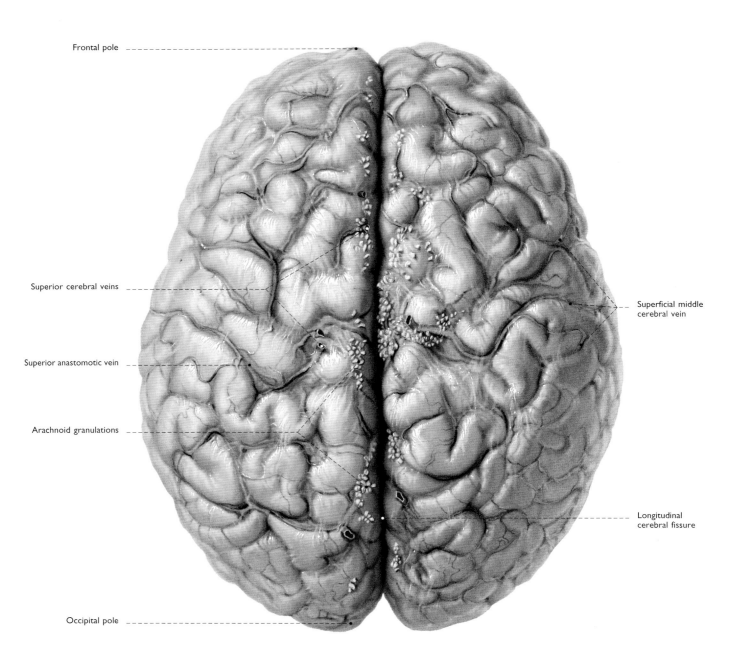

Frontal pole

Superior cerebral veins

Superior anastomotic vein

Arachnoid granulations

Occipital pole

Superficial middle cerebral vein

Longitudinal cerebral fissure

296 Brain with leptomeninx (100%)
Superior aspect

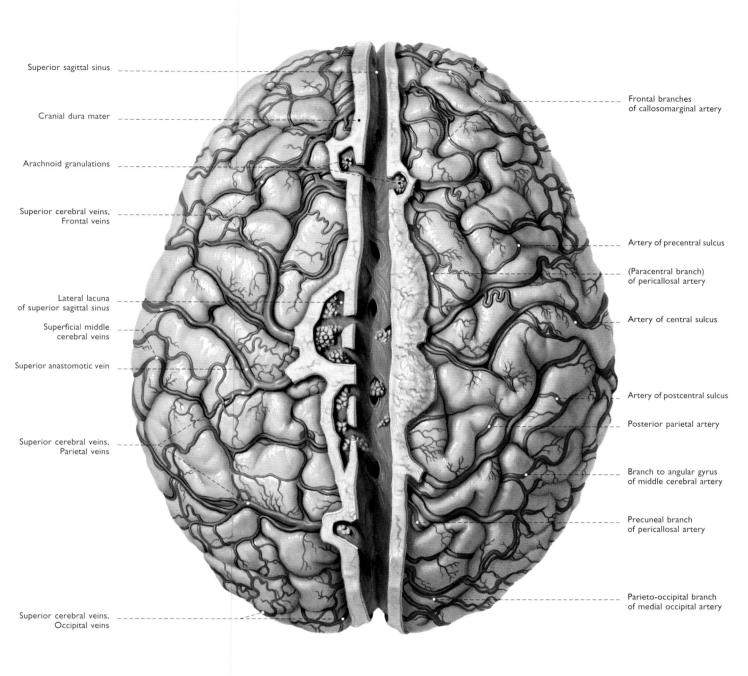

Superior sagittal sinus

Cranial dura mater

Arachnoid granulations

Superior cerebral veins,
Frontal veins

Lateral lacuna
of superior sagittal sinus

Superficial middle
cerebral veins

Superior anastomotic vein

Superior cerebral veins,
Parietal veins

Superior cerebral veins,
Occipital veins

Frontal branches
of callosomarginal artery

Artery of precentral sulcus

(Paracentral branch)
of pericallosal artery

Artery of central sulcus

Artery of postcentral sulcus

Posterior parietal artery

Branch to angular gyrus
of middle cerebral artery

Precuneal branch
of pericallosal artery

Parieto-occipital branch
of medial occipital artery

297   Superficial arteries and veins
of the cerebral hemispheres (100%)
Superior aspect

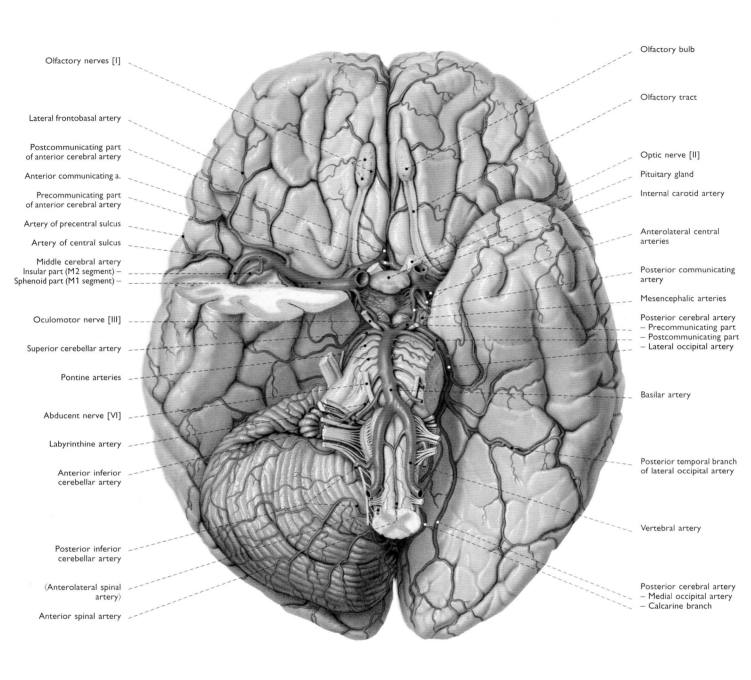

Olfactory nerves [I]

Lateral frontobasal artery

Postcommunicating part
of anterior cerebral artery

Anterior communicating a.

Precommunicating part
of anterior cerebral artery

Artery of precentral sulcus

Artery of central sulcus

Middle cerebral artery
Insular part (M2 segment) –
Sphenoid part (M1 segment) –

Oculomotor nerve [III]

Superior cerebellar artery

Pontine arteries

Abducent nerve [VI]

Labyrinthine artery

Anterior inferior
cerebellar artery

Posterior inferior
cerebellar artery

⟨Anterolateral spinal
artery⟩

Anterior spinal artery

Olfactory bulb

Olfactory tract

Optic nerve [II]

Pituitary gland

Internal carotid artery

Anterolateral central
arteries

Posterior communicating
artery

Mesencephalic arteries

Posterior cerebral artery
– Precommunicating part
– Postcommunicating part
– Lateral occipital artery

Basilar artery

Posterior temporal branch
of lateral occipital artery

Vertebral artery

Posterior cerebral artery
– Medial occipital artery
– Calcarine branch

298 Arteries of the brain (100%)
Inferior aspect

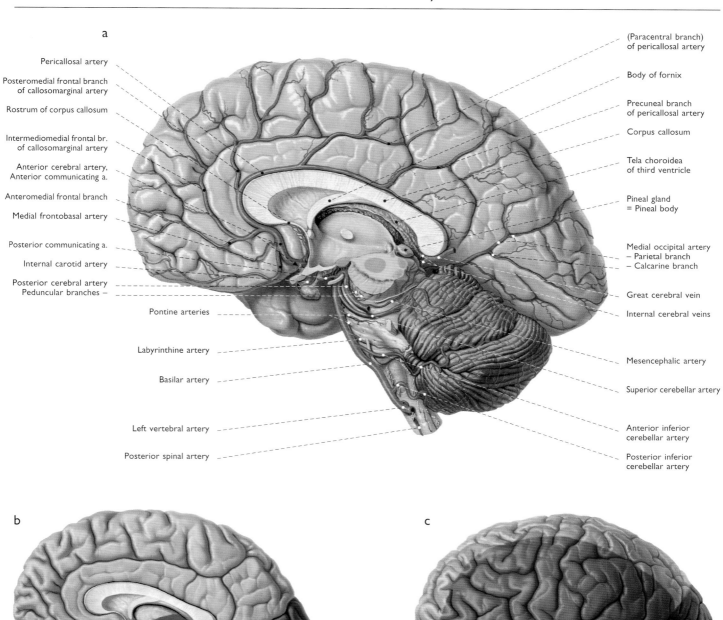

a

Pericallosal artery

Posteromedial frontal branch
of callosomarginal artery

Rostrum of corpus callosum

Intermediomedial frontal br.
of callosomarginal artery

Anterior cerebral artery,
Anterior communicating a.

Anteromedial frontal branch

Medial frontobasal artery

Posterior communicating a.

Internal carotid artery

Posterior cerebral artery
Peduncular branches —

Pontine arteries

Labyrinthine artery

Basilar artery

Left vertebral artery

Posterior spinal artery

(Paracentral branch)
of pericallosal artery

Body of fornix

Precuneal branch
of pericallosal artery

Corpus callosum

Tela choroidea
of third ventricle

Pineal gland
= Pineal body

Medial occipital artery
– Parietal branch
– Calcarine branch

Great cerebral vein

Internal cerebral veins

Mesencephalic artery

Superior cerebellar artery

Anterior inferior
cerebellar artery

Posterior inferior
cerebellar artery

b

c

| Anterior cerebral artery | Middle cerebral artery | Posterior cerebral artery |

299 Arteries of the brain

a Medial aspect of the right cerebral hemisphere and lateral aspect
   of the left cerebellar hemisphere (80%)

b, c Circulation areas of the anterior (**yellow**), middle (**red**),
      and posterior (**brown**) cerebral arteries at the cerebral cortex (50%)

b Medial aspect

c Lateral aspect

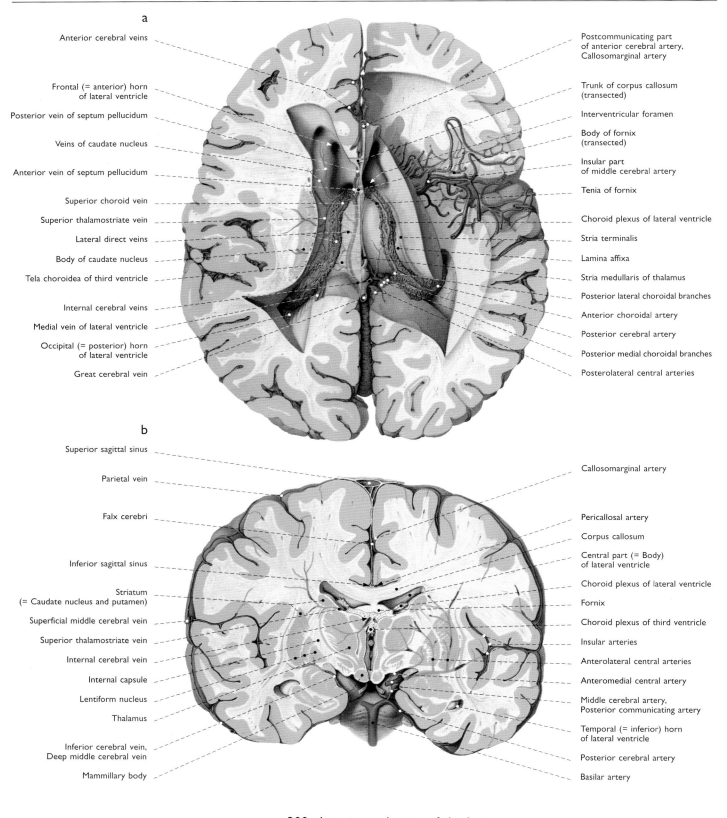

a

Anterior cerebral veins

Frontal (= anterior) horn of lateral ventricle

Posterior vein of septum pellucidum

Veins of caudate nucleus

Anterior vein of septum pellucidum

Superior choroid vein

Superior thalamostriate vein

Lateral direct veins

Body of caudate nucleus

Tela choroidea of third ventricle

Internal cerebral veins

Medial vein of lateral ventricle

Occipital (= posterior) horn of lateral ventricle

Great cerebral vein

Postcommunicating part of anterior cerebral artery, Callosomarginal artery

Trunk of corpus callosum (transected)

Interventricular foramen

Body of fornix (transected)

Insular part of middle cerebral artery

Tenia of fornix

Choroid plexus of lateral ventricle

Stria terminalis

Lamina affixa

Stria medullaris of thalamus

Posterior lateral choroidal branches

Anterior choroidal artery

Posterior cerebral artery

Posterior medial choroidal branches

Posterolateral central arteries

b

Superior sagittal sinus

Parietal vein

Falx cerebri

Inferior sagittal sinus

Striatum (= Caudate nucleus and putamen)

Superficial middle cerebral vein

Superior thalamostriate vein

Internal cerebral vein

Internal capsule

Lentiform nucleus

Thalamus

Inferior cerebral vein, Deep middle cerebral vein

Mammillary body

Callosomarginal artery

Pericallosal artery

Corpus callosum

Central part (= Body) of lateral ventricle

Choroid plexus of lateral ventricle

Fornix

Choroid plexus of third ventricle

Insular arteries

Anterolateral central arteries

Anteromedial central artery

Middle cerebral artery, Posterior communicating artery

Temporal (= inferior) horn of lateral ventricle

Posterior cerebral artery

Basilar artery

300   Arteries and veins of the brain (70%)

  a   Horizontal section through the upper parts of the lateral ventricle. The corpus callosum, the fornix, and parts of the cerebral hemispheres were removed. Superior aspect

  b   Coronal section at the level of the mammillary bodies, frontal aspect

a

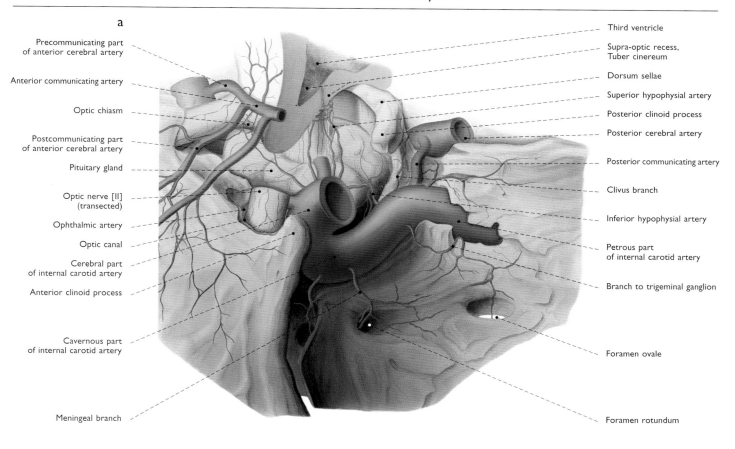

Precommunicating part
of anterior cerebral artery

Anterior communicating artery

Optic chiasm

Postcommunicating part
of anterior cerebral artery

Pituitary gland

Optic nerve [II]
(transected)

Ophthalmic artery

Optic canal

Cerebral part
of internal carotid artery

Anterior clinoid process

Cavernous part
of internal carotid artery

Meningeal branch

Third ventricle

Supra-optic recess,
Tuber cinereum

Dorsum sellae

Superior hypophysial artery

Posterior clinoid process

Posterior cerebral artery

Posterior communicating artery

Clivus branch

Inferior hypophysial artery

Petrous part
of internal carotid artery

Branch to trigeminal ganglion

Foramen ovale

Foramen rotundum

b

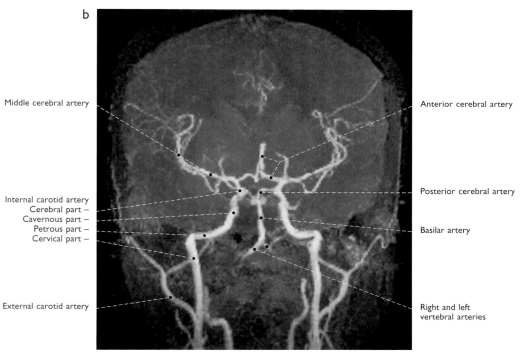

Middle cerebral artery

Internal carotid artery
Cerebral part –
Cavernous part –
Petrous part –
Cervical part –

External carotid artery

Anterior cerebral artery

Posterior cerebral artery

Basilar artery

Right and left
vertebral arteries

301   Arteries of the brain

a   Hypophysial arteries (300%), left superior aspect
b   Coronal magnetic resonance angiogram (MRA)
     of the arteries of brain (50%), frontal aspect

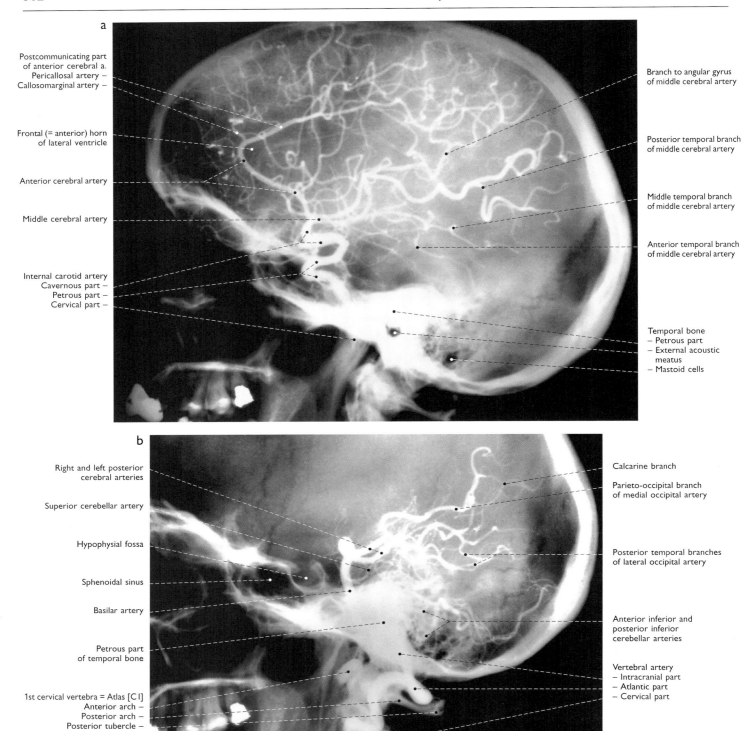

a

Postcommunicating part
of anterior cerebral a.
Pericallosal artery –
Callosomarginal artery –

Frontal (= anterior) horn
of lateral ventricle

Anterior cerebral artery

Middle cerebral artery

Internal carotid artery
Cavernous part –
Petrous part –
Cervical part –

Branch to angular gyrus
of middle cerebral artery

Posterior temporal branch
of middle cerebral artery

Middle temporal branch
of middle cerebral artery

Anterior temporal branch
of middle cerebral artery

Temporal bone
– Petrous part
– External acoustic
  meatus
– Mastoid cells

b

Right and left posterior
cerebral arteries

Superior cerebellar artery

Hypophysial fossa

Sphenoidal sinus

Basilar artery

Petrous part
of temporal bone

1st cervical vertebra = Atlas [C I]
Anterior arch –
Posterior arch –
Posterior tubercle –

Calcarine branch

Parieto-occipital branch
of medial occipital artery

Posterior temporal branches
of lateral occipital artery

Anterior inferior and
posterior inferior
cerebellar arteries

Vertebral artery
– Intracranial part
– Atlantic part
– Cervical part

302 Arteries of the brain (75%)

    Lateral radiographs
a Selective arteriogram of the internal carotid artery
b Selective arteriogram of the vertebral artery

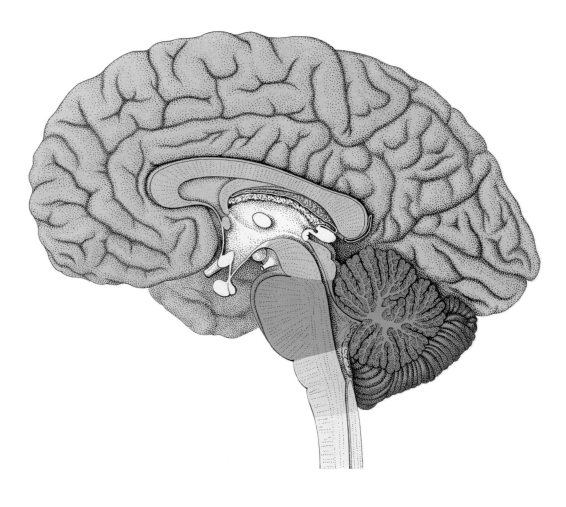

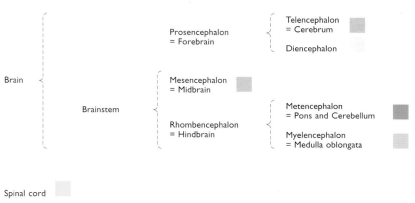

Brain

Prosencephalon = Forebrain

Telencephalon = Cerebrum

Diencephalon

Brainstem

Mesencephalon = Midbrain

Rhombencephalon = Hindbrain

Metencephalon = Pons and Cerebellum

Myelencephalon = Medulla oblongata

Spinal cord

303 Division of the central nervous system

Schematic representation of the right hemisphere,
medial aspect of a median section

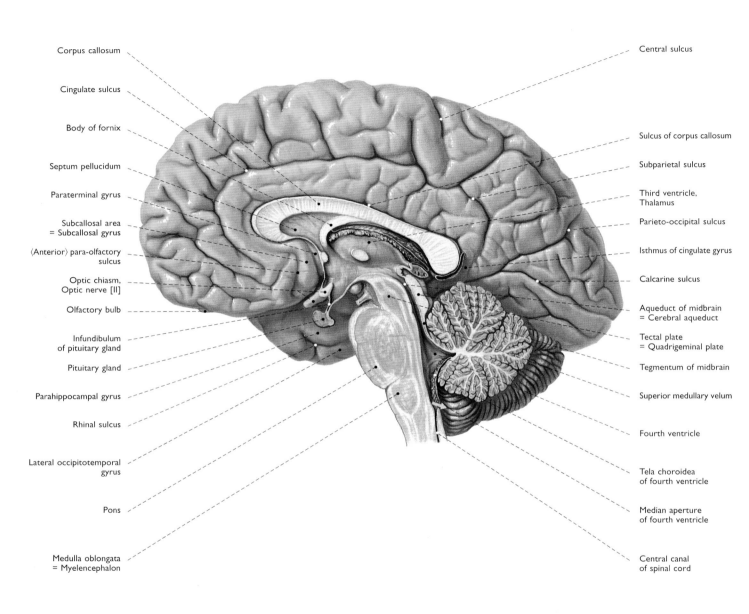

Corpus callosum

Cingulate sulcus

Body of fornix

Septum pellucidum

Paraterminal gyrus

Subcallosal area
= Subcallosal gyrus

(Anterior) para-olfactory
sulcus

Optic chiasm,
Optic nerve [II]

Olfactory bulb

Infundibulum
of pituitary gland

Pituitary gland

Parahippocampal gyrus

Rhinal sulcus

Lateral occipitotemporal
gyrus

Pons

Medulla oblongata
= Myelencephalon

Central sulcus

Sulcus of corpus callosum

Subparietal sulcus

Third ventricle,
Thalamus

Parieto-occipital sulcus

Isthmus of cingulate gyrus

Calcarine sulcus

Aqueduct of midbrain
= Cerebral aqueduct

Tectal plate
= Quadrigeminal plate

Tegmentum of midbrain

Superior medullary velum

Fourth ventricle

Tela choroidea
of fourth ventricle

Median aperture
of fourth ventricle

Central canal
of spinal cord

304 Brain (80%)
Median section,
medial aspect of the right hemisphere

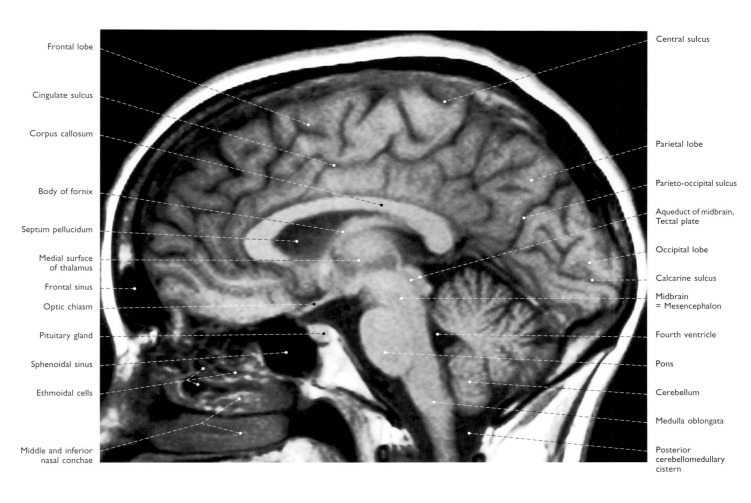

Frontal lobe

Cingulate sulcus

Corpus callosum

Body of fornix

Septum pellucidum

Medial surface
of thalamus

Frontal sinus

Optic chiasm

Pituitary gland

Sphenoidal sinus

Ethmoidal cells

Middle and inferior
nasal conchae

Central sulcus

Parietal lobe

Parieto-occipital sulcus

Aqueduct of midbrain,
Tectal plate

Occipital lobe

Calcarine sulcus

Midbrain
= Mesencephalon

Fourth ventricle

Pons

Cerebellum

Medulla oblongata

Posterior
cerebellomedullary
cistern

305 Brain (80%)
Sagittal paramedian magnetic resonance image
(MRI, T_1-weighted)

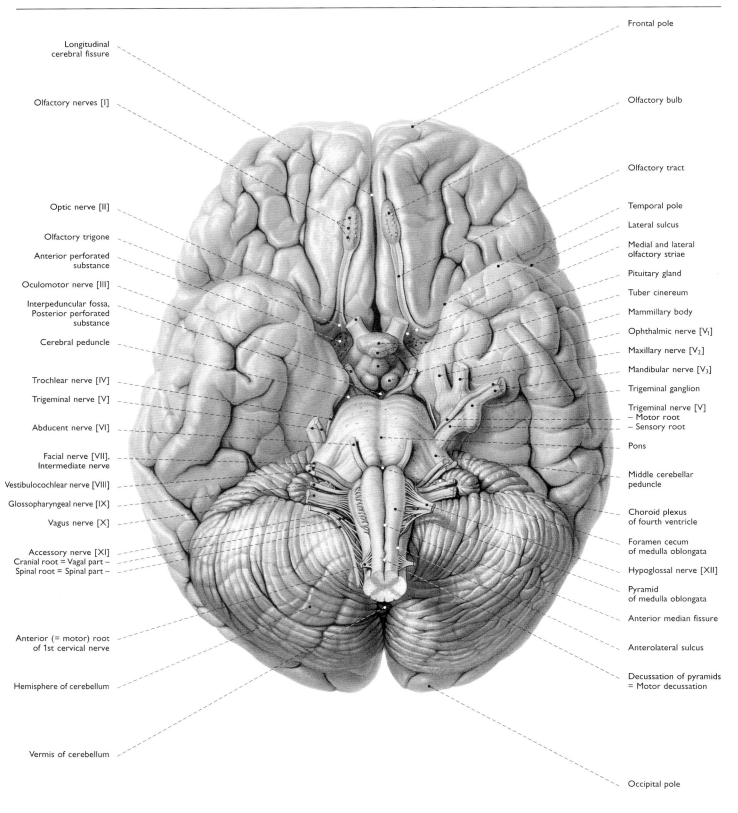

Longitudinal cerebral fissure

Olfactory nerves [I]

Optic nerve [II]

Olfactory trigone

Anterior perforated substance

Oculomotor nerve [III]

Interpeduncular fossa, Posterior perforated substance

Cerebral peduncle

Trochlear nerve [IV]

Trigeminal nerve [V]

Abducent nerve [VI]

Facial nerve [VII], Intermediate nerve

Vestibulocochlear nerve [VIII]

Glossopharyngeal nerve [IX]

Vagus nerve [X]

Accessory nerve [XI]
Cranial root = Vagal part –
Spinal root = Spinal part –

Anterior (= motor) root of 1st cervical nerve

Hemisphere of cerebellum

Vermis of cerebellum

Frontal pole

Olfactory bulb

Olfactory tract

Temporal pole

Lateral sulcus

Medial and lateral olfactory striae

Pituitary gland

Tuber cinereum

Mammillary body

Ophthalmic nerve [V₁]

Maxillary nerve [V₂]

Mandibular nerve [V₃]

Trigeminal ganglion

Trigeminal nerve [V]
– Motor root
– Sensory root

Pons

Middle cerebellar peduncle

Choroid plexus of fourth ventricle

Foramen cecum of medulla oblongata

Hypoglossal nerve [XII]

Pyramid of medulla oblongata

Anterior median fissure

Anterolateral sulcus

Decussation of pyramids = Motor decussation

Occipital pole

306 Brain and cranial nerves (100%)
Inferior aspect

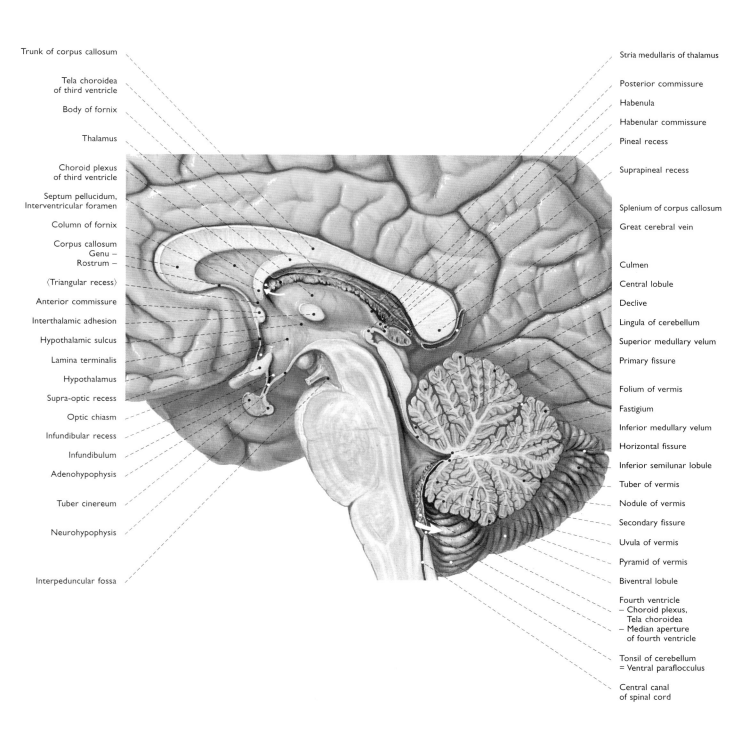

Trunk of corpus callosum

Tela choroidea
of third ventricle

Body of fornix

Thalamus

Choroid plexus
of third ventricle

Septum pellucidum,
Interventricular foramen

Column of fornix

Corpus callosum
Genu –
Rostrum –

⟨Triangular recess⟩

Anterior commissure

Interthalamic adhesion

Hypothalamic sulcus

Lamina terminalis

Hypothalamus

Supra-optic recess

Optic chiasm

Infundibular recess

Infundibulum

Adenohypophysis

Tuber cinereum

Neurohypophysis

Interpeduncular fossa

Stria medullaris of thalamus

Posterior commissure

Habenula

Habenular commissure

Pineal recess

Suprapineal recess

Splenium of corpus callosum

Great cerebral vein

Culmen

Central lobule

Declive

Lingula of cerebellum

Superior medullary velum

Primary fissure

Folium of vermis

Fastigium

Inferior medullary velum

Horizontal fissure

Inferior semilunar lobule

Tuber of vermis

Nodule of vermis

Secondary fissure

Uvula of vermis

Pyramid of vermis

Biventral lobule

Fourth ventricle
– Choroid plexus,
   Tela choroidea
– Median aperture
   of fourth ventricle

Tonsil of cerebellum
= Ventral paraflocculus

Central canal
of spinal cord

307 Brainstem, third and fourth ventricles (110%)
Median section, medial aspect of the right hemisphere

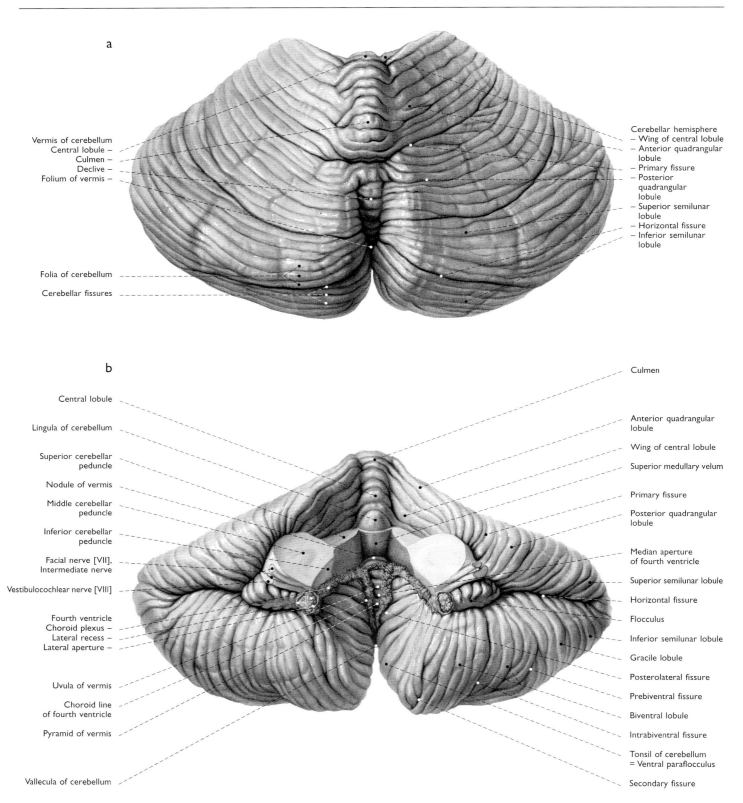

a

Vermis of cerebellum
Central lobule –
Culmen –
Declive –
Folium of vermis –

Folia of cerebellum

Cerebellar fissures

Cerebellar hemisphere
– Wing of central lobule
– Anterior quadrangular lobule
– Primary fissure
– Posterior quadrangular lobule
– Superior semilunar lobule
– Horizontal fissure
– Inferior semilunar lobule

b

Central lobule

Lingula of cerebellum

Superior cerebellar peduncle

Nodule of vermis

Middle cerebellar peduncle

Inferior cerebellar peduncle

Facial nerve [VII], Intermediate nerve

Vestibulocochlear nerve [VIII]

Fourth ventricle
Choroid plexus –
Lateral recess –
Lateral aperture –

Uvula of vermis

Choroid line of fourth ventricle

Pyramid of vermis

Vallecula of cerebellum

Culmen

Anterior quadrangular lobule

Wing of central lobule

Superior medullary velum

Primary fissure

Posterior quadrangular lobule

Median aperture of fourth ventricle

Superior semilunar lobule

Horizontal fissure

Flocculus

Inferior semilunar lobule

Gracile lobule

Posterolateral fissure

Prebiventral fissure

Biventral lobule

Intrabiventral fissure

Tonsil of cerebellum = Ventral paraflocculus

Secondary fissure

308 Cerebellum (120%)

  a   Occipitoparietal aspect
  b   The cerebellar peduncles were transected. Ventral aspect

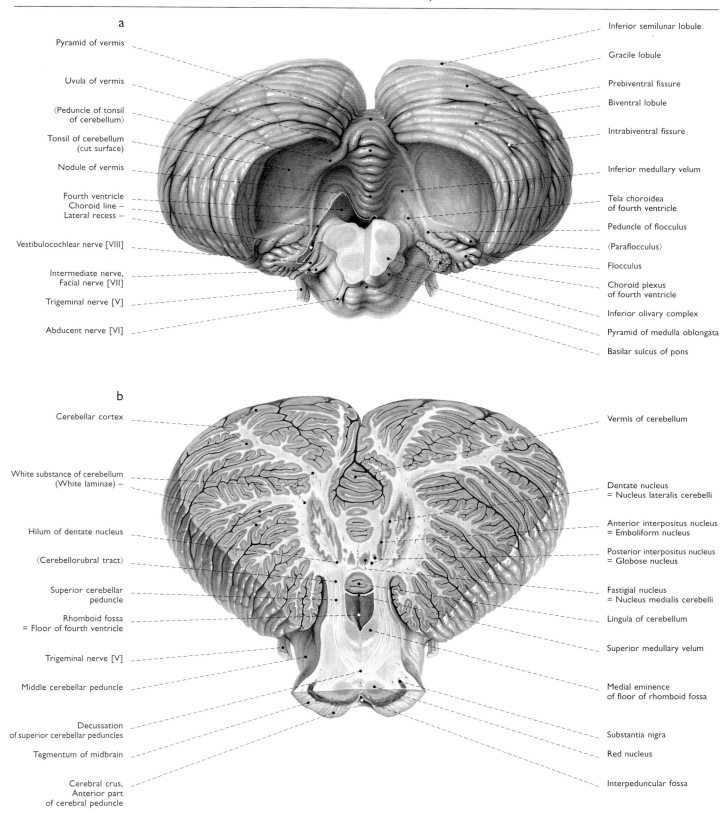

a

Pyramid of vermis

Uvula of vermis

⟨Peduncle of tonsil of cerebellum⟩

Tonsil of cerebellum (cut surface)

Nodule of vermis

Fourth ventricle
Choroid line –
Lateral recess –

Vestibulocochlear nerve [VIII]

Intermediate nerve,
Facial nerve [VII]

Trigeminal nerve [V]

Abducent nerve [VI]

Inferior semilunar lobule

Gracile lobule

Prebiventral fissure

Biventral lobule

Intrabiventral fissure

Inferior medullary velum

Tela choroidea of fourth ventricle

Peduncle of flocculus

⟨Paraflocculus⟩

Flocculus

Choroid plexus of fourth ventricle

Inferior olivary complex

Pyramid of medulla oblongata

Basilar sulcus of pons

b

Cerebellar cortex

White substance of cerebellum (White laminae) –

Hilum of dentate nucleus

⟨Cerebellorubral tract⟩

Superior cerebellar peduncle

Rhomboid fossa = Floor of fourth ventricle

Trigeminal nerve [V]

Middle cerebellar peduncle

Decussation of superior cerebellar peduncles

Tegmentum of midbrain

Cerebral crus, Anterior part of cerebral peduncle

Vermis of cerebellum

Dentate nucleus = Nucleus lateralis cerebelli

Anterior interpositus nucleus = Emboliform nucleus

Posterior interpositus nucleus = Globose nucleus

Fastigial nucleus = Nucleus medialis cerebelli

Lingula of cerebellum

Superior medullary velum

Medial eminence of floor of rhomboid fossa

Substantia nigra

Red nucleus

Interpeduncular fossa

309　Cerebellum 100%)
a　The tonsils of cerebellum were removed. Inferior aspect
b　Section through the cerebellum and midbrain, superior aspect

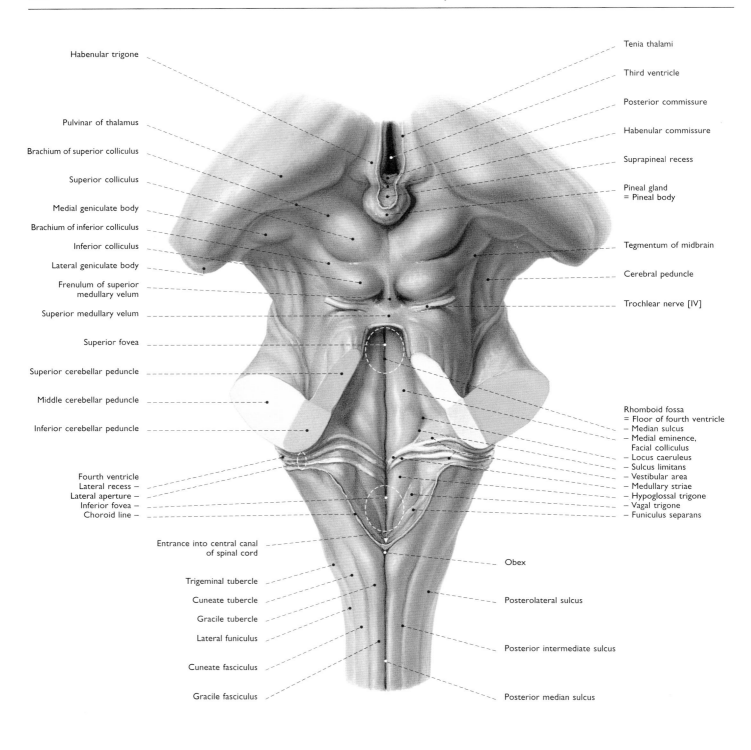

Habenular trigone

Pulvinar of thalamus

Brachium of superior colliculus

Superior colliculus

Medial geniculate body

Brachium of inferior colliculus

Inferior colliculus

Lateral geniculate body

Frenulum of superior
medullary velum

Superior medullary velum

Superior fovea

Superior cerebellar peduncle

Middle cerebellar peduncle

Inferior cerebellar peduncle

Fourth ventricle
Lateral recess −
Lateral aperture −
Inferior fovea −
Choroid line −

Entrance into central canal
of spinal cord

Trigeminal tubercle

Cuneate tubercle

Gracile tubercle

Lateral funiculus

Cuneate fasciculus

Gracile fasciculus

Tenia thalami

Third ventricle

Posterior commissure

Habenular commissure

Suprapineal recess

Pineal gland
= Pineal body

Tegmentum of midbrain

Cerebral peduncle

Trochlear nerve [IV]

Rhomboid fossa
= Floor of fourth ventricle
− Median sulcus
− Medial eminence,
  Facial colliculus
− Locus caeruleus
− Sulcus limitans
− Vestibular area
− Medullary striae
− Hypoglossal trigone
− Vagal trigone
− Funiculus separans

Obex

Posterolateral sulcus

Posterior intermediate sulcus

Posterior median sulcus

310 Brainstem and fourth ventricle (180%)
Dorsal aspect

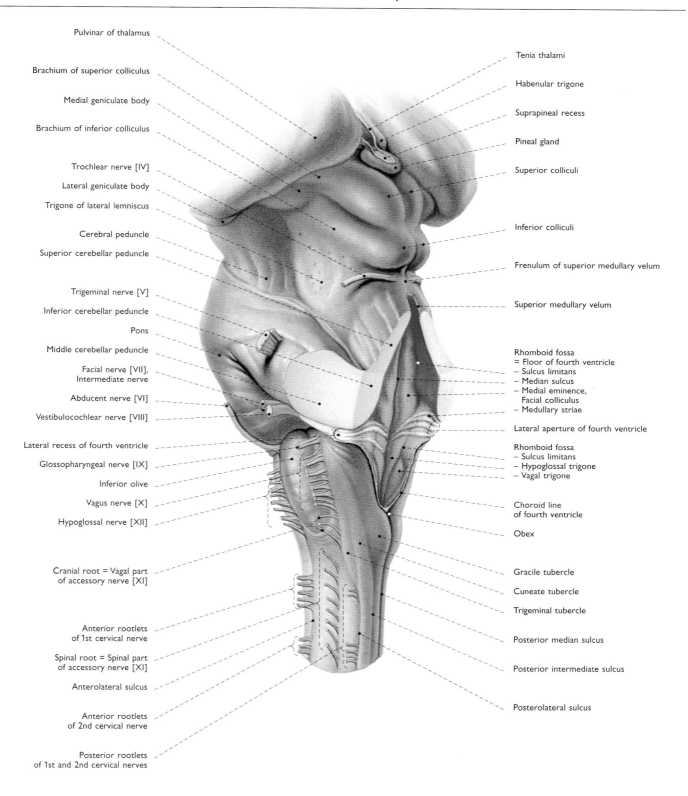

Pulvinar of thalamus

Brachium of superior colliculus

Medial geniculate body

Brachium of inferior colliculus

Trochlear nerve [IV]

Lateral geniculate body

Trigone of lateral lemniscus

Cerebral peduncle

Superior cerebellar peduncle

Trigeminal nerve [V]

Inferior cerebellar peduncle

Pons

Middle cerebellar peduncle

Facial nerve [VII], Intermediate nerve

Abducent nerve [VI]

Vestibulocochlear nerve [VIII]

Lateral recess of fourth ventricle

Glossopharyngeal nerve [IX]

Inferior olive

Vagus nerve [X]

Hypoglossal nerve [XII]

Cranial root = Vagal part of accessory nerve [XI]

Anterior rootlets of 1st cervical nerve

Spinal root = Spinal part of accessory nerve [XI]

Anterolateral sulcus

Anterior rootlets of 2nd cervical nerve

Posterior rootlets of 1st and 2nd cervical nerves

Tenia thalami

Habenular trigone

Suprapineal recess

Pineal gland

Superior colliculi

Inferior colliculi

Frenulum of superior medullary velum

Superior medullary velum

Rhomboid fossa
= Floor of fourth ventricle
– Sulcus limitans
– Median sulcus
– Medial eminence,
   Facial colliculus
– Medullary striae

Lateral aperture of fourth ventricle

Rhomboid fossa
– Sulcus limitans
– Hypoglossal trigone
– Vagal trigone

Choroid line
of fourth ventricle

Obex

Gracile tubercle

Cuneate tubercle

Trigeminal tubercle

Posterior median sulcus

Posterior intermediate sulcus

Posterolateral sulcus

311 Brainstem and fourth ventricle (180%)
Left dorsolateral aspect

a

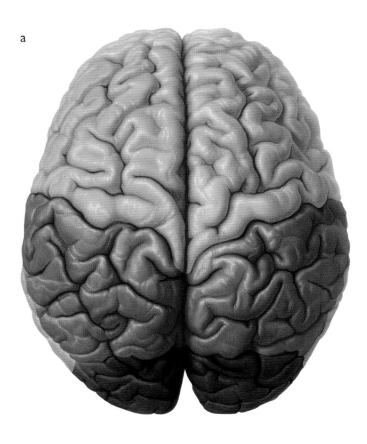

Frontal lobe
Parietal lobe
Occipital lobe
Temporal lobe
Limbic lobe

b

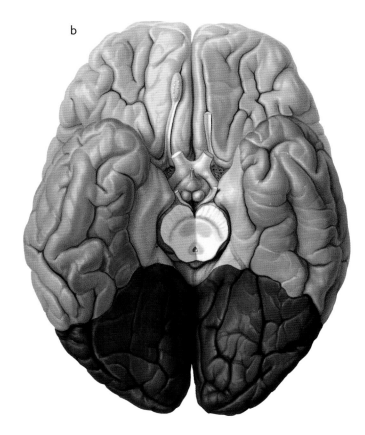

312 Cerebral lobes (70%)

The diverse cerebral lobes are indicated by different colors.
a Superior aspect
b Inferior aspect

a

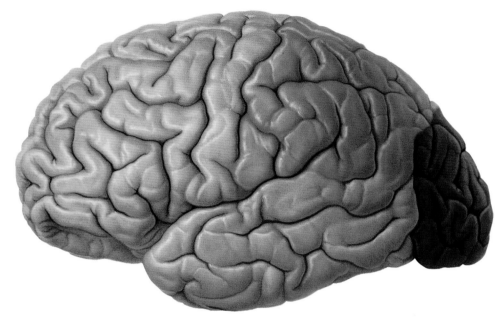

Frontal lobe
Parietal lobe
Occipital lobe
Temporal lobe
Limbic lobe

b

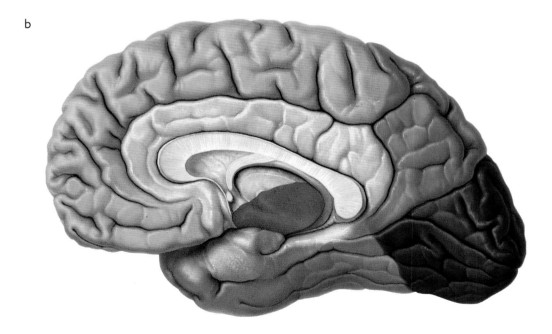

313 Cerebral lobes (80%)

The diverse cerebral lobes are indicated by different colors.
a   Left lateral aspect of the left hemisphere
b   Medial aspect of the right hemisphere

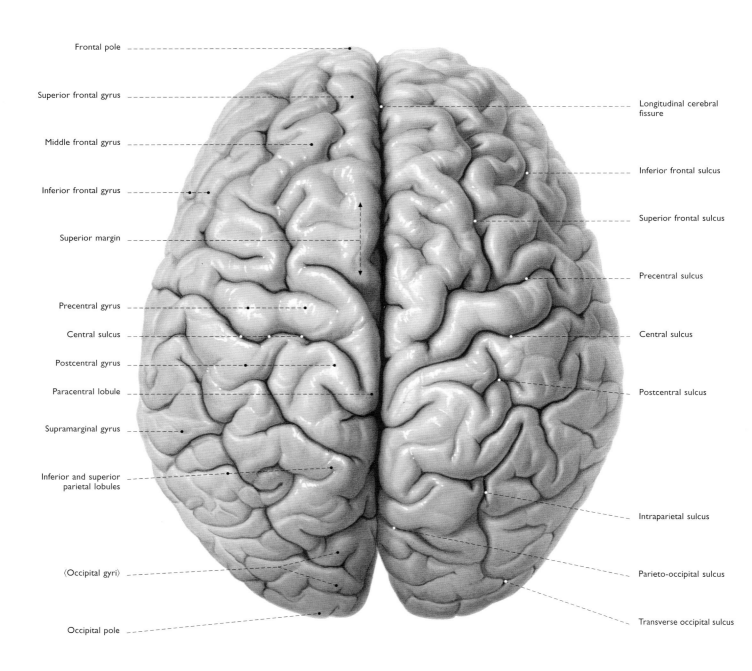

Frontal pole

Superior frontal gyrus

Middle frontal gyrus

Inferior frontal gyrus

Superior margin

Precentral gyrus

Central sulcus

Postcentral gyrus

Paracentral lobule

Supramarginal gyrus

Inferior and superior parietal lobules

⟨Occipital gyri⟩

Occipital pole

Longitudinal cerebral fissure

Inferior frontal sulcus

Superior frontal sulcus

Precentral sulcus

Central sulcus

Postcentral sulcus

Intraparietal sulcus

Parieto-occipital sulcus

Transverse occipital sulcus

314 Cerebral hemispheres (100%)
Superior aspect

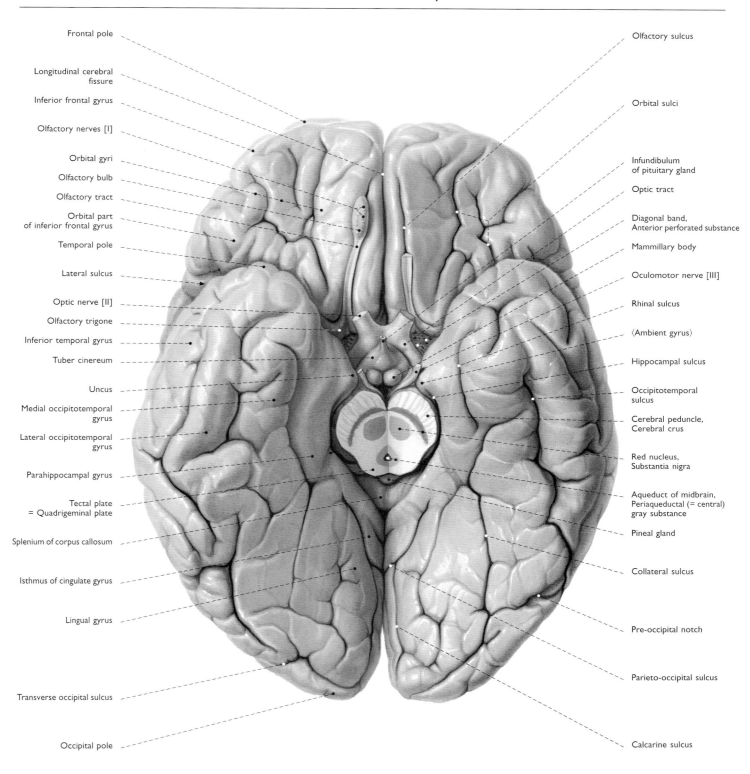

Frontal pole

Longitudinal cerebral fissure

Inferior frontal gyrus

Olfactory nerves [I]

Orbital gyri

Olfactory bulb

Olfactory tract

Orbital part of inferior frontal gyrus

Temporal pole

Lateral sulcus

Optic nerve [II]

Olfactory trigone

Inferior temporal gyrus

Tuber cinereum

Uncus

Medial occipitotemporal gyrus

Lateral occipitotemporal gyrus

Parahippocampal gyrus

Tectal plate = Quadrigeminal plate

Splenium of corpus callosum

Isthmus of cingulate gyrus

Lingual gyrus

Transverse occipital sulcus

Occipital pole

Olfactory sulcus

Orbital sulci

Infundibulum of pituitary gland

Optic tract

Diagonal band, Anterior perforated substance

Mammillary body

Oculomotor nerve [III]

Rhinal sulcus

⟨Ambient gyrus⟩

Hippocampal sulcus

Occipitotemporal sulcus

Cerebral peduncle, Cerebral crus

Red nucleus, Substantia nigra

Aqueduct of midbrain, Periaqueductal (= central) gray substance

Pineal gland

Collateral sulcus

Pre-occipital notch

Parieto-occipital sulcus

Calcarine sulcus

315 Cerebral hemispheres (100%)
The midbrain was transected. Inferior aspect

a

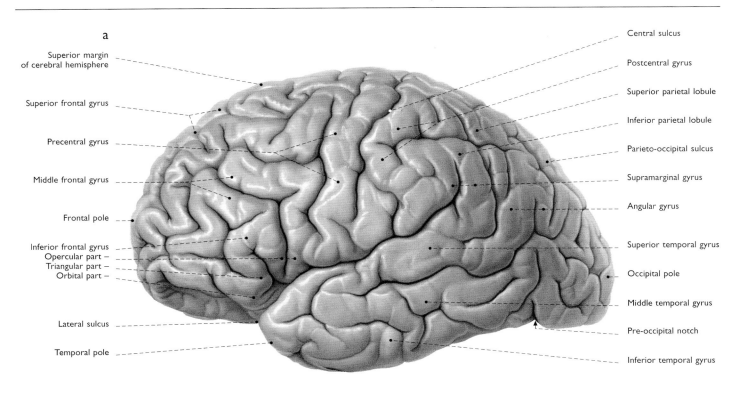

Superior margin
of cerebral hemisphere

Superior frontal gyrus

Precentral gyrus

Middle frontal gyrus

Frontal pole

Inferior frontal gyrus
Opercular part —
Triangular part —
Orbital part —

Lateral sulcus

Temporal pole

Central sulcus

Postcentral gyrus

Superior parietal lobule

Inferior parietal lobule

Parieto-occipital sulcus

Supramarginal gyrus

Angular gyrus

Superior temporal gyrus

Occipital pole

Middle temporal gyrus

Pre-occipital notch

Inferior temporal gyrus

b

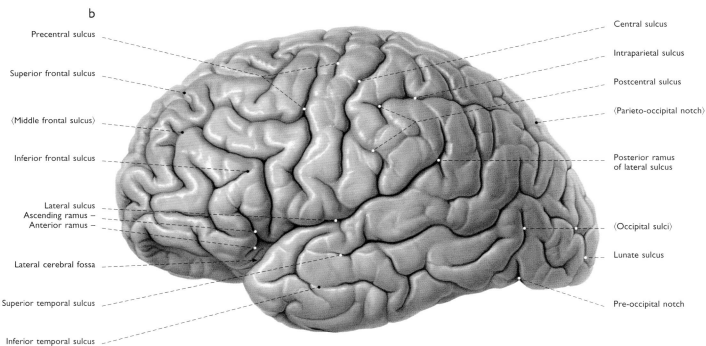

Precentral sulcus

Superior frontal sulcus

〈Middle frontal sulcus〉

Inferior frontal sulcus

Lateral sulcus
Ascending ramus —
Anterior ramus —

Lateral cerebral fossa

Superior temporal sulcus

Inferior temporal sulcus

Central sulcus

Intraparietal sulcus

Postcentral sulcus

〈Parieto-occipital notch〉

Posterior ramus
of lateral sulcus

〈Occipital sulci〉

Lunate sulcus

Pre-occipital notch

316 Left cerebral hemisphere (80%)
Left lateral aspect
Lettering of the
a   gyri
b   sulci

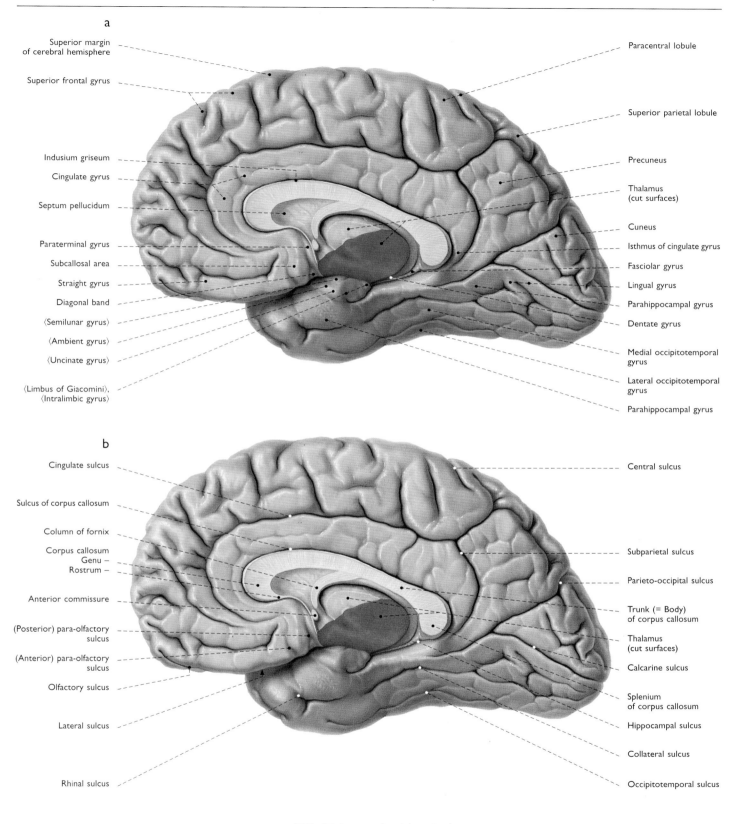

a

Superior margin of cerebral hemisphere
Superior frontal gyrus
Indusium griseum
Cingulate gyrus
Septum pellucidum
Paraterminal gyrus
Subcallosal area
Straight gyrus
Diagonal band
⟨Semilunar gyrus⟩
⟨Ambient gyrus⟩
⟨Uncinate gyrus⟩
⟨Limbus of Giacomini⟩, ⟨Intralimbic gyrus⟩

Paracentral lobule
Superior parietal lobule
Precuneus
Thalamus (cut surfaces)
Cuneus
Isthmus of cingulate gyrus
Fasciolar gyrus
Lingual gyrus
Parahippocampal gyrus
Dentate gyrus
Medial occipitotemporal gyrus
Lateral occipitotemporal gyrus
Parahippocampal gyrus

b

Cingulate sulcus
Sulcus of corpus callosum
Column of fornix
Corpus callosum Genu – Rostrum –
Anterior commissure
(Posterior) para-olfactory sulcus
(Anterior) para-olfactory sulcus
Olfactory sulcus
Lateral sulcus
Rhinal sulcus

Central sulcus
Subparietal sulcus
Parieto-occipital sulcus
Trunk (= Body) of corpus callosum
Thalamus (cut surfaces)
Calcarine sulcus
Splenium of corpus callosum
Hippocampal sulcus
Collateral sulcus
Occipitotemporal sulcus

317 Right cerebral hemisphere (80%)
Medial aspect of a median section. The corpus callosum and the diencephalon were transected. Lettering of the
a gyri
b sulci

a

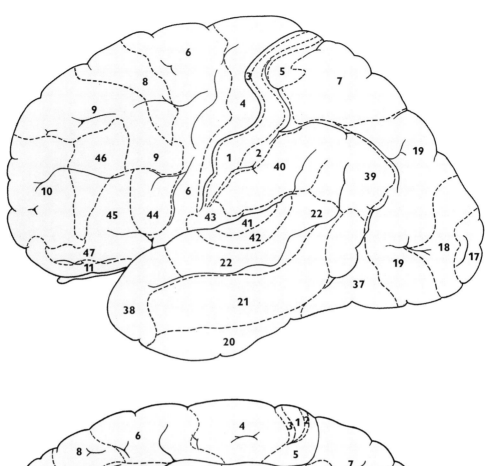

b

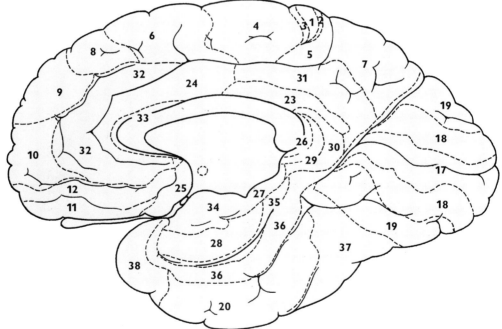

318 Cerebral cortex (80%)
     Brodmann's areas 1–47
   a Left hemisphere, lateral aspect
   b Right hemisphere, medial aspect

a

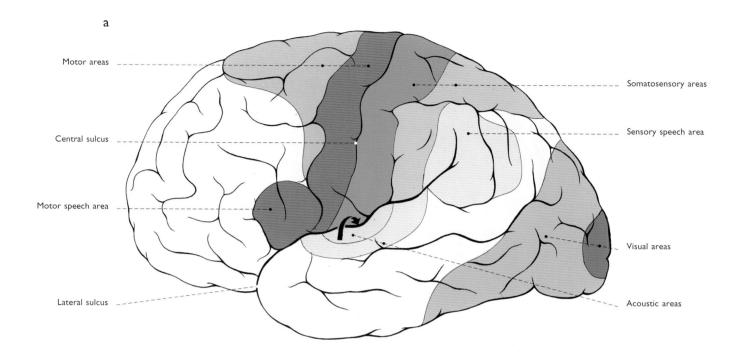

Motor areas

Central sulcus

Motor speech area

Lateral sulcus

Somatosensory areas

Sensory speech area

Visual areas

Acoustic areas

b

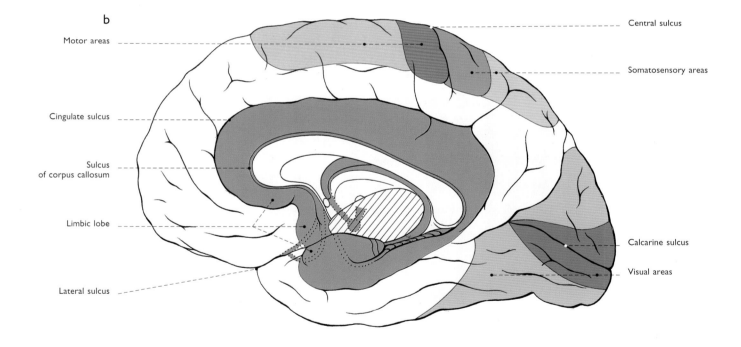

Motor areas

Cingulate sulcus

Sulcus
of corpus callosum

Limbic lobe

Lateral sulcus

Central sulcus

Somatosensory areas

Calcarine sulcus

Visual areas

319 Cerebral cortex (80%)

Main first (dark) and second (light) functional areas
a Left hemisphere, lateral aspect
b Right hemisphere, medial aspect

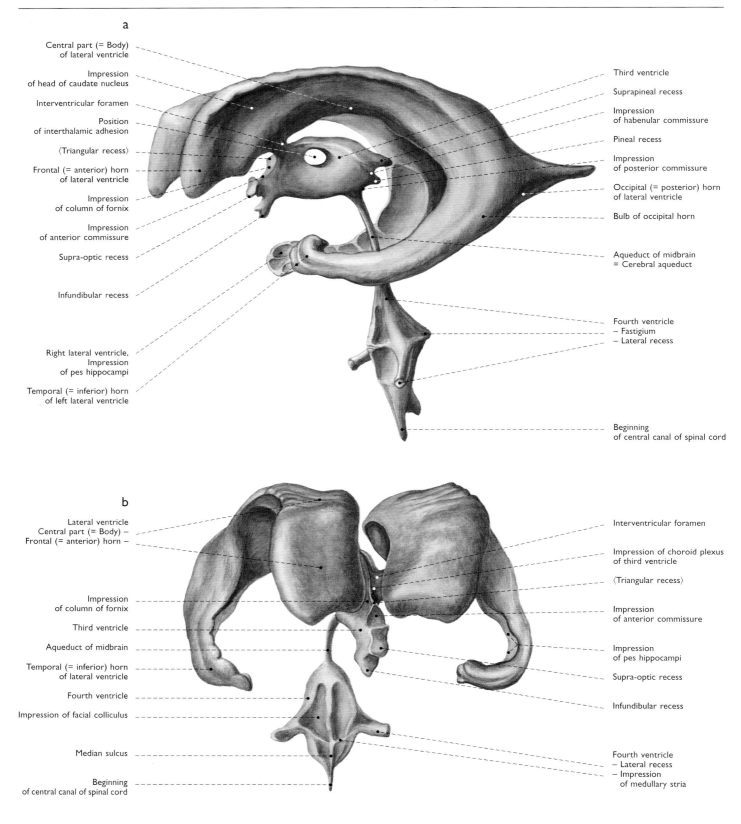

a

Central part (= Body) of lateral ventricle

Impression of head of caudate nucleus

Interventricular foramen

Position of interthalamic adhesion

⟨Triangular recess⟩

Frontal (= anterior) horn of lateral ventricle

Impression of column of fornix

Impression of anterior commissure

Supra-optic recess

Infundibular recess

Right lateral ventricle, Impression of pes hippocampi

Temporal (= inferior) horn of left lateral ventricle

Third ventricle

Suprapineal recess

Impression of habenular commissure

Pineal recess

Impression of posterior commissure

Occipital (= posterior) horn of lateral ventricle

Bulb of occipital horn

Aqueduct of midbrain = Cerebral aqueduct

Fourth ventricle
– Fastigium
– Lateral recess

Beginning of central canal of spinal cord

b

Lateral ventricle
Central part (= Body) –
Frontal (= anterior) horn –

Impression of column of fornix

Third ventricle

Aqueduct of midbrain

Temporal (= inferior) horn of lateral ventricle

Fourth ventricle

Impression of facial colliculus

Median sulcus

Beginning of central canal of spinal cord

Interventricular foramen

Impression of choroid plexus of third ventricle

⟨Triangular recess⟩

Impression of anterior commissure

Impression of pes hippocampi

Supra-optic recess

Infundibular recess

Fourth ventricle
– Lateral recess
– Impression of medullary stria

320 Ventricular system of the brain

Cast of the ventricular system (120%)
a Left lateral aspect
b Frontal aspect

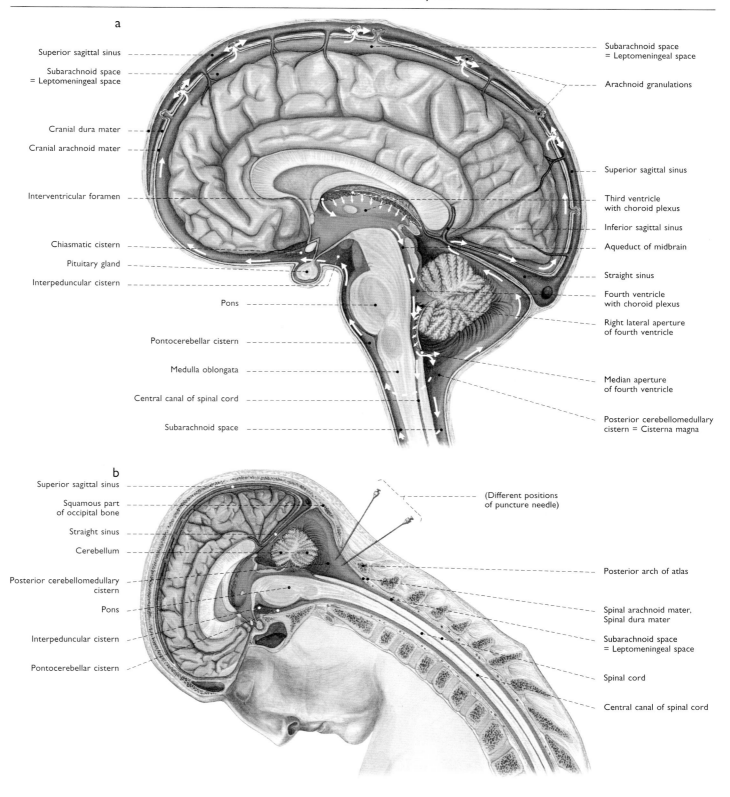

a

Superior sagittal sinus

Subarachnoid space = Leptomeningeal space

Cranial dura mater

Cranial arachnoid mater

Interventricular foramen

Chiasmatic cistern

Pituitary gland

Interpeduncular cistern

Pons

Pontocerebellar cistern

Medulla oblongata

Central canal of spinal cord

Subarachnoid space

Subarachnoid space = Leptomeningeal space

Arachnoid granulations

Superior sagittal sinus

Third ventricle with choroid plexus

Inferior sagittal sinus

Aqueduct of midbrain

Straight sinus

Fourth ventricle with choroid plexus

Right lateral aperture of fourth ventricle

Median aperture of fourth ventricle

Posterior cerebellomedullary cistern = Cisterna magna

b

Superior sagittal sinus

Squamous part of occipital bone

Straight sinus

Cerebellum

Posterior cerebellomedullary cistern

Pons

Interpeduncular cistern

Pontocerebellar cistern

(Different positions of puncture needle)

Posterior arch of atlas

Spinal arachnoid mater, Spinal dura mater

Subarachnoid space = Leptomeningeal space

Spinal cord

Central canal of spinal cord

321 Subarachnoid space, subarachnoid cisterns, and cerebrospinal fluid

a Circulation of the cerebrospinal fluid (60%)
b Puncture of the posterior cerebellomedullary cistern (suboccipital puncture) (35%)

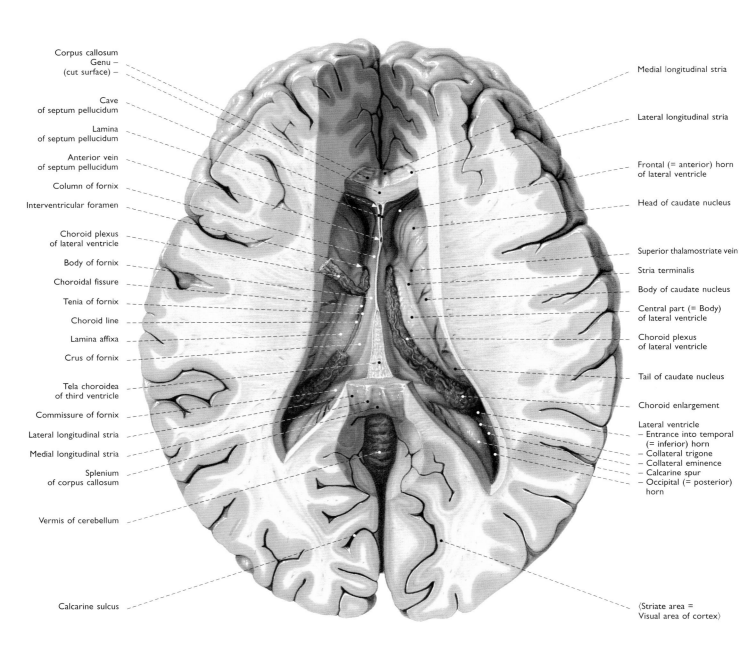

Corpus callosum
Genu –
(cut surface) –

Cave
of septum pellucidum

Lamina
of septum pellucidum

Anterior vein
of septum pellucidum

Column of fornix

Interventricular foramen

Choroid plexus
of lateral ventricle

Body of fornix

Choroidal fissure

Tenia of fornix

Choroid line

Lamina affixa

Crus of fornix

Tela choroidea
of third ventricle

Commissure of fornix

Lateral longitudinal stria

Medial longitudinal stria

Splenium
of corpus callosum

Vermis of cerebellum

Calcarine sulcus

Medial longitudinal stria

Lateral longitudinal stria

Frontal (= anterior) horn
of lateral ventricle

Head of caudate nucleus

Superior thalamostriate vein

Stria terminalis

Body of caudate nucleus

Central part (= Body)
of lateral ventricle

Choroid plexus
of lateral ventricle

Tail of caudate nucleus

Choroid enlargement

Lateral ventricle
– Entrance into temporal
  (= inferior) horn
– Collateral trigone
– Collateral eminence
– Calcarine spur
– Occipital (= posterior)
  horn

⟨Striate area =
Visual area of cortex⟩

322 Lateral ventricles of the brain (100%)
The lateral ventricles were opened from above,
the trunk of the corpus callosum was removed.
Superior aspect of a horizontal section

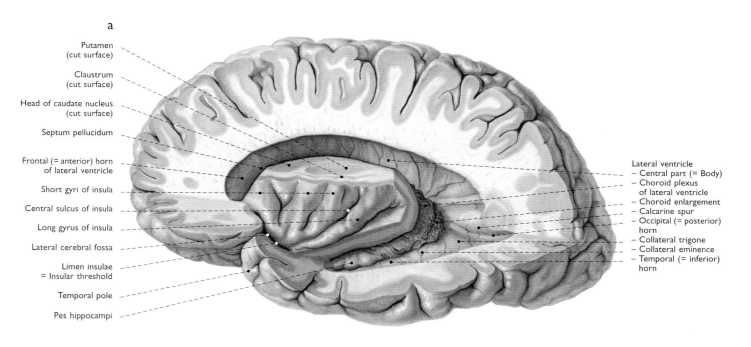

a

Putamen
(cut surface)

Claustrum
(cut surface)

Head of caudate nucleus
(cut surface)

Septum pellucidum

Frontal (= anterior) horn
of lateral ventricle

Short gyri of insula

Central sulcus of insula

Long gyrus of insula

Lateral cerebral fossa

Limen insulae
= Insular threshold

Temporal pole

Pes hippocampi

Lateral ventricle
– Central part (= Body)
– Choroid plexus
of lateral ventricle
– Choroid enlargement
– Calcarine spur
– Occipital (= posterior)
horn
– Collateral trigone
– Collateral eminence
– Temporal (= inferior)
horn

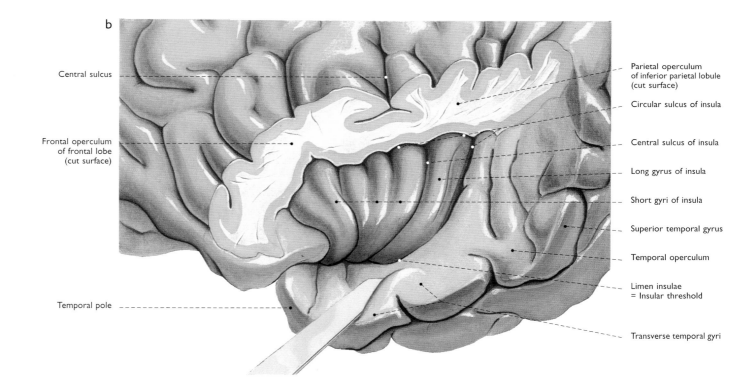

b

Central sulcus

Frontal operculum
of frontal lobe
(cut surface)

Temporal pole

Parietal operculum
of inferior parietal lobule
(cut surface)

Circular sulcus of insula

Central sulcus of insula

Long gyrus of insula

Short gyri of insula

Superior temporal gyrus

Temporal operculum

Limen insulae
= Insular threshold

Transverse temporal gyri

323 Lateral ventricle and insula

a The lateral ventricle of the left hemisphere
was opened (80%). Left lateral aspect

b Parts of the frontal, parietal, and temporal lobes
of the left hemisphere were removed (100%).
Left lateral aspect

a

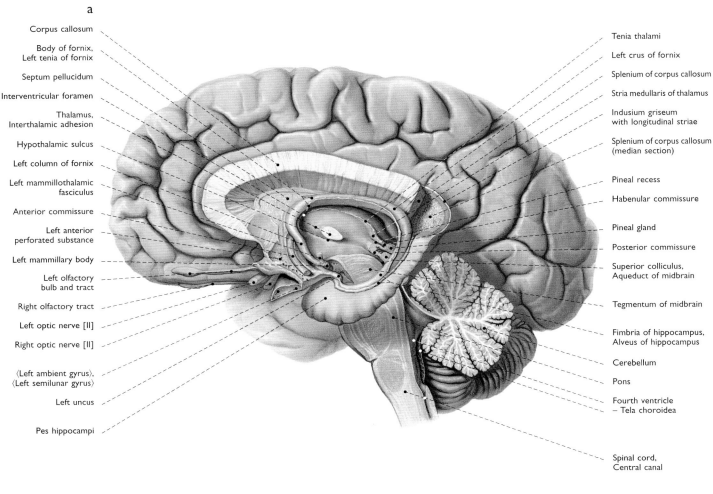

Corpus callosum

Body of fornix,
Left tenia of fornix

Septum pellucidum

Interventricular foramen

Thalamus,
Interthalamic adhesion

Hypothalamic sulcus

Left column of fornix

Left mammillothalamic
fasciculus

Anterior commissure

Left anterior
perforated substance

Left mammillary body

Left olfactory
bulb and tract

Right olfactory tract

Left optic nerve [II]

Right optic nerve [II]

⟨Left ambient gyrus⟩,
⟨Left semilunar gyrus⟩

Left uncus

Pes hippocampi

Tenia thalami

Left crus of fornix

Splenium of corpus callosum

Stria medullaris of thalamus

Indusium griseum
with longitudinal striae

Splenium of corpus callosum
(median section)

Pineal recess

Habenular commissure

Pineal gland

Posterior commissure

Superior colliculus,
Aqueduct of midbrain

Tegmentum of midbrain

Fimbria of hippocampus,
Alveus of hippocampus

Cerebellum

Pons

Fourth ventricle
– Tela choroidea

Spinal cord,
Central canal

b

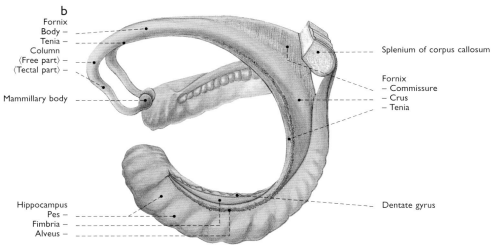

Fornix
Body –
Tenia –
Column
⟨Free part⟩ –
⟨Tectal part⟩ –

Mammillary body

Hippocampus
Pes –
Fimbria –
Alveus –

Splenium of corpus callosum

Fornix
– Commissure
– Crus
– Tenia

Dentate gyrus

324 Fornix and hippocampus

a Dissection of the left cerebral hemisphere.
The right hemisphere is intact, the brainstem was sectioned
in the median plane (80%). Left lateral aspect

b Fornices and hippocampi of both sides (120%),
three-dimensional schematic representation,
left parietolateral aspect

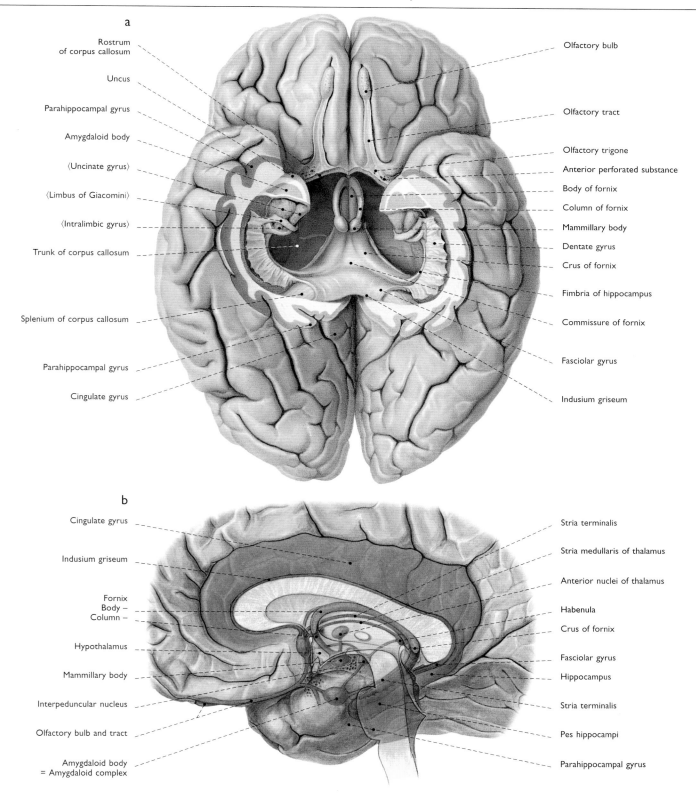

a

Rostrum of corpus callosum

Uncus

Parahippocampal gyrus

Amygdaloid body

⟨Uncinate gyrus⟩

⟨Limbus of Giacomini⟩

⟨Intralimbic gyrus⟩

Trunk of corpus callosum

Splenium of corpus callosum

Parahippocampal gyrus

Cingulate gyrus

Olfactory bulb

Olfactory tract

Olfactory trigone

Anterior perforated substance

Body of fornix

Column of fornix

Mammillary body

Dentate gyrus

Crus of fornix

Fimbria of hippocampus

Commissure of fornix

Fasciolar gyrus

Indusium griseum

b

Cingulate gyrus

Indusium griseum

Fornix
Body –
Column –

Hypothalamus

Mammillary body

Interpeduncular nucleus

Olfactory bulb and tract

Amygdaloid body
= Amygdaloid complex

Stria terminalis

Stria medullaris of thalamus

Anterior nuclei of thalamus

Habenula

Crus of fornix

Fasciolar gyrus

Hippocampus

Stria terminalis

Pes hippocampi

Parahippocampal gyrus

325 Fornix and limbic system

a The undersurface of the brain was partly dissected
in order to show the fornix and some other elements
of the limbic system (80%). Inferior aspect

b The structures of the limbic system are emphasized
by brown color (100%). Medial aspect of the right hemisphere

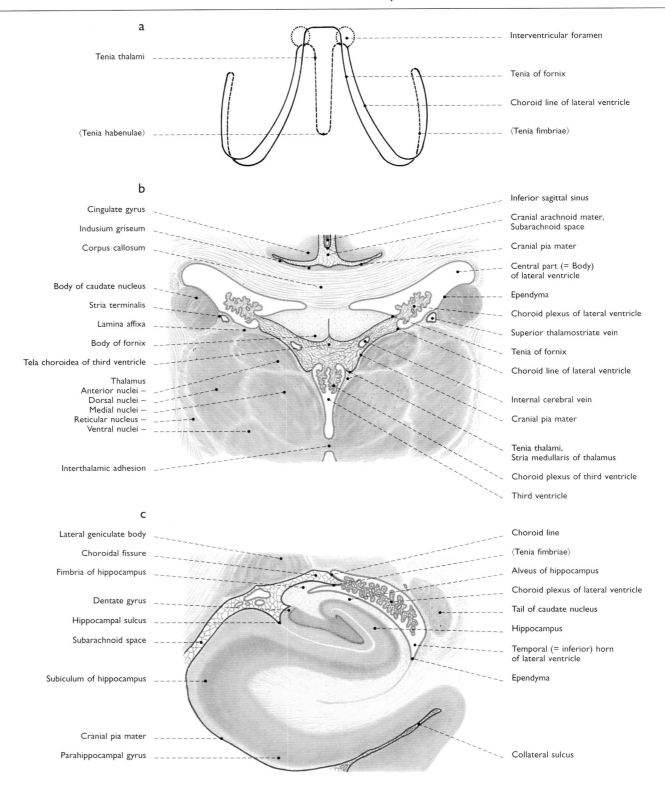

a

Tenia thalami

⟨Tenia habenulae⟩

Interventricular foramen

Tenia of fornix

Choroid line of lateral ventricle

⟨Tenia fimbriae⟩

b

Cingulate gyrus
Indusium griseum
Corpus callosum

Body of caudate nucleus
Stria terminalis
Lamina affixa
Body of fornix
Tela choroidea of third ventricle
Thalamus
Anterior nuclei −
Dorsal nuclei −
Medial nuclei −
Reticular nucleus −
Ventral nuclei −

Interthalamic adhesion

Inferior sagittal sinus
Cranial arachnoid mater,
Subarachnoid space
Cranial pia mater
Central part (= Body)
of lateral ventricle
Ependyma
Choroid plexus of lateral ventricle
Superior thalamostriate vein
Tenia of fornix
Choroid line of lateral ventricle
Internal cerebral vein
Cranial pia mater
Tenia thalami,
Stria medullaris of thalamus
Choroid plexus of third ventricle
Third ventricle

c

Lateral geniculate body
Choroidal fissure
Fimbria of hippocampus
Dentate gyrus
Hippocampal sulcus
Subarachnoid space
Subiculum of hippocampus
Cranial pia mater
Parahippocampal gyrus

Choroid line
⟨Tenia fimbriae⟩
Alveus of hippocampus
Choroid plexus of lateral ventricle
Tail of caudate nucleus
Hippocampus
Temporal (= inferior) horn
of lateral ventricle
Ependyma
Collateral sulcus

326 Choroid plexuses of the forebrain

Schematic representations
a Lines of tearing of the choroid plexuses of both sides, superior aspect
b, c Occipital aspect of coronal sections through
b the central part of both lateral ventricles and the third ventricle (200%)
c the temporal horn of the right lateral ventricle (300%)

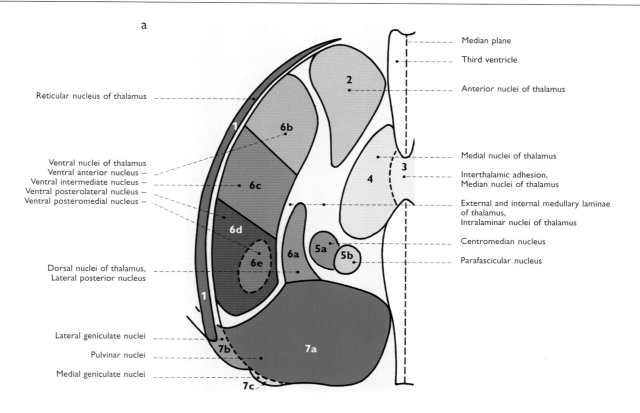

a

Reticular nucleus of thalamus

Median plane
Third ventricle
Anterior nuclei of thalamus

Medial nuclei of thalamus

Interthalamic adhesion,
Median nuclei of thalamus

Ventral nuclei of thalamus
Ventral anterior nucleus –
Ventral intermediate nucleus –
Ventral posterolateral nucleus –
Ventral posteromedial nucleus –

External and internal medullary laminae
of thalamus,
Intralaminar nuclei of thalamus

Centromedian nucleus

Parafascicular nucleus

Dorsal nuclei of thalamus,
Lateral posterior nucleus

Lateral geniculate nuclei

Pulvinar nuclei

Medial geniculate nuclei

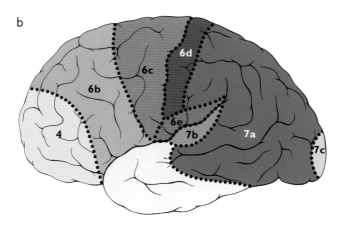

b

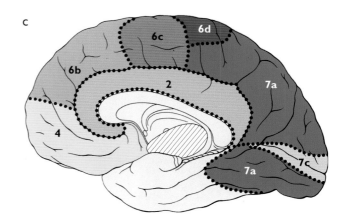

c

327 Thalamus

The nuclei of thalamus and their projection onto the cerebral cortex.
Identical numbers indicate the nuclei and their functionally connected
areas of cerebral cortex. The nuclei 1, 3 and 6a seem to be without
specific projection to the cerebral cortex.

a   Main nuclear masses of the left thalamus, schematic representation,
    superior aspect of a horizontal section

b   Fields of thalamic projection onto the superolateral surface
    of cerebral hemisphere, left lateral aspect of the left hemisphere

c   Fields of thalamic projection onto the medial surface
    of cerebral hemisphere, medial aspect of the right hemisphere

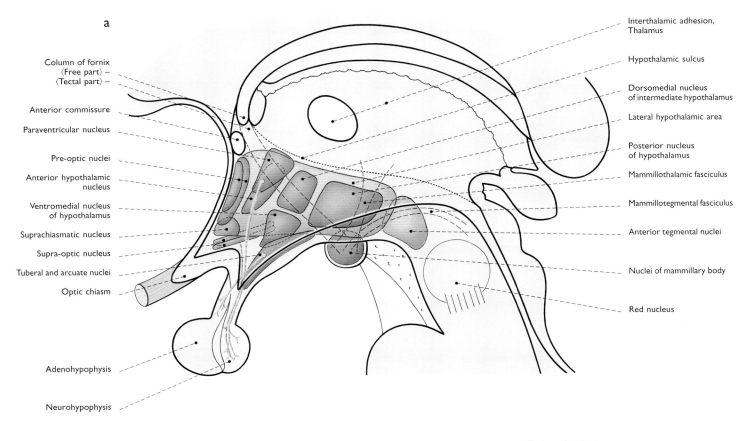

a

Column of fornix
⟨Free part⟩ —
⟨Tectal part⟩ —

Anterior commissure

Paraventricular nucleus

Pre-optic nuclei

Anterior hypothalamic
nucleus

Ventromedial nucleus
of hypothalamus

Suprachiasmatic nucleus

Supra-optic nucleus

Tuberal and arcuate nuclei

Optic chiasm

Adenohypophysis

Neurohypophysis

Interthalamic adhesion,
Thalamus

Hypothalamic sulcus

Dorsomedial nucleus
of intermediate hypothalamus

Lateral hypothalamic area

Posterior nucleus
of hypothalamus

Mammillothalamic fasciculus

Mammillotegmental fasciculus

Anterior tegmental nuclei

Nuclei of mammillary body

Red nucleus

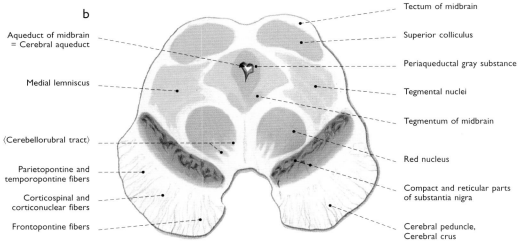

b

Aqueduct of midbrain
= Cerebral aqueduct

Medial lemniscus

⟨Cerebellorubral tract⟩

Parietopontine and
temporopontine fibers

Corticospinal and
corticonuclear fibers

Frontopontine fibers

Tectum of midbrain

Superior colliculus

Periaqueductal gray substance

Tegmental nuclei

Tegmentum of midbrain

Red nucleus

Compact and reticular parts
of substantia nigra

Cerebral peduncle,
Cerebral crus

328 Hypothalamus and midbrain (250%)

  a Nuclei of the hypothalamus, schematic representation,
     medial aspect
  b Oblique section through the midbrain (= mesencephalon)
     at the level of the superior colliculi

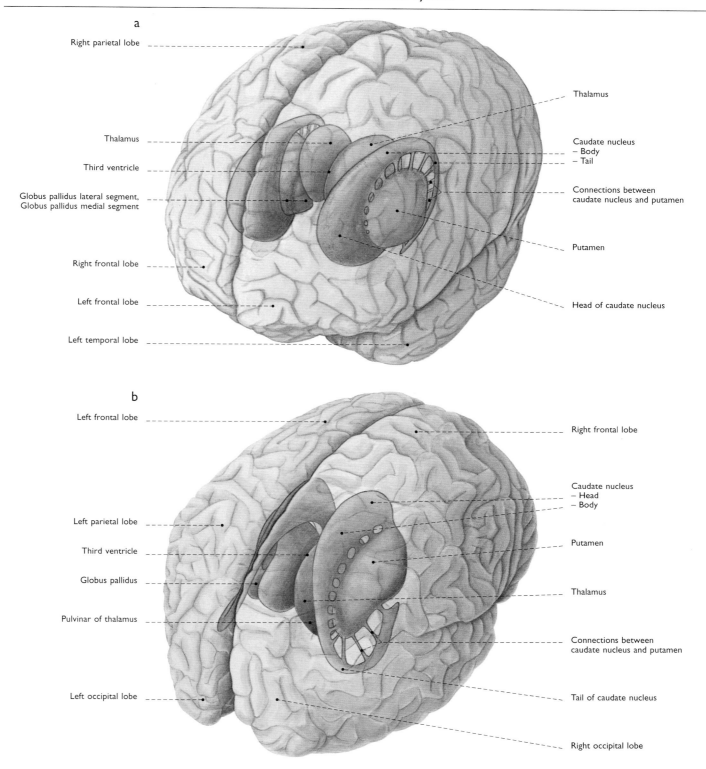

a

Right parietal lobe

Thalamus

Third ventricle

Globus pallidus lateral segment,
Globus pallidus medial segment

Right frontal lobe

Left frontal lobe

Left temporal lobe

Thalamus

Caudate nucleus
– Body
– Tail

Connections between
caudate nucleus and putamen

Putamen

Head of caudate nucleus

b

Left frontal lobe

Left parietal lobe

Third ventricle

Globus pallidus

Pulvinar of thalamus

Left occipital lobe

Right frontal lobe

Caudate nucleus
– Head
– Body

Putamen

Thalamus

Connections between
caudate nucleus and putamen

Tail of caudate nucleus

Right occipital lobe

329 Nuclei of the forebrain (70%)
Thalamus, striatum (= caudate nucleus and putamen),
and lentiform nucleus (= putamen and globus pallidus)
are shown in the interior of the two cerebral hemispheres
(corpus striatum = caudate nucleus, putamen, and globus pallidus).
Schematized three-dimensional representations
a Left lateral anterior superior aspect
(left frontoparietolateral aspect)
b Right lateral posterior superior aspect
(right occipitoparietolateral aspect)

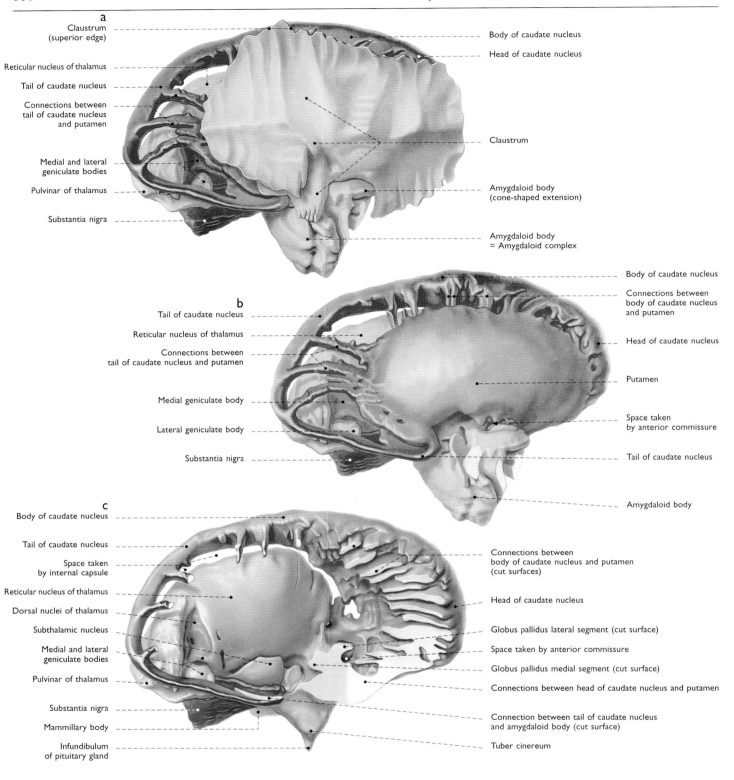

a

Claustrum (superior edge)

Reticular nucleus of thalamus

Tail of caudate nucleus

Connections between tail of caudate nucleus and putamen

Medial and lateral geniculate bodies

Pulvinar of thalamus

Substantia nigra

Body of caudate nucleus

Head of caudate nucleus

Claustrum

Amygdaloid body (cone-shaped extension)

Amygdaloid body = Amygdaloid complex

b

Tail of caudate nucleus

Reticular nucleus of thalamus

Connections between tail of caudate nucleus and putamen

Medial geniculate body

Lateral geniculate body

Substantia nigra

Body of caudate nucleus

Connections between body of caudate nucleus and putamen

Head of caudate nucleus

Putamen

Space taken by anterior commissure

Tail of caudate nucleus

Amygdaloid body

c

Body of caudate nucleus

Tail of caudate nucleus

Space taken by internal capsule

Reticular nucleus of thalamus

Dorsal nuclei of thalamus

Subthalamic nucleus

Medial and lateral geniculate bodies

Pulvinar of thalamus

Substantia nigra

Mammillary body

Infundibulum of pituitary gland

Connections between body of caudate nucleus and putamen (cut surfaces)

Head of caudate nucleus

Globus pallidus lateral segment (cut surface)

Space taken by anterior commissure

Globus pallidus medial segment (cut surface)

Connections between head of caudate nucleus and putamen

Connection between tail of caudate nucleus and amygdaloid body (cut surface)

Tuber cinereum

330 Nuclei of the forebrain and midbrain

Collapsible model of reconstruction of the basal nuclei of the right half of brain (Anatomical Collection, Basel) (150%), right lateral aspect

a Claustrum and caudate nucleus
b Putamen and caudate nucleus after removal of the claustrum
c Thalamus and caudate nucleus after removal of claustrum, lentiform nucleus, and amygdaloid body

a

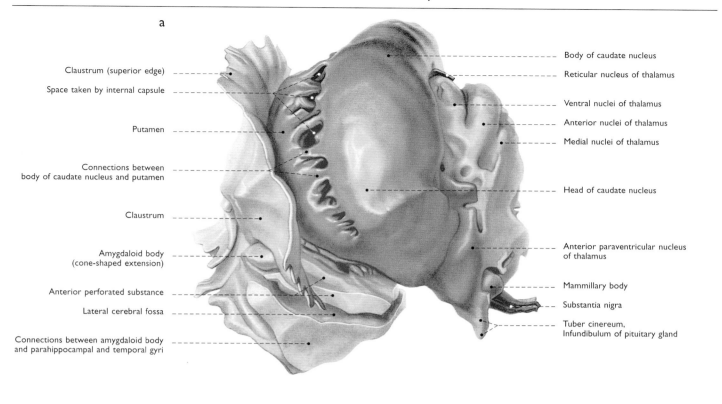

Claustrum (superior edge) — Body of caudate nucleus

Space taken by internal capsule — Reticular nucleus of thalamus

Putamen — Ventral nuclei of thalamus

— Anterior nuclei of thalamus

— Medial nuclei of thalamus

Connections between
body of caudate nucleus and putamen

Claustrum — Head of caudate nucleus

Amygdaloid body
(cone-shaped extension) — Anterior paraventricular nucleus
of thalamus

Anterior perforated substance — Mammillary body

Lateral cerebral fossa — Substantia nigra

— Tuber cinereum,
Infundibulum of pituitary gland

Connections between amygdaloid body
and parahippocampal and temporal gyri

b

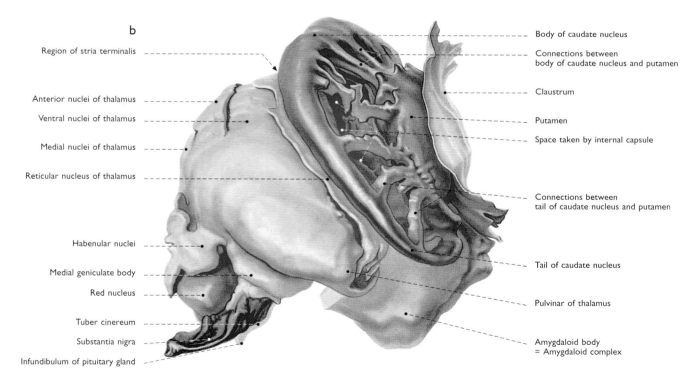

Region of stria terminalis — Body of caudate nucleus

— Connections between
body of caudate nucleus and putamen

— Claustrum

Anterior nuclei of thalamus

Ventral nuclei of thalamus — Putamen

Medial nuclei of thalamus — Space taken by internal capsule

Reticular nucleus of thalamus

— Connections between
tail of caudate nucleus and putamen

Habenular nuclei

Medial geniculate body — Tail of caudate nucleus

Red nucleus

Tuber cinereum — Pulvinar of thalamus

Substantia nigra — Amygdaloid body
= Amygdaloid complex

Infundibulum of pituitary gland

331 Nuclei of the forebrain and midbrain
Collapsible model of reconstruction of the basal nuclei
of the right half of brain (Anatomical Collection, Basel) (200%)
a Frontal aspect
b Occipital aspect

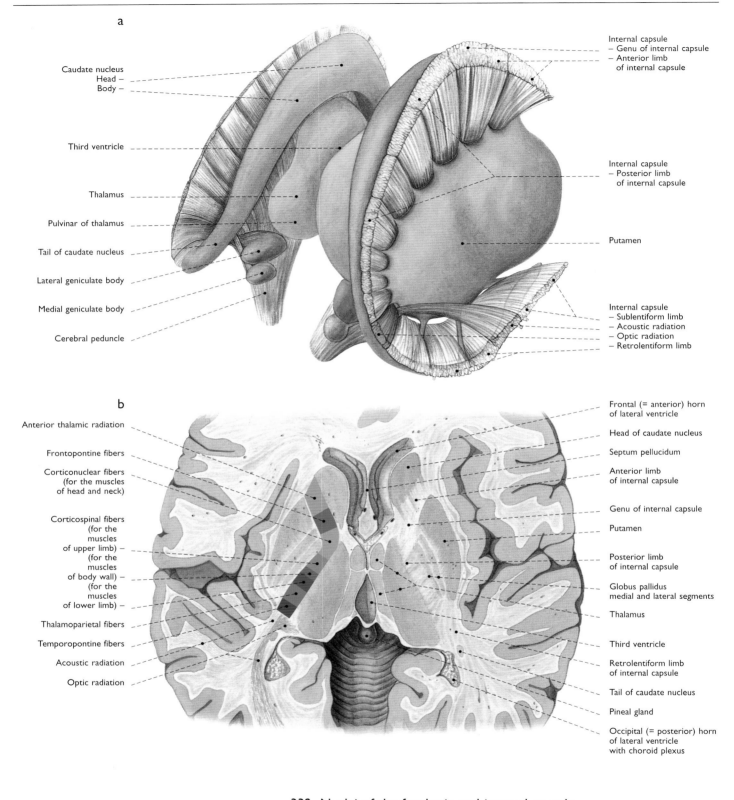

a

Caudate nucleus
Head –
Body –

Third ventricle

Thalamus

Pulvinar of thalamus

Tail of caudate nucleus

Lateral geniculate body

Medial geniculate body

Cerebral peduncle

Internal capsule
– Genu of internal capsule
– Anterior limb
  of internal capsule

Internal capsule
– Posterior limb
  of internal capsule

Putamen

Internal capsule
– Sublentiform limb
– Acoustic radiation
– Optic radiation
– Retrolentiform limb

b

Anterior thalamic radiation

Frontopontine fibers

Corticonuclear fibers
(for the muscles
of head and neck)

Corticospinal fibers
(for the
muscles
of upper limb) –
(for the
muscles
of body wall) –
(for the
muscles
of lower limb) –

Thalamoparietal fibers

Temporopontine fibers

Acoustic radiation

Optic radiation

Frontal (= anterior) horn
of lateral ventricle

Head of caudate nucleus

Septum pellucidum

Anterior limb
of internal capsule

Genu of internal capsule

Putamen

Posterior limb
of internal capsule

Globus pallidus
medial and lateral segments

Thalamus

Third ventricle

Retrolentiform limb
of internal capsule

Tail of caudate nucleus

Pineal gland

Occipital (= posterior) horn
of lateral ventricle
with choroid plexus

332 Nuclei of the forebrain and internal capsule

a Thalamus, striatum (= caudate nucleus and putamen),
   and lentiform nucleus (= putamen and globus pallidus)
   with the internal capsule (250%), right occipitolateral aspect
b Horizontal section through the internal capsule and adjacent nuclei
   (corpus striatum = caudate nucleus, putamen, and globus pallidus).
   On the left side, the main components of the internal capsule
   are marked by different colors (90%). Superior aspect

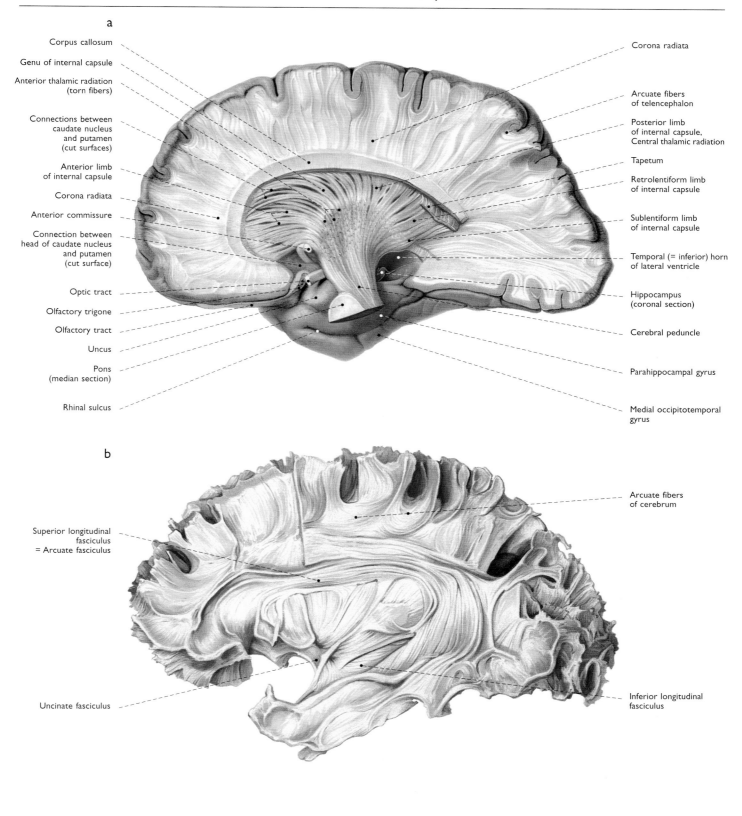

a

Corpus callosum

Genu of internal capsule

Anterior thalamic radiation
(torn fibers)

Connections between
caudate nucleus
and putamen
(cut surfaces)

Anterior limb
of internal capsule

Corona radiata

Anterior commissure

Connection between
head of caudate nucleus
and putamen
(cut surface)

Optic tract

Olfactory trigone

Olfactory tract

Uncus

Pons
(median section)

Rhinal sulcus

Corona radiata

Arcuate fibers
of telencephalon

Posterior limb
of internal capsule,
Central thalamic radiation

Tapetum

Retrolentiform limb
of internal capsule

Sublentiform limb
of internal capsule

Temporal (= inferior) horn
of lateral ventricle

Hippocampus
(coronal section)

Cerebral peduncle

Parahippocampal gyrus

Medial occipitotemporal
gyrus

b

Superior longitudinal
fasciculus
= Arcuate fasciculus

Arcuate fibers
of cerebrum

Uncinate fasciculus

Inferior longitudinal
fasciculus

333 Nerve fascicles of the cerebrum (80%)

a   Internal capsule with corona radiata of the right half
of brain. The caudate nucleus and the thalamus
were removed. Medial aspect of the right half

b   Association tracts of the left half of brain, left lateral aspect

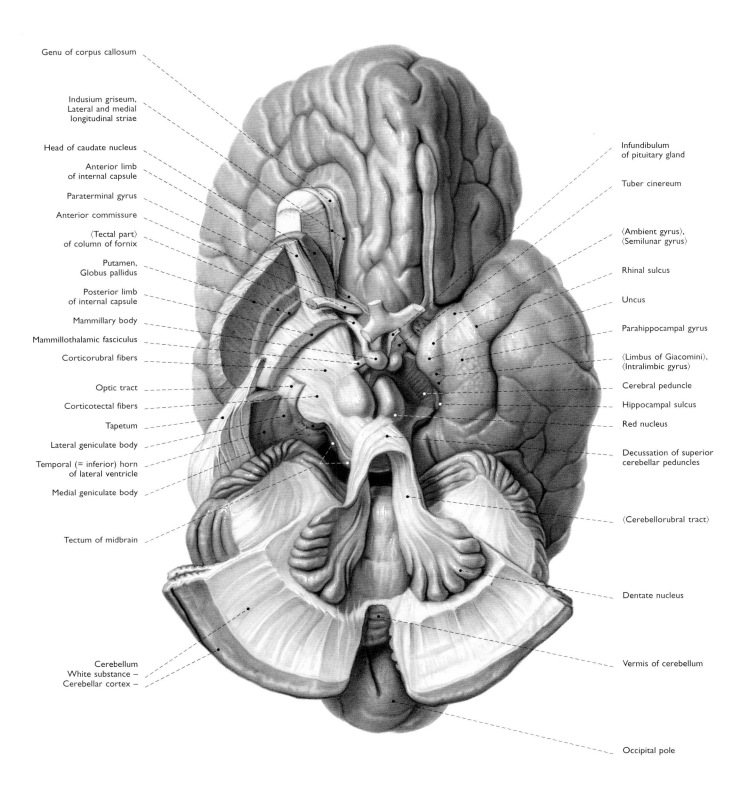

Genu of corpus callosum

Indusium griseum,
Lateral and medial
longitudinal striae

Head of caudate nucleus

Anterior limb
of internal capsule

Paraterminal gyrus

Anterior commissure

⟨Tectal part⟩
of column of fornix

Putamen,
Globus pallidus

Posterior limb
of internal capsule

Mammillary body

Mammillothalamic fasciculus

Corticorubral fibers

Optic tract

Corticotectal fibers

Tapetum

Lateral geniculate body

Temporal (= inferior) horn
of lateral ventricle

Medial geniculate body

Tectum of midbrain

Cerebellum
White substance –
Cerebellar cortex –

Infundibulum
of pituitary gland

Tuber cinereum

⟨Ambient gyrus⟩,
⟨Semilunar gyrus⟩

Rhinal sulcus

Uncus

Parahippocampal gyrus

⟨Limbus of Giacomini⟩,
⟨Intralimbic gyrus⟩

Cerebral peduncle

Hippocampal sulcus

Red nucleus

Decussation of superior
cerebellar peduncles

⟨Cerebellorubral tract⟩

Dentate nucleus

Vermis of cerebellum

Occipital pole

334   Cerebellorubral connections (100%)

Dissection revealing the cerebellorubral tract (decussation of Stilling)
and several fiber systems in the mesencephalic and diencephalic regions,
inferior aspect

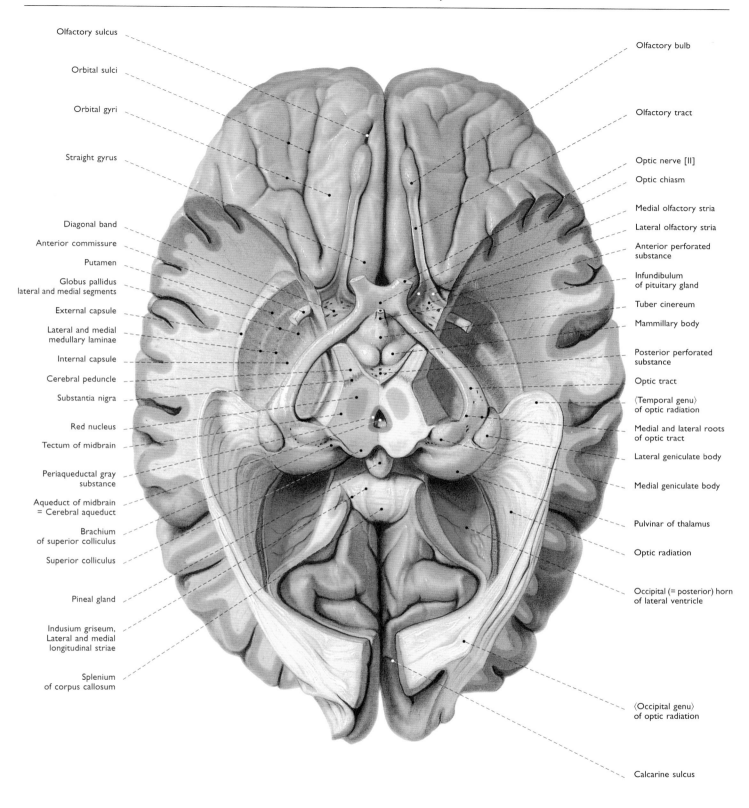

Olfactory sulcus

Orbital sulci

Orbital gyri

Straight gyrus

Diagonal band

Anterior commissure

Putamen

Globus pallidus
lateral and medial segments

External capsule

Lateral and medial
medullary laminae

Internal capsule

Cerebral peduncle

Substantia nigra

Red nucleus

Tectum of midbrain

Periaqueductal gray
substance

Aqueduct of midbrain
= Cerebral aqueduct

Brachium
of superior colliculus

Superior colliculus

Pineal gland

Indusium griseum,
Lateral and medial
longitudinal striae

Splenium
of corpus callosum

Olfactory bulb

Olfactory tract

Optic nerve [II]

Optic chiasm

Medial olfactory stria

Lateral olfactory stria

Anterior perforated
substance

Infundibulum
of pituitary gland

Tuber cinereum

Mammillary body

Posterior perforated
substance

Optic tract

⟨Temporal genu⟩
of optic radiation

Medial and lateral roots
of optic tract

Lateral geniculate body

Medial geniculate body

Pulvinar of thalamus

Optic radiation

Occipital (= posterior) horn
of lateral ventricle

⟨Occipital genu⟩
of optic radiation

Calcarine sulcus

335   Visual pathway (100%)
Dissection showing the optic radiation. The fibers pass
from the optic chiasm to the visual area of cortex.
Inferior aspect

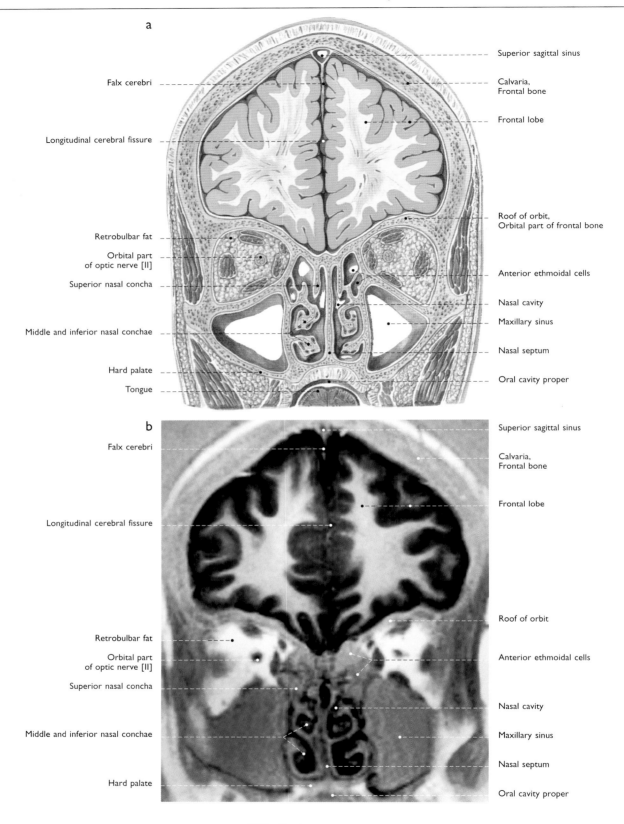

a

Falx cerebri

Longitudinal cerebral fissure

Retrobulbar fat

Orbital part
of optic nerve [II]

Superior nasal concha

Middle and inferior nasal conchae

Hard palate

Tongue

Superior sagittal sinus

Calvaria,
Frontal bone

Frontal lobe

Roof of orbit,
Orbital part of frontal bone

Anterior ethmoidal cells

Nasal cavity

Maxillary sinus

Nasal septum

Oral cavity proper

b

Falx cerebri

Longitudinal cerebral fissure

Retrobulbar fat

Orbital part
of optic nerve [II]

Superior nasal concha

Middle and inferior nasal conchae

Hard palate

Superior sagittal sinus

Calvaria,
Frontal bone

Frontal lobe

Roof of orbit

Anterior ethmoidal cells

Nasal cavity

Maxillary sinus

Nasal septum

Oral cavity proper

336 Brain (75%)

Coronal sections through the frontal lobes of cerebrum,
adjacent bones of cranium, and the orbital and nasal cavities,
frontal aspect
a Anatomical section (painted)
b Magnetic resonance image (MRI, T_1-weighted)

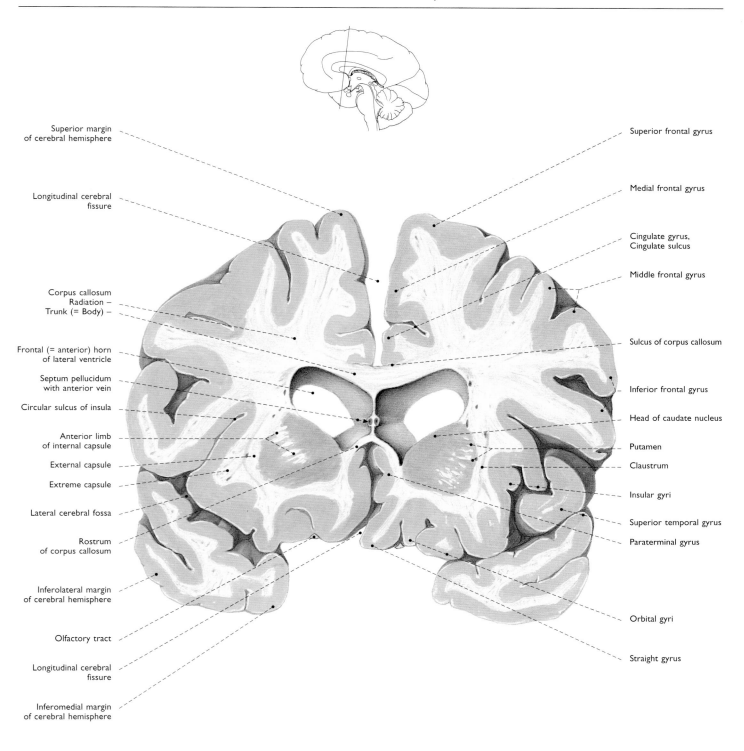

Superior margin
of cerebral hemisphere

Longitudinal cerebral
fissure

Corpus callosum
Radiation –
Trunk (= Body) –

Frontal (= anterior) horn
of lateral ventricle

Septum pellucidum
with anterior vein

Circular sulcus of insula

Anterior limb
of internal capsule

External capsule

Extreme capsule

Lateral cerebral fossa

Rostrum
of corpus callosum

Inferolateral margin
of cerebral hemisphere

Olfactory tract

Longitudinal cerebral
fissure

Inferomedial margin
of cerebral hemisphere

Superior frontal gyrus

Medial frontal gyrus

Cingulate gyrus,
Cingulate sulcus

Middle frontal gyrus

Sulcus of corpus callosum

Inferior frontal gyrus

Head of caudate nucleus

Putamen

Claustrum

Insular gyri

Superior temporal gyrus

Paraterminal gyrus

Orbital gyri

Straight gyrus

337 Brain (100%)
Coronal section in the plane of the frontal horn
of the lateral ventricles, occipital aspect

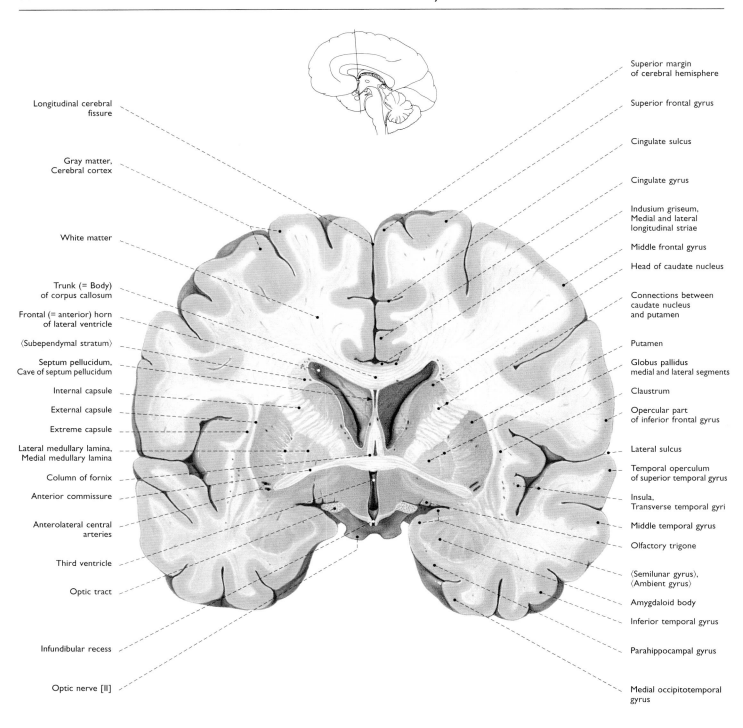

Longitudinal cerebral fissure

Gray matter, Cerebral cortex

White matter

Trunk (= Body) of corpus callosum

Frontal (= anterior) horn of lateral ventricle

⟨Subependymal stratum⟩

Septum pellucidum, Cave of septum pellucidum

Internal capsule

External capsule

Extreme capsule

Lateral medullary lamina, Medial medullary lamina

Column of fornix

Anterior commissure

Anterolateral central arteries

Third ventricle

Optic tract

Infundibular recess

Optic nerve [II]

Superior margin of cerebral hemisphere

Superior frontal gyrus

Cingulate sulcus

Cingulate gyrus

Indusium griseum, Medial and lateral longitudinal striae

Middle frontal gyrus

Head of caudate nucleus

Connections between caudate nucleus and putamen

Putamen

Globus pallidus medial and lateral segments

Claustrum

Opercular part of inferior frontal gyrus

Lateral sulcus

Temporal operculum of superior temporal gyrus

Insula, Transverse temporal gyri

Middle temporal gyrus

Olfactory trigone

⟨Semilunar gyrus⟩, ⟨Ambient gyrus⟩

Amygdaloid body

Inferior temporal gyrus

Parahippocampal gyrus

Medial occipitotemporal gyrus

338 Brain (100%)
Coronal section in the plane of the anterior commissure, occipital aspect

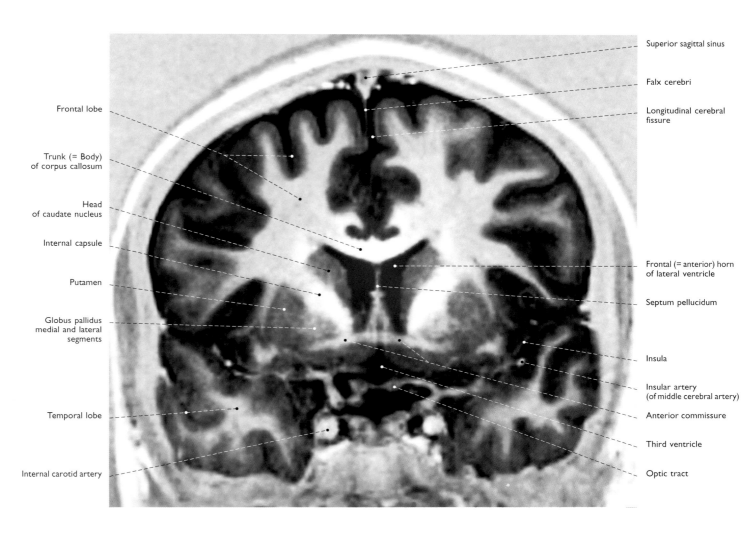

Superior sagittal sinus

Falx cerebri

Longitudinal cerebral
fissure

Frontal lobe

Trunk (= Body)
of corpus callosum

Head
of caudate nucleus

Internal capsule

Putamen

Globus pallidus
medial and lateral
segments

Temporal lobe

Internal carotid artery

Frontal (= anterior) horn
of lateral ventricle

Septum pellucidum

Insula

Insular artery
(of middle cerebral artery)

Anterior commissure

Third ventricle

Optic tract

339 Brain (100%)
Coronal magnetic resonance image (MRI, T$_1$-weighted)
in the plane of the anterior commissure, in correspondence to fig. 338

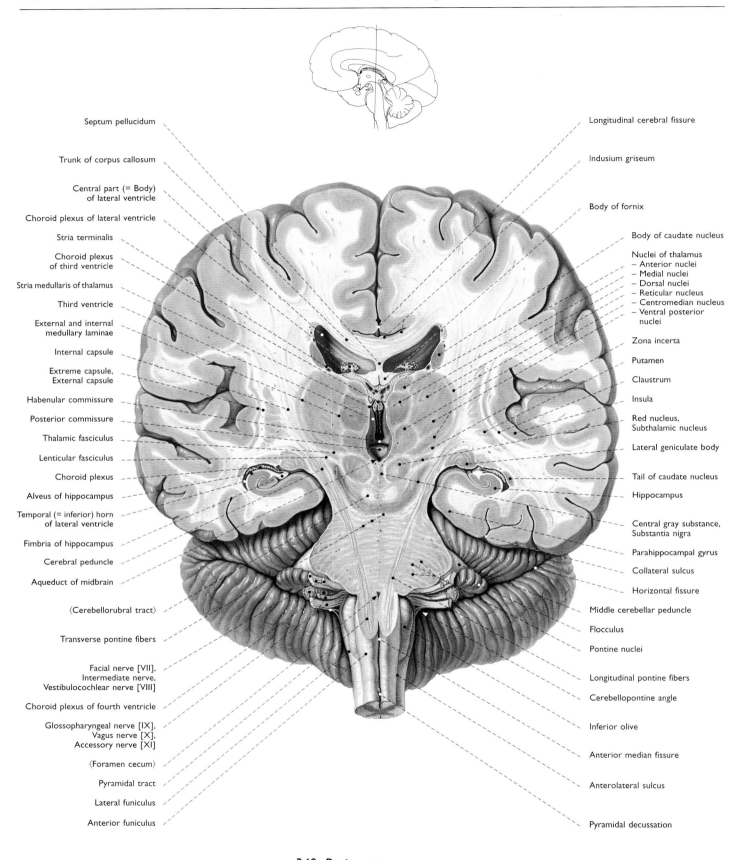

Septum pellucidum

Trunk of corpus callosum

Central part (= Body) of lateral ventricle

Choroid plexus of lateral ventricle

Stria terminalis

Choroid plexus of third ventricle

Stria medullaris of thalamus

Third ventricle

External and internal medullary laminae

Internal capsule

Extreme capsule, External capsule

Habenular commissure

Posterior commissure

Thalamic fasciculus

Lenticular fasciculus

Choroid plexus

Alveus of hippocampus

Temporal (= inferior) horn of lateral ventricle

Fimbria of hippocampus

Cerebral peduncle

Aqueduct of midbrain

⟨Cerebellorubral tract⟩

Transverse pontine fibers

Facial nerve [VII], Intermediate nerve, Vestibulocochlear nerve [VIII]

Choroid plexus of fourth ventricle

Glossopharyngeal nerve [IX], Vagus nerve [X], Accessory nerve [XI]

⟨Foramen cecum⟩

Pyramidal tract

Lateral funiculus

Anterior funiculus

Longitudinal cerebral fissure

Indusium griseum

Body of fornix

Body of caudate nucleus

Nuclei of thalamus
– Anterior nuclei
– Medial nuclei
– Dorsal nuclei
– Reticular nucleus
– Centromedian nucleus
– Ventral posterior nuclei

Zona incerta

Putamen

Claustrum

Insula

Red nucleus, Subthalamic nucleus

Lateral geniculate body

Tail of caudate nucleus

Hippocampus

Central gray substance, Substantia nigra

Parahippocampal gyrus

Collateral sulcus

Horizontal fissure

Middle cerebellar peduncle

Flocculus

Pontine nuclei

Longitudinal pontine fibers

Cerebellopontine angle

Inferior olive

Anterior median fissure

Anterolateral sulcus

Pyramidal decussation

340 Brain (100%)
Coronal section in the plane of the cerebral peduncles, frontal aspect

Longitudinal cerebral
fissure

Superior sagittal sinus

Parietal lobe

Central part (= Body)
of lateral ventricle

Trunk (= Body)
of corpus callosum

Internal cerebral vein

Body
of caudate nucleus

Thalamus

Third ventricle

Internal capsule

Putamen

Temporal (= inferior)
horn of lateral ventricle

Temporal lobe

Hippocampus

Red nucleus

Cerebral peduncle

Pons

Trigeminal nerve [V]

Pontocerebellar
cistern

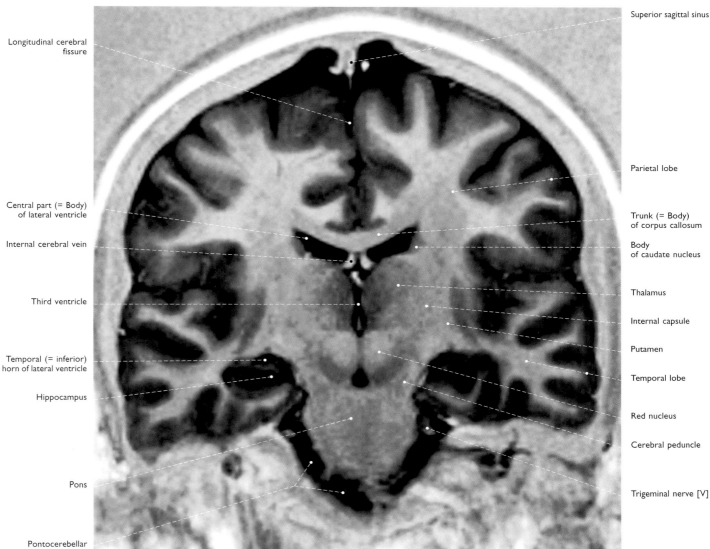

341 Brain (100%)
Coronal magnetic resonance image (MRI, T$_1$-weighted)
in the plane of the cerebral peduncles, in correspondence to fig. 340

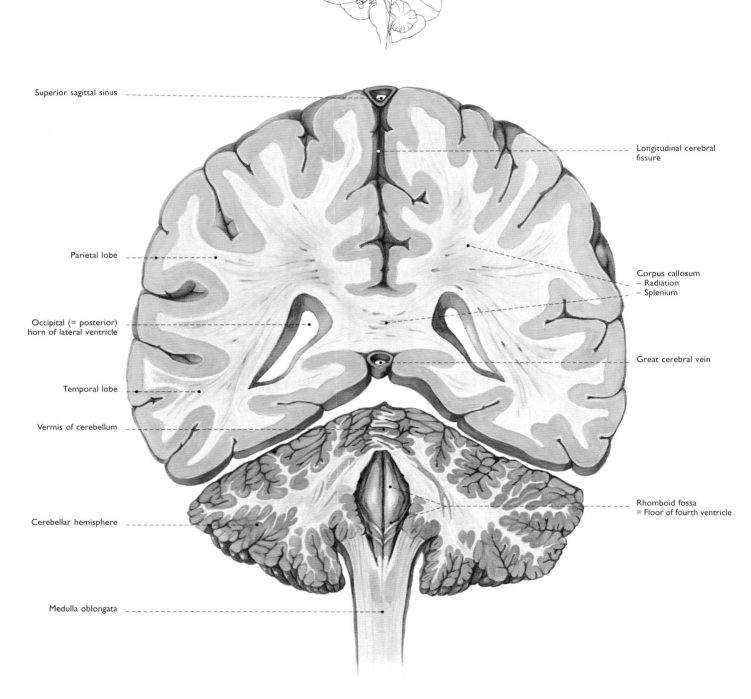

Superior sagittal sinus

Parietal lobe

Occipital (= posterior) horn of lateral ventricle

Temporal lobe

Vermis of cerebellum

Cerebellar hemisphere

Medulla oblongata

Longitudinal cerebral fissure

Corpus callosum
– Radiation
– Splenium

Great cerebral vein

Rhomboid fossa
= Floor of fourth ventricle

342 Brain (100%)

Coronal section in the plane of the occipital horn
of the lateral ventricles and the fourth ventricle,
occipital aspect

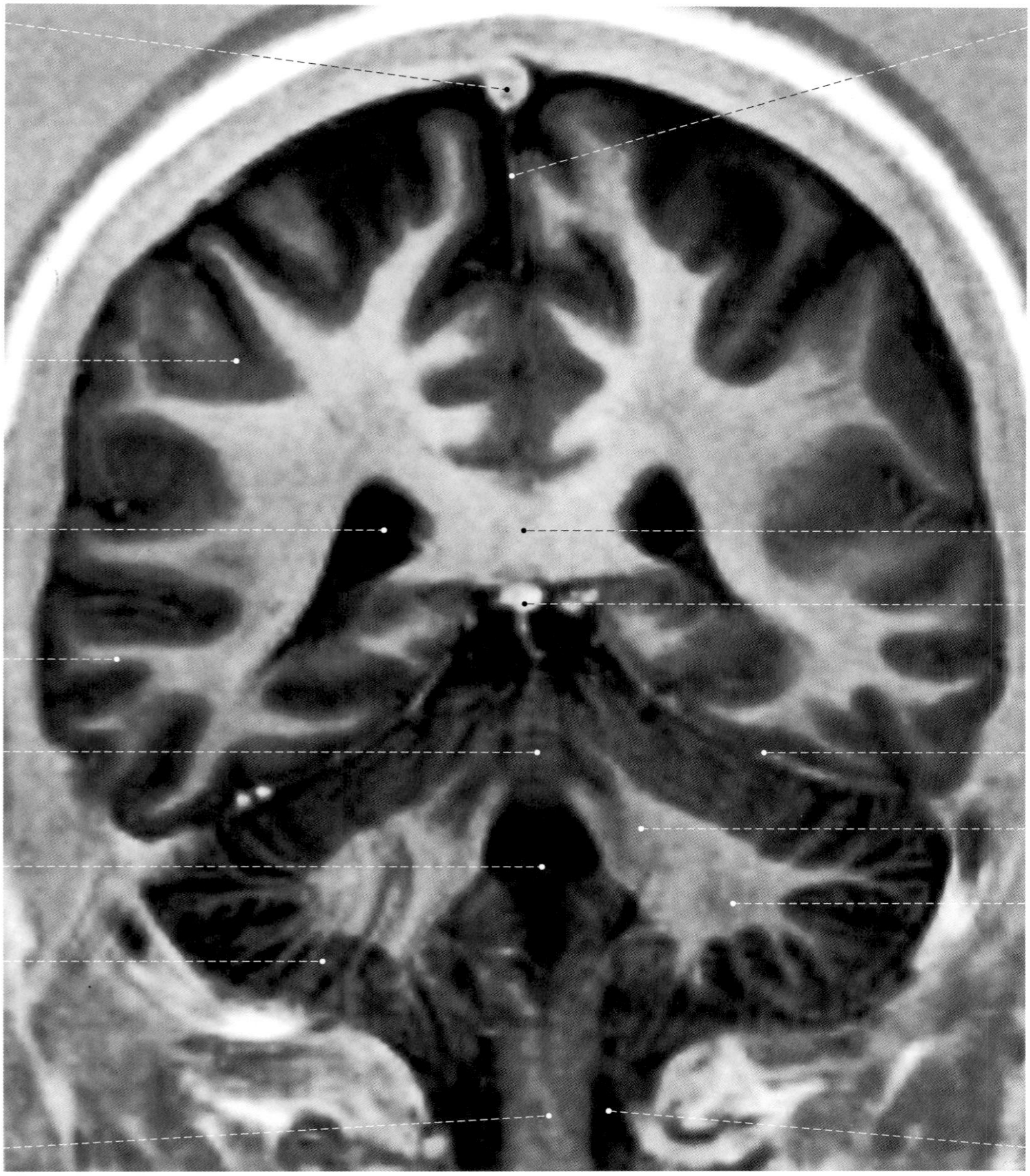

Superior sagittal sinus

Longitudinal cerebral fissure with falx cerebri

Parietal lobe

Occipital (= posterior) horn of lateral ventricle

Splenium of corpus callosum

Great cerebral vein

Temporal lobe

Vermis of cerebellum

Tentorium cerebelli

Fourth ventricle

Superior cerebellar peduncle

Cerebellar hemisphere

Middle cerebellar peduncle

Medulla oblongata

Posterior cerebello-medullary cistern = Cisterna magna

343 Brain (100%)
Coronal magnetic resonance image (MRI, T$_1$-weighted)
in the plane of the occipital horn of the lateral ventricles
and the fourth ventricle, in correspondence to fig. 342

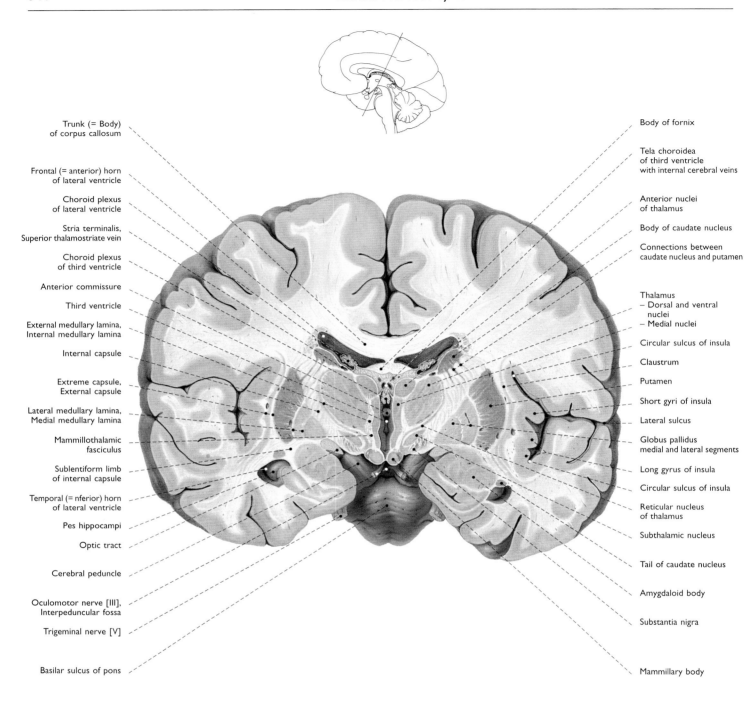

Trunk (= Body)
of corpus callosum

Frontal (= anterior) horn
of lateral ventricle

Choroid plexus
of lateral ventricle

Stria terminalis,
Superior thalamostriate vein

Choroid plexus
of third ventricle

Anterior commissure

Third ventricle

External medullary lamina,
Internal medullary lamina

Internal capsule

Extreme capsule,
External capsule

Lateral medullary lamina,
Medial medullary lamina

Mammillothalamic
fasciculus

Sublentiform limb
of internal capsule

Temporal (= nferior) horn
of lateral ventricle

Pes hippocampi

Optic tract

Cerebral peduncle

Oculomotor nerve [III],
Interpeduncular fossa

Trigeminal nerve [V]

Basilar sulcus of pons

Body of fornix

Tela choroidea
of third ventricle
with internal cerebral veins

Anterior nuclei
of thalamus

Body of caudate nucleus

Connections between
caudate nucleus and putamen

Thalamus
– Dorsal and ventral
nuclei
– Medial nuclei

Circular sulcus of insula

Claustrum

Putamen

Short gyri of insula

Lateral sulcus

Globus pallidus
medial and lateral segments

Long gyrus of insula

Circular sulcus of insula

Reticular nucleus
of thalamus

Subthalamic nucleus

Tail of caudate nucleus

Amygdaloid body

Substantia nigra

Mammillary body

344 Brain (100%)
Coronal section in the plane of the mammillary bodies,
frontal aspect

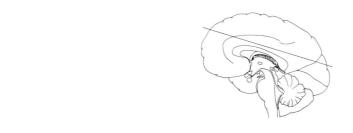

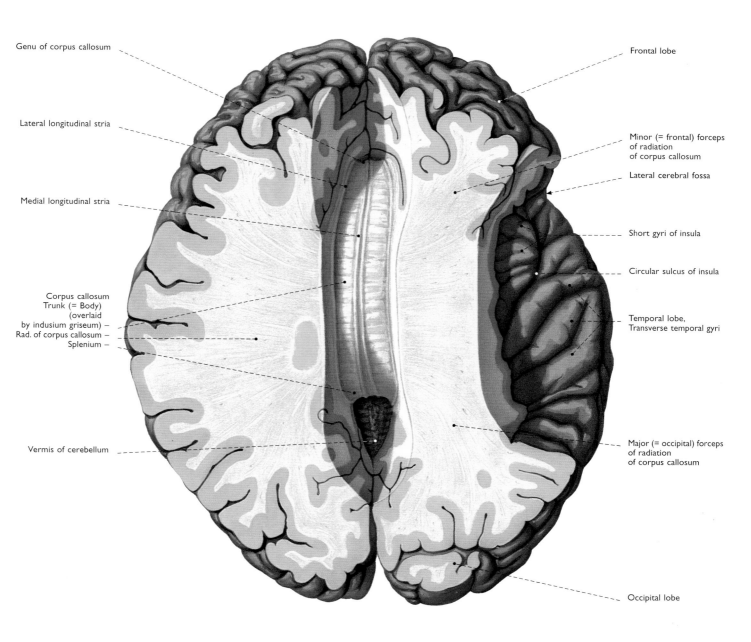

Genu of corpus callosum

Lateral longitudinal stria

Medial longitudinal stria

Corpus callosum
Trunk (= Body)
(overlaid
by indusium griseum) —
Rad. of corpus callosum —
Splenium —

Vermis of cerebellum

Frontal lobe

Minor (= frontal) forceps
of radiation
of corpus callosum

Lateral cerebral fossa

Short gyri of insula

Circular sulcus of insula

Temporal lobe,
Transverse temporal gyri

Major (= occipital) forceps
of radiation
of corpus callosum

Occipital lobe

345   Brain (100%)

Horizontal section above the corpus callosum.
The upper surface of the temporal lobe and the insula
were exposed in the right hemisphere. Superior aspect

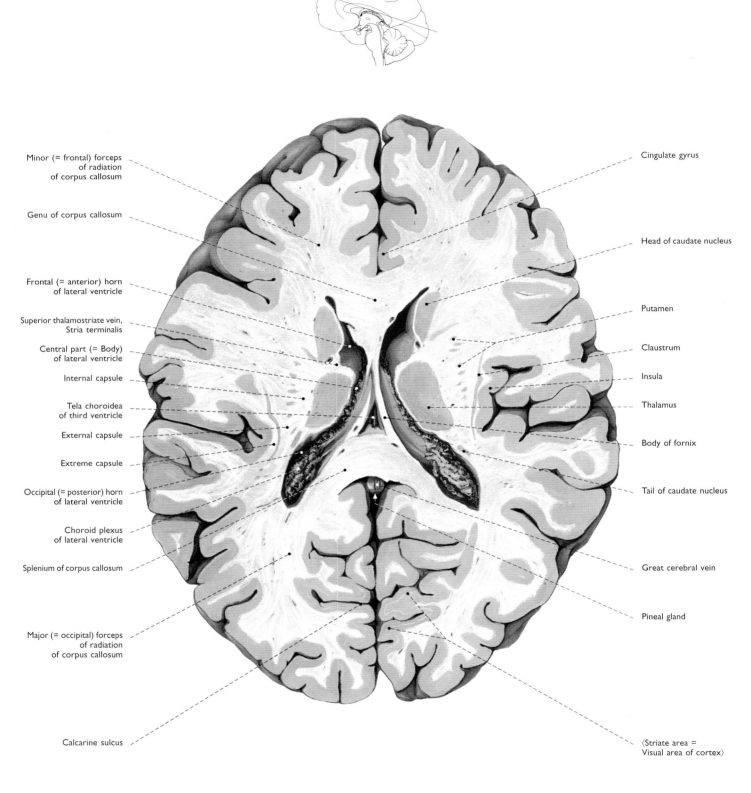

Minor (= frontal) forceps
of radiation
of corpus callosum

Genu of corpus callosum

Frontal (= anterior) horn
of lateral ventricle

Superior thalamostriate vein,
Stria terminalis

Central part (= Body)
of lateral ventricle

Internal capsule

Tela choroidea
of third ventricle

External capsule

Extreme capsule

Occipital (= posterior) horn
of lateral ventricle

Choroid plexus
of lateral ventricle

Splenium of corpus callosum

Major (= occipital) forceps
of radiation
of corpus callosum

Calcarine sulcus

Cingulate gyrus

Head of caudate nucleus

Putamen

Claustrum

Insula

Thalamus

Body of fornix

Tail of caudate nucleus

Great cerebral vein

Pineal gland

⟨Striate area =
Visual area of cortex⟩

346 Brain (100%)
Transverse section at the level of the body
of fornix, and the frontal and occipital horns
of the lateral ventricles, superior aspect

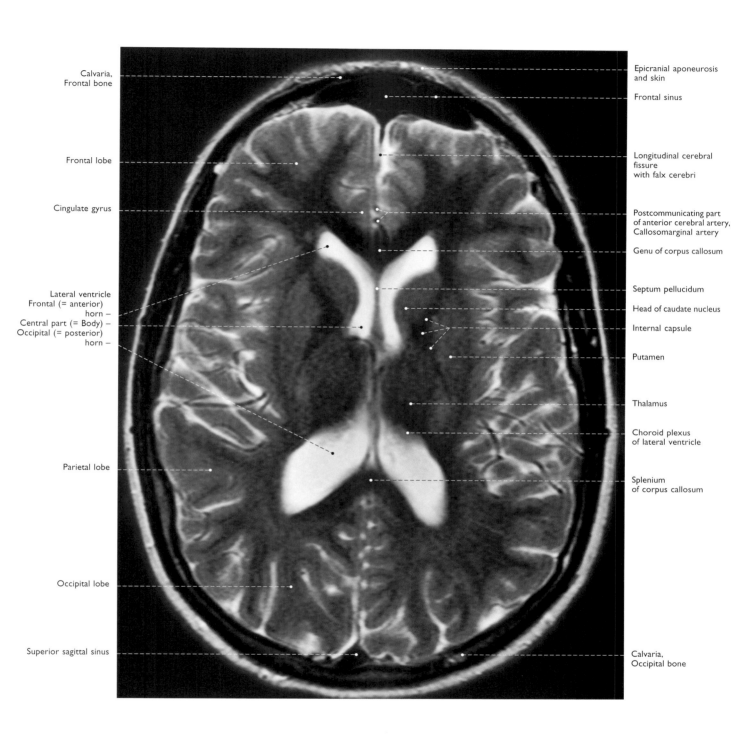

Calvaria,
Frontal bone

Frontal lobe

Cingulate gyrus

Lateral ventricle
Frontal (= anterior)
horn –
Central part (= Body) –
Occipital (= posterior)
horn –

Parietal lobe

Occipital lobe

Superior sagittal sinus

Epicranial aponeurosis
and skin

Frontal sinus

Longitudinal cerebral
fissure
with falx cerebri

Postcommunicating part
of anterior cerebral artery,
Callosomarginal artery

Genu of corpus callosum

Septum pellucidum

Head of caudate nucleus

Internal capsule

Putamen

Thalamus

Choroid plexus
of lateral ventricle

Splenium
of corpus callosum

Calvaria,
Occipital bone

347 Brain (100%)

Transverse magnetic resonance image (MRI, T$_2$-weighted)
at the level of the frontal and occipital horns of the lateral ventricles,
in correspondence to fig. 346, inferior aspect

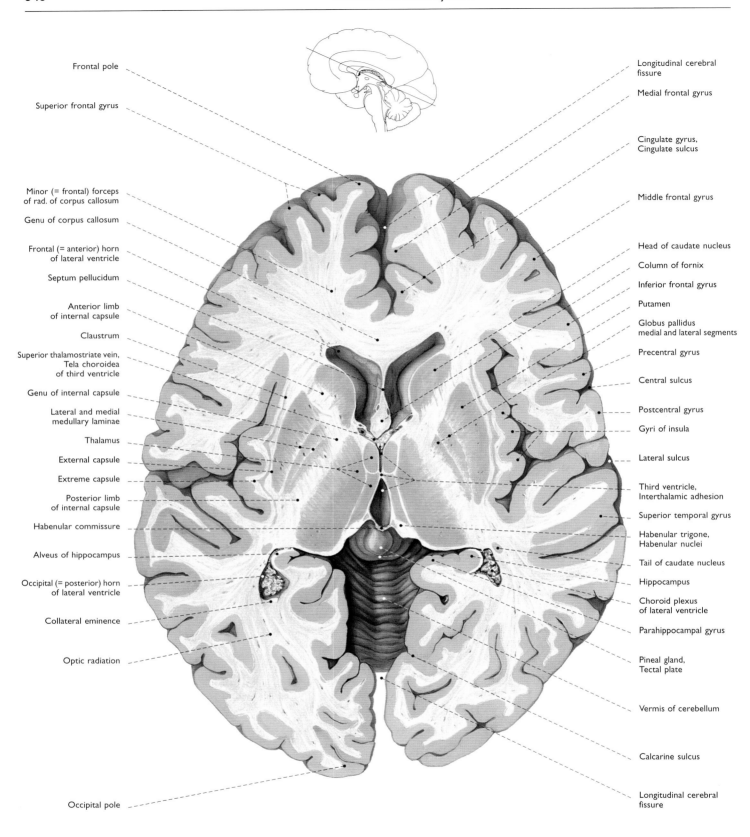

Frontal pole

Superior frontal gyrus

Minor (= frontal) forceps
of rad. of corpus callosum

Genu of corpus callosum

Frontal (= anterior) horn
of lateral ventricle

Septum pellucidum

Anterior limb
of internal capsule

Claustrum

Superior thalamostriate vein,
Tela choroidea
of third ventricle

Genu of internal capsule

Lateral and medial
medullary laminae

Thalamus

External capsule

Extreme capsule

Posterior limb
of internal capsule

Habenular commissure

Alveus of hippocampus

Occipital (= posterior) horn
of lateral ventricle

Collateral eminence

Optic radiation

Occipital pole

Longitudinal cerebral
fissure

Medial frontal gyrus

Cingulate gyrus,
Cingulate sulcus

Middle frontal gyrus

Head of caudate nucleus

Column of fornix

Inferior frontal gyrus

Putamen

Globus pallidus
medial and lateral segments

Precentral gyrus

Central sulcus

Postcentral gyrus

Gyri of insula

Lateral sulcus

Third ventricle,
Interthalamic adhesion

Superior temporal gyrus

Habenular trigone,
Habenular nuclei

Tail of caudate nucleus

Hippocampus

Choroid plexus
of lateral ventricle

Parahippocampal gyrus

Pineal gland,
Tectal plate

Vermis of cerebellum

Calcarine sulcus

Longitudinal cerebral
fissure

348 Brain (100%)

Transverse section at the level of the third ventricle,
the frontal and occipital horns of the lateral ventricles,
and the pineal gland, superior aspect

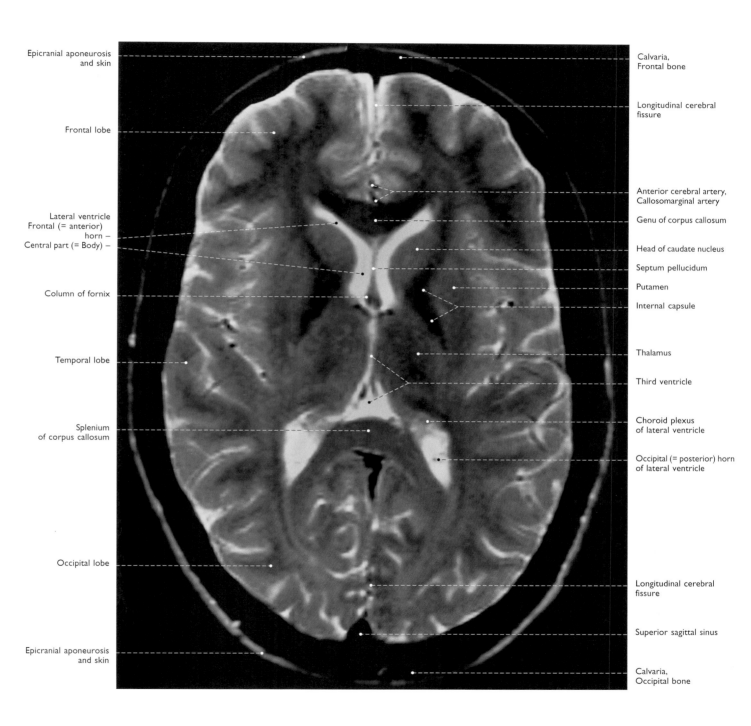

Epicranial aponeurosis and skin

Frontal lobe

Lateral ventricle
Frontal (= anterior) horn —
Central part (= Body) —

Column of fornix

Temporal lobe

Splenium of corpus callosum

Occipital lobe

Epicranial aponeurosis and skin

Calvaria, Frontal bone

Longitudinal cerebral fissure

Anterior cerebral artery, Callosomarginal artery

Genu of corpus callosum

Head of caudate nucleus

Septum pellucidum

Putamen

Internal capsule

Thalamus

Third ventricle

Choroid plexus of lateral ventricle

Occipital (= posterior) horn of lateral ventricle

Longitudinal cerebral fissure

Superior sagittal sinus

Calvaria, Occipital bone

349 Brain (100%)
Transverse magnetic resonance image (MRI, T_2-weighted)
at the level of the third ventricle, and the frontal and occipital horns
of the lateral ventricles, in correspondence to fig. 348, inferior aspect

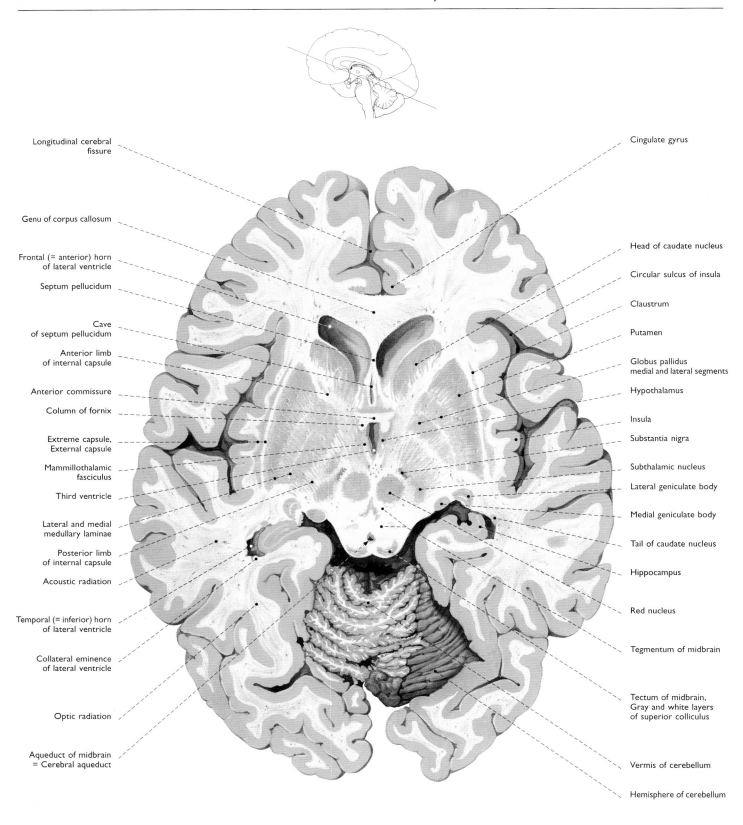

Longitudinal cerebral fissure

Genu of corpus callosum

Frontal (= anterior) horn of lateral ventricle

Septum pellucidum

Cave of septum pellucidum

Anterior limb of internal capsule

Anterior commissure

Column of fornix

Extreme capsule, External capsule

Mammillothalamic fasciculus

Third ventricle

Lateral and medial medullary laminae

Posterior limb of internal capsule

Acoustic radiation

Temporal (= inferior) horn of lateral ventricle

Collateral eminence of lateral ventricle

Optic radiation

Aqueduct of midbrain = Cerebral aqueduct

Cingulate gyrus

Head of caudate nucleus

Circular sulcus of insula

Claustrum

Putamen

Globus pallidus medial and lateral segments

Hypothalamus

Insula

Substantia nigra

Subthalamic nucleus

Lateral geniculate body

Medial geniculate body

Tail of caudate nucleus

Hippocampus

Red nucleus

Tegmentum of midbrain

Tectum of midbrain, Gray and white layers of superior colliculus

Vermis of cerebellum

Hemisphere of cerebellum

350 Brain (100%)
Transverse section at the level of the anterior commissure, superior aspect

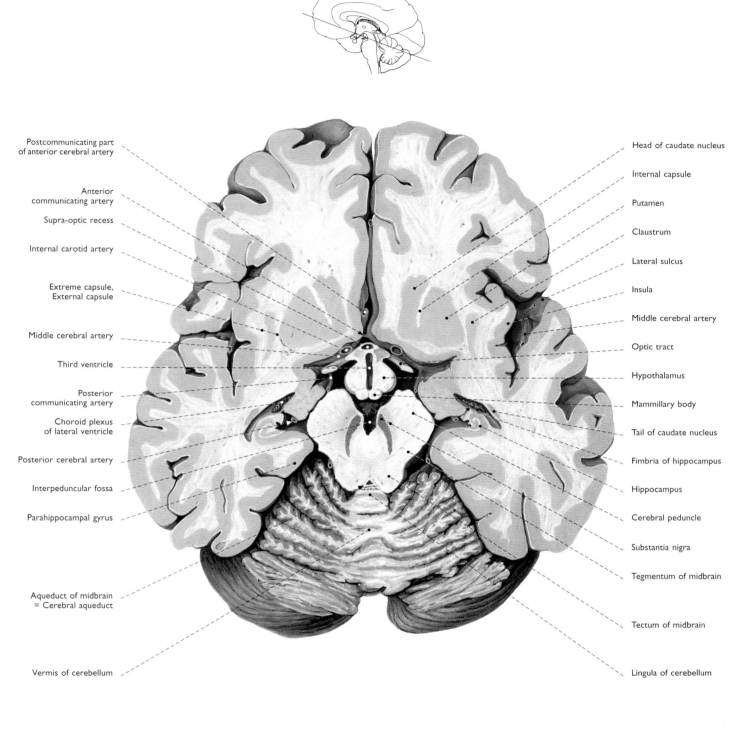

Postcommunicating part of anterior cerebral artery

Anterior communicating artery

Supra-optic recess

Internal carotid artery

Extreme capsule, External capsule

Middle cerebral artery

Third ventricle

Posterior communicating artery

Choroid plexus of lateral ventricle

Posterior cerebral artery

Interpeduncular fossa

Parahippocampal gyrus

Aqueduct of midbrain = Cerebral aqueduct

Vermis of cerebellum

Head of caudate nucleus

Internal capsule

Putamen

Claustrum

Lateral sulcus

Insula

Middle cerebral artery

Optic tract

Hypothalamus

Mammillary body

Tail of caudate nucleus

Fimbria of hippocampus

Hippocampus

Cerebral peduncle

Substantia nigra

Tegmentum of midbrain

Tectum of midbrain

Lingula of cerebellum

351 Brain (100%)
Transverse section at the level of the midbrain
and the mammillary bodies, superior aspect

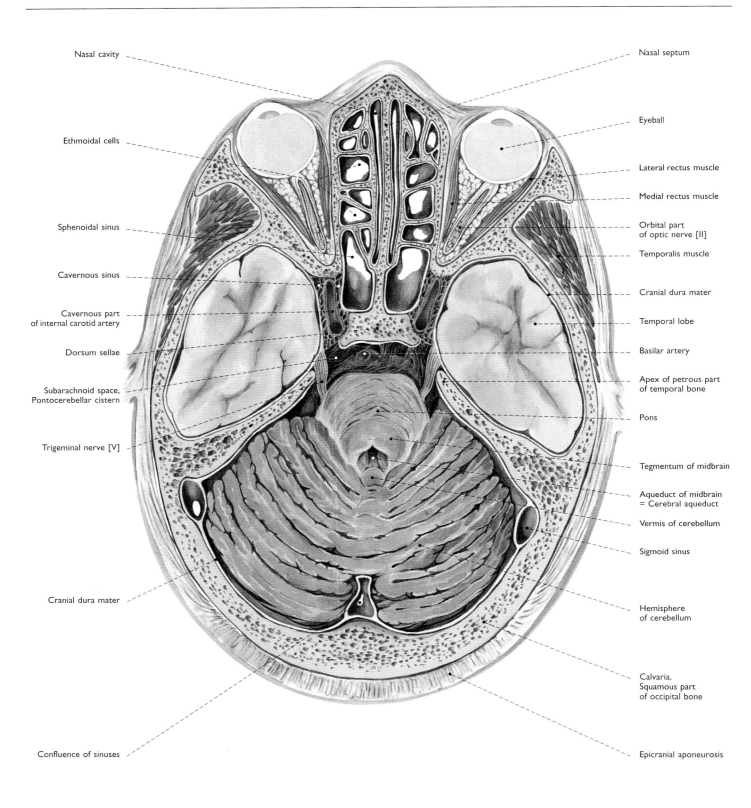

Nasal cavity

Ethmoidal cells

Sphenoidal sinus

Cavernous sinus

Cavernous part
of internal carotid artery

Dorsum sellae

Subarachnoid space,
Pontocerebellar cistern

Trigeminal nerve [V]

Cranial dura mater

Confluence of sinuses

Nasal septum

Eyeball

Lateral rectus muscle

Medial rectus muscle

Orbital part
of optic nerve [II]

Temporalis muscle

Cranial dura mater

Temporal lobe

Basilar artery

Apex of petrous part
of temporal bone

Pons

Tegmentum of midbrain

Aqueduct of midbrain
= Cerebral aqueduct

Vermis of cerebellum

Sigmoid sinus

Hemisphere
of cerebellum

Calvaria,
Squamous part
of occipital bone

Epicranial aponeurosis

352 Brain (100%)

Transverse section through the head and brain at the level
of the optic nerves, the dorsum sellae, the pons, and
the aqueduct of midbrain, superior aspect

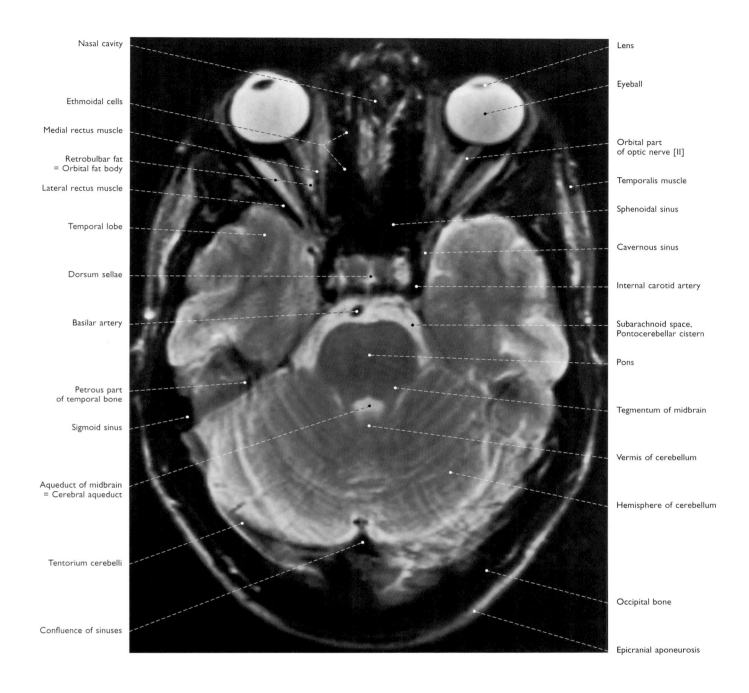

Nasal cavity

Ethmoidal cells

Medial rectus muscle

Retrobulbar fat
= Orbital fat body

Lateral rectus muscle

Temporal lobe

Dorsum sellae

Basilar artery

Petrous part
of temporal bone

Sigmoid sinus

Aqueduct of midbrain
= Cerebral aqueduct

Tentorium cerebelli

Confluence of sinuses

Lens

Eyeball

Orbital part
of optic nerve [II]

Temporalis muscle

Sphenoidal sinus

Cavernous sinus

Internal carotid artery

Subarachnoid space,
Pontocerebellar cistern

Pons

Tegmentum of midbrain

Vermis of cerebellum

Hemisphere of cerebellum

Occipital bone

Epicranial aponeurosis

353 Brain (100%)
Transverse magnetic resonance image (MRI, T$_2$-weighted)
at the level of the optic nerves, the dorsum sellae, the pons,
and the aqueduct of midbrain, in correspondence to fig. 352,
inferior aspect

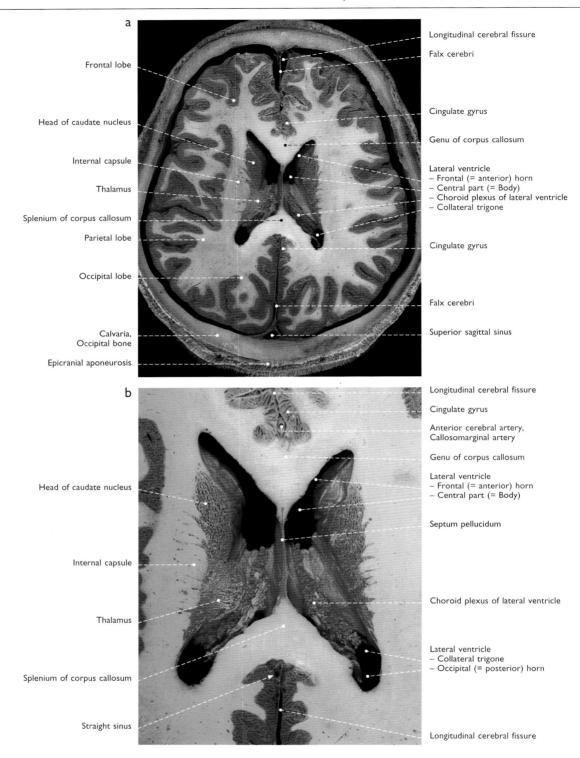

a

Frontal lobe

Head of caudate nucleus

Internal capsule

Thalamus

Splenium of corpus callosum

Parietal lobe

Occipital lobe

Calvaria,
Occipital bone

Epicranial aponeurosis

Longitudinal cerebral fissure

Falx cerebri

Cingulate gyrus

Genu of corpus callosum

Lateral ventricle
– Frontal (= anterior) horn
– Central part (= Body)
– Choroid plexus of lateral ventricle
– Collateral trigone

Cingulate gyrus

Falx cerebri

Superior sagittal sinus

b

Head of caudate nucleus

Internal capsule

Thalamus

Splenium of corpus callosum

Straight sinus

Longitudinal cerebral fissure

Cingulate gyrus

Anterior cerebral artery,
Callosomarginal artery

Genu of corpus callosum

Lateral ventricle
– Frontal (= anterior) horn
– Central part (= Body)

Septum pellucidum

Choroid plexus of lateral ventricle

Lateral ventricle
– Collateral trigone
– Occipital (= posterior) horn

Longitudinal cerebral fissure

354 Brain

Anatomical transverse section of the head and brain
at an upper level through the central part and the frontal
and occipital horns of the lateral ventricles, superior aspect
a Cross section through the whole head (50%)
b Magnification of central parts of the brain (110%)

a

Frontal lobe

Genu of corpus callosum

Septum pellucidum

Head of caudate nucleus

Anterior limb of internal capsule

Putamen

Thalamus

Posterior limb of internal capsule

Third ventricle

Optic radiation

Calcarine sulcus

Calvaria,
Occipital bone

Epicranial aponeurosis

Longitudinal cerebral fissure

Falx cerebri

Cingulate gyrus

Lateral ventricle
– Frontal (= anterior) horn
– Central part (= Body)

Insula

Lateral sulcus

Lateral ventricle
– Choroid plexus of lateral ventricle
– Occipital (= posterior) horn

Occipital lobe

Superior sagittal sinus

b

Cingulate gyrus

Lateral ventricle
Frontal (= anterior) horn –
Central part (= Body) –

Extreme capsule,
External capsule

Claustrum

Internal capsule
Anterior limb of internal capsule –
Genu of internal capsule –
Posterior limb of internal capsule –

Thalamus

Internal cerebral veins

Splenium of corpus callosum

Choroid plexus of lateral ventricle

Occipital (= posterior) horn
of lateral ventricle

Straight sinus

Longitudinal cerebral fissure

Anterior cerebral artery,
Callosomarginal artery

Genu of corpus callosum

Head of caudate nucleus

Septum pellucidum

Putamen

Claustrum

Interventricular foramen

Column of fornix

Third ventricle

Tail of caudate nucleus

Cingulate gyrus

Falx cerebri

Longitudinal cerebral fissure

355 Brain

Anatomical transverse section (more caudal than in fig. 354)
through the head and brain at the level of the third ventricle,
upper parts of the internal capsule, and the frontal and
occipital horns of the lateral ventricles, superior aspect
a Cross section through the whole head (50%)
b Magnification of central parts of the brain (110%)

a

Calvaria,
Frontal bone

Frontal lobe

Head of caudate nucleus

Internal capsule

Putamen

Globus pallidus
lateral and medial segments

Thalamus

Tail of caudate nucleus

Lateral ventricle
Collateral trigone –
Choroid plexus of lateral ventricle –
Occipital (= posterior) horn –

Longitudinal cerebral fissure

Falx cerebri

Superior sagittal sinus

Longitudinal cerebral fissure

Postcommunicating part
of anterior cerebral artery

Lateral ventricle

Column of fornix

Third ventricle

Interthalamic adhesion

Third ventricle

Optic radiation

Temporal lobe

Occipital lobe

Calvaria,
Occipital bone

Epicranial aponeurosis

b

Anterior cerebral artery

Longitudinal cerebral fissure

Internal capsule
Anterior limb of internal capsule –
Genu of internal capsule –

Third ventricle

Globus pallidus
lateral and medial segments

Posterior limb of internal capsule

Third ventricle

Pineal gland

Tail of caudate nucleus

Splenium of corpus callosum

Lateral ventricle
Choroid plexus of lateral ventricle –
Occipital (= posterior) horn –

Falx cerebri

Longitudinal cerebral fissure

Head of caudate nucleus

Central part (= Body)
of lateral ventricle

Column of fornix

Extreme capsule

Claustrum

External capsule

Putamen

Interthalamic adhesion

Thalamus

Hippocampus

Vermis of cerebellum

Tentorium cerebelli

Straight sinus

356 Brain

Anatomical transverse section (more caudal than in fig. 355)
through the head and brain at the level of lower parts
of the third ventricle, the internal capsule, and the occipital
horn of lateral ventricles, superior aspect
a   Cross section through the whole head (50%)
b   Magnification of central parts of the brain (110%)

a

Calvaria,
Frontal bone

Orbital part
of frontal bone

Frontal sinus

Frontal lobe

Third ventricle

Longitudinal cerebral fissure

Aqueduct of midbrain

Temporal lobe

Tectum of midbrain

Temporal (= inferior) horn
of lateral ventricle

Optic radiation

Hippocampus

Vermis of cerebellum

Straight sinus

Occipital lobe

Longitudinal cerebral fissure

Falx cerebri

Calvaria,
Occipital bone

Superior sagittal sinus

Epicranial aponeurosis

b

Cingulate gyrus

Subcallosal area

Postcommunicating part
of anterior cerebral artery

Third ventricle

Head of caudate nucleus

Red nucleus

Putamen

Aqueduct of midbrain

Posterior limb of internal capsule

Cisterna ambiens

Medial and lateral geniculate bodies

Temporal (= inferior) horn
of lateral ventricle

Hippocampus

Superior colliculus
of tectum of midbrain

Vermis of cerebellum

Tentorium cerebelli

Falx cerebri

Longitudinal cerebral fissure

Straight sinus

357 Brain

Anatomical transverse section (more caudal than in fig. 356)
through the head and brain at the level of the roof of orbit,
the aqueduct of midbrain, and the vermis of cerebellum, superior aspect
a Cross section through the whole head (50%)
b Magnification of central parts of the brain (110%)

a

Nose

Eyeball

Anterior ethmoidal cells

Retrobulbar fat

Temporalis muscle

Frontal lobe

Optic nerve [II]

Optic chiasm

Temporal lobe

Internal carotid artery

Infundibulum of pituitary gland

Temporal (= inferior) horn of lateral ventricle

Hippocampus

Basilar artery

Tegmentum of midbrain

Aqueduct of midbrain

Vermis of cerebellum

Tentorium cerebelli

Hemisphere of cerebellum

Longitudinal cerebral fissure with falx cerebri

Straight sinus

Calvaria, Occipital bone

Occipital lobe

Superior sagittal sinus

Epicranial aponeurosis

b

Anterior cerebral artery, Middle cerebral artery

Intracranial part of optic nerve [II]

Right internal carotid artery

Left internal carotid artery

Posterior communicating artery

Infundibulum of pituitary gland

Basilar artery

Interpeduncular cistern

Oculomotor nerve [III]

Posterior cerebral artery

Cerebral peduncle, Cerebral crus

Tegmentum of midbrain

Aqueduct of midbrain

Tectum of midbrain

Vermis of cerebellum

Hemisphere of cerebellum

Occipital lobe

Tentorium cerebelli

Straight sinus

Falx cerebri in the longitudinal cerebral fissure

358 Brain

Anatomical transverse section (more caudal than in fig. 357) through the head and brain at the level of the optic chiasm, the aqueduct of midbrain, and upper parts of the cerebellum, superior aspect

a   Cross section through the whole head (50%)
b   Magnification of central parts of the brain (110%)

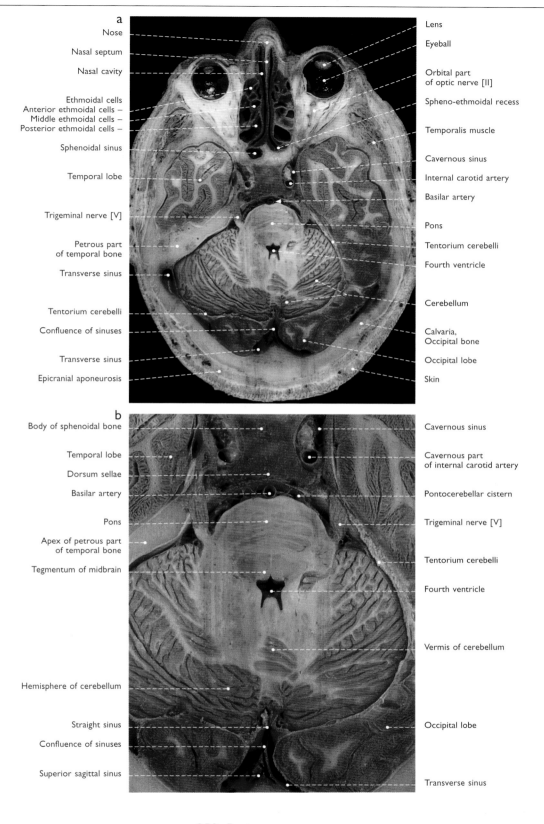

a

Nose

Nasal septum

Nasal cavity

Ethmoidal cells
Anterior ethmoidal cells –
Middle ethmoidal cells –
Posterior ethmoidal cells –

Sphenoidal sinus

Temporal lobe

Trigeminal nerve [V]

Petrous part
of temporal bone

Transverse sinus

Tentorium cerebelli

Confluence of sinuses

Transverse sinus

Epicranial aponeurosis

Lens

Eyeball

Orbital part
of optic nerve [II]

Spheno-ethmoidal recess

Temporalis muscle

Cavernous sinus

Internal carotid artery

Basilar artery

Pons

Tentorium cerebelli

Fourth ventricle

Cerebellum

Calvaria,
Occipital bone

Occipital lobe

Skin

b

Body of sphenoidal bone

Temporal lobe

Dorsum sellae

Basilar artery

Pons

Apex of petrous part
of temporal bone

Tegmentum of midbrain

Hemisphere of cerebellum

Straight sinus

Confluence of sinuses

Superior sagittal sinus

Cavernous sinus

Cavernous part
of internal carotid artery

Pontocerebellar cistern

Trigeminal nerve [V]

Tentorium cerebelli

Fourth ventricle

Vermis of cerebellum

Occipital lobe

Transverse sinus

359 Brain

Anatomical transverse section (more caudal than in fig. 358) through
the head and brain at the level of the optic nerves, the cavernous sinuses,
the pons, the fourth ventricle, and the cerebellum, superior aspect
a   Cross section through the whole head (50%)
b   Magnification of central parts of the brain (110%)

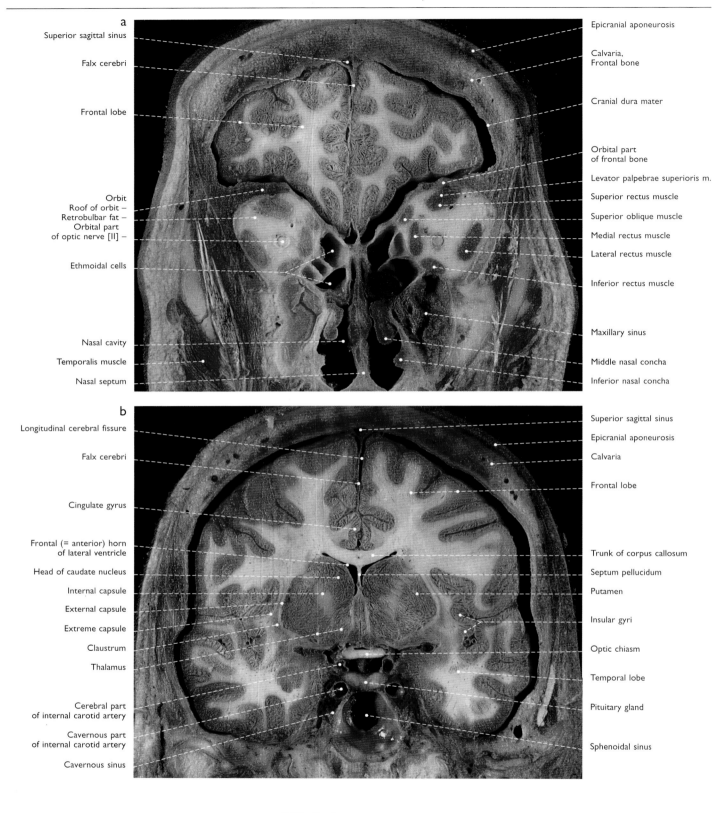

a

Superior sagittal sinus

Falx cerebri

Frontal lobe

Orbit
Roof of orbit –
Retrobulbar fat –
Orbital part
of optic nerve [II] –

Ethmoidal cells

Nasal cavity

Temporalis muscle

Nasal septum

Epicranial aponeurosis

Calvaria,
Frontal bone

Cranial dura mater

Orbital part
of frontal bone

Levator palpebrae superioris m.

Superior rectus muscle

Superior oblique muscle

Medial rectus muscle

Lateral rectus muscle

Inferior rectus muscle

Maxillary sinus

Middle nasal concha

Inferior nasal concha

b

Longitudinal cerebral fissure

Falx cerebri

Cingulate gyrus

Frontal (= anterior) horn
of lateral ventricle

Head of caudate nucleus

Internal capsule

External capsule

Extreme capsule

Claustrum

Thalamus

Cerebral part
of internal carotid artery

Cavernous part
of internal carotid artery

Cavernous sinus

Superior sagittal sinus

Epicranial aponeurosis

Calvaria

Frontal lobe

Trunk of corpus callosum

Septum pellucidum

Putamen

Insular gyri

Optic chiasm

Temporal lobe

Pituitary gland

Sphenoidal sinus

360 Brain (80%)

Occipital aspect
Coronal anatomical sections of the head and brain (80%)
a   in a plane through the frontal lobes of cerebrum and the orbits
     behind the eyeballs
b   in a plane through the optic chiasm, the frontal horn
     of the lateral ventricles, and the head of the caudate nuclei

a

Falx cerebri

Cingulate gyrus

Central part (= Body)
of lateral ventricle

Body of fornix

Third ventricle

Lateral sulcus

Putamen

Temporal lobe

Hippocampus

Parahippocampal gyrus

Tympanic cavity
with auditory ossicles

External acoustic meatus

Superior sagittal sinus

Longitudinal cerebral fissure

Calvaria

Epicranial aponeurosis
and skin

Body of caudate nucleus

Insula

Internal capsule

Thalamus

Aqueduct of midbrain

Longitudinal pontine fibers

Pons

Cochlea

External acoustic meatus

Basilar artery

b

Superior sagittal sinus

Longitudinal cerebral fissure

Falx cerebri

Parietal lobe

Lateral sulcus

Temporal lobe

Thalamus

Hippocampus,
Pineal gland

Parahippocampal gyrus

Aqueduct of midbrain

Mastoid cells of temporal bone

Epicranial aponeurosis
and skin

Calvaria

Cingulate gyrus

Splenium of corpus callosum

Lateral ventricle

Choroid plexus of lateral ventricle

Internal cerebral vein

Tail of caudate nucleus

Temporal (= inferior) horn
of lateral ventricle

Tectum of midbrain

Tentorium cerebelli

Hemisphere of cerebellum

Middle cerebellar peduncle

Medulla oblongata

361 Brain (80%)

Occipital aspect
Coronal anatomical sections of the head and brain (80%)
a in a plane through the central part of the lateral ventricles,
   the third ventricle, and the pons
b in a plane through the pineal gland, the aqueduct of midbrain,
   and the middle cerebellar peduncles

a

Frontal lobe

Cranial dura mater

Middle cerebral artery

Lateral sulcus

Frontal sinus

Superior rectus muscle

Orbital part
of optic nerve [II]

Superior eyelid

Eyeball

Inferior eyelid

Inferior rectus muscle

Temporal lobe

Maxillary sinus

Precentral gyrus

Central sulcus

Postcentral gyrus

Parietal lobe

Epicranial aponeurosis

Calvaria,
Occipital bone

Putamen

Lateral ventricle
– Collateral trigone
with choroid plexus
– Occipital (= posterior)
horn

Hippocampus

Occipital lobe

Tentorium cerebelli

Hemisphere of cerebellum

Petrous part
of temporal bone

b

Frontal lobe

Cranial dura mater

Lateral sulcus

Anterior cranial fossa

Temporal lobe

Temporalis muscle

Petrous part
of temporal bone

Precentral gyrus

Central sulcus

Postcentral gyrus

Parietal lobe

Calvaria,
Occipital bone

Epicranial aponeurosis
and skin

Occipital lobe

Tentorium cerebelli

Transverse sinus

Hemisphere of cerebellum

362 Brain (70%)

Sagittal anatomical sections through the right half
of head and brain
a in a paramedian plane through the right eyeball,
the putamen, and the temporal horn of the right lateral ventricle
b in a more lateral plane through the lateral angle of the right orbit,
the lateral sulcus of cerebrum, and lateral parts of the cerebellum.
Medial aspect of the lateral parts of head

Visual Organ and Orbital Cavity

a

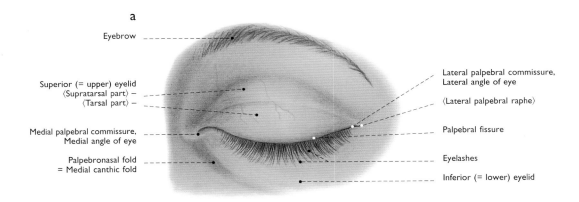

Eyebrow

Superior (= upper) eyelid
⟨Supratarsal part⟩ –
⟨Tarsal part⟩ –

Medial palpebral commissure,
Medial angle of eye

Palpebronasal fold
= Medial canthic fold

Lateral palpebral commissure,
Lateral angle of eye

⟨Lateral palpebral raphe⟩

Palpebral fissure

Eyelashes

Inferior (= lower) eyelid

b

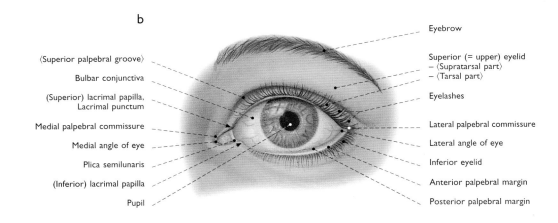

⟨Superior palpebral groove⟩

Bulbar conjunctiva

(Superior) lacrimal papilla,
Lacrimal punctum

Medial palpebral commissure

Medial angle of eye

Plica semilunaris

(Inferior) lacrimal papilla

Pupil

Eyebrow

Superior (= upper) eyelid
– ⟨Supratarsal part⟩
– ⟨Tarsal part⟩

Eyelashes

Lateral palpebral commissure

Lateral angle of eye

Inferior eyelid

Anterior palpebral margin

Posterior palpebral margin

c

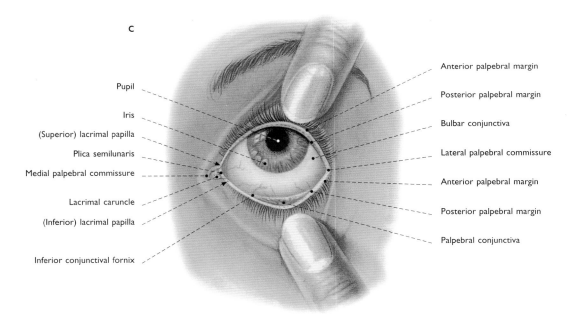

Pupil

Iris

(Superior) lacrimal papilla

Plica semilunaris

Medial palpebral commissure

Lacrimal caruncle

(Inferior) lacrimal papilla

Inferior conjunctival fornix

Anterior palpebral margin

Posterior palpebral margin

Bulbar conjunctiva

Lateral palpebral commissure

Anterior palpebral margin

Posterior palpebral margin

Palpebral conjunctiva

364 Eye (110%)
Frontal aspect
a Eyelids of the left eye closed
b Eyelids of the left eye open
c Upper eyelid of the left eye drawn upwards
and lower eyelid slightly everted

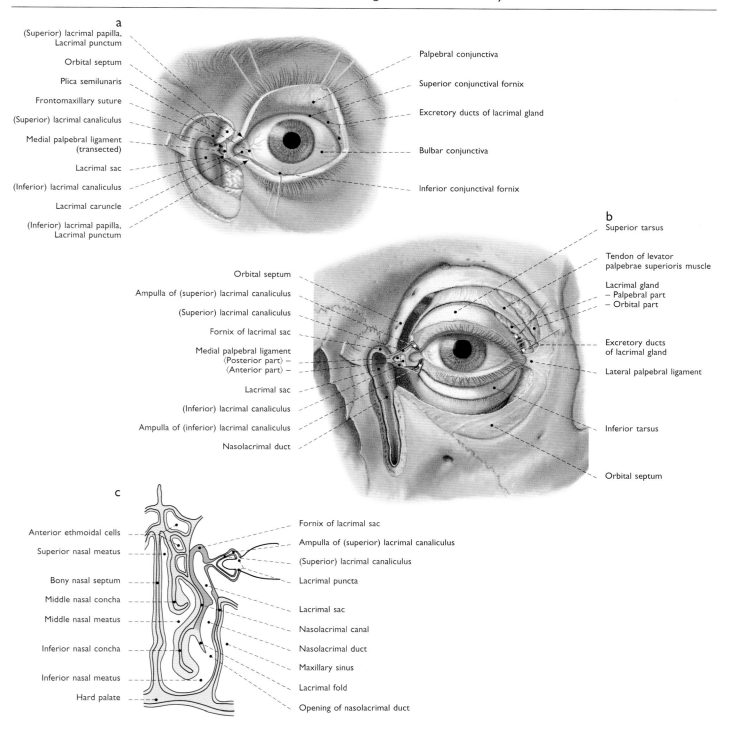

a

(Superior) lacrimal papilla, Lacrimal punctum

Orbital septum

Plica semilunaris

Frontomaxillary suture

(Superior) lacrimal canaliculus

Medial palpebral ligament (transected)

Lacrimal sac

(Inferior) lacrimal canaliculus

Lacrimal caruncle

(Inferior) lacrimal papilla, Lacrimal punctum

Palpebral conjunctiva

Superior conjunctival fornix

Excretory ducts of lacrimal gland

Bulbar conjunctiva

Inferior conjunctival fornix

b

Superior tarsus

Tendon of levator palpebrae superioris muscle

Lacrimal gland
– Palpebral part
– Orbital part

Excretory ducts of lacrimal gland

Lateral palpebral ligament

Inferior tarsus

Orbital septum

Orbital septum

Ampulla of (superior) lacrimal canaliculus

(Superior) lacrimal canaliculus

Fornix of lacrimal sac

Medial palpebral ligament
⟨Posterior part⟩ –
⟨Anterior part⟩ –

Lacrimal sac

(Inferior) lacrimal canaliculus

Ampulla of (inferior) lacrimal canaliculus

Nasolacrimal duct

c

Anterior ethmoidal cells

Superior nasal meatus

Bony nasal septum

Middle nasal concha

Middle nasal meatus

Inferior nasal concha

Inferior nasal meatus

Hard palate

Fornix of lacrimal sac

Ampulla of (superior) lacrimal canaliculus

(Superior) lacrimal canaliculus

Lacrimal puncta

Lacrimal sac

Nasolacrimal canal

Nasolacrimal duct

Maxillary sinus

Lacrimal fold

Opening of nasolacrimal duct

365 Lacrimal apparatus

Frontal aspect

a The lacrimal apparatus of the left eye was exposed. The upper eyelid was pulled upwards by sutures, while the lower eyelid was drawn slightly downwards (90%).

b Left orbit and its contents after removal of facial muscles. The tendon of the levator palpebrae superioris muscle was divided by a bow-shaped incision. The lacrimal apparatus was exposed and opened (90%).

c Schematized coronal section through the lacrimal ducts, the nasolacrimal duct, and the nasal cavity of the left side (100%)

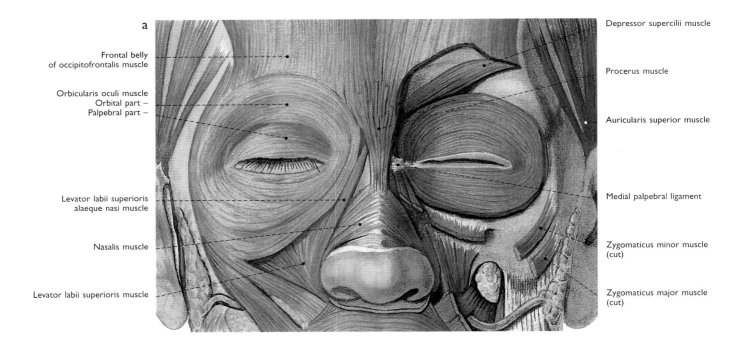

a

Frontal belly
of occipitofrontalis muscle

Orbicularis oculi muscle
Orbital part –
Palpebral part –

Levator labii superioris
alaeque nasi muscle

Nasalis muscle

Levator labii superioris muscle

Depressor supercilii muscle

Procerus muscle

Auricularis superior muscle

Medial palpebral ligament

Zygomaticus minor muscle
(cut)

Zygomaticus major muscle
(cut)

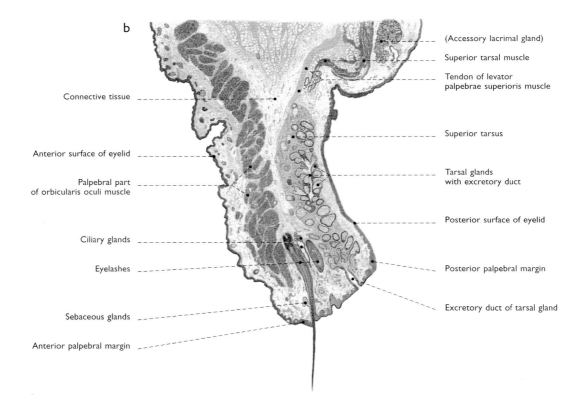

b

Connective tissue

Anterior surface of eyelid

Palpebral part
of orbicularis oculi muscle

Ciliary glands

Eyelashes

Sebaceous glands

Anterior palpebral margin

(Accessory lacrimal gland)

Superior tarsal muscle

Tendon of levator
palpebrae superioris muscle

Superior tarsus

Tarsal glands
with excretory duct

Posterior surface of eyelid

Posterior palpebral margin

Excretory duct of tarsal gland

366   Orbital region

a   Facial muscles around the eyes (75%),
frontal aspect

b   Sagittal section through the upper eyelid (700%),
medial aspect

a

Crista galli

Ethmoidal labyrinth

(Innominate line)

Zygomatic bone

Maxillary sinus

Nasal septum

Frontal sinus

Supra-orbital margin

Medial wall of orbit

Superior orbital fissure

Infra-orbital margin

Infra-orbital canal

Inferior nasal meatus

b

Frontal notch

Frontal bone

Trochlear fovea

Anterior and posterior
ethmoidal foramina

Frontomaxillary suture

Maxilla
Frontal process –
Anterior lacrimal crest –
Lacrimal notch –

Fossa for lacrimal sac

Lacrimal bone

Ethmoidal bone

Maxilla
Orbital surface –
Infra-orbital margin –
⟨Infra-orbital suture⟩ –
Infra-orbital foramen –
Body of maxilla –

Frontal bone
– Supra-orbital foramen
– Supra-orbital margin
– Fossa for lacrimal gland
– Orbital surface
– Zygomatic process

Sphenoidal bone
– Lesser wing
– Optic canal
– Greater wing

Superior orbital fissure

Zygomatic bone
– Frontal process
– Orbital surface

Inferior orbital fissure

Zygomaticofacial foramen

Infra-orbital groove

Lateral surface
of zygomatic bone

Zygomaticomaxillary suture

367 Orbital cavity (110%)
a Postero-anterior radiograph of both orbits
b Left osseous orbit, frontal aspect.
   Individual bones are indicated by different colors.

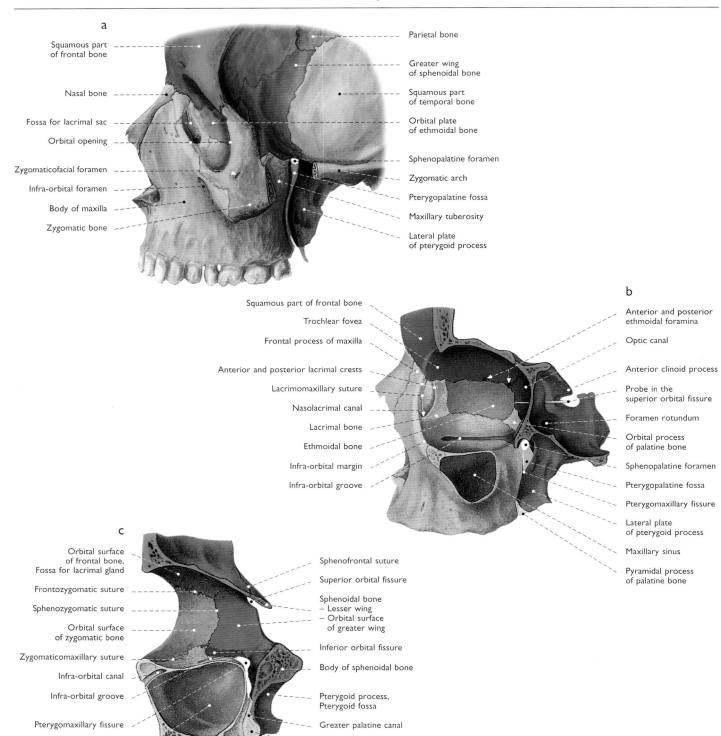

a
Squamous part of frontal bone
Nasal bone
Fossa for lacrimal sac
Orbital opening
Zygomaticofacial foramen
Infra-orbital foramen
Body of maxilla
Zygomatic bone

Parietal bone
Greater wing of sphenoidal bone
Squamous part of temporal bone
Orbital plate of ethmoidal bone
Sphenopalatine foramen
Zygomatic arch
Pterygopalatine fossa
Maxillary tuberosity
Lateral plate of pterygoid process

Squamous part of frontal bone
Trochlear fovea
Frontal process of maxilla
Anterior and posterior lacrimal crests
Lacrimomaxillary suture
Nasolacrimal canal
Lacrimal bone
Ethmoidal bone
Infra-orbital margin
Infra-orbital groove

b
Anterior and posterior ethmoidal foramina
Optic canal
Anterior clinoid process
Probe in the superior orbital fissure
Foramen rotundum
Orbital process of palatine bone
Sphenopalatine foramen
Pterygopalatine fossa
Pterygomaxillary fissure
Lateral plate of pterygoid process
Maxillary sinus
Pyramidal process of palatine bone

c
Orbital surface of frontal bone, Fossa for lacrimal gland
Frontozygomatic suture
Sphenozygomatic suture
Orbital surface of zygomatic bone
Zygomaticomaxillary suture
Infra-orbital canal
Infra-orbital groove
Pterygomaxillary fissure
Maxillary sinus

Sphenofrontal suture
Superior orbital fissure
Sphenoidal bone
– Lesser wing
– Orbital surface of greater wing
Inferior orbital fissure
Body of sphenoidal bone
Pterygoid process, Pterygoid fossa
Greater palatine canal
Pyramidal process of palatine bone

368 Walls of the orbital cavity (65%)
Individual bones are indicated by different colors.
a Lateral wall of the left orbit and adjacent bones, left lateral aspect
b Medial wall of the left orbit and adjacent bones, left lateral aspect
c Lateral wall of the right orbit and adjacent bones, medial aspect

a

Anterior cranial fossa

Frontal sinus

Orbit

Anterior ethmoidal cells

Bony nasal cavity

Infra-orbital canal

Maxillary hiatus

Maxillary sinus

Alveolar process
of maxilla

Molar tooth

Crista galli

Orbit
– Orbital surface of frontal bone
– Superior orbital fissure
– Orbital plate
of ethmoidal bone
– Orbital surface of maxilla
– Inferior orbital fissure

Middle nasal concha

Bony nasal septum

Inferior nasal concha

Palatine process
of maxilla

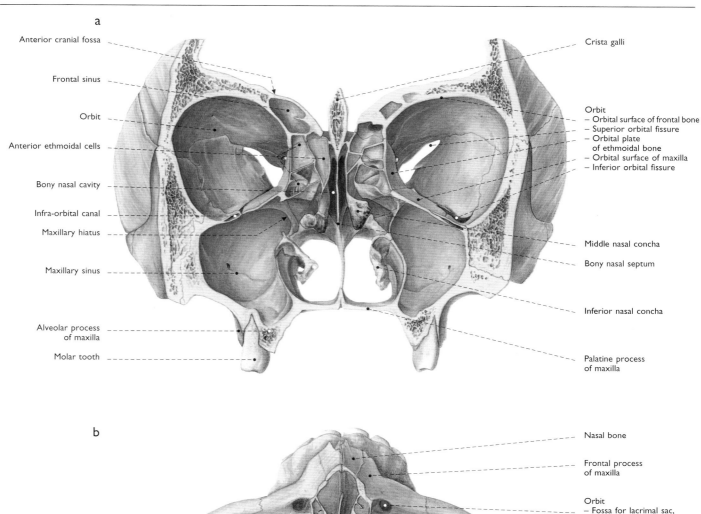

b

Anterior and middle
ethmoidal cells

Posterior ethmoidal cells

Sphenoidal sinus

Nasal bone

Frontal process
of maxilla

Orbit
– Fossa for lacrimal sac,
Entrance into
nasolacrimal duct
– Orbital surface of maxilla
– Orbital plate of ethmoidal
bone
– Inferior orbital fissure

Bony nasal cavity

Bony nasal septum

Middle cranial fossa

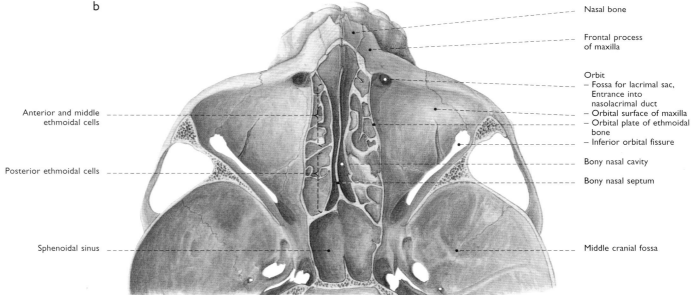

369 Orbital cavity (85%)

Sections through the osseous walls of the orbits,
the nasal cavity, and paranasal sinuses
a Coronal section through the viscerocranium,
frontal aspect
b Transverse section through the middle parts of the orbits,
the nasal cavity, the ethmoidal labyrinth, and sphenoidal sinuses,
superior aspect

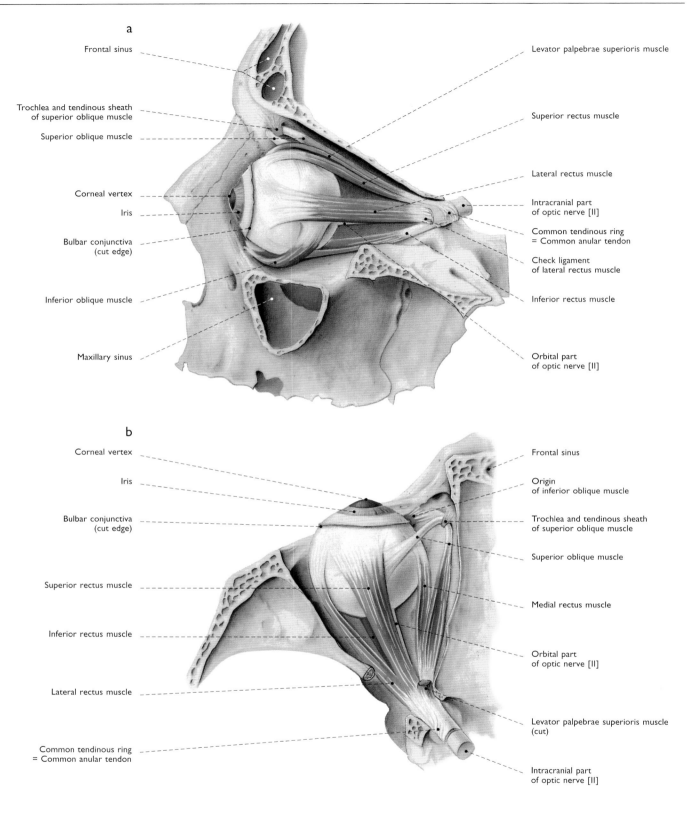

a

Frontal sinus

Trochlea and tendinous sheath
of superior oblique muscle

Superior oblique muscle

Corneal vertex

Iris

Bulbar conjunctiva
(cut edge)

Inferior oblique muscle

Maxillary sinus

Levator palpebrae superioris muscle

Superior rectus muscle

Lateral rectus muscle

Intracranial part
of optic nerve [II]

Common tendinous ring
= Common anular tendon

Check ligament
of lateral rectus muscle

Inferior rectus muscle

Orbital part
of optic nerve [II]

b

Corneal vertex

Iris

Bulbar conjunctiva
(cut edge)

Superior rectus muscle

Inferior rectus muscle

Lateral rectus muscle

Common tendinous ring
= Common anular tendon

Frontal sinus

Origin
of inferior oblique muscle

Trochlea and tendinous sheath
of superior oblique muscle

Superior oblique muscle

Medial rectus muscle

Orbital part
of optic nerve [II]

Levator palpebrae superioris muscle
(cut)

Intracranial part
of optic nerve [II]

370 Extra-ocular (= extrinsic) muscles
of the left eyeball (100%)
a The lateral wall of the left orbit was removed.
Left lateral aspect of the left eyeball
b The roof of orbit was removed.
Superior aspect of the left eyeball

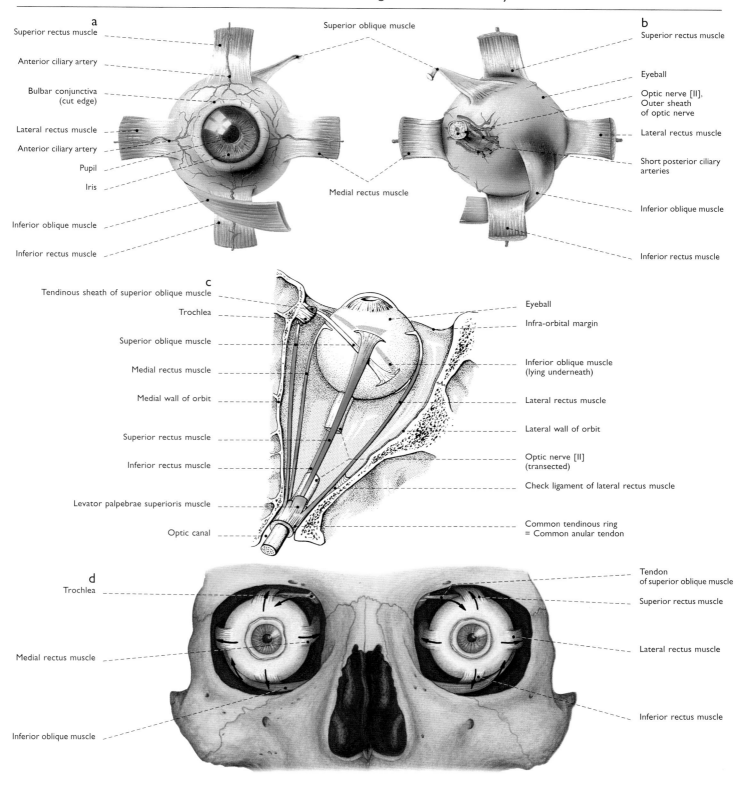

a
Superior rectus muscle
Anterior ciliary artery
Bulbar conjunctiva (cut edge)
Lateral rectus muscle
Anterior ciliary artery
Pupil
Iris
Inferior oblique muscle
Inferior rectus muscle

Superior oblique muscle

Medial rectus muscle

b
Superior rectus muscle
Eyeball
Optic nerve [II], Outer sheath of optic nerve
Lateral rectus muscle
Short posterior ciliary arteries
Inferior oblique muscle
Inferior rectus muscle

c
Tendinous sheath of superior oblique muscle
Trochlea
Superior oblique muscle
Medial rectus muscle
Medial wall of orbit
Superior rectus muscle
Inferior rectus muscle
Levator palpebrae superioris muscle
Optic canal

Eyeball
Infra-orbital margin
Inferior oblique muscle (lying underneath)
Lateral rectus muscle
Lateral wall of orbit
Optic nerve [II] (transected)
Check ligament of lateral rectus muscle
Common tendinous ring = Common anular tendon

d
Trochlea
Medial rectus muscle
Inferior oblique muscle

Tendon of superior oblique muscle
Superior rectus muscle
Lateral rectus muscle
Inferior rectus muscle

371 Extra-ocular (= extrinsic) muscles of the eyeball
a Frontal aspect of the right eyeball (125%)
b Dorsal aspect of the right eyeball (125%)
c Superior aspect of the right orbit (100%), schematic representation
d Frontal aspect of the osseous orbits and both eyeballs with muscle insertions (80%). The arrows indicate ocular movements after muscle contraction.

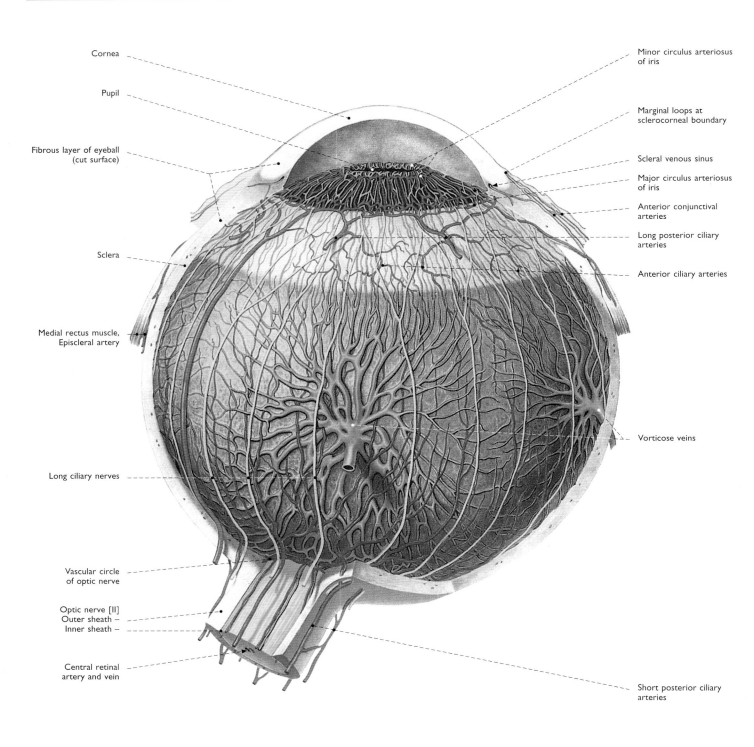

Cornea

Pupil

Fibrous layer of eyeball
(cut surface)

Sclera

Medial rectus muscle,
Episcleral artery

Long ciliary nerves

Vascular circle
of optic nerve

Optic nerve [II]
Outer sheath —
Inner sheath —

Central retinal
artery and vein

Minor circulus arteriosus
of iris

Marginal loops at
sclerocorneal boundary

Scleral venous sinus

Major circulus arteriosus
of iris

Anterior conjunctival
arteries

Long posterior ciliary
arteries

Anterior ciliary arteries

Vorticose veins

Short posterior ciliary
arteries

372 Blood vessels of the eyeball (500%)
The upper part of the fibrous layer of the right eyeball
was removed nearly completely. Superior aspect

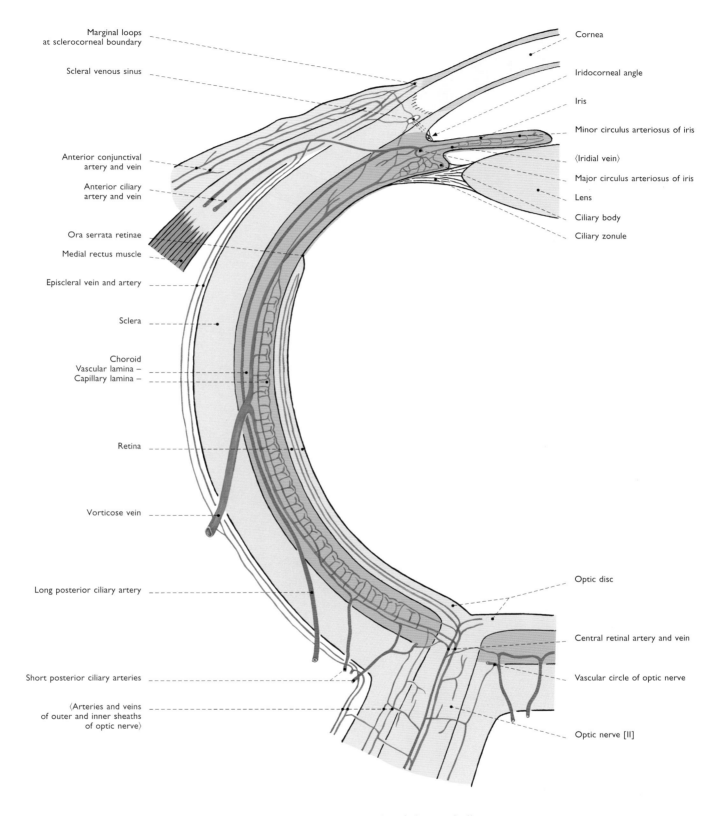

Marginal loops
at sclerocorneal boundary

Scleral venous sinus

Anterior conjunctival
artery and vein

Anterior ciliary
artery and vein

Ora serrata retinae

Medial rectus muscle

Episcleral vein and artery

Sclera

Choroid
Vascular lamina –
Capillary lamina –

Retina

Vorticose vein

Long posterior ciliary artery

Short posterior ciliary arteries

〈Arteries and veins
of outer and inner sheaths
of optic nerve〉

Cornea

Iridocorneal angle

Iris

Minor circulus arteriosus of iris

〈Iridial vein〉

Major circulus arteriosus of iris

Lens

Ciliary body

Ciliary zonule

Optic disc

Central retinal artery and vein

Vascular circle of optic nerve

Optic nerve [II]

373 Blood vessels of the eyeball (700%)

Transverse section through the right eyeball incised along
the equatorial plane and schematic representation
of the blood vessels in the nasal part of the eyeball,
superior aspect

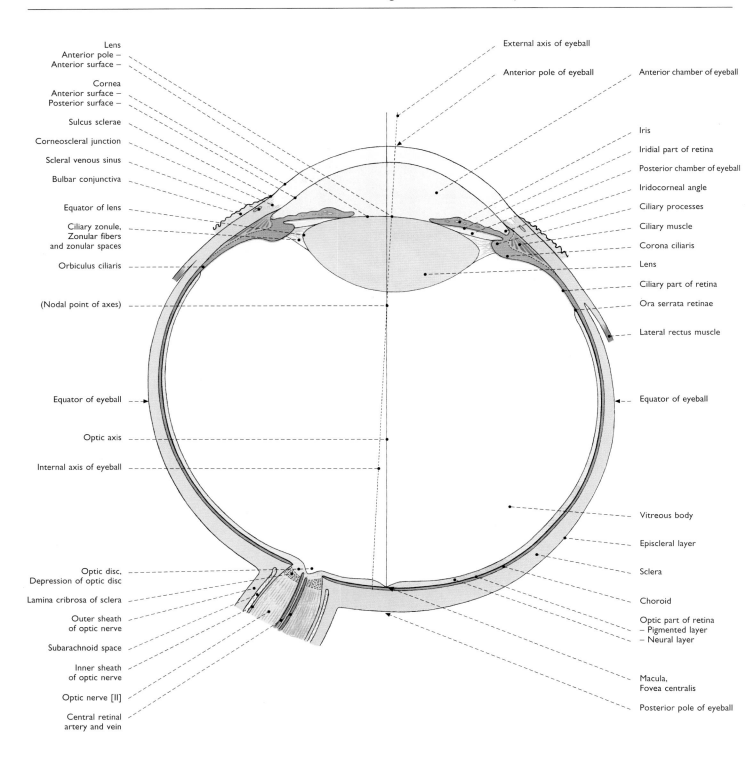

Lens
Anterior pole –
Anterior surface –

Cornea
Anterior surface –
Posterior surface –

Sulcus sclerae

Corneoscleral junction

Scleral venous sinus

Bulbar conjunctiva

Equator of lens

Ciliary zonule,
Zonular fibers
and zonular spaces

Orbiculus ciliaris

(Nodal point of axes)

Equator of eyeball

Optic axis

Internal axis of eyeball

Optic disc,
Depression of optic disc

Lamina cribrosa of sclera

Outer sheath
of optic nerve

Subarachnoid space

Inner sheath
of optic nerve

Optic nerve [II]

Central retinal
artery and vein

External axis of eyeball

Anterior pole of eyeball

Anterior chamber of eyeball

Iris

Iridial part of retina

Posterior chamber of eyeball

Iridocorneal angle

Ciliary processes

Ciliary muscle

Corona ciliaris

Lens

Ciliary part of retina

Ora serrata retinae

Lateral rectus muscle

Equator of eyeball

Vitreous body

Episcleral layer

Sclera

Choroid

Optic part of retina
– Pigmented layer
– Neural layer

Macula,
Fovea centralis

Posterior pole of eyeball

374 Eyeball (500%)
Schematized transverse section through the right eyeball
of an adult with normal vision, superior aspect

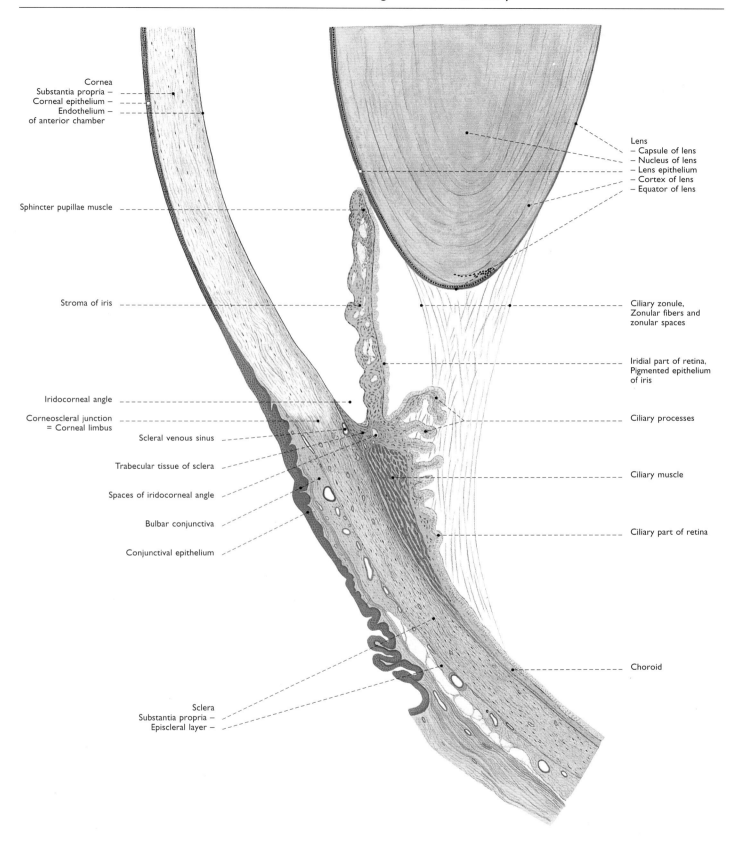

Cornea
Substantia propria –
Corneal epithelium –
Endothelium –
of anterior chamber

Sphincter pupillae muscle

Stroma of iris

Iridocorneal angle

Corneoscleral junction
= Corneal limbus

Scleral venous sinus

Trabecular tissue of sclera

Spaces of iridocorneal angle

Bulbar conjunctiva

Conjunctival epithelium

Sclera
Substantia propria –
Episcleral layer –

Lens
– Capsule of lens
– Nucleus of lens
– Lens epithelium
– Cortex of lens
– Equator of lens

Ciliary zonule,
Zonular fibers and
zonular spaces

Iridial part of retina,
Pigmented epithelium
of iris

Ciliary processes

Ciliary muscle

Ciliary part of retina

Choroid

375 Eyeball
Meridional section through the anterior part
of the eyeball (2 000%)

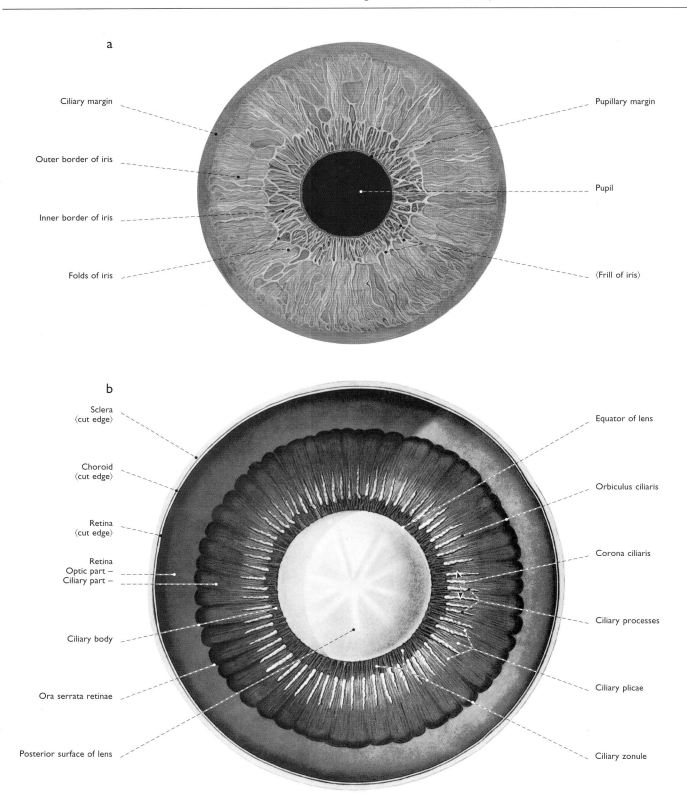

a

Ciliary margin

Outer border of iris

Inner border of iris

Folds of iris

Pupillary margin

Pupil

⟨Frill of iris⟩

b

Sclera
⟨cut edge⟩

Choroid
⟨cut edge⟩

Retina
⟨cut edge⟩

Retina
Optic part —
Ciliary part —

Ciliary body

Ora serrata retinae

Posterior surface of lens

Equator of lens

Orbiculus ciliaris

Corona ciliaris

Ciliary processes

Ciliary plicae

Ciliary zonule

376 Iris and ciliary body
a   Ventral aspect after removal of the cornea (700%)
b   Dorsal aspect after removal of the vitreous body (400%)

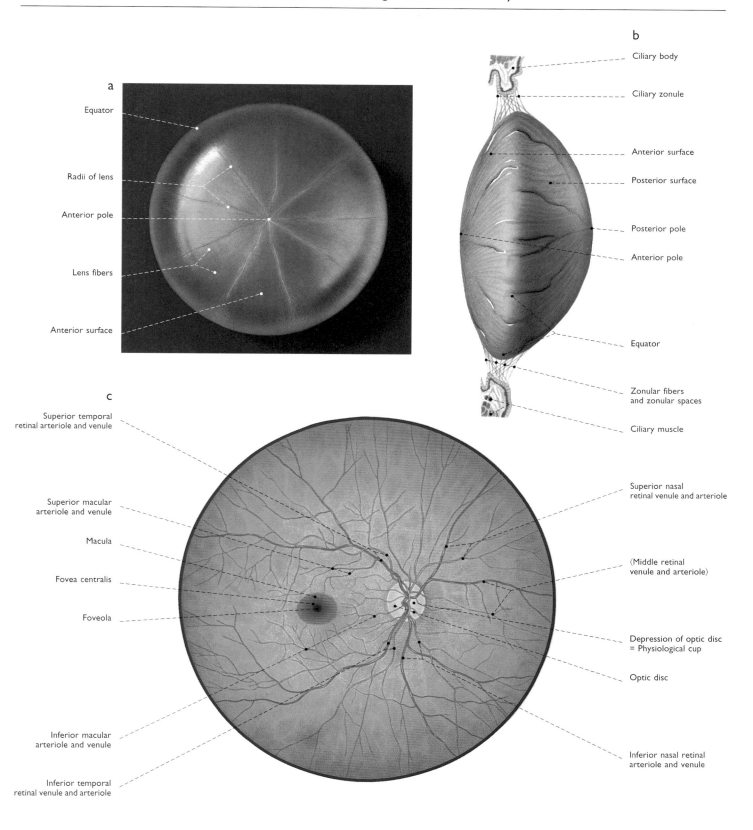

a

Equator

Radii of lens

Anterior pole

Lens fibers

Anterior surface

b

Ciliary body

Ciliary zonule

Anterior surface

Posterior surface

Posterior pole

Anterior pole

Equator

Zonular fibers
and zonular spaces

Ciliary muscle

c

Superior temporal
retinal arteriole and venule

Superior macular
arteriole and venule

Macula

Fovea centralis

Foveola

Inferior macular
arteriole and venule

Inferior temporal
retinal venule and arteriole

Superior nasal
retinal venule and arteriole

⟨Middle retinal
venule and arteriole⟩

Depression of optic disc
= Physiological cup

Optic disc

Inferior nasal retinal
arteriole and venule

377 Lens and retina (600%)

a Lens, the lens star showing several rays, frontal aspect
b Lens, lateral aspect
c Retina of the right eye, ophthalmoscopic view

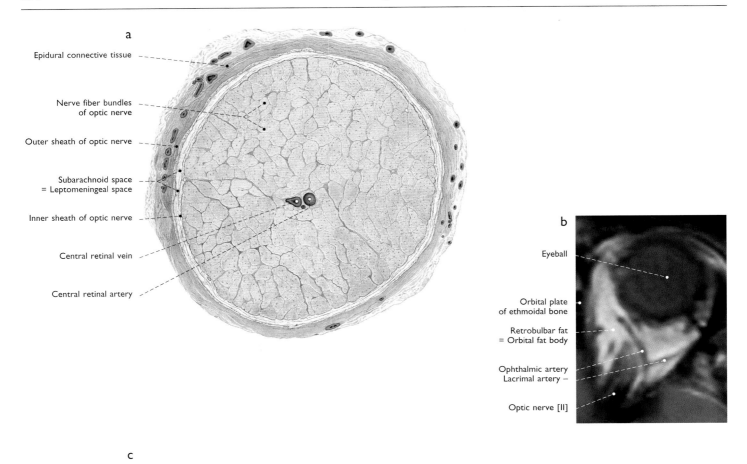

a

Epidural connective tissue

Nerve fiber bundles
of optic nerve

Outer sheath of optic nerve

Subarachnoid space
= Leptomeningeal space

Inner sheath of optic nerve

Central retinal vein

Central retinal artery

b

Eyeball

Orbital plate
of ethmoidal bone

Retrobulbar fat
= Orbital fat body

Ophthalmic artery
Lacrimal artery

Optic nerve [II]

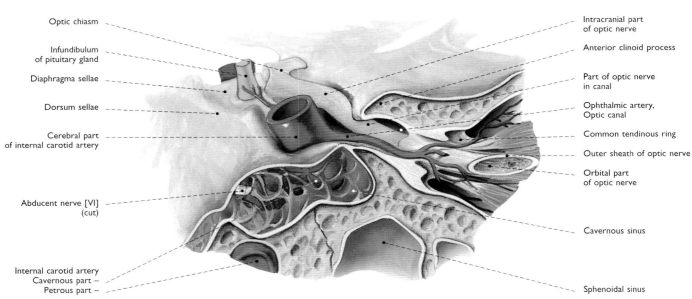

c

Optic chiasm

Infundibulum
of pituitary gland

Diaphragma sellae

Dorsum sellae

Cerebral part
of internal carotid artery

Abducent nerve [VI]
(cut)

Internal carotid artery
Cavernous part
Petrous part

Intracranial part
of optic nerve

Anterior clinoid process

Part of optic nerve
in canal

Ophthalmic artery,
Optic canal

Common tendinous ring

Outer sheath of optic nerve

Orbital part
of optic nerve

Cavernous sinus

Sphenoidal sinus

378 Optic nerve and ophthalmic artery

a Optic nerve of the right eye, cross section close
to the eyeball (1 600%), frontal aspect
b Optic nerve, eyeball, and ophthalmic artery,
transverse magnetic resonance image
(MRI, T_1-weighted) (100%)
c Oblique section through the optic canal
of the right orbit (250%), right lateral aspect

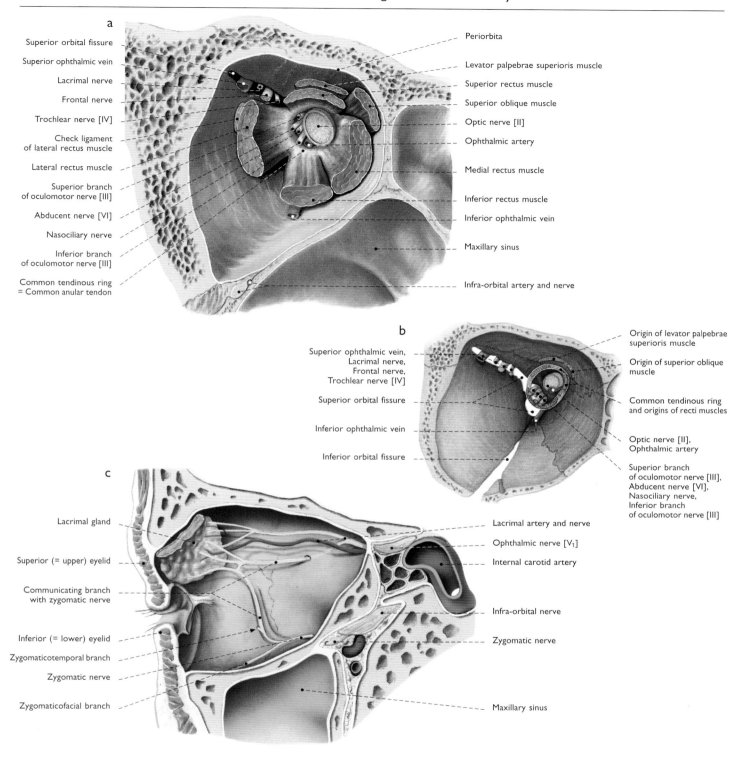

a
Superior orbital fissure
Superior ophthalmic vein
Lacrimal nerve
Frontal nerve
Trochlear nerve [IV]
Check ligament
of lateral rectus muscle
Lateral rectus muscle
Superior branch
of oculomotor nerve [III]
Abducent nerve [VI]
Nasociliary nerve
Inferior branch
of oculomotor nerve [III]
Common tendinous ring
= Common anular tendon

Periorbita
Levator palpebrae superioris muscle
Superior rectus muscle
Superior oblique muscle
Optic nerve [II]
Ophthalmic artery
Medial rectus muscle
Inferior rectus muscle
Inferior ophthalmic vein
Maxillary sinus
Infra-orbital artery and nerve

b
Superior ophthalmic vein,
Lacrimal nerve,
Frontal nerve,
Trochlear nerve [IV]
Superior orbital fissure
Inferior ophthalmic vein
Inferior orbital fissure

Origin of levator palpebrae
superioris muscle
Origin of superior oblique
muscle
Common tendinous ring
and origins of recti muscles
Optic nerve [II],
Ophthalmic artery
Superior branch
of oculomotor nerve [III],
Abducent nerve [VI],
Nasociliary nerve,
Inferior branch
of oculomotor nerve [III]

c
Lacrimal gland
Superior (= upper) eyelid
Communicating branch
with zygomatic nerve
Inferior (= lower) eyelid
Zygomaticotemporal branch
Zygomatic nerve
Zygomaticofacial branch

Lacrimal artery and nerve
Ophthalmic nerve [V$_1$]
Internal carotid artery
Infra-orbital nerve
Zygomatic nerve
Maxillary sinus

379 Right orbital cavity
a Coronal section. The common tendinous ring and the origins
   of the extra-ocular muscles are shown (150%). Frontal aspect
b Coronal section. The extra-ocular muscles were transected close
   to their origins, the nerves and blood vessels were cut close
   to their points of entry into or exit from the orbit, respectively (150%).
   Frontal aspect
c Sagittal section. The lateral wall of the right orbit is shown
   after removal of the eyeball (100%). Medial aspect

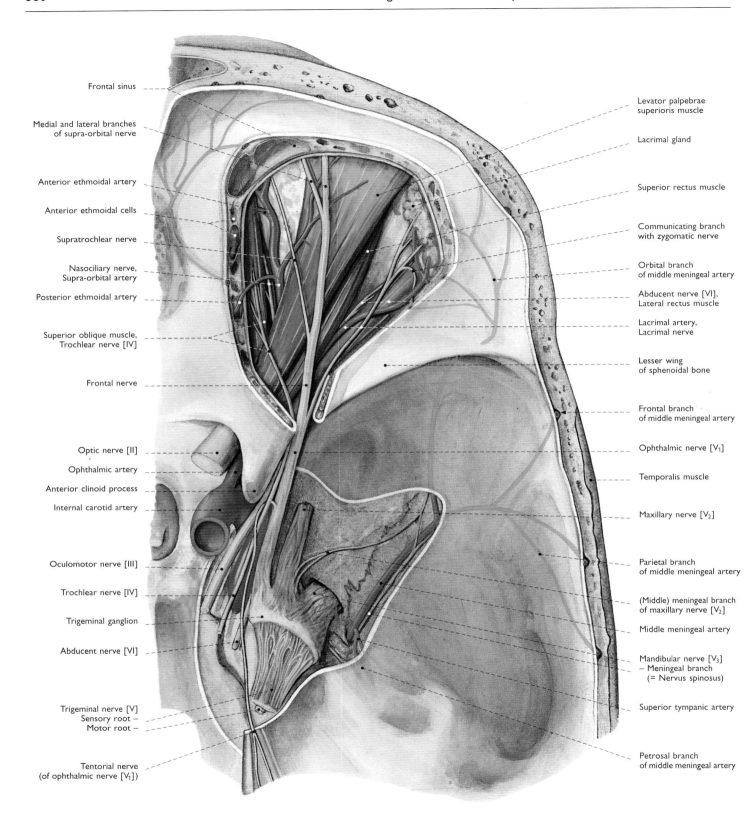

Frontal sinus

Medial and lateral branches
of supra-orbital nerve

Anterior ethmoidal artery

Anterior ethmoidal cells

Supratrochlear nerve

Nasociliary nerve,
Supra-orbital artery

Posterior ethmoidal artery

Superior oblique muscle,
Trochlear nerve [IV]

Frontal nerve

Optic nerve [II]

Ophthalmic artery

Anterior clinoid process

Internal carotid artery

Oculomotor nerve [III]

Trochlear nerve [IV]

Trigeminal ganglion

Abducent nerve [VI]

Trigeminal nerve [V]
Sensory root –
Motor root –

Tentorial nerve
(of ophthalmic nerve [V₁])

Levator palpebrae
superioris muscle

Lacrimal gland

Superior rectus muscle

Communicating branch
with zygomatic nerve

Orbital branch
of middle meningeal artery

Abducent nerve [VI],
Lateral rectus muscle

Lacrimal artery,
Lacrimal nerve

Lesser wing
of sphenoidal bone

Frontal branch
of middle meningeal artery

Ophthalmic nerve [V₁]

Temporalis muscle

Maxillary nerve [V₂]

Parietal branch
of middle meningeal artery

(Middle) meningeal branch
of maxillary nerve [V₂]

Middle meningeal artery

Mandibular nerve [V₃]
– Meningeal branch
(= Nervus spinosus)

Superior tympanic artery

Petrosal branch
of middle meningeal artery

380   Right orbital cavity and middle cranial fossa (200%)
The roof of orbit and the cranial dura mater beyond the right orbit
were removed, the right cavernous sinus was opened. Superior aspect

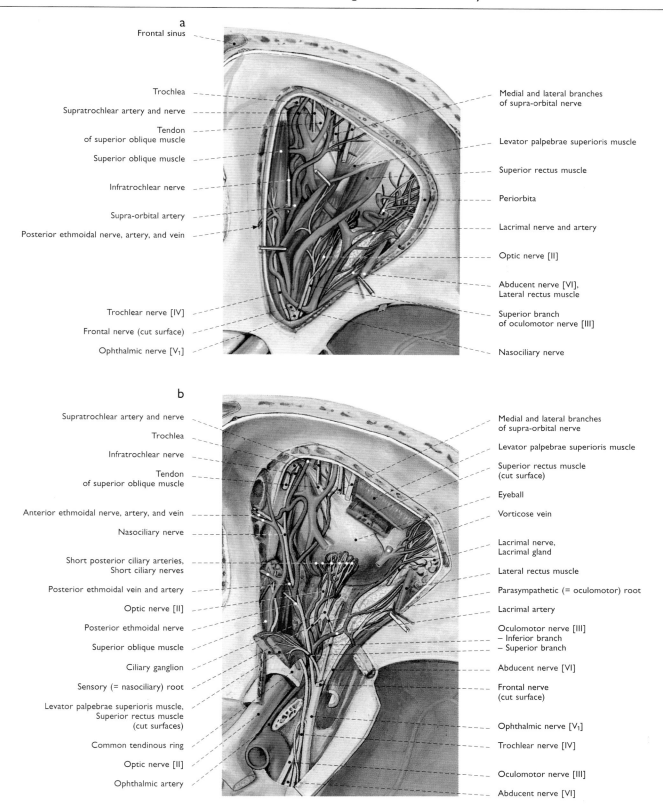

a

Frontal sinus

Trochlea

Supratrochlear artery and nerve

Tendon of superior oblique muscle

Superior oblique muscle

Infratrochlear nerve

Supra-orbital artery

Posterior ethmoidal nerve, artery, and vein

Trochlear nerve [IV]

Frontal nerve (cut surface)

Ophthalmic nerve [V₁]

Medial and lateral branches of supra-orbital nerve

Levator palpebrae superioris muscle

Superior rectus muscle

Periorbita

Lacrimal nerve and artery

Optic nerve [II]

Abducent nerve [VI], Lateral rectus muscle

Superior branch of oculomotor nerve [III]

Nasociliary nerve

b

Supratrochlear artery and nerve

Trochlea

Infratrochlear nerve

Tendon of superior oblique muscle

Anterior ethmoidal nerve, artery, and vein

Nasociliary nerve

Short posterior ciliary arteries, Short ciliary nerves

Posterior ethmoidal vein and artery

Optic nerve [II]

Posterior ethmoidal nerve

Superior oblique muscle

Ciliary ganglion

Sensory (= nasociliary) root

Levator palpebrae superioris muscle, Superior rectus muscle (cut surfaces)

Common tendinous ring

Optic nerve [II]

Ophthalmic artery

Medial and lateral branches of supra-orbital nerve

Levator palpebrae superioris muscle

Superior rectus muscle (cut surface)

Eyeball

Vorticose vein

Lacrimal nerve, Lacrimal gland

Lateral rectus muscle

Parasympathetic (= oculomotor) root

Lacrimal artery

Oculomotor nerve [III] – Inferior branch – Superior branch

Abducent nerve [VI]

Frontal nerve (cut surface)

Ophthalmic nerve [V₁]

Trochlear nerve [IV]

Oculomotor nerve [III]

Abducent nerve [VI]

381 Right orbital cavity (140%)

The roof of orbit was removed. Superior aspect
a   Superficial dissection
b   Deeper dissection just above the optic nerve. The upper extra-ocular muscles were transected and removed.

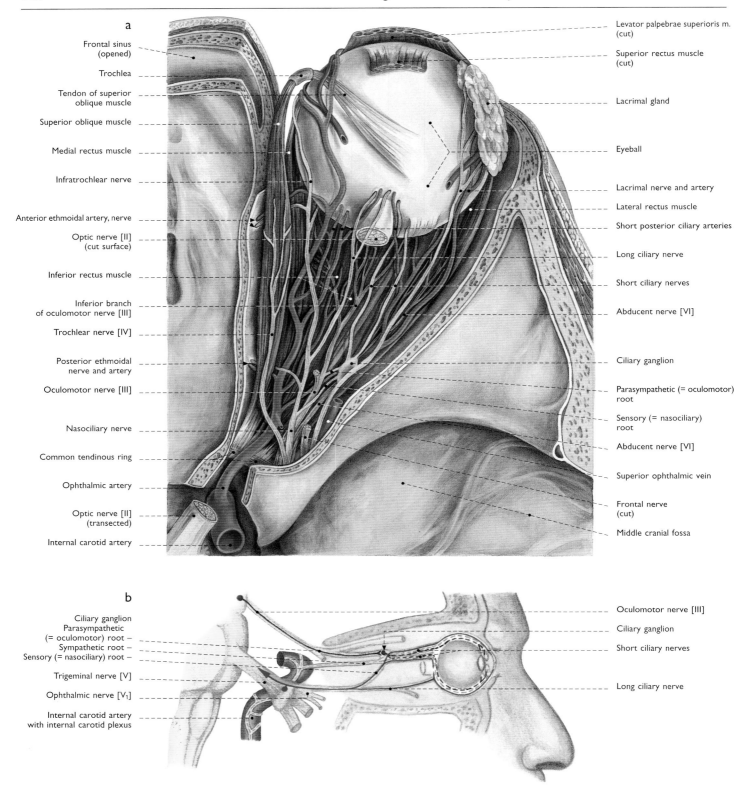

a

Frontal sinus (opened)
Trochlea
Tendon of superior oblique muscle
Superior oblique muscle
Medial rectus muscle
Infratrochlear nerve
Anterior ethmoidal artery, nerve
Optic nerve [II] (cut surface)
Inferior rectus muscle
Inferior branch of oculomotor nerve [III]
Trochlear nerve [IV]
Posterior ethmoidal nerve and artery
Oculomotor nerve [III]
Nasociliary nerve
Common tendinous ring
Ophthalmic artery
Optic nerve [II] (transected)
Internal carotid artery

Levator palpebrae superioris m. (cut)
Superior rectus muscle (cut)
Lacrimal gland
Eyeball
Lacrimal nerve and artery
Lateral rectus muscle
Short posterior ciliary arteries
Long ciliary nerve
Short ciliary nerves
Abducent nerve [VI]
Ciliary ganglion
Parasympathetic (= oculomotor) root
Sensory (= nasociliary) root
Abducent nerve [VI]
Superior ophthalmic vein
Frontal nerve (cut)
Middle cranial fossa

b

Ciliary ganglion
Parasympathetic (= oculomotor) root –
Sympathetic root –
Sensory (= nasociliary) root –
Trigeminal nerve [V]
Ophthalmic nerve [V₁]
Internal carotid artery with internal carotid plexus

Oculomotor nerve [III]
Ciliary ganglion
Short ciliary nerves
Long ciliary nerve

382 Right orbital cavity

a Deep dissection. The roof of orbit was completely removed, the upper extra-ocular muscles and the optic nerve were transected and removed (150%). Superior aspect
b Ciliary ganglion and autonomic innervation of the eyeball (80%), schematic representation, right lateral aspect

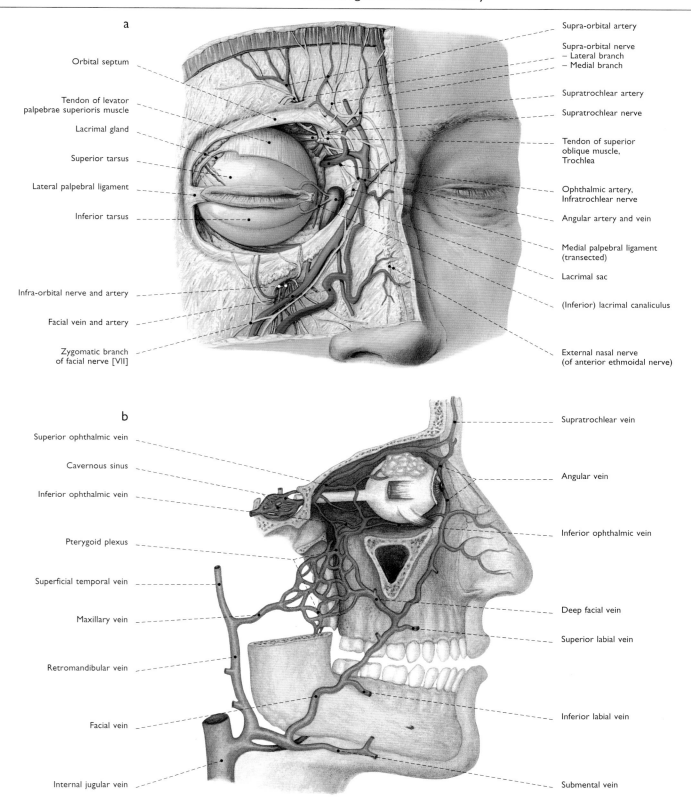

a

Orbital septum

Tendon of levator palpebrae superioris muscle

Lacrimal gland

Superior tarsus

Lateral palpebral ligament

Inferior tarsus

Infra-orbital nerve and artery

Facial vein and artery

Zygomatic branch of facial nerve [VII]

Supra-orbital artery

Supra-orbital nerve
– Lateral branch
– Medial branch

Supratrochlear artery

Supratrochlear nerve

Tendon of superior oblique muscle, Trochlea

Ophthalmic artery, Infratrochlear nerve

Angular artery and vein

Medial palpebral ligament (transected)

Lacrimal sac

(Inferior) lacrimal canaliculus

External nasal nerve (of anterior ethmoidal nerve)

b

Superior ophthalmic vein

Cavernous sinus

Inferior ophthalmic vein

Pterygoid plexus

Superficial temporal vein

Maxillary vein

Retromandibular vein

Facial vein

Internal jugular vein

Supratrochlear vein

Angular vein

Inferior ophthalmic vein

Deep facial vein

Superior labial vein

Inferior labial vein

Submental vein

383 Right orbital region

a Gross anatomy of the right orbital region (90%)
b Drainage of the orbital veins. The lateral wall of the right orbit and parts of the ramus of mandible were removed, the right maxillary sinus is opened (80%). Right lateral aspect

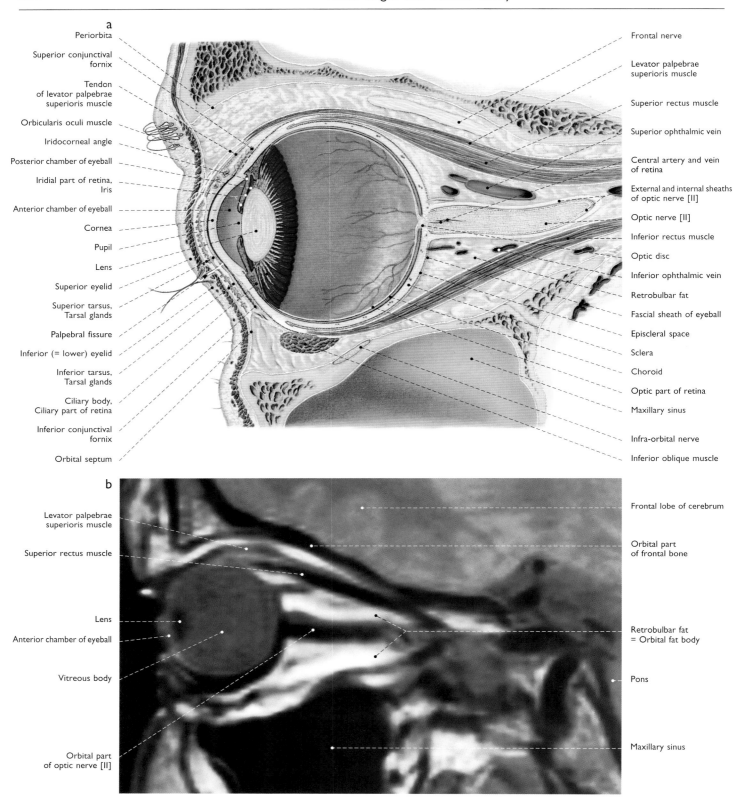

a

Periorbita

Superior conjunctival fornix

Tendon of levator palpebrae superioris muscle

Orbicularis oculi muscle

Iridocorneal angle

Posterior chamber of eyeball

Iridial part of retina, Iris

Anterior chamber of eyeball

Cornea

Pupil

Lens

Superior eyelid

Superior tarsus, Tarsal glands

Palpebral fissure

Inferior (= lower) eyelid

Inferior tarsus, Tarsal glands

Ciliary body, Ciliary part of retina

Inferior conjunctival fornix

Orbital septum

Frontal nerve

Levator palpebrae superioris muscle

Superior rectus muscle

Superior ophthalmic vein

Central artery and vein of retina

External and internal sheaths of optic nerve [II]

Optic nerve [II]

Inferior rectus muscle

Optic disc

Inferior ophthalmic vein

Retrobulbar fat

Fascial sheath of eyeball

Episcleral space

Sclera

Choroid

Optic part of retina

Maxillary sinus

Infra-orbital nerve

Inferior oblique muscle

b

Levator palpebrae superioris muscle

Superior rectus muscle

Lens

Anterior chamber of eyeball

Vitreous body

Orbital part of optic nerve [II]

Frontal lobe of cerebrum

Orbital part of frontal bone

Retrobulbar fat = Orbital fat body

Pons

Maxillary sinus

384 Orbital cavity

Oblique vertical sections along the axis of the optic nerve through the right orbit, medial aspect

a Anatomical section (200%)
b Magnetic resonance image (MRI, T_1-weighted) (140%)

a

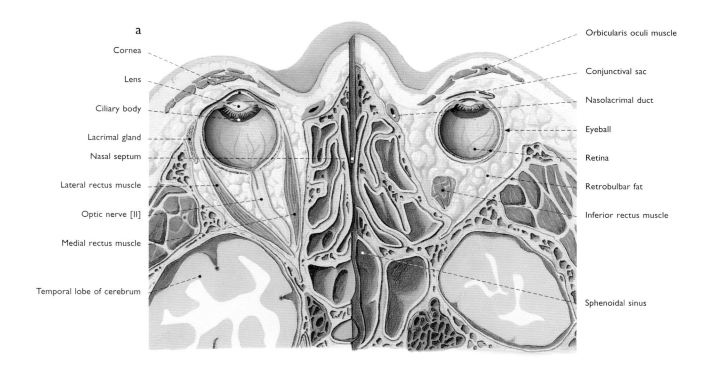

Cornea
Lens
Ciliary body
Lacrimal gland
Nasal septum
Lateral rectus muscle
Optic nerve [II]
Medial rectus muscle
Temporal lobe of cerebrum

Orbicularis oculi muscle
Conjunctival sac
Nasolacrimal duct
Eyeball
Retina
Retrobulbar fat
Inferior rectus muscle
Sphenoidal sinus

b

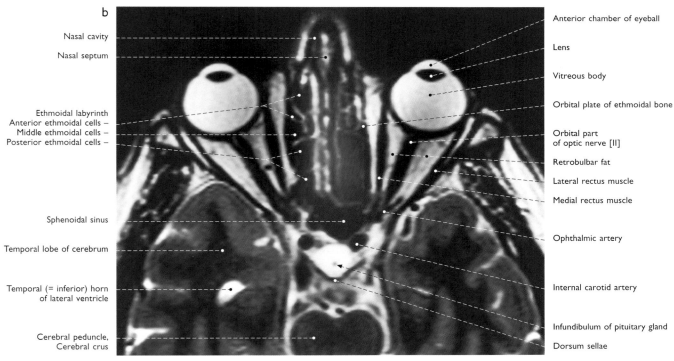

Nasal cavity
Nasal septum
Ethmoidal labyrinth
Anterior ethmoidal cells –
Middle ethmoidal cells –
Posterior ethmoidal cells –
Sphenoidal sinus
Temporal lobe of cerebrum
Temporal (= inferior) horn
of lateral ventricle
Cerebral peduncle,
Cerebral crus

Anterior chamber of eyeball
Lens
Vitreous body
Orbital plate of ethmoidal bone
Orbital part
of optic nerve [II]
Retrobulbar fat
Lateral rectus muscle
Medial rectus muscle
Ophthalmic artery
Internal carotid artery
Infundibulum of pituitary gland
Dorsum sellae

385 Orbital cavity 90%)
a Stepped anatomical transverse section through both orbits
   and eyeballs, superior aspect
b Transverse magnetic resonance image (MRI, T$_2$-weighted)
   through both orbits, eyeballs, and optic nerves, inferior aspect

a

Frontal lobe of cerebrum

Frontal sinus

Levator palpebrae superioris muscle

Superior rectus muscle

Eyeball

Lacrimal gland

Medial rectus muscle

Anterior ethmoidal cells

Inferior oblique muscle

Retrobulbar fat = Orbital fat body

Inferior rectus muscle

Middle and inferior nasal conchae

Nasal septum

Maxillary sinus

Oral cavity proper

Nasal cavity

Hard palate

b

Frontal lobe of cerebrum

Levator palpebrae superioris muscle, Superior rectus muscle

Roof of orbit

Superior oblique muscle

Lacrimal gland

Frontal sinus

Eyeball

Eyeball

Anterior ethmoidal cells

Medial rectus muscle

Retrobulbar fat = Orbital fat body

Inferior oblique muscle, Inferior rectus muscle

Middle and inferior nasal conchae

Maxillary sinus

Nasal cavity

Nasal septum

Hard palate

Oral cavity proper

386 Orbital cavity (100%)

Coronal sections through ventral parts of both orbits, the nasal cavities, and the paranasal sinuses, frontal aspect

a   Anatomical section

b   Magnetic resonance image (MRI, T$_1$-weighted)

a

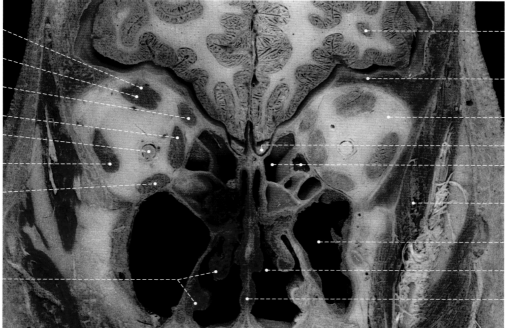

Levator palpebrae superioris muscle

Superior rectus muscle

Superior oblique muscle

Medial rectus muscle

Orbital part of optic nerve [II]

Lateral rectus muscle

Inferior rectus muscle

Middle and inferior nasal conchae

Frontal lobe of cerebrum

Roof of orbit, Orbital part of frontal bone

Retrobulbar fat = Orbital fat body

Olfactory tract

Posterior ethmoidal cells

Temporalis muscle

Maxillary sinus

Nasal cavity

Nasal septum

b

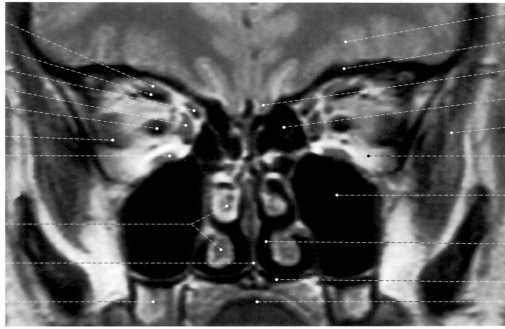

Levator palpebrae superioris muscle

Superior rectus muscle

Superior oblique muscle

Medial rectus muscle

Orbital part of optic nerve [II]

Lateral rectus muscle

Inferior rectus muscle

Middle and inferior nasal conchae

Nasal septum

Molar tooth

Frontal lobe of cerebrum

Roof of orbit

Olfactory tract

Posterior ethmoidal cells

Temporalis muscle

Retrobulbar fat = Orbital fat body

Maxillary sinus

Nasal cavity

Hard palate

Oral cavity proper

387 Orbital cavity (100%)
Coronal sections through dorsal parts of both orbits,
the nasal cavities, and the paranasal sinuses, frontal aspect
a Anatomical section
b Magnetic resonance image (MRI, T$_1$-weighted)

Vestibulocochlear Organ

a

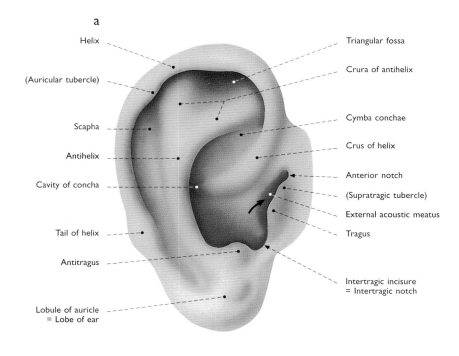

Helix	Triangular fossa
(Auricular tubercle)	Crura of antihelix
Scapha	Cymba conchae
Antihelix	Crus of helix
Cavity of concha	Anterior notch
	(Supratragic tubercle)
	External acoustic meatus
	Tragus
Tail of helix	
Antitragus	Intertragic incisure = Intertragic notch
Lobule of auricle = Lobe of ear	

b

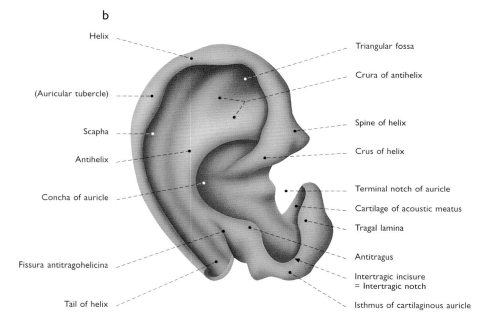

Helix	Triangular fossa
(Auricular tubercle)	Crura of antihelix
Scapha	Spine of helix
Antihelix	Crus of helix
Concha of auricle	Terminal notch of auricle
	Cartilage of acoustic meatus
	Tragal lamina
Fissura antitragohelicina	Antitragus
	Intertragic incisure = Intertragic notch
Tail of helix	Isthmus of cartilaginous auricle

390 External ear (110%)

Right external ear, lateral aspect
a   Auricle = pinna
b   Auricular cartilage

a

Squamous part
of temporal bone

Temporalis muscle

Auricular cartilage

(Bony) external
acoustic meatus

Cartilaginous external
acoustic meatus

Cartilage of acoustic meatus

Tympanic part
of temporal bone

Tympanic membrane

Tegmental wall,
Epitympanic recess

Superior ligament of incus

Superior ligament of malleus,
Head of malleus

Facial nerve [VII]

Chorda tympani,
Anterior fold of malleus

Cochlear duct

Tensor tympani muscle

Scala vestibuli,
Scala tympani

Head of stapes

Long limb of incus

Handle of malleus

Promontory

Round window,
Secondary tympanic membrane

Tympanic cavity,
⟨Hypotympanic recess⟩

Internal carotid artery

b

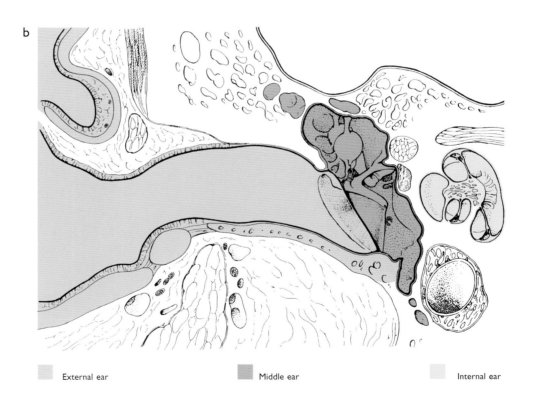

External ear   Middle ear   Internal ear

391 Ear (300%)

a, b   Coronal section through the external, middle,
       and internal ear of the right side, frontal aspect
b   The parts of the external, middle, and internal ear
       are indicated by different colors.

a

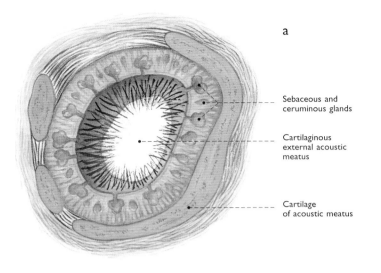

Sebaceous and
ceruminous glands

Cartilaginous
external acoustic
meatus

Cartilage
of acoustic meatus

b

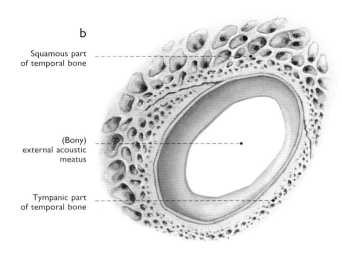

Squamous part
of temporal bone

(Bony)
external acoustic
meatus

Tympanic part
of temporal bone

c

Branches of
deep auricular artery

Posterior fold of malleus

Pars flaccida

Anterior fold of malleus

Malleolar prominence,
Lateral process of malleus

Malleolar stria,
Handle of malleus

Pars tensa

Fibrocartilaginous ring

Umbo of tympanic membrane

External acoustic meatus

(Cone of reflected light)

d

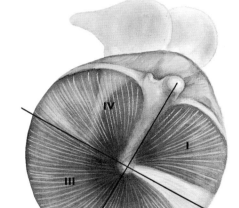

392 External acoustic meatus and
tympanic membrane of the right ear
Lateral aspect
a, b Cross sections through the
a cartilaginous and
b noncartilaginous parts
of the right external acoustic meatus (500%)
c View of the right tympanic membrane (= eardrum)
as seen through an otoscope in a living subject (700%)
d Division of the right tympanic membrane into quadrants,
schematic representation

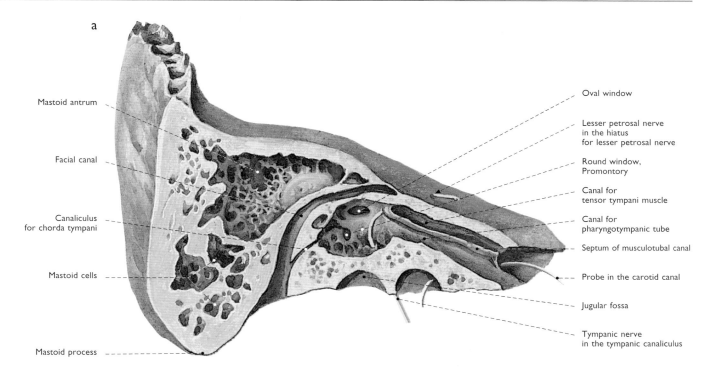

a

Mastoid antrum

Facial canal

Canaliculus
for chorda tympani

Mastoid cells

Mastoid process

Oval window

Lesser petrosal nerve
in the hiatus
for lesser petrosal nerve

Round window,
Promontory

Canal for
tensor tympani muscle

Canal for
pharyngotympanic tube

Septum of musculotubal canal

Probe in the carotid canal

Jugular fossa

Tympanic nerve
in the tympanic canaliculus

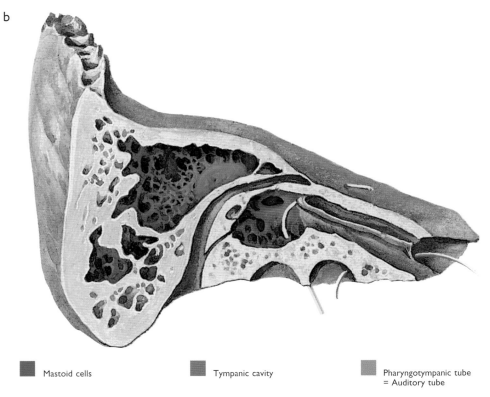

b

Mastoid cells

Tympanic cavity

Pharyngotympanic tube
= Auditory tube

393   Right temporal bone

a, b   Vertical section through the petrous bone parallel to its long axis.
The tympanic cavity and the facial canal were opened (100%).
Frontolateral aspect

b   The three parts of the middle ear are indicated by different colors
(mastoid cells **dark-brown**, tympanic cavity **red**,
pharyngotympanic tube **light-brown**).

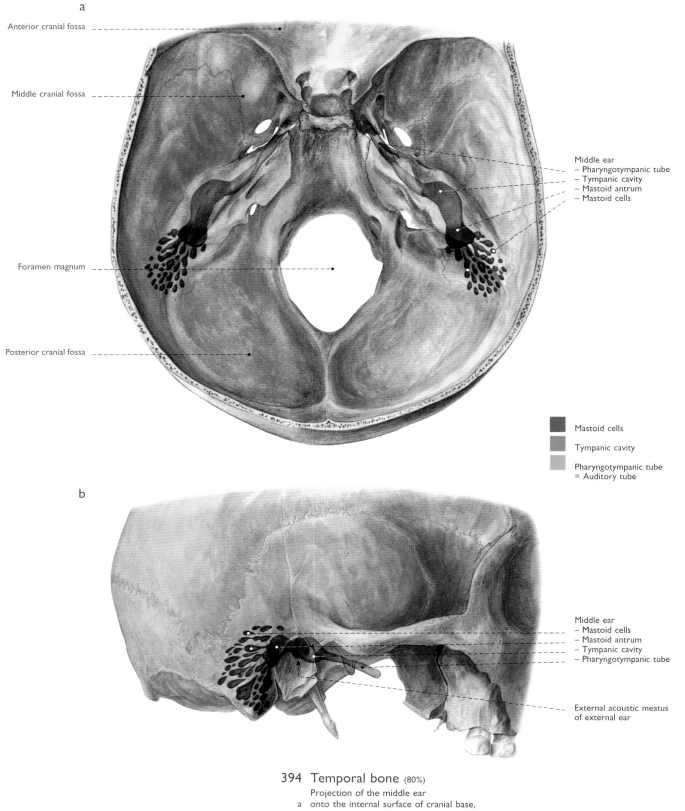

a

Anterior cranial fossa

Middle cranial fossa

Foramen magnum

Posterior cranial fossa

Middle ear
– Pharyngotympanic tube
– Tympanic cavity
– Mastoid antrum
– Mastoid cells

■ Mastoid cells

■ Tympanic cavity

■ Pharyngotympanic tube
= Auditory tube

b

Middle ear
– Mastoid cells
– Mastoid antrum
– Tympanic cavity
– Pharyngotympanic tube

External acoustic meatus
of external ear

394 Temporal bone (80%)
Projection of the middle ear
a onto the internal surface of cranial base,
  superior aspect
b onto the lateral external surface of cranium,
  right lateral aspect
  The three parts of the middle ear are indicated
  by different colors (mastoid cells **dark-brown**,
  tympanic cavity **red**, pharyngotympanic tube **light-brown**).

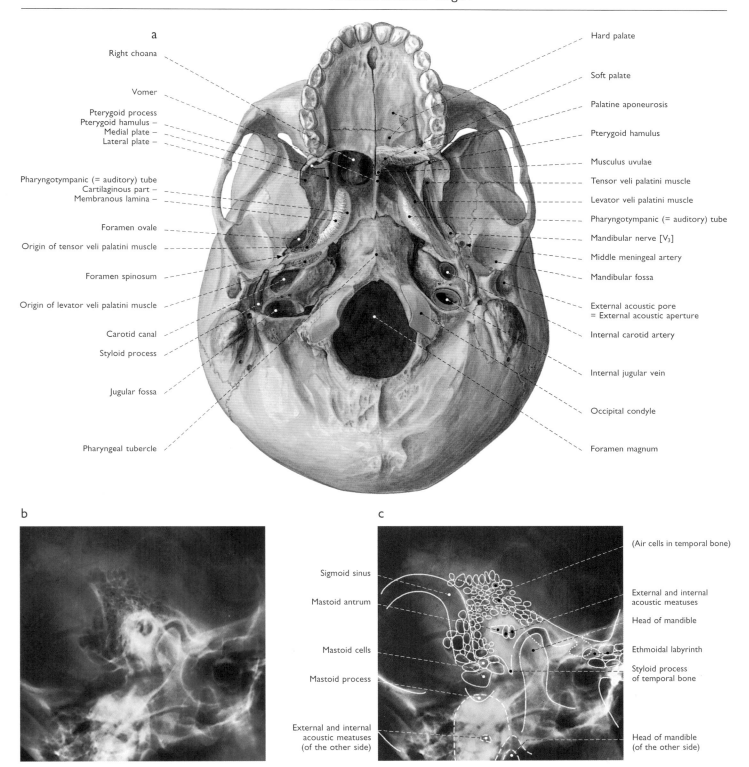

a

Right choana

Vomer

Pterygoid process
Pterygoid hamulus –
Medial plate –
Lateral plate –

Pharyngotympanic (= auditory) tube
Cartilaginous part –
Membranous lamina –

Foramen ovale

Origin of tensor veli palatini muscle

Foramen spinosum

Origin of levator veli palatini muscle

Carotid canal

Styloid process

Jugular fossa

Pharyngeal tubercle

Hard palate

Soft palate

Palatine aponeurosis

Pterygoid hamulus

Musculus uvulae

Tensor veli palatini muscle

Levator veli palatini muscle

Pharyngotympanic (= auditory) tube

Mandibular nerve [V₃]

Middle meningeal artery

Mandibular fossa

External acoustic pore
= External acoustic aperture

Internal carotid artery

Internal jugular vein

Occipital condyle

Foramen magnum

b

c

Sigmoid sinus

Mastoid antrum

Mastoid cells

Mastoid process

External and internal
acoustic meatuses
(of the other side)

(Air cells in temporal bone)

External and internal
acoustic meatuses

Head of mandible

Ethmoidal labyrinth

Styloid process
of temporal bone

Head of mandible
(of the other side)

395 Temporal bone (100%)

a External surface of cranial base with pharyngotympanic tubes.
The muscles of soft palate are shown on the left half of cranium,
the areas of attachment of the levator and tensor veli palatini muscles
on the right half (70%). Inferior aspect

b Parietolateral radiograph of the petrous part of temporal bones
according to Schüller

c Explanatory drawing as to fig. b

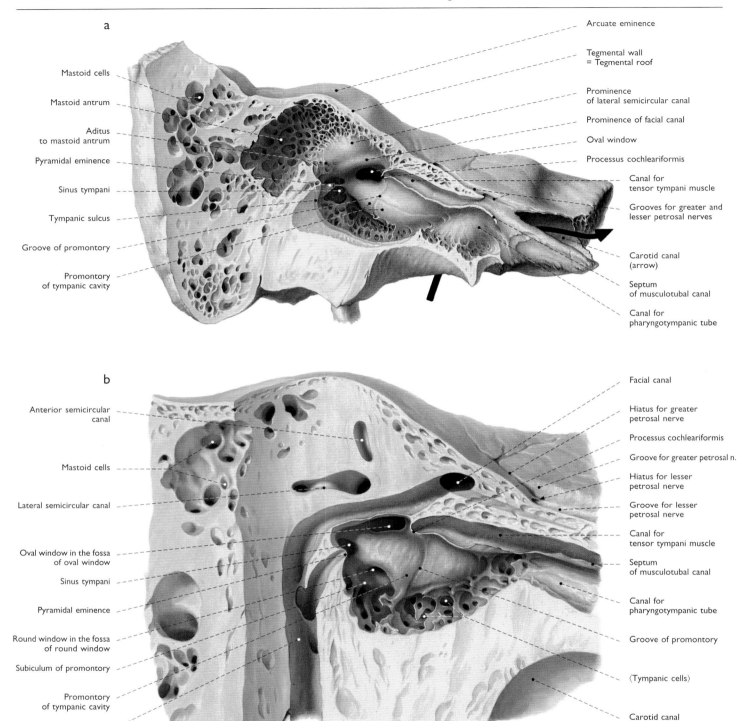

a

Mastoid cells

Mastoid antrum

Aditus
to mastoid antrum

Pyramidal eminence

Sinus tympani

Tympanic sulcus

Groove of promontory

Promontory
of tympanic cavity

Arcuate eminence

Tegmental wall
= Tegmental roof

Prominence
of lateral semicircular canal

Prominence of facial canal

Oval window

Processus cochleariformis

Canal for
tensor tympani muscle

Grooves for greater and
lesser petrosal nerves

Carotid canal
(arrow)

Septum
of musculotubal canal

Canal for
pharyngotympanic tube

b

Anterior semicircular
canal

Mastoid cells

Lateral semicircular canal

Oval window in the fossa
of oval window

Sinus tympani

Pyramidal eminence

Round window in the fossa
of round window

Subiculum of promontory

Promontory
of tympanic cavity

Facial canal

Facial canal

Hiatus for greater
petrosal nerve

Processus cochleariformis

Groove for greater petrosal n.

Hiatus for lesser
petrosal nerve

Groove for lesser
petrosal nerve

Canal for
tensor tympani muscle

Septum
of musculotubal canal

Canal for
pharyngotympanic tube

Groove of promontory

⟨Tympanic cells⟩

Carotid canal

396 Right tympanic cavity
Frontolateral aspect of the labyrinthine (= medial) wall
of tympanic cavity. The oval window was opened by removing
the stapes. The mucous membrane was taken away.
a Vertical section through the petrous part of temporal bone
parallel to its longitudinal axis (200%)
b Section through the tympanic cavity parallel to its labyrinthine wall.
The facial canal was opened and the facial nerve removed (500%).

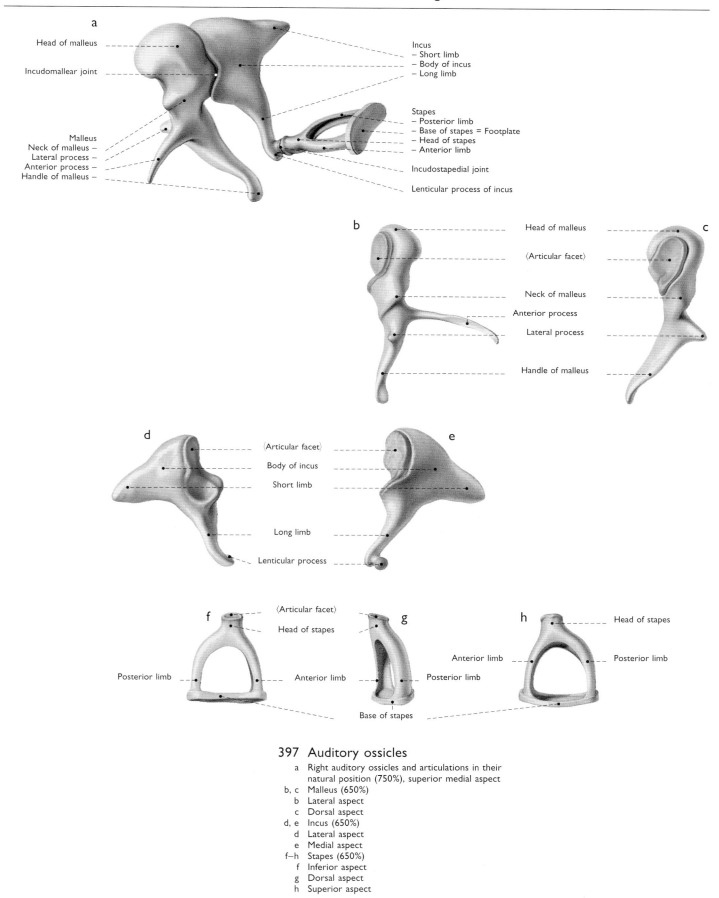

a

Head of malleus

Incudomallear joint

Malleus
Neck of malleus –
Lateral process –
Anterior process –
Handle of malleus –

Incus
– Short limb
– Body of incus
– Long limb

Stapes
– Posterior limb
– Base of stapes = Footplate
– Head of stapes
– Anterior limb

Incudostapedial joint

Lenticular process of incus

b

Head of malleus

⟨Articular facet⟩

Neck of malleus

Anterior process

Lateral process

Handle of malleus

c

d

⟨Articular facet⟩

Body of incus

Short limb

Long limb

Lenticular process

e

f

⟨Articular facet⟩

Head of stapes

Posterior limb

Anterior limb

g

Posterior limb

Base of stapes

h

Head of stapes

Anterior limb

Posterior limb

397   Auditory ossicles

a   Right auditory ossicles and articulations in their natural position (750%), superior medial aspect

b, c   Malleus (650%)

b   Lateral aspect

c   Dorsal aspect

d, e   Incus (650%)

d   Lateral aspect

e   Medial aspect

f–h   Stapes (650%)

f   Inferior aspect

g   Dorsal aspect

h   Superior aspect

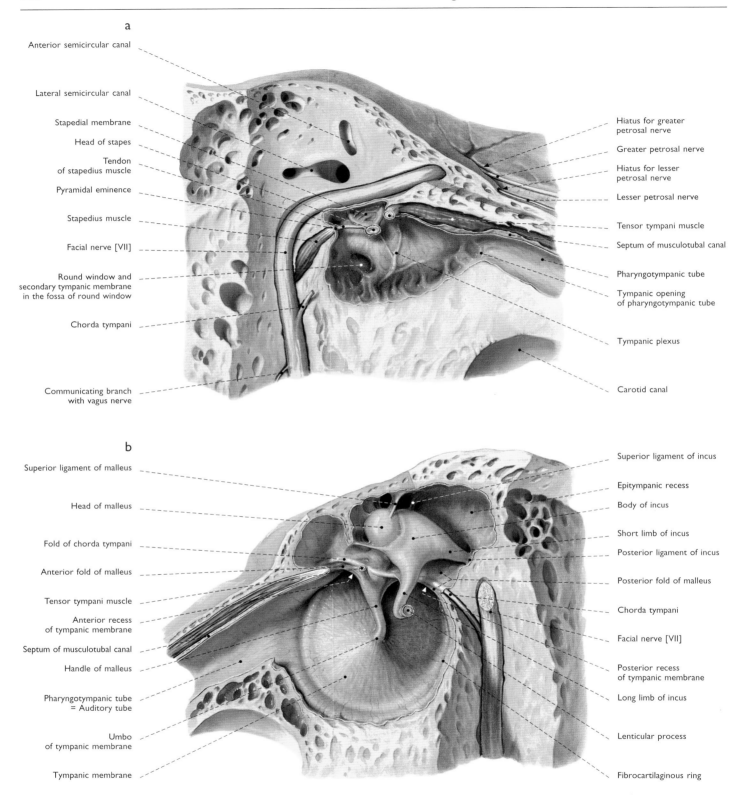

a

Anterior semicircular canal

Lateral semicircular canal

Stapedial membrane

Head of stapes

Tendon of stapedius muscle

Pyramidal eminence

Stapedius muscle

Facial nerve [VII]

Round window and secondary tympanic membrane in the fossa of round window

Chorda tympani

Communicating branch with vagus nerve

Hiatus for greater petrosal nerve

Greater petrosal nerve

Hiatus for lesser petrosal nerve

Lesser petrosal nerve

Tensor tympani muscle

Septum of musculotubal canal

Pharyngotympanic tube

Tympanic opening of pharyngotympanic tube

Tympanic plexus

Carotid canal

b

Superior ligament of malleus

Head of malleus

Fold of chorda tympani

Anterior fold of malleus

Tensor tympani muscle

Anterior recess of tympanic membrane

Septum of musculotubal canal

Handle of malleus

Pharyngotympanic tube = Auditory tube

Umbo of tympanic membrane

Tympanic membrane

Superior ligament of incus

Epitympanic recess

Body of incus

Short limb of incus

Posterior ligament of incus

Posterior fold of malleus

Chorda tympani

Facial nerve [VII]

Posterior recess of tympanic membrane

Long limb of incus

Lenticular process

Fibrocartilaginous ring

398 Right tympanic cavity (450%)

a   Section through the tympanic cavity parallel to its labyrinthine (= medial) wall, frontolateral aspect of the labyrinthine wall

b   Section through the tympanic cavity parallel to its membranous (= lateral) wall, medial aspect of the membranous wall

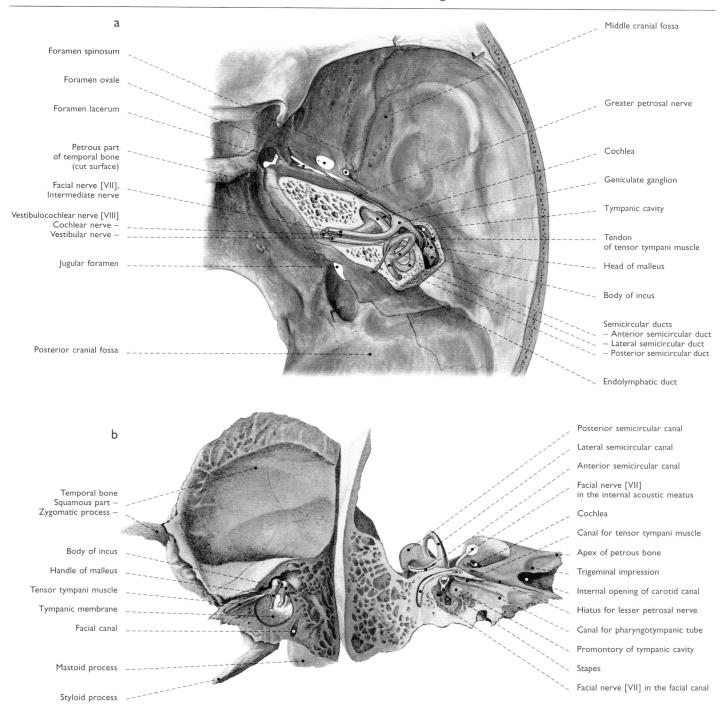

a

Foramen spinosum

Foramen ovale

Foramen lacerum

Petrous part
of temporal bone
(cut surface)

Facial nerve [VII],
Intermediate nerve

Vestibulocochlear nerve [VIII]
Cochlear nerve –
Vestibular nerve –

Jugular foramen

Posterior cranial fossa

Middle cranial fossa

Greater petrosal nerve

Cochlea

Geniculate ganglion

Tympanic cavity

Tendon
of tensor tympani muscle

Head of malleus

Body of incus

Semicircular ducts
– Anterior semicircular duct
– Lateral semicircular duct
– Posterior semicircular duct

Endolymphatic duct

b

Temporal bone
Squamous part –
Zygomatic process –

Body of incus

Handle of malleus

Tensor tympani muscle

Tympanic membrane

Facial canal

Mastoid process

Styloid process

Posterior semicircular canal

Lateral semicircular canal

Anterior semicircular canal

Facial nerve [VII]
in the internal acoustic meatus

Cochlea

Canal for tensor tympani muscle

Apex of petrous bone

Trigeminal impression

Internal opening of carotid canal

Hiatus for lesser petrosal nerve

Canal for pharyngotympanic tube

Promontory of tympanic cavity

Stapes

Facial nerve [VII] in the facial canal

399   Temporal bone and facial canal (100%)

  a   Transverse section through the petrous part of the right temporal bone
      in the plane of the internal acoustic meatus. Exposure of the cochlear duct,
      the semicircular ducts, and the facial and vestibulocochlear nerves.
      The facial canal and the tympanic cavity were opened. Superior aspect
  b   Vertical section through the middle ear, the facial canal, and the mastoid cells
      of the petrous part of the right temporal bone. The lateral part was turned outwards.
      The semicircular canals and the cochlea were exposed. Frontolateral aspect

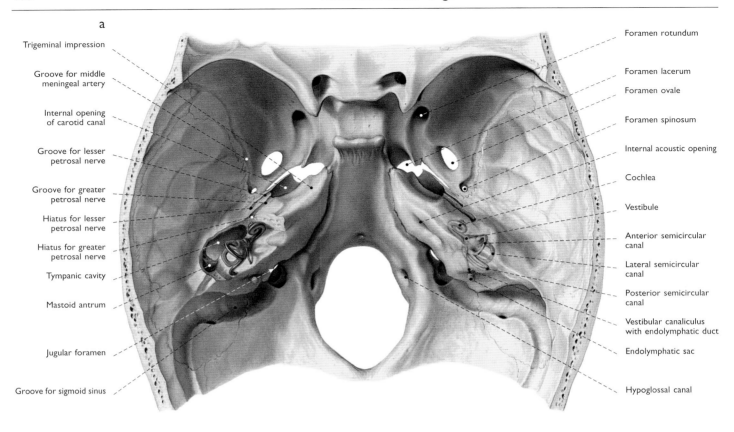

a

Trigeminal impression

Groove for middle meningeal artery

Internal opening of carotid canal

Groove for lesser petrosal nerve

Groove for greater petrosal nerve

Hiatus for lesser petrosal nerve

Hiatus for greater petrosal nerve

Tympanic cavity

Mastoid antrum

Jugular foramen

Groove for sigmoid sinus

Foramen rotundum

Foramen lacerum

Foramen ovale

Foramen spinosum

Internal acoustic opening

Cochlea

Vestibule

Anterior semicircular canal

Lateral semicircular canal

Posterior semicircular canal

Vestibular canaliculus with endolymphatic duct

Endolymphatic sac

Hypoglossal canal

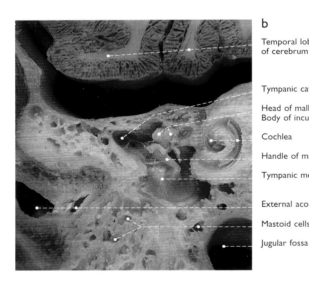

b

Temporal lobe of cerebrum

Tympanic cavity

Head of malleus, Body of incus

Cochlea

Handle of malleus

Tympanic membrane

External acoustic meatus

Mastoid cells

Jugular fossa

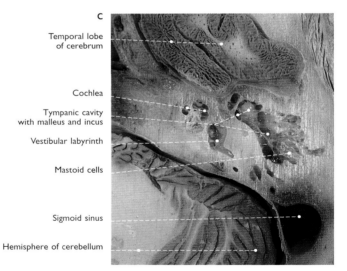

c

Temporal lobe of cerebrum

Cochlea

Tympanic cavity with malleus and incus

Vestibular labyrinth

Mastoid cells

Sigmoid sinus

Hemisphere of cerebellum

400   Bony labyrinth

a   Internal surface of cranial base. On the right side, the bony labyrinth is shown in projection onto the superior surface of the petrous part of temporal bone, on the left side, a cast of the bony labyrinth in its natural position (100%). Superior aspect

b, c   Anatomical sections through the petrous part of the right temporal bone, the tympanic cavity, and the cochlea

b   Coronal section (180%), frontal aspect

c   Transverse section (130%), superior aspect

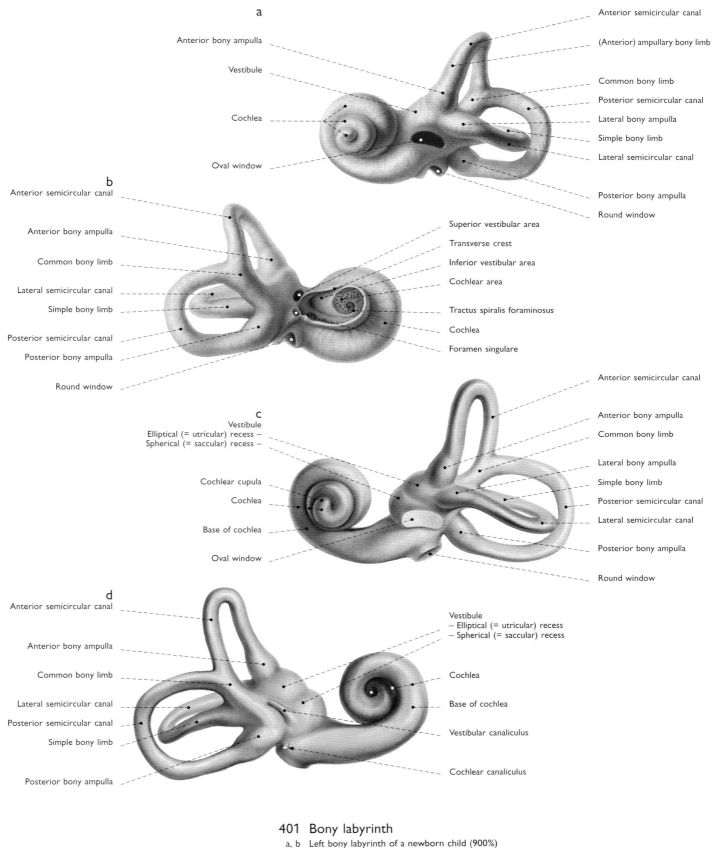

a

Anterior bony ampulla

Vestibule

Cochlea

Oval window

Anterior semicircular canal

(Anterior) ampullary bony limb

Common bony limb

Posterior semicircular canal

Lateral bony ampulla

Simple bony limb

Lateral semicircular canal

Posterior bony ampulla

Round window

b

Anterior semicircular canal

Anterior bony ampulla

Common bony limb

Lateral semicircular canal

Simple bony limb

Posterior semicircular canal

Posterior bony ampulla

Round window

Superior vestibular area

Transverse crest

Inferior vestibular area

Cochlear area

Tractus spiralis foraminosus

Cochlea

Foramen singulare

c

Vestibule
Elliptical (= utricular) recess –
Spherical (= saccular) recess –

Cochlear cupula

Cochlea

Base of cochlea

Oval window

Anterior semicircular canal

Anterior bony ampulla

Common bony limb

Lateral bony ampulla

Simple bony limb

Posterior semicircular canal

Lateral semicircular canal

Posterior bony ampulla

Round window

d

Anterior semicircular canal

Anterior bony ampulla

Common bony limb

Lateral semicircular canal

Posterior semicircular canal

Simple bony limb

Posterior bony ampulla

Vestibule
– Elliptical (= utricular) recess
– Spherical (= saccular) recess

Cochlea

Base of cochlea

Vestibular canaliculus

Cochlear canaliculus

401 Bony labyrinth

a, b Left bony labyrinth of a newborn child (900%)
c, d Left bony labyrinth of an adult (400%), cast preparation
a, c Frontolateral aspect
b, d Dorsomedial aspect

a

Facial canal

Superior vestibular area

Spiral canal of modiolus

Cochlear area,
Tractus spiralis foraminosus

Scala tympani

Osseous spiral lamina

Secondary spiral lamina

Jugular fossa

Styloid process

Anterior bony ampulla

Lateral bony ampulla

Oval window

Entrance to scala vestibuli

Lateral semicircular canal

Osseous spiral lamina

Secondary spiral lamina

Posterior bony ampulla

Groove for sigmoid sinus

b

Anterior semicircular canal

Anterior bony ampulla

Lateral bony ampulla

Lateral semicircular canal

Common bony limb

Elliptical (= utricular) recess

Simple bony limb

Posterior bony ampulla

Facial canal

Tympanic cavity

Cochlear recess

Round window,
Scala tympani

Promontory

Macula cribrosa superior

Vestibular canaliculus

Facial canal

Spherical (= saccular) recess

Groove for greater
petrosal nerve

Scala tympani

Osseous spiral lamina

Scala vestibuli

Lamina of modiolus

Hamulus of spiral lamina

Osseous spiral lamina

Secondary spiral lamina

Tympanic canaliculus

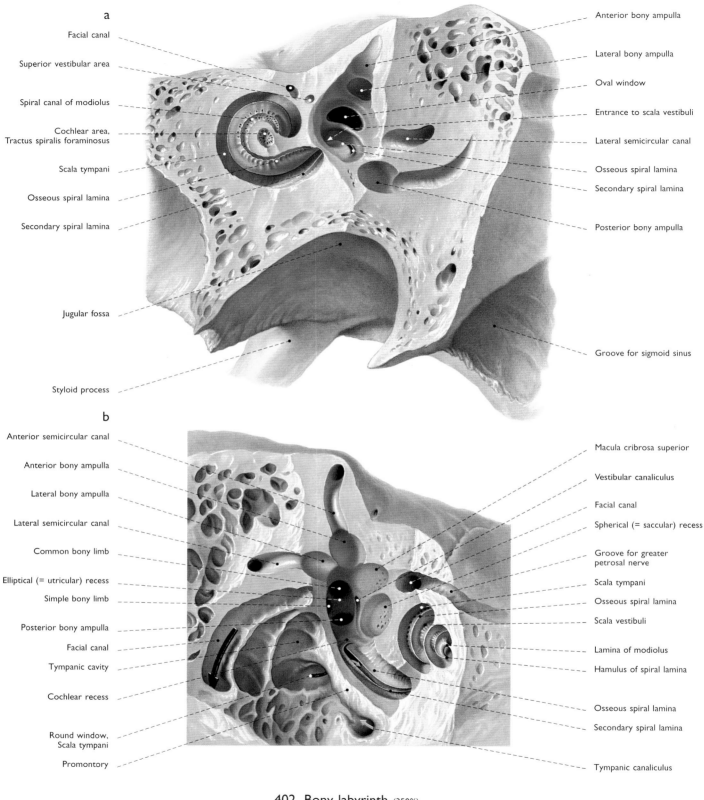

402   Bony labyrinth (350%)

Vestibule, cochlea, and parts of the semicircular canals
of the petrous part of the right temporal bone

a   revealed and opened by dissection of the petrous bone from medial,
    dorsomedial aspect

b   exposed and opened by dissection of the petrous bone from lateral,
    frontolateral aspect

a

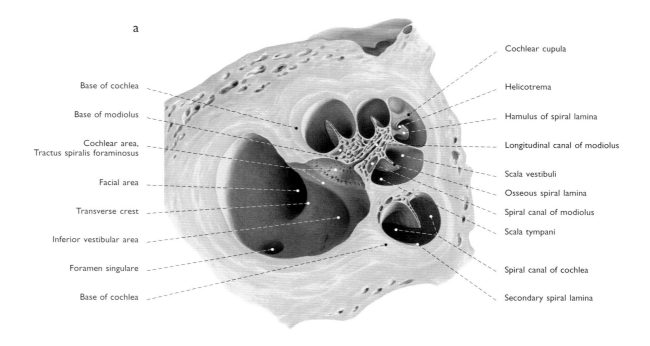

Base of cochlea

Base of modiolus

Cochlear area,
Tractus spiralis foraminosus

Facial area

Transverse crest

Inferior vestibular area

Foramen singulare

Base of cochlea

Cochlear cupula

Helicotrema

Hamulus of spiral lamina

Longitudinal canal of modiolus

Scala vestibuli

Osseous spiral lamina

Spiral canal of modiolus

Scala tympani

Spiral canal of cochlea

Secondary spiral lamina

b

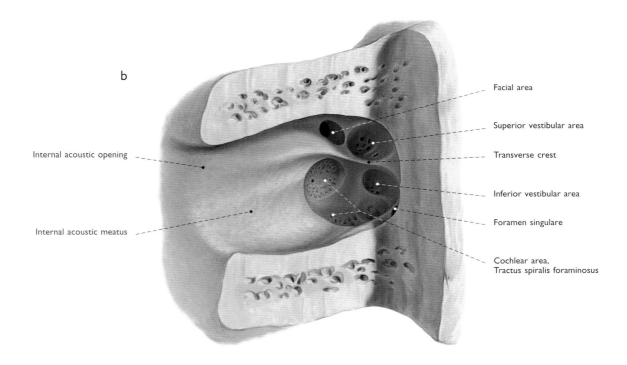

Internal acoustic opening

Internal acoustic meatus

Facial area

Superior vestibular area

Transverse crest

Inferior vestibular area

Foramen singulare

Cochlear area,
Tractus spiralis foraminosus

403 Internal ear (500%)

a   The cochlea and the fundus of the internal acoustic meatus
were opened by an axial bisection through the right cochlea.
Superior aspect

b   Internal acoustic meatus after removal of the dorsomedial wall
of the right internal acoustic meatus, medial aspect

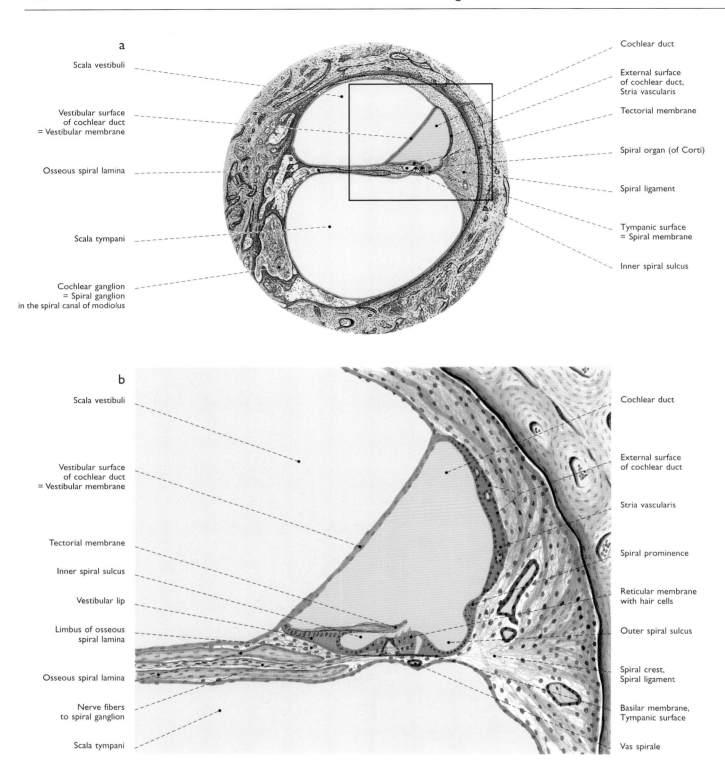

a

Scala vestibuli

Vestibular surface
of cochlear duct
= Vestibular membrane

Osseous spiral lamina

Scala tympani

Cochlear ganglion
= Spiral ganglion
in the spiral canal of modiolus

Cochlear duct

External surface
of cochlear duct,
Stria vascularis

Tectorial membrane

Spiral organ (of Corti)

Spiral ligament

Tympanic surface
= Spiral membrane

Inner spiral sulcus

b

Scala vestibuli

Vestibular surface
of cochlear duct
= Vestibular membrane

Tectorial membrane

Inner spiral sulcus

Vestibular lip

Limbus of osseous
spiral lamina

Osseous spiral lamina

Nerve fibers
to spiral ganglion

Scala tympani

Cochlear duct

External surface
of cochlear duct

Stria vascularis

Spiral prominence

Reticular membrane
with hair cells

Outer spiral sulcus

Spiral crest,
Spiral ligament

Basilar membrane,
Tympanic surface

Vas spirale

404 Cochlea, cochlear duct, and spiral organ of Corti
a Transverse section through one of the coils of cochlea (2000%)
b Enlargement of an area similar to the rectangle in fig. a showing
a cross section through the cochlear duct (8000%)

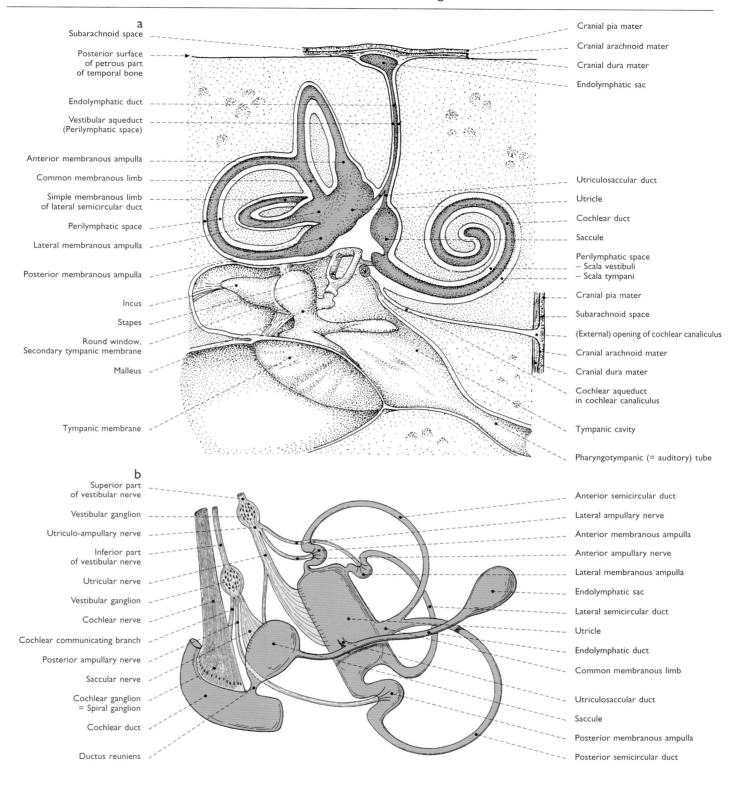

a
Subarachnoid space
Posterior surface of petrous part of temporal bone
Endolymphatic duct
Vestibular aqueduct (Perilymphatic space)
Anterior membranous ampulla
Common membranous limb
Simple membranous limb of lateral semicircular duct
Perilymphatic space
Lateral membranous ampulla
Posterior membranous ampulla
Incus
Stapes
Round window, Secondary tympanic membrane
Malleus
Tympanic membrane

Cranial pia mater
Cranial arachnoid mater
Cranial dura mater
Endolymphatic sac
Utriculosaccular duct
Utricle
Cochlear duct
Saccule
Perilymphatic space
– Scala vestibuli
– Scala tympani
Cranial pia mater
Subarachnoid space
(External) opening of cochlear canaliculus
Cranial arachnoid mater
Cranial dura mater
Cochlear aqueduct in cochlear canaliculus
Tympanic cavity
Pharyngotympanic (= auditory) tube

b
Superior part of vestibular nerve
Vestibular ganglion
Utriculo-ampullary nerve
Inferior part of vestibular nerve
Utricular nerve
Vestibular ganglion
Cochlear nerve
Cochlear communicating branch
Posterior ampullary nerve
Saccular nerve
Cochlear ganglion = Spiral ganglion
Cochlear duct
Ductus reuniens

Anterior semicircular duct
Lateral ampullary nerve
Anterior membranous ampulla
Anterior ampullary nerve
Lateral membranous ampulla
Endolymphatic sac
Lateral semicircular duct
Utricle
Endolymphatic duct
Common membranous limb
Utriculosaccular duct
Saccule
Posterior membranous ampulla
Posterior semicircular duct

405   Membranous labyrinth and vestibulocochlear nerve

Schematic representations
a   Membranous labyrinth. The membranous labyrinth filled with endolymph is represented in light-green color, the surrounding perilymphatic spaces are given in white color.
b   Ramification of the vestibulocochlear nerve (N. VIII)

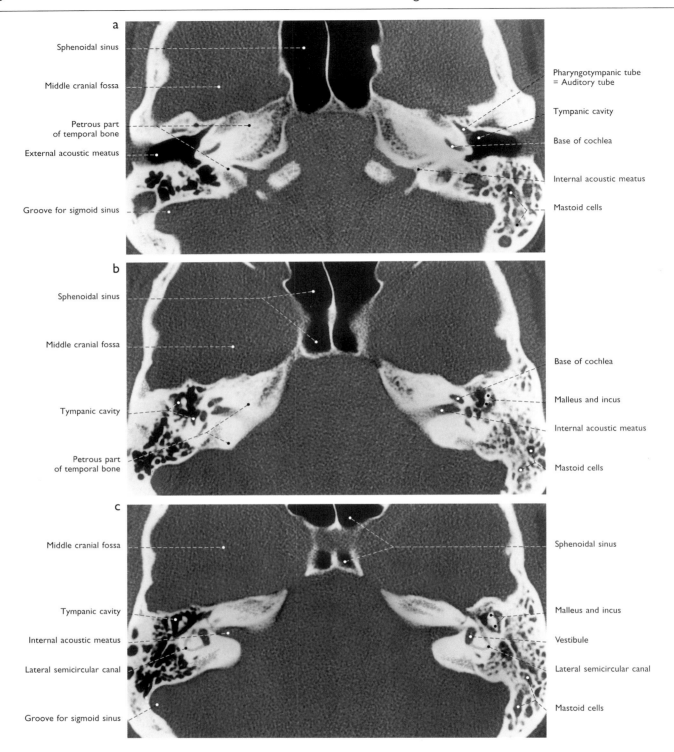

a

Sphenoidal sinus

Middle cranial fossa

Petrous part of temporal bone

External acoustic meatus

Groove for sigmoid sinus

Pharyngotympanic tube = Auditory tube

Tympanic cavity

Base of cochlea

Internal acoustic meatus

Mastoid cells

b

Sphenoidal sinus

Middle cranial fossa

Tympanic cavity

Petrous part of temporal bone

Base of cochlea

Malleus and incus

Internal acoustic meatus

Mastoid cells

c

Middle cranial fossa

Tympanic cavity

Internal acoustic meatus

Lateral semicircular canal

Groove for sigmoid sinus

Sphenoidal sinus

Malleus and incus

Vestibule

Lateral semicircular canal

Mastoid cells

406 Petrous part of temporal bone (85%)

Horizontal computed tomograms (CT) through caudal parts of the petrous part of temporal bone, inferior aspect

a Section through the external acoustic meatus, the pharyngotympanic tube, and the base of cochlea

b Section (a little more cranial than fig. a) through the tympanic cavity, the base of cochlea, and the internal acoustic meatus

c Section (a little more cranial than fig. b) through the tympanic cavity, the lateral semicircular canal, the vestibule, and the internal acoustic meatus

a

Sphenoidal sinus

Middle cranial fossa

Petrous part
of temporal bone

Lateral semicircular canal

Internal acoustic meatus

Epitympanic recess
of tympanic cavity

Groove for sigmoid sinus

Mastoid cells

Posterior cranial fossa

b

Middle cranial fossa

Dorsum sellae

Petrous part
of temporal bone

Epitympanic recess
of tympanic cavity

Posterior semicircular canal

Mastoid cells

Posterior cranial fossa

c

Dorsum sellae

Middle cranial fossa

Petrous part
of temporal bone

Anterior semicircular canal

Mastoid cells

Posterior cranial fossa

407 Petrous part of temporal bone (85%)

Horizontal computed tomograms (CT) through cranial parts
of the petrous part of temporal bone, inferior aspect

a Section through the epitympanic recess, the lateral semicircular canal,
and mastoid cells

b Section (a little more cranial than fig. a) through the epitympanic recess,
the posterior semicircular canal, and mastoid cells

c Section (a little more cranial than fig. b) through
the anterior semicircular canal and mastoid cells

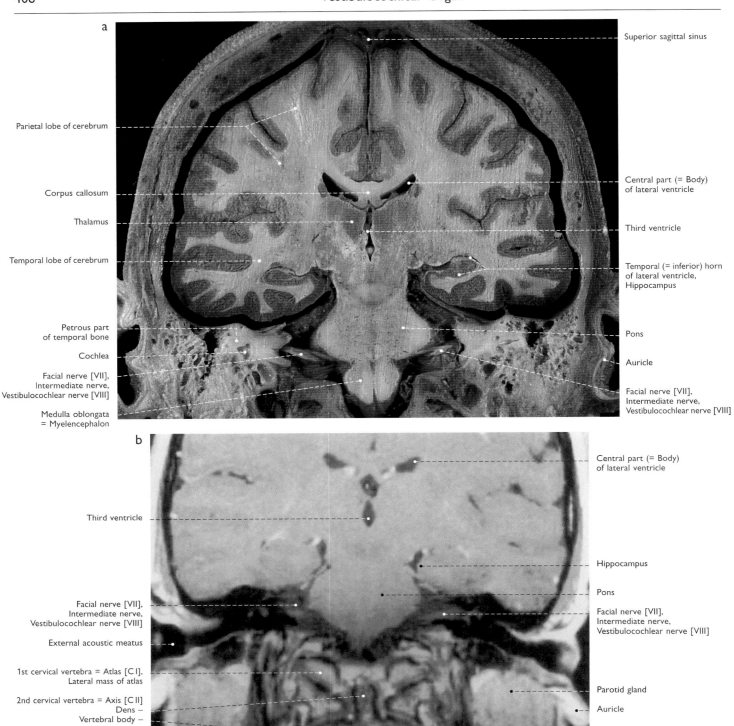

a

Parietal lobe of cerebrum

Corpus callosum

Thalamus

Temporal lobe of cerebrum

Petrous part
of temporal bone

Cochlea

Facial nerve [VII],
Intermediate nerve,
Vestibulocochlear nerve [VIII]

Medulla oblongata
= Myelencephalon

Superior sagittal sinus

Central part (= Body)
of lateral ventricle

Third ventricle

Temporal (= inferior) horn
of lateral ventricle,
Hippocampus

Pons

Auricle

Facial nerve [VII],
Intermediate nerve,
Vestibulocochlear nerve [VIII]

b

Third ventricle

Facial nerve [VII],
Intermediate nerve,
Vestibulocochlear nerve [VIII]

External acoustic meatus

1st cervical vertebra = Atlas [C I],
Lateral mass of atlas

2nd cervical vertebra = Axis [C II]
Dens —
Vertebral body —

Central part (= Body)
of lateral ventricle

Hippocampus

Pons

Facial nerve [VII],
Intermediate nerve,
Vestibulocochlear nerve [VIII]

Parotid gland

Auricle

**408 Temporal bone and
vestibulocochlear nerve** (100%)

Coronal sections through the parietal lobes of cerebrum,
the petrous part of temporal bones, and the pons
a Anatomical section, occipital aspect
b Computed tomogram (CT), frontal aspect

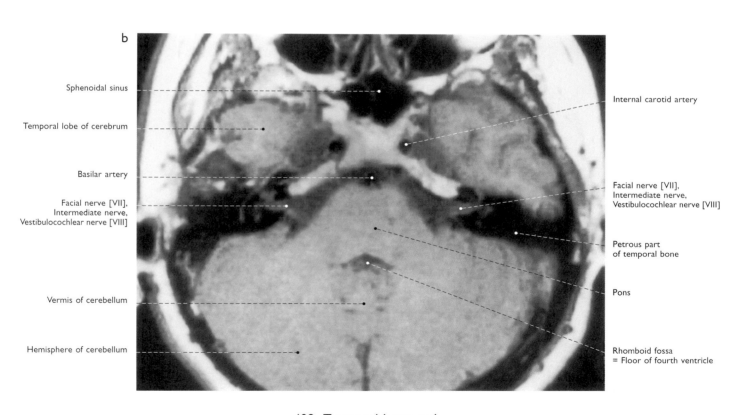

a

Basilar artery

Cochlea

Internal acoustic meatus
with facial nerve [VII],
intermediate nerve,
and vestibulocochlear
nerve [VIII]

Sigmoid sinus

Vermis of cerebellum

Calvaria,
Occipital bone

Epicranial aponeurosis

Internal occipital
protuberance

Pons

Cochlea

Facial nerve [VII],
Intermediate nerve,
Vestibulocochlear nerve [VIII]

Posterior semicircular
canal

Rhomboid fossa
= Floor of fourth ventricle

Hemisphere of cerebellum

(Tumor in the cerebellum)

Transverse sinus

b

Sphenoidal sinus

Temporal lobe of cerebrum

Basilar artery

Facial nerve [VII],
Intermediate nerve,
Vestibulocochlear nerve [VIII]

Vermis of cerebellum

Hemisphere of cerebellum

Internal carotid artery

Facial nerve [VII],
Intermediate nerve,
Vestibulocochlear nerve [VIII]

Petrous part
of temporal bone

Pons

Rhomboid fossa
= Floor of fourth ventricle

**409 Temporal bone and
vestibulocochlear nerve** (100%)
Transverse sections through the temporal lobes of cerebrum,
the petrous part of temporal bones, the pons, and the cerebellum,
inferior aspect
a Anatomical section
b Computed tomogram (CT)

Subject Index

Volume numbering is given in bold print, followed by page numbers.
Adjectives generally precede nouns (as in the index of the Terminologia Anatomica).
Brackets in the text of illustrations were omitted in the subject index.